SMALL
ANIMAL
ORTHOPEDICS

SMALL ANIMAL ORTHOPEDICS

MARVIN L. OLMSTEAD, D.V.M., M.S.

Diplomate ACVS
Professor of Small Animal Orthopedics
Department of Veterinary Clinical Sciences
College of Veterinary Medicine
The Ohio State University
Columbus, Ohio

With Artwork by

FELECIA J. PARAS

Biomedical Visuals
Columbus, Ohio

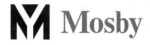 Mosby

St. Louis Baltimore Boston Carlsbad Chicago Naples New York Philadelphia Portland
London Madrid Mexico City Singapore Sydney Tokyo Toronto Wiesbaden

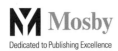

Mosby
Dedicated to Publishing Excellence

A Times Mirror
Company

Publisher: Don Ladig
Editor: Linda L. Duncan
Developmental Editor: Jo Salway
Project Manager: Patricia Tannian
Production Editor: Melissa Mraz
Senior Book Designer: Gail Morey Hudson
Cover Design: Teresa Breckwoldt
Manufacturing Supervisor: Karen Lewis
Illustrator: Felecia Paras, Biomedical Visuals

Printed in the United States of America
Composition by Shepherd, Inc.
Printing and Binding by Maple-Vail Book Mfg Group

Mosby-Year Book, Inc.
11830 Westline Industrial Drive
St. Louis, Missouri 63146

Library of Congress Cataloging in Publication Data

Olmstead, Marvin L.
    Small animal orthopedics / Marvin L. Olmstead: with artwork by
  Felecia J. Paras
        p.   cm.
    Includes bibliographical references and index.
    ISBN 0-8016-5874-8
        1. Dogs—Surgery.   2. Dogs—Fractures—Treatment.   3. Cats—Surgery.
4. Cats—Fractures—Treatment.   5. Veterinary orthopedics.   6. Fractures in
animals—Treatment.   I. Title.
SF991.O58   1995
636.089'747—dc20   95-15902
                                                        CIP

95 96 97 98 99 / 9 8 7 6 5 4 3 2 1

Contributors

LAWRENCE W. ANSON, D.V.M.
Diplomate ACVS
Veterinary Surgical Associates
Akron-Cleveland, Ohio

JEAN F. BARDET, D.V.M.
Diplomate ECVS
Neuilly Sur Seine, France

C. WILLIAM BETTS, D.V.M.
Diplomate ACVS
Veterinary Surgical Referral Practice
Raleigh, North Carolina

MARK S. BLOOMBERG, D.V.M., M.S.
Diplomate ACVS
Collins Professor and Chairman
Department of Small Animal Clinical Sciences
Chief of Staff, Small Animal Teaching Hospital
Director, Center for Veterinary Sports Medicine
College of Veterinary Medicine
University of Florida
Gainesville, Florida

SABINA BRÜSE, Dr. med vet
Sonnenberg
Hohr-Grenhaus, Germany

STEVEN C. BUDSBERG, D.V.M., M.S.
Diplomate ACVS
Associate Professor of Surgery
Department of Small Animal Medicine
College of Veterinary Medicine
University of Georgia
Athens, Georgia

JONATHAN H. CHAMBERS, D.V.M.
Diplomate ACVS
Professor and Chief of Staff
Small Animal Surgery
Department of Small Animal Medicine
College of Veterinary Medicine
University of Georgia
Athens, Georgia

CHARLES E. DeCAMP, D.V.M., M.S.
Diplomate ACVS
Associate Professor of Surgery
Veterinary Clinical Center
Michigan State University
East Lansing, Michigan

ERICK L. EGGER, D.V.M.
Diplomate ACVS
Associate Professor of Surgery
College of Veterinary Medicine
Colorado State University
Fort Collins, Colorado

DONALD A. HULSE, D.V.M.
Professor
Department of Small Animal Medical Sciences
College of Veterinary Medicine
Texas A & M University
College Station, Texas

WILLIAM HYMAN, Sc.D.
Professor
Section of Bioengineering
College of Industrial Engineering
Texas A & M University
College Station, Texas

ANN L. JOHNSON, D.V.M.
Diplomate ACVS
Professor
Department of Veterinary Clinical Medicine
College of Veterinary Medicine
University of Illinois
Urbana, Illinois

KENNETH A. JOHNSON, M.V.Sc., Ph.D., F.A.C.V.S.
Diplomate ACVS
Associate Professor
School of Veterinary Medicine
University of Wisconsin-Madison
Madison, Wisconsin

PAUL MANLEY, D.V.M., M.Sc.
Diplomate ACVS
Associate Professor
School of Veterinary Medicine
University of Wisconsin-Madison
Madison, Wisconsin

MARVIN L. OLMSTEAD, D.V.M., M.S.
Diplomate ACVS
Professor of Small Animal Orthopedics
Department of Veterinary Clinical Sciences
College of Veterinary Medicine
The Ohio State University
Columbus, Ohio

RODNEY L. PAGE, D.V.M., M.S.
Diplomate ACVIM (Medicine/Oncology)
Professor of Medicine/Oncology
College of Veterinary Medicine
North Carolina State University
Raleigh, North Carolina

W. DIETER PRIEUR, Dr. med. vet
Head, AO Vet Centre (Retired)
Altenweg Muhle
Liesenich, Germany

STEVEN C. SCHRADER, D.V.M.
Diplomate ACVS
Associate Professor
Department of Veterinary Clinical Sciences
College of Veterinary Medicine
The Ohio State University
Columbus, Ohio

PETER K. SHIRES, BVSc, MS
Diplomate ACVS
Professor
Department of Small Animal Clinical Sciences
Virginia Polytechnic Institute and State University
Virginia-Maryland Regional College of Veterinary Medicine
Blacksburg, Virginia

TODD A. TOBIAS, D.V.M., M.S.
Diplomate ACVS
Assistant Professor of Surgery
Chief, Small Animal Surgery
College of Veterinary Medicine
Mississippi State University
Starkville, Mississippi

THOMAS M. TURNER, D.V.M.
Assistant Professor
Department of Orthopedic Surgery
Rush-Presbyterian-St. Luke's Medical Center
Chicago, Illinois
Staff Surgeon
Berwyn Veterinary Associates
Berwyn, Illinois

LARRY J. WALLACE, D.V.M.
Diplomate ACVS
Professor of Orthopedic Surgery
Department of Small Animal Clinical Sciences
College of Veterinary Medicine
University of Minnesota
St. Paul, Minnesota

STEVEN E. WEISBRODE, V.M.D., Ph.D.
Diplomate ACVP
Professor
Department of Veterinary Biosciences
College of Veterinary Medicine
The Ohio State University
Columbus, Ohio

FOR
HEATHER

Preface

For over 22 years I have been teaching veterinary orthopedics to both veterinary students and veterinarians. During that time I have learned much from those I have taught and from the patients I have treated. If the time ever comes that I stop climbing the orthopedic learning curve, I will have to find something else to do with my life. That day has not arrived and I hope it never will. Reading the chapters of this textbook has certainly been a learning experience for me. I chose my coauthors because I knew they would present their subject in a concise, practical manner. I wanted their material to be well founded in science but I did not want the science to overwhelm the art of the subject. Now that I have seen what has been written, it is clear my coauthors have all done an outstanding job meeting my goals. For all the hard work so many have put into this book, I am extremely grateful.

It is my hope that the readers of this textbook will receive a sound orthopedic base from the information presented. Since disease conditions and orthopedic injuries are many and vary in their presentation, finding a description in any textbook that exactly fits every aspect of the patients that veterinarians encounter is unlikely. However, the principles of fracture repair, orthopedic reconstructive surgery, and musculoskeletal disease diagnosis and management can be applied even when the case is not "textbook." The information provided within these pages should allow a sound treatment plan to be developed, as well as an alternative plan for those times when the first plan cannot be successfully implemented.

Each patient offers an opportunity for learning, even if we have seen the condition or done the surgery 1000 times before. With each patient we have an opportunity to improve that animal's quality of life. Our obligation must be to make a correct diagnosis, institute a proper treatment plan, execute the indicated surgery with respect for tissues, and provide managed convalescence. I sincerely hope the orthopedic principles and techniques found in this textbook help veterinarians successfully resolve their patients' orthopedic problems.

Marvin L. Olmstead, D.V.M., M.S.

Contents

SMALL
ANIMAL
ORTHOPEDICS

I

INTRODUCTION TO MUSCULOSKELETAL SURGERY

1

Diagnosis: Historical, Physical, and Ancillary Examinations

STEVEN C. SCHRADER
W. DIETER PRIEUR
SABINA BRUSE

Practicing veterinarians are frequently asked to examine animals that are lame. Lameness may be the result of pathology or injury to bone, cartilage, muscle, tendon, ligament, or neurovascular structures; as such, lameness may be manifested in a variety of ways and to varying degrees. Careful historical and physical examinations are necessary to differentiate one cause of lameness from another; they help establish the diagnosis, that is, they allow the veterinarian to formulate a reasonable method of treatment and offer the client an accurate prognosis.

Veterinarians must know the age of onset, breed prevalence, and clinical findings associated with various disorders, as well as be able to conduct appropriate historical and physical examinations. Diagnosis can often be made with no further investigation if the veterinarian has an accurate history, is knowledgeable about the various disorders that cause lameness, and has the ability to perform and interpret the physical examination.

Radiographic and laboratory examinations may help to further define the problem or to confirm the clinical diagnosis. The limitations of radiographic and laboratory examinations should be understood; the results of such examinations should always be interpreted with the clinical findings in mind. A radiographic diagnosis of degenerative joint disease secondary to hip dysplasia may lead to inappropriate treatment if coexisting stifle instability secondary to rupture of the cranial cruciate ligament was overlooked during physical examination. The diagnosis and treatment of lameness in dogs and cats are hardly ever based on laboratory tests alone. A positive *Borrelia burgdorferi* titer may have little clinical significance when detected in a dog that lives in an area where this spirochete is endemic; detection of rheumatoid factor does not necessarily mean the animal has rheumatoid arthritis.

SIGNALMENT

Knowledge of the animal's age, breed, and gender (signalment), helps the veterinarian determine the probability that the animal's lameness is caused by one disorder or another (Tables 1-1 and 1-2). An awareness of the disorders that are common in certain breeds and the age at which clinical manifestations are noted may help focus the physical examination. A heightened awareness that certain disorders are probable helps prevent them from being overlooked as the cause of lameness; however, biases should never be so strong that they preclude a thorough examination or otherwise obstruct the diagnostic process.

HISTORICAL EXAMINATION

The historical features of many of the disorders that cause lameness are similar; nevertheless, historical examination coupled with signalment helps the veterinarian formulate a short list of plausible diagnoses. For example, although it is possible for a 7-year-old German shepherd dog with non-weight-bearing lameness of the forelimb to have panosteitis, it is not likely due to the dog's advanced age (see Chapter 20). Likewise, an 8-month-old German shepherd dog with similar signs is much more likely to have panosteitis than osteochondritis dissecans (OCD) of the humeral head (see Chapter 21). Panosteitis is more prevalent in young German shepherd dogs, and OCD rarely causes such severe lameness.

Owners should be questioned concerning past and concurrent problems; the onset, character, and intensity of the clinical signs; progression or course of the problem; and response to medications or other therapies. Facts should be gathered concerning any past or current problems even if they do not appear to be associated with lameness. Many of the inflammatory joint disorders have systemic manifestations (see Chapter 21); a past history of tumor removal may heighten the clinical suspicion concerning neoplasia as a cause of lameness.

Onset

Knowledge about the onset of clinical signs (abrupt versus protracted or insidious versus overt) and the character of the lameness may allow the veterinarian to decide which diagnoses are reasonable. A rottweiler with an insidious onset of a weight-bearing lameness of a rear limb is more likely to have a partial than complete rupture of the cranial cruciate ligament (see Chapter 18). A complete rupture of this ligament is more likely to result in an acute onset of overt lameness; the affected limb is initially held with the stifle in a flexed position.

Character of Gait Disturbance

Historical inquiry concerning the character of the gait disturbance may help the veterinarian differentiate between neurological and skeletal causes of lameness. Gait disturbance associated with spinal cord disease is typified by awkward or uncoordinated movements, and the animal usually does not exhibit any reluctance to use the limb. Owners often complain that the limb(s) appears weak; that the animal cannot, versus will not, stand, walk, run, or jump. Animals with skeletal disease (including disease of the spine) tend to have lameness that is characterized by deliberate movement. There is no apparent proprioceptive deficit or voluntary motor weakness. These animals appear to be reluctant to use the limb; they seem unwilling to stand, walk, or jump instead of unable to function.

Peripheral nerve disease may cause the animal to hold the affected limb off the floor or ground while it is stationary, but there may be little or no gait disturbance when the animal walks or runs (Fig. 1-1). Such historical

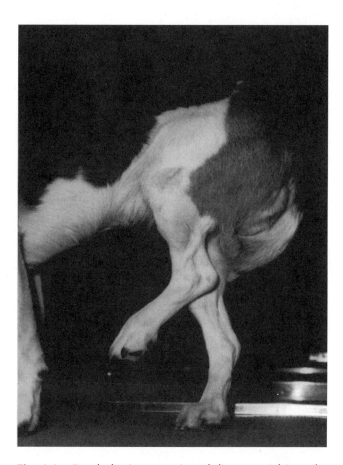

Fig. 1-1 Beagle having extrusion of disc material into the spinal canal between the sixth and seventh lumbar vertebrae. The dog is lifting the left rear limb as a result of attenuation of nerve roots by disc material. This is an example of a "root signature."

information would not be typical of skeletal disease alone. As such, careful examination of the axillary and inguinal regions and the associated vertebral column is mandatory whenever such clinical signs are described. Lameness, excessive licking or chewing, or other clinical signs associated with nerve root disease (so-called root signatures) may develop in dogs with intervertebral disc extrusion, intradiscal osteomyelitis (discospondylitis), spinal fractures or luxation, and neoplasia (neurofibroma).

Clinical Course and Response to Treatment

Knowing the course or progression of clinical signs and whether there has been any response to medication or other treatments provides an insight as to the diagnosis and probable effectiveness of the therapeutic options that might be considered. If the rottweiler described in a preceding paragraph experienced an acute exacerbation of lameness 5 months after onset, it would be reasonable to assume that the partial cruciate ligament rupture suddenly became complete or that the medial meniscus was entrapped and was subsequently torn as a result of persistent stifle instability (see Chapter 18).

Lameness and joint swelling associated with inflammatory joint disease, for example, systemic lupus erythematosus and idiopathic immune-mediated arthritis (see Chapter 21), will generally not subside with administration of aspirin or other nonsteroidal antiinflammatory drugs (NSAIDs); the response to corticosteroid administration is usually dramatic. Likewise, animals with spinal cord or nerve root disease are more likely to have a favorable response when given corticosteroids than with NSAID therapy.

Knowledge about the course of the disorder and the effectiveness of previously tried treatments often affects the diagnostic and therapeutic plans and the prognosis. The veterinarian is more likely to recommend ancillary diagnostic testing when lameness is persistent or progressive or when so-called conservative or symptomatic treatments have failed. Alternative methods of management are sought when therapies fail or when the veterinarian is consulted for the second or third time. Persistence or progression of lameness despite appropriate therapy suggests an unfavorable prognosis. Serial reexamination is necessary whenever the character or course of the disease seems to be changing. This helps to prevent overlooking new or coexisting problems. A dog having degenerative joint disease of the hip and an acute exacerbation of lameness might have ruptured the cruciate ligament, sustained some other injury, or had an infection develop in the hip that was predisposed by joint disease and corticosteroid administration.

PHYSICAL EXAMINATION
General Considerations

Physical examination begins when the owner and pet are first encountered in the waiting area. If the animal is able to walk, the owner should lead the pet into the examination room. This allows the veterinarian to begin to assess the animal's gait, stance, and attitude.

The animal should be given a few moments to become familiar with the examination room and with the veterinarian before the physical examination is begun. Large breed dogs can be examined on the floor rather than lifted onto the examination table. The owner should be allowed to stroke and talk to the animal while the examination is being performed. If the animal assumes a defensive posture or in any way becomes intractable, a trained assistant should be asked to restrain the pet. It is sometimes necessary to isolate the pet from the owner, other animals, and other distractions in order to complete the examination. Clinical experience will dictate when this is necessary.

The veterinarian should avoid sedating the patient that is ill tempered or ill behaved, although this is not always possible. It is sometimes helpful to take such animals away from the owner and do the examination in a quiet place. Leaving the animal on the floor and avoiding firm restraint, muzzles, or excessive manipulation of the affected part may allow at least a cursory examination to be performed. Examination of the affected (painful) part should be performed last. After the problem has been localized or a probable cause identified, sedation may be performed to allow further examination.

General Physical Examinations

A general physical examination should always precede examinations of the spine or limbs. Several musculoskeletal disorders have systemic manifestations, and decisions concerning treatment and prognosis of musculoskeletal lesions may be influenced by coexisting problems. Although surgical intervention is usually recommended in dogs having a rupture of the cranial cruciate ligament, it may not be warranted in a small dog that is also coughing secondary to congestive heart failure. Rectal examination may allow detection of the cause of rear limb lameness. Rectal examination should always be performed when pelvic or inguinal trauma has been sustained.

Neurological Examinations

A cursory examination of the spinal column and assessment of the neurological status of the affected limb should precede other examinations of the extremity. This ensures that neurological examination is always

Table 1-1 Signalment and Historical Features of Various Causes of Lameness in Immature Dogs and Cats*†

Clinical prevalence	Disorder	Breed/Species Prevalence					Sex Predisposition	Onset of Signs	Course of Lameness or Deformity	Other signs	Comments
		Breeds of Dog				Cat					
		Small	Medium	Large	Giant						
Common	Hip dysplasia	-	+	++	++	-	-	Slow	W/P	-	Particularly common in breeds having endomorphic traits. Almost always bilateral. Affected dogs have variable degree of dysfunction.
	Medial patellar luxation	++	-	+	+	-	Female?	Slow	I/P	-	Usually congenital/developmental. Usually bilateral. Bone and joint deformities may develop with persistent luxation in young animals.
	Panosteitis	-	-	++	++	-	Male	Rapid	V/SL	±	Clinically, affects forelimb more often than rear limb. Many dogs have multiple limb involvement. Especially common in German shepard dog. May be anorectic.
Occasional	Osteochondritis dissecans	-	-	++	++	-	Male	Slow	W/P	-	Frequently bilateral. Especially common in dogs having endomorphic features and working/hunting breeds.
	Legg-Calvé-Perthes	++	-	-	-	-	-	Slow	P	-	10%-15% bilateral.
	Hypertrophic osteodystrophy	-	-	++	++	-	-	Rapid	V/SL	±	Multiple limbs affected. May be very painful, anorectic, febrile.
	Fragmented coronoid process	-	-	++	++	-	Male?	Slow	W/P	-	May be bilateral. Especially common in Rottweiler and retrievers.
	Ununited anconeal process	-	+	++	+	-	Male	Slow	W/P	-	Less common than fragmented coronoid process. Especially common in German shepherd dog. Associated with elbow incongruity in basset hound and English bulldog.
	Lateral patellar luxation	-	-	+	++	-	-	Slow	I/P	-	May be associated with other development abnormalities such as hip dysplasia.
	Carpal weakness/instability	-	+	++	+	-	-	Rapid	V/SL	-	Occurs at weaning; 8-16 weeks of age. Forepaws buckle over, animal walks on lateral aspect of paw. Doberman, Great Dane, Shar-pei.

Table 1-1 Signalment and Historical Features of Various Causes of Lameness in Immature Dogs and Cats*† (continued)

Clinical prevalence	Disorder	Breed/Species Prevalence					Sex predisposition	Onset of signs	Course of lameness or deformity	Other signs	Comments
		Breeds of Dog				Cat					
		Small	Medium	Large	Giant						
Occasional (continued)	Forelimb shortening/deformity	−	+	++	++	−	−	Slow	P	−	Usually the result of physeal injury (asynchronous radial-ulnar growth). Clinical implications greatest in large breed dogs. May cause secondary elbow/carpal incongruity.
Rare	Craniomandibular osteopathy	++	+	+	+	−	−	Slow	V	+	Especially common in terrier breeds. Involvement of long bones of the limb is unusual but documented.
	Retained cartilage core	−	−	+	++	−	−	Slow	V	−	May be associated with slowly progressive limb deformity. Most commonly found in distal ulna.
	Bacterial arthritis	−	−	++	++	−	−	Rapid	P	+	Usually hematogenous; sometimes polyarticular. Other organs often involved.
	Bone cysts	−	−	++	+	−	−	Slow	P/SL	−	Onset of signs may be rapid if fracture occurs. Doberman pinscher, German shepherd, Old English sheepdog.
	Neoplasia	−	−	++	++	−	−	Slow	P	±	Osteosarcoma, chondrosarcoma, osteocartilaginous exostosis.
	Secondary hyperparathyroidism	+	+	+	+	+	−	Slow	P	±	Nutritional: all-meat diets. Onset may be rapid if pathological fracture occurs.
	Constitutional disorders	+	+	+	+	+	±			±	Mucopolysaccharidosis, congenital hypothyroidism, ectrodactyly, etc. Achondro/hypochondroplasia common but considered normal in many breeds.

−, Least common; +, occasional; ++, most common relative to other animals. W, wax-wane; P, progressive; I, intermittent; V, variable; SL, self-limiting.

* Fractures, traumatic joint dislocation, soft tissue injuries have been excluded; such injuries are common in immature animals.

† Disorders that affect joints may cause lameness after the animal has reached skeletal maturity.

Table 1-2   Signalment and Historical Features of Various Causes of Lameness in Mature Dogs and Cats*

Clinical prevalence	Disorder	Breed/Species Prevalence					Sex predisposition	Onset of signs	Course of lameness or deformity	Other signs	Comments
		Breeds of Dog				Cat					
		Small	Medium	Large	Giant						
Common	Noninflammatory/degenerative joint disease†	-	+	++	+	-	-	Slow	W/P	-	Present in all breeds of dogs and cats; clinical manifestations most common in larger dogs. May affect one or multiple joints.
	Cruciate ligament and meniscal injury	++	++	++	+	-	-	Rapid	Initially Improves then W/P	-	May occur with inflammatory joint disorders.
Occasional	Idiopathic inflammatory joint disease	+	++	++	+	-	-	Rapid	W/V	±	Probably immune-mediated; usually multiple joints are affected.
	Patellar luxation	++	-	+	+	-	-	Usually slow	I/P	-	See Table 1-1. Most traumatic luxations result in acute onset of lameness; are unilateral.
	Nerve root disorders	++	++	-	-	-	-	Rapid	W/P	±	Usually the result of intervertebral disc herniation; dachshund, cocker spaniel, beagle. Neurofibroma: older dogs
	Neoplasia	-	+	++	++	-	-	Slow	P	±	Primary neoplasms of bone, cartilage, synovium are most common.
Rare	Hypertrophic osteopathy	+	+	+	+	-	-	Slow to rapid	P	+	Usually associated with intrathoracic lesions.
	Hypervitaminosis A	-	-	-	-	++	-	Slow	P	+	Associated with all-liver diets.
	Rheumatoid arthritis	++	+	-	-	-	-	Slow	P	±	Most clinically evident in carpus, tarsus, small joints of paws. Symmetrical disease. Shetland sheepdog, collie.
	Systemic lupus erythematosus	-	+	+	-	-	-	Usually rapid	W/P	+	Multiple joints/other systems affected.
	Erosive feline polyarthritis	-	-	-	-	++	-	Slow	P	±	Similar to canine rheumatoid arthritis.
	Proliferative feline polyarthritis	-	-	-	-	++	Male	Rapid	P	+	Etiology linked with feline leukemia and feline syncytium-forming virus infections.
	Bacterial arthritis‡	-	-	++	+	-	-	Rapid		±	Usually monoarticular. Predisposed by preexisting joint disease.

-, Least common; +, occasional; ++, most common relative to other animals. W, wax-wane; P, progressive; I, intermittent; V, variable; SL, self-limiting.
*Fractures and most traumatic joint and soft tissue injuries excluded.
†Often the sequela of disorders present in immature dogs (Table 1-1).
‡Hematogenous.

performed. Spinal cord lesions may produce tetraparesis, hemiparesis, or paraparesis. Lesions that are located within the cervical or lumbar intumescence or that affect the nerves of the brachial or lumbosacral plexus are especially prone to disturb gait as the result of pain or paresis.

Spinal pain. The presence of spinal pain is suggestive of extradural lesions such as disc, neoplasia, discospondylitis, and fracture-luxation injuries. In such cases a painful response is most consistently obtained by direct palpation of the individual vertebra. In the cervical region this is accomplished by applying digital pressure to the ventrolateral aspect of the bone (Fig. 1-2). In the thoracolumbar region digital pressure is applied to the epaxial muscles that lie adjacent to the dorsal spinous process and over the laminae of the respective vertebra (Fig. 1-3). Cats are normally more responsive than dogs when digital pressure is applied to the lumbar and sacral vertebrae (Fig. 1-4).

Proprioceptive deficits. Proprioceptive deficits can be detected by using the knuckling test. The paw is carefully turned over while the animal is standing. If the animal fails to instantaneously right the paw and continues to bear weight on the dorsum of the overturned digits, the clinician can assume that the animal has lost some

conscious proprioceptive sense (Fig. 1-5). Animals with proprioceptive deficits may have a shuffling gait with the paw contacting the floor as it is advanced. In chronic cases the nails may be worn short and the skin on the dorsum of the digits may appear abraded. Animals with

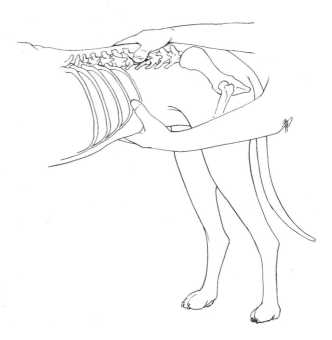

Fig. 1-3 Digital pressure applied via the thumb to the epaxial muscles that overlie the facets, laminae, and dorsal spinous processes of the thoracolumbar vertebrae for detection of spinal hyperpathia. The hyperpathic zone can be established by alternately beginning at the cranial and caudal extent of the thoracolumbar spine and proceeding in the opposite direction until a response is elicited.

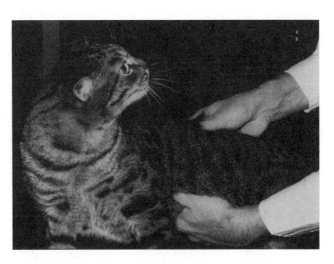

Fig. 1-4 Normal cat responding to moderate digital pressure applied over the lumbar spine. Cats are usually much more responsive to palpation over the thoracolumbar and sacral vertebrae than dogs. This difference must be considered when interpreting the results of physical examination.

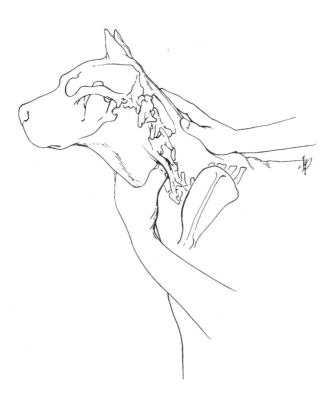

Fig. 1-2 Digital pressure applied to the ventrolateral aspect of the cervical vertebrae for detection of spinal hyperpathia. The trachea lies between the thumb and fingers.

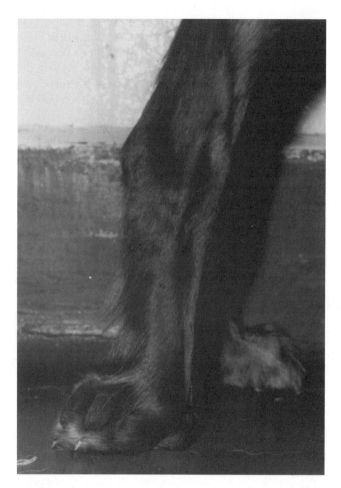

Fig. 1–5 Proprioceptive deficit in the rear limb of an Irish setter. Sustained weight-bearing on the dorsal surface of the overturned paw confirms the presence of neurologic disease.

pelvic or humeral fractures or other traumatically induced injuries may not right an overturned paw immediately. This is the result of pain, not paresis. Such animals rarely bear much weight on the overturned paw; this helps the veterinarian distinguish this response from a "true" proprioceptive deficit.

Voluntary motor ability and reflex testing. Detection of spinal pain or proprioceptive deficits dictates that a more thorough neurological examination be performed. Loss of voluntary motor ability suggests neurologic rather than musculoskeletal disease. The limb appears weak, and movement may appear awkward or uncoordinated. Muscle tone status and reflex testing help to differentiate upper motor neuron (suprasegmental) from lower motor neuron (segmental) spinal cord lesions. Flexor (withdrawal), patellar tendon, and crossed extensor reflexes are helpful in localizing the lesion. The triceps and biceps tendon reflexes and the panniculus reflex are less helpful because they can be inconsistent or are otherwise more difficult to interpret.

Sensory status. The sensory status of the paw should be evaluated whenever a neurological cause of lameness is suspected. Damage to peripheral nerves may be associated with fractures, especially fractures of the ilium or sacroiliac injuries. The sensory status is determined by applying a noxious stimulus to the region of the paw innervated by the radial, ulnar, and median nerves (forepaw) and the sciatic and femoral nerves (hindpaw) (Fig. 1-6). A flexor (withdrawal) response suggests that the local reflex arc is intact; a conscious response from the animal confirms that it perceives the stimulus. The presence of a flexor reflex should never be construed as conscious perception of pain.

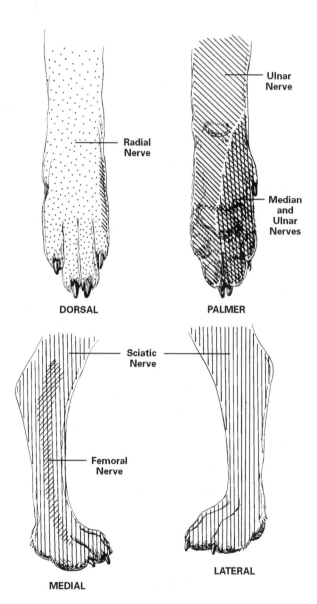

Fig. 1–6 Cutaneous innervation of the forepaw (*upper*) and rear paw (*lower*) of the dog.

Modified from deLahunta A: *Veterinary neuroanatomy and clinical neurology*, Philadelphia, 1977, WB Saunders.

Axillary and Inguinal Examinations

Examination of the axillary and inguinal areas should be a routine part of physical examination. These examinations should follow the cursory neurological examination to ensure that they are not forgotten. Careful palpation may allow detection of tumor or enlarged lymph nodes and, in the inguinal region, allow characterization of the femoral pulse. Unfortunately, early detection of axillary masses such as neurofibroma of the brachial plexus or neoplasia of the rib(s) is usually difficult. Even relatively large masses may be hard to detect in the axillary area. In the late stages, animals with axillary or rib masses may appear to be in pain and are reluctant to bear weight on the limb, especially while standing still (Fig. 1-7). The pain may be difficult to localize; it may be misinterpreted as spinal in origin.

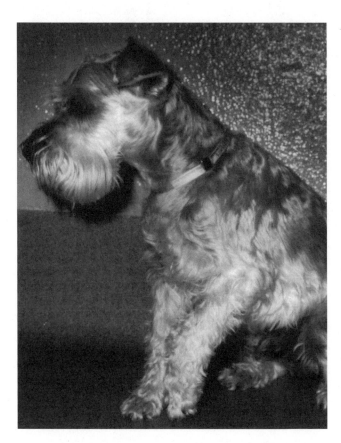

Fig. 1–7 Eleven-year-old schnauzer having a neurofibroma of the brachial plexus causing left front limb lameness. The dog places weight on the limb while walking but not while stationary. Physical examination of the front limb should include palpation of the axillary region and the first few ribs. Small axillary masses are especially difficult to detect; this dog had been lame for 1½ years before the tumor was detected.

Examination of the Limbs

Examination of the extremities begins after other portions of the physical examination have been completed. Manipulation of the affected limb should be left until last to avoid annoying the animal. Cats are usually more difficult to examine than dogs; they are not conditioned to stand still, and they are less tolerant of manipulation and firm restraint. Most animals can be examined if the veterinarian can modify the method of examination to accommodate the circumstance.

Visual Examination

General considerations. Certain visual clues help the veterinarian determine the site of involvement. Body weight may be shifted to the normal (unaffected) limb. In such cases the normal limb may be held closer to the midline or under the body while the affected limb is held out to the side or away from the body. Because more weight is carried by them, the toes of the normal limb may appear to spread further apart than the toes of the affected limb. The back arches dorsally as weight is shifted to the front or rear limbs. The elbows appear abducted, and the head and neck are held low in animals that are shifting weight off the rear limbs. Conversely, the rear limb stance is wide based and there may be a "bowlegged" appearance when weight is being shifted to the rear limbs. Dogs with severe hip dysplasia or with bilateral rupture of the cranial cruciate ligament appear to lean forward as they walk; the head and neck go down, the back arches dorsally, and the elbows appear abducted.

Differences in the length of the nails may suggest limb dysfunction. The nails of the affected limb may be longer than those of the opposite side when the animal is not bearing full weight on the limb or when deformity of the paw or limb precludes normal weight distribution. The nails may be excessively short when the limb is not lifted high enough to avoid scuffing as the limb is advanced. Hairless areas over joints caused by constant licking or chewing of the extremity may be a clue that the animal is experiencing pain or paresthesia.

Gait and stance. Gait and stance analysis provides additional information concerning the location of the abnormality. Gait is assessed as the animal is led into the examination room or up and down a hospital corridor. Allowing the animal to move about in a fenced area or outside the hospital may help eliminate distractions that might otherwise obscure a subtle problem. It is usually necessary to forgo this portion of the examination in cats and other animals that are not accustomed to being led.

Detection of gait and stance abnormalities can be quite challenging. Cats tend to seek out a secluded area and, once found, refuse to move. Cats and dogs can be encouraged to walk by placing them a few feet from where they want to be and observing them as they walk into their cage or box or into a secluded corner to hide (Fig. 1-8). Subtle lameness may be more difficult to detect in very small dogs, which move their limbs relatively more rapidly than large dogs. Lameness may be impossible to observe when the dog is excited or easily distracted and will not walk in a straight line. In addition, there are conformational differences among breeds; the chow chow and Akita have very straight or erect rear limb stance, whereas some German shepherd dogs normally assume a more markedly flexed posture. The veterinarian must be familiar with such differences.

The degree of weight-bearing and type of limb carriage may help the veterinarian differentiate one cause of lameness from another. Fractures, nerve root disease, and lacerations of the digital pads often cause the animal to completely lift the limb off the floor. Dogs with stifle injuries (cruciate ligament rupture) initially hold the limb up toward the body in a flexed position (Fig. 1-9), a position rarely assumed by dogs with hip injuries. Intermittent or episodic non-weight-bearing lameness may be observed in dogs having patellar instability or nerve root disease. The former become non-weight-bearing while running; the latter tend to lift the limb off the floor when standing still.

Gait should be observed at the walk and trot. The presence of a "head bob" is suggestive of lameness. The head and neck move upward as the affected forelimb touches the floor and downward when the affected rear limb touches down. This motion helps to reduce the load carried by the limb. In addition, the stride is shortened on the affected side; the animal appears to unload the affected limb more quickly than it does the normal one. In effect, the animal spends less time on the affected limb. Shuffling gaits or movements that are uncoordinated and allow the limb to cross over the midline and into the pathway of the opposite limb (crossing-over) suggest neurological disease (Fig. 1-10). In such cases the owner or veterinarian can usually hear the digits interfere with the floor as the limb is advanced. Audible clicks are sometimes heard in young dogs with hip instability (hip dysplasia) or in dogs that have a medial meniscal tear secondary to rupture of the cranial cruciate ligament.

Palpation and Manipulation

General considerations. Following gait analysis, palpation and manipulation of the affected limb(s) are used to determine the specific site and character of the problem. A complete knowledge of structure and function helps the veterinarian decide how to perform specific tests and how to interpret the results. A cranial

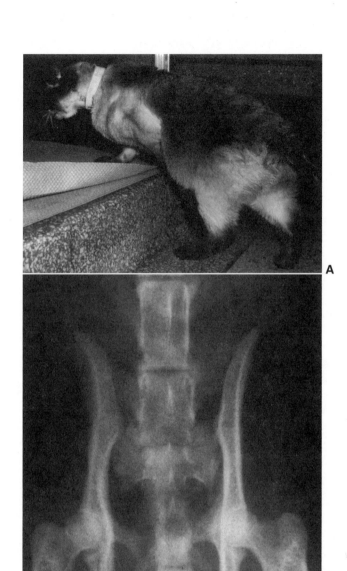

Fig. 1-8 A, Siamese cat immediately after bilateral sacroiliac luxation. Cats and dogs can be encouraged to walk by placing them a short distance from food, their cage, or a secluded area of the room. Observation of gait is important in diagnosis and in formulating a treatment plan. This cat recovered without reduction or fixation of the sacroiliac injuries. **B,** Radiograph of the pelvis of the cat in **A** with luxation of the sacroiliac joints. The pelvic inlet is foreshortened, but there was minimal narrowing of the pelvic inlet and canal on rectal examination.

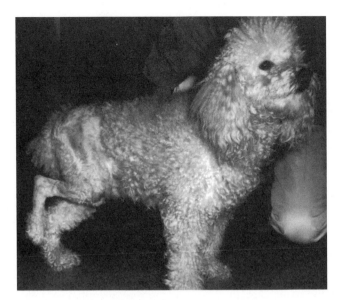

Fig. 1-9 Poodle with rupture of the cranial cruciate ligament. The affected limb is held with the stifle in a flexed position and the paw off the floor. This is typical of (acute) stifle injuries. This position is rarely assumed by dogs having hip disease. Limb carriage may provide important diagnostic clues to the veterinarian.

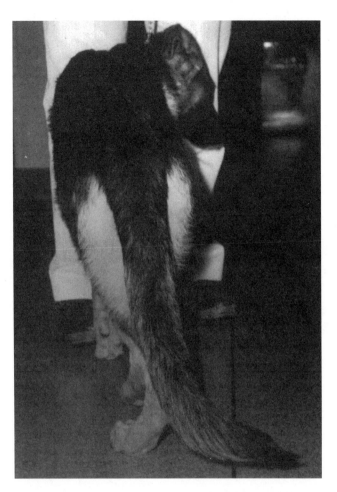

Fig. 1-10 The rear limbs of this German shepherd dog appear to cross over the midline and into the path of the opposite limb while the dog is walking. This suggests the presence of neurological disease or other cause of rear limb weakness rather than bone or joint disease.

drawer sign may not be detected in patients with partial rupture of the cranial cruciate ligament until the stifle is placed in a partially flexed position. Understanding the anatomy of the cranial cruciate ligament helps explain this phenomenon (see Chapter 18).

Comparing one side with the other (normal versus abnormal) helps the veterinarian detect specific abnormalities. This type of comparison may also help compensate for lack of experience and for differences that may exist between various breeds and species. For example, the anatomical features of the chondrodystrophoid breeds of dogs are distorted relative to other breeds.

Standing animal. Physical examination of the limbs should begin with the dog or cat standing and with the limbs in a symmetrical position. Simultaneous palpation of the right and left front or rear limbs helps the examiner detect swelling, muscle atrophy, and deformity of bone or joint. Simultaneous palpation of opposite limbs is best accomplished by standing over or kneeling in front of or behind the animal (Fig. 1-11).

Palpation of the joints with the animal standing helps the veterinarian detect effusion and subtle differences in the character of the periarticular soft tissues that might otherwise be overlooked. Elbow and stifle effusion and thickening of periarticular soft tissues can usually be detected by moving the thumb and forefinger up and down over the medial and lateral aspects of the joints

just caudal to the epicondylar region of the humerus and to each side to the straight patellar tendon, respectively. With chronic rupture of the cranial cruciate ligament, inflammatory joint disease, or other disorders of the stifle, the lateral and medial margins of the patellar tendon become less distinct. Tarsal effusion or swelling is detected by moving the thumb and forefinger of each hand up and down over the medial and lateral aspect of each calcaneus just caudal to the medial and lateral malleoli. Carpal joint swelling is easiest to detect over the dorsal surface of the joint.

It is sometimes possible to differentiate between effusion and capsular thickening by palpation alone. Digital pressure, alternately applied over the medial and lateral aspects of the joint, may redistribute fluid from one side of the joint to the other. This suggests that an effusion is present. Effusions are more common with inflammatory than with noninflammatory joint disorders (see Chapter 21). It is difficult to detect effusion or capsular thickening

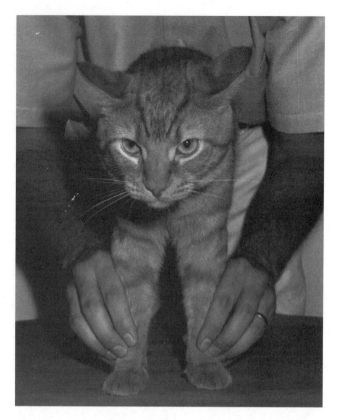

Fig. 1-11   Detection of subtle joint swelling, muscle atrophy, or deformity of bone or joint is facilitated by simultaneous palpation of opposite limbs while the dog or cat is standing.

From Schrader SC, Sherding RG: *The cat: diseases and clinical management*, New York, 1989, Churchill Livingstone.

of the hip and shoulder, since these joints are surrounded by a substantial amount of muscle.

Individual limbs. Once the limbs have been examined with the animal in a standing position, the remainder of the evaluation can be performed on the side of involvement with the animal standing or in lateral recumbency. Many veterinarians start the examination at the level of the digits (paw) and proceed proximally. Response to palpation or manipulation and joint range of motion are assessed at this time. Many of the specific tests, like those used to detect stifle and hip instability, are generally performed while the animal is held in lateral recumbency.

As before, the veterinarian must consider the animal's temperament when interpreting the response obtained to palpation or manipulation of the limb; for example, Doberman pinschers tend to have a more stoic nature than rottweilers. Again, it is helpful to compare the reaction obtained on one side with that obtained on the other. The method of examination should be discrete enough to avoid evoking a response from an adjacent area or joint.

The veterinarian must have the ability to detect a painful area when and wherever it exists. Because the presence of pain is a consistent indicator of disease, the animal should be given every opportunity to express a painful response during the examination. Such reaction may be abolished by overzealous restraint, application of a muzzle, or sedation. Palpation and manipulation need not be excessively forceful or rough to elicit a painful response. Palpation should be precise; bone, joint, and soft tissues need to be evaluated. Direct pressure applied over the medial coronoid process of the ulna (just distal to the medial epicondyle of the humerus between the digital flexor and flexor carpi radialis muscles) is a useful method of eliciting a painful response in dogs having fragmented coronoid process (Fig. 1-12).

Animals with joint disease usually resist manipulation or exhibit a painful response when the joint is moved in the same direction as joint motion is limited. Animals with disease of the carpal joint usually have a reduced range of flexion and resist forced flexion of the joint (Fig. 1-13). In normal dogs and cats the carpus can usually be flexed so that the metacarpal pad touches the caudal aspect of the antebrachium. Forced extension is a good way to elicit a painful response from a diseased

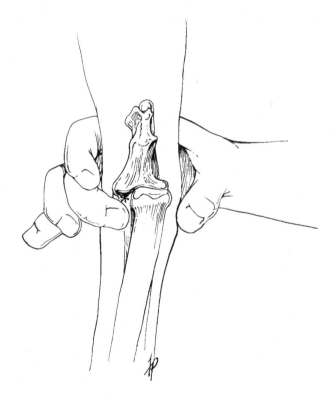

Fig. 1-12   A painful response can sometimes be elicited in dogs with fragmented medial coronoid process by direct application of pressure to the soft tissues overlying the affected structure (*asterisk*). Careful palpation often helps the veterinarian determine which area of the limb or spine needs further evaluation (by radiographs or arthrocentesis).

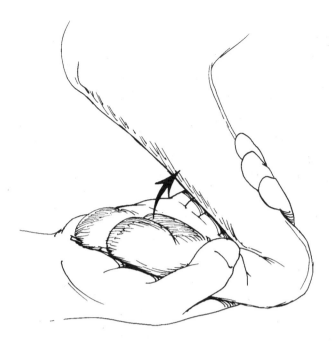

Fig. 1-13 Forced flexion of the carpus helps the veterinarian determine range of motion and detect the presence of pain in the joint. Dogs and cats with carpal disease tend to have limited range of flexion and begin to struggle or withdraw the limb when the limit of flexion is reached. This method of examining the carpus is specific; more proximal structures are not affected by the maneuver.

elbow, shoulder, tarsus, stifle, or hip. In addition, a consistent method of eliciting a painful reaction from the diseased hip is to abduct the femur. Dogs with degenerative joint disease secondary to hip dysplasia and small dogs with Legg-Calvé-Perthes disease may have relatively good range of hip flexion and extension but only a limited degree of pain-free abduction. In addition, crepitus is more consistently detected while the hip and shoulder are being abducted or rotated than with flexion and extension. Table 1-3 lists the normal values for joint range of motion in dogs and cats.

Detection of bone pain facilitates early detection of neoplasia and diagnosis of fractures, bone infections, and panosteitis. It is usually possible to apply direct digital pressure to the bones, for example, along the medial aspect of the radius and tibia and the caudal aspect of the ulna. Direct palpation of the humerus and femur is more difficult; however, the lateral aspect of both bones can be palpated at the junction between the flexor and extensor muscles of the brachium and thigh, respectively. The veterinarian should avoid application of digital pressure on the radial nerve as it courses over the lateral aspect of the humerus.

Pain or paresis may result in muscle atrophy. The degree of muscle wasting depends on the cause, severity, and duration of the disability. Muscle atrophy caused

by denervation tends to be more acute, severe, and discrete than atrophy caused by disuse of the limb. Although the presence of muscle atrophy provides a clue as to which limb is most clinically affected, it does not usually provide a specific diagnosis. Disuse atrophy is often diffuse rather than localized and is rarely detected during the first 3 weeks of lameness; its presence usually implies chronic disability. Muscle atrophy is best confirmed by simultaneous palpation of opposite limbs and is usually easier to detect when muscle groups rather than individual muscles are palpated.

Specific methods. The practicing veterinarian needs to master several specific methods of physical examination. These specific methods of palpation or manipulation are illustrated in Figs. 1-2 and 1-3 and Figs. 1-12 through 1-20.

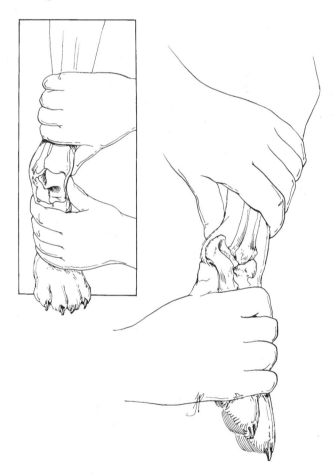

Fig. 1-14 Disruption of the lateral collateral ligament(s) of the tibiotarsal joint can be detected by placing the joint in full extension (*right*) and simultaneously applying pressure to the medial aspect of the joint (*upper left*). The joint will open on the lateral side when the ligament(s) has been stretched, torn, or avulsed. Pressure is applied to the lateral surface to evaluate the medial collateral ligament. Similar methods are used to evaluate the callateral ligaments at the carpus, elbow, and stifle.

Table 1-3 Joint Range of Motion in Dogs and Cats[*]

Joint	Range of Motion (Degrees)	
	Dog	Cat
SHOULDER		
Flexion	60-70	60-70
Extension	65-75	90
Hyperextension	0	20-30
Adduction	40-50	20-30
Abduction	40-50	80-90
Internal rotation	40-50	30-40
External rotation	40-50	30-40
ELBOW		
Flexion	70-75	50-60
Extension	70-75	80-90
Hyperextension	0	0-5
Supination	80-90	90-110
Pronation	40-50	40-50
CARPUS		
Flexion	155-160	130-140
Extension	20-30	30-40
Ulnar deviation	15-20	10-15
Radial deviation	15-20	35-40
HIP		
Flexion	70-80	50-60
Extension	80-90	100-110
Adduction	30-40	20-30
Abduction	70-80	60-70
Internal rotation	50-60	35-45
External rotation	80-90	80-90
STIFLE		
Flexion	65-75	50-60
Extension	65-75	90
Hyperextension	0	10-20
TARSUS		
Flexion	65-75	50-60
Extension	90-110	90-110
Inversion	40-50	10-20
Eversion	40-50	30-40

From Newton CD: Normal joint range of motion in the dog and cat—Appendix B. In Newton CD, Nunamaker DM, editors: *Textbook of small animal orthopaedics*, Philadelphia, 1985, JB Lippincott.
[*]Average of 10 mixed-breed dogs and 10 domestic short-haired cats.

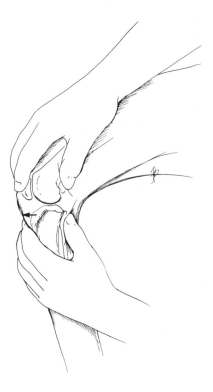

Fig. 1-15 Cranial "drawer" test for stifle joint stability (lateral view). The index fingers of opposite hands are placed on the patella and tibial tuberosity while the thumbs are positioned over the caudal aspect of the lateral femoral condyle (lateral fabella) and the fibular head, respectively. With the stifle in various degrees of flexion and the distal femur held immobile, force is applied in a cranial direction to the proximal tibia/fibula (*arrow*). Cranial displacement of the tibia/fibula relative to the femoral condyles suggests that the cranial cruciate ligament has been disrupted (positive drawer sign). Only a limited amount of cranial displacement may be detected with partial disruption of the cranial cruciate ligament or when periarticular fibrosis has had time to develop. Force is applied in a caudal direction to detect disruption of the caudal cruciate ligament (caudal drawer test); however, because disruption of the caudal cruciate ligament allows spontaneous caudal displacement of the tibia/fibula relative to the femoral condyles, a false positive cranial drawer sign may be detected when the cranial drawer test is done. (It is difficult to feel the subtle degree of caudal subluxation associated with caudal cruciate ligament disruption; the bony relationships seem normal to the examiner.) Any cranial movement of the tibia/fibula that is detected with caudal cruciate disruption will come to an abrupt stop when the intact cranial cruciate ligament becomes taut. Cranial movement detected with cranial cruciate ligament disruption will not end so abruptly.

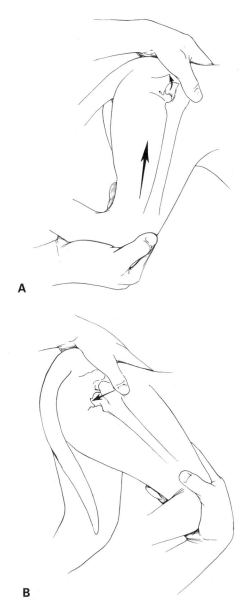

A

B

Fig. 1-16   **A,** Barlow test of hip joint stability. With the dog in lateral recumbency, the stifle in moderate flexion, and the hip joint slightly adducted, one hand pushes the femur (femoral head) proximally while the thumb of the other hand is used to determine if dorsolateral displacement of the greater trochanter occurs (Barlow sign). (There will be no apparent displacement of the trochanter when the femoral head is already subluxated at the time pressure is applied to the distal femur.) **B,** Ortolani test of hip joint stability. This is a reduction maneuver, in contrast to Barlow test (**A**) and Barden test (see Fig. 1–17). Reduction is accomplished by abducting the femur. Ortolani sign is detected as a "click" or "clunk" as the subluxated femoral head drops into the acetabulum (the greater trochanter moves distal and medially). It is common to refer to the combined subluxation and reduction maneuvers of Barlow and Ortolani as the Ortolani test. In fact, the former (Barlow) should always precede the latter (Ortolani) to help ensure that the unstable femoral head is subluxated before the reduction maneuver is attempted.

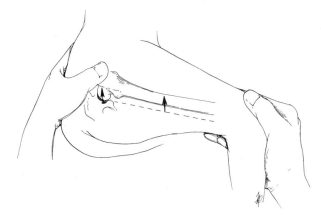

Fig. 1-17   Barden test for hip joint stability. With the dog in lateral recumbency, the fingertips of one hand "lift" the femur (femoral head) while the thumb of the other hand is used to determine if lateral displacement of the greater trochanter occurs (Barden sign). The Barden, Barlow (see Fig. 1–16, A), and Ortolani (see Fig. 1–16, B) signs tend to become more difficult to detect over time because of continued periarticular fibrosis and remodeling of the acetabulum and femoral head. Thus these tests are most useful for detection of hip joint instability in young growing dogs.

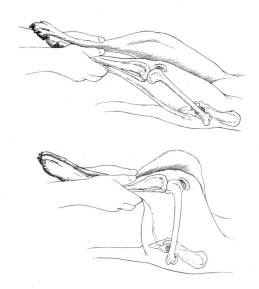

Fig. 1-18   Two methods of detecting apparent leg length discrepancy in dogs and cats with craniodorsal luxation of the hip. With the first method (*upper*), traction is applied to the limbs with the animal in dorsal recumbency. The affected limb appears shorter than the other. With the second method (*lower*) the length of the limb from the rump to the stifle is compared. The rump to stifle distance appears shorter on the affected side. Unanesthetized animals with dislocation of the hip will resist attempts to apply traction to the limbs; the second method of evaluation (*lower*) is better tolerated and just as accurate as the first.

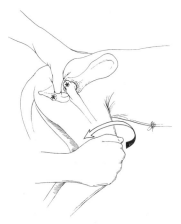

Fig. 1-19 The so-called thumb test for hip joint luxation. Whenever the femoral head is within the acetabulum, external rotation of the femur will cause the femoral head to pivot within the acetabulum and the thumb to be squeezed between the tuber ischium and the greater trochanter. With craniodorsal luxation of the hip, the distance between the tuber ischium and greater trochanter is increased and the femoral head no longer pivots within the acetabulum as the femur is rotated; external rotation will not produce the sensation that the thumb is being compressed between the tuber ischium and the greater trochanter. Craniodorsal hip luxation is easily detected by performing the thumb test and the tests depicted in Fig. 1–18.

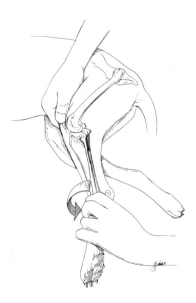

Fig. 1-20 Test for patellar stability. Medial luxation of the patella is encouraged by digital pressure (thumb) applied to the lateral aspect of the bone and simultaneous internal rotation of the lower leg. The test should be performed with the stifle in various degrees of flexion and extension. Lateral luxation of the patella (not shown) would be encouraged by digital pressure (fingertips) applied to the medial aspect of the bone; that is, the fingertips are used to "pull" the patella laterally as the lower leg is rotated externally. This test should also be performed with the stifle in various degrees of flexion and extension.

RADIOLOGIC EXAMINATION

Radiologic examination is an important adjunct to the historical and physical examinations in the diagnostic process. Good-quality craniocaudal and mediolateral views are generally sufficient for examination of the limbs. Oblique views or "stress" views may be indicated to allow better visualization of the lesion or to further define the problem (Fig. 1-21). Radiographs of the opposite limb may help the veterinarian detect subtle differences and determine whether or not a lesion exists (Fig. 1-22). Special imaging techniques (tomograms, bone scans) are rarely necessary in determining the cause of lameness.

Radiographs should be made to document or confirm the results of physical examination, not supplant it. The practice of making radiographs of the entire limb when there are no clinical clues as to which area is affected is often a fruitless venture; time and money are wasted and the veterinarian's credibility may be undermined. When the physical examination has failed to disclose any abnormality, the dog or cat should be more carefully examined or perhaps reexamined in 1 to 3 weeks if the problem persists.

Limitations of Radiological Examination

Numerous limitations are associated with radiographic examination. Bony lesions usually take some time to develop, and with many disorders, early radiographic changes are nonspecific. The bony changes associated with septic arthritis do not become apparent for 14 to 17 days (Fig. 1-23). Early diagnosis of this problem depends on physical examination and subsequent joint fluid analysis. Treatment should begin before bony changes become evident. The nonerosive immune-mediated arthropathies produce few or no bony lesions even when of chronic duration. Preexisting radiographic abnormalities may obscure abnormalities associated with a second process. Periarticular osteophytes and subchondral remodeling associated with degenerative joint disease may obscure the bony changes that develop with neoplasia or infection (Fig. 1-24). In skeletally mature dogs, monoarticular septic arthritis occurs with some frequency in joints where there is preexisting degenerative joint disease. The early radiographic changes associated with septic arthritis are not easily identified in such cases. The fact that most animals with septic joint disease have an acute onset of severe lameness and appear to be in great pain when the affected joint is manipulated should suggest that something in addition to degenerative joint disease might exist. The clinician must always consider the historical and physical findings when interpreting radiographs. Whenever the radiographic diagnosis is in conflict with the clinical scenario, further investigation is indicated.

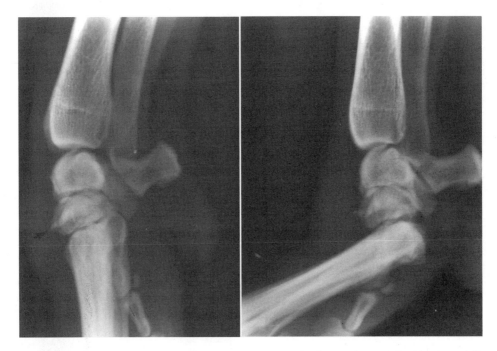

Fig. 1-21   *Left,* Mediolateral radiograph of the carpus of a dog made immediately after a fall. There is diffuse soft tissue swelling about the carpus and a small fragment of bone cranial to the distal row of carpal bones (*arrow*). *Right,* Forced (hyper) extension of the joint results in subluxation of the carpometacarpal joint. The radiograph confirms that the joint is unstable and that the palmar supporting soft tissues have been disrupted. Stress views may provide an insight to diagnosis and therapy.

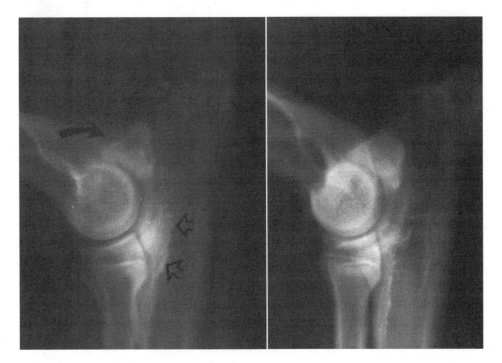

Fig. 1-22   *Left,* Mediolateral radiograph of the elbow of a dog with fragmented medial coronoid process. There is increased bone density and apparent narrowing of the medullary canal of the ulna just caudal to the level of the medial and lateral coronoid processes and the adjacent trochlear notch (*open arrows*). In addition, there is a small amount of new-bone formation on the dorsal surface of the anconeal process (*curved solid arrow*). *Right,* The opposite elbow appears normal. Such comparisons may help the veterinarian to detect abnormalities and to correctly interpret their significance.

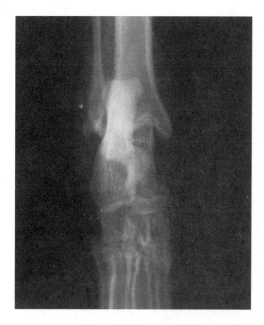

Fig. 1-23 Bacterial arthritis of the tibiotarsal joint of a cat. The periarticular soft tissues are swollen, but as yet there are no visible changes in the subchondral bone that would suggest the presence of infection. Radiographic changes may be absent or nonspecific in the early stages of certain disorders.

From Schrader SC, Sherding RG: *The cat: diseases and clinical management*, New York, 1989, Churchill Livingstone.

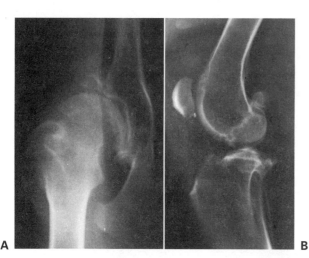

A   B

Fig. 1-24 **A,** Lymphosarcoma of the femoral head and neck in an aged German shepherd dog having preexisting degenerative joint disease (DJD) of the hip. The dog underwent femoral head and neck excisional arthroplasty as treatment for DJD. Histopathologic evaluation was sought when the affected bone was found to be soft and discolored at the time it was being removed. **B,** Septic arthritis of the stifle in an aged dog with preexisting degenerative joint disease. The dog had sustained a rupture of the cranial cruciate ligament several years before the onset of infection. The presence of periarticular osteophytes and subchondral remodeling may obscure the bony changes associated with infection (**B**) or neoplasia (**A**) and preclude an accurate diagnosis. Careful interpretation of historical and physical findings helps to ensure that the proper diagnosis will be made.

Finally, the severity of clinical signs cannot consistently be predicted from examination of radiographs. As such, therapeutic decisions are based primarily on the historical and physical findings rather than the degree of radiographic change. Many dogs with apparently severe degenerative joint disease of the hip or spine seem to function well; dogs having nonerosive inflammatory joint disease may exhibit marked lameness but have little or no radiographic evidence of joint disease. Of all the radiographic abnormalities, the presence of muscle atrophy provides the radiologist with the most information concerning the functional status of the animal. The presence of asymmetrical muscle mass in animals with bilateral joint disease provides the radiologist with valuable clinical insight (Fig. 1-25).

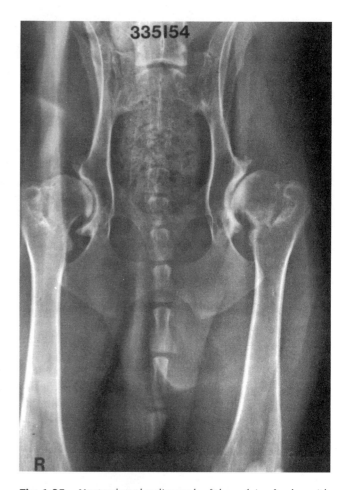

Fig. 1-25 Ventrodorsal radiograph of the pelvis of a dog with hip dysplasia and secondary degenerative joint disease. There is asymmetrical muscle mass about the femurs consistent with the diagnosis of disuse atrophy of the right limb. Indeed, the dog had been lame on the right rear limb for several months. No obvious lameness had been observed on the left side. Asymmetrical muscle mass provides the radiologist with valuable clinical insight. The severity of bone remodeling that is associated with degenerative joint disease does not always correspond with the degree of clinical dysfunction.

ARTHROCENTESIS AND JOINT FLUID ANALYSIS

Central to the diagnosis and treatment of lameness is the question of whether joint disease is present and, if so, if the disorder is inflammatory or noninflammatory (see Chapter 21). Complete physical and historical examinations help the clinician formulate a sound clinical opinion concerning these issues; joint fluid analysis helps confirm or deny the clinical supposition. Joint fluid analysis helps the veterinarian to differentiate inflammatory from noninflammatory disorders and infectious from noninfectious joint disease (Table 1-4). It may be useful in monitoring the clinical course (response to treatment) of various inflammatory joint diseases.

In addition to the preceding, arthrocentesis and fluid analysis can be used to confirm the presence of joint disease when the veterinarian is unsure that lameness is joint related or that a specific joint is swollen or distended. Normal joint fluid is clear and viscid, and only a small amount of fluid can be collected from a normal joint. Obtaining a large amount of fluid or finding fluid that lacks viscosity, is discolored, or is turbid confirms that the joint in question is indeed affected and that the disorder probably has an inflammatory component. Obtaining a large amount of fluid helps the veterinarian differentiate periarticular and joint capsular thickening from joint effusion. Certain joint disorders are more likely to be associated with one than the other (see Chapter 21).

Joint fluid analysis provides information that can help the veterinarian determine the diagnosis when radiographic changes have not had time to develop or when such changes are subtle or nonspecific. This is often the case with inflammatory joint disorders such as septic arthritis, systemic lupus erythematosus (SLE), and rheumatoid arthritis. Joint fluid analysis is a more sensitive test than palpation for detecting the presence of inflammation. Analysis of joint fluid may suggest continuation of the inflammatory process even though joint swelling and lameness appear to have resolved with treatment.

Results of joint fluid analysis should always be viewed in concert with clinical, radiographic, and other findings. It might be difficult to differentiate one inflammatory or noninflammatory disorder from another purely on the basis of joint fluid analysis. All of the various inflammatory disorders are characterized by high numbers of white blood cells (Table 1-4); these cells directly or indirectly affect clarity, color, and viscosity of the fluid. In addition, joint fluid analysis occasionally fails to provide an insight into the cause of joint disease. Even septic arthritis may be difficult to confirm when no degenerative neutrophils or bacteria are seen and when cultures fail to grow the microorganism (see Chapter 21).

Collection

The methods used for collection of joint fluid are similar in the dog and cat. Some sites used for arthrocentesis are illustrated by Fig. 1-26. It is usually not necessary to use chemical restraint or local anesthesia unless the animal is fractious or especially apprehensive. The hair should be clipped from the site and the area cleaned. Contrary to popular belief, it is not necessary to perform a surgical scrub or to wear sterile gloves as long as the procedure is done with reasonable attention to cleanliness. A

Table 1-4   Classification of Joint Disease Based on Joint Fluid Analysis

	Noninflammatory			Inflammatory	
	Degenerative	**Hemarthrosis (trauma)**	**Neoplastic**	**Infectious**	**Noninfectious**
Color	Pale yellow	Red	Yellow to bloodtinged	Yellow to sanguineous	Yellow to sanguineous
Turbidity	Clear-slight	Blood-tinged	Slight to moderate	Turbid to purulent	Slight to turbid
Viscosity	Normal	Reduced	Reduced	Reduced	Reduced
Mucin clot	Normal	Fair	Normal	Poor	Poor to fair
Red cells	Few	Many	Few to moderate	Moderate	Few to moderate
White cells	Few	Moderate	Moderate	Many	Many
Neutrophils	Few	Moderate	Moderate	Many	Moderate to many
Toxic change	None	None	None	Mild to prominent	None to mild
Neoplastic cells	—	—	+*	—	—
Microorganisms	—	—	—	+†	—
Fluid/blood glucose ratio	Normal (0.8–1.0)	Normal (1.0)	Low (0.5–0.8)	Very low (<0.5)	Low (0.5–0.8)

Modified from Wilkins RJ: Joint serology. In Bojrab MJ, editor: *Pathophysiology in small animal surgery*, Philadelphia, 1981, Lea & Febiger.
*Neoplastic cells not always detected.
†Microorganisms not always detected.

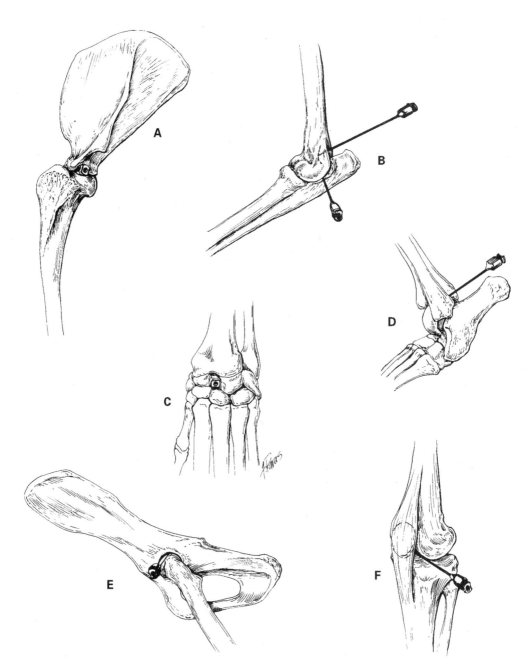

Fig. 1-26 Schematic representation of the sites recommended for arthrocentesis of various joints of the domestic cat. **A,** Lateral view of the shoulder joint. The needle is advanced from lateral to medial just caudodistal to the distal tip of the acromion. **B,** Lateral view of the elbow joint. The needle is advanced in a craniomedial direction through the anconeus muscle and into the joint. Alternatively, the needle is directed medial to the lateral epicondylar ridge and into the olecranon fossa while the elbow is held in a moderate degree of flexion. **C,** Cranial view of the carpus. The needle is advanced from cranial to caudal between the tendons of insertion of the extensor carpi radialis and common digital extensor muscles and into the radiocarpal joint. **D,** Lateral view of the tarsal joint. The needle is inserted into the caudal portion of the joint immediately medial to the lateral malleolus or immediately lateral to the medial malleolus. The joint is held in slight flexion to facilitate entry into the joint. **E,** Lateral view of the hip joint. The needle is advanced in a lateral to medial direction into the craniodorsal portion of the joint. The greater trochanter is used for orientation. **F,** Craniolateral view of the stifle joint. The needle is advanced in a caudomedial direction to enter the joint immediately lateral and distal to the distal tip of the patella. Similar methods are used for arthrocentesis in the dog.

From Schrader SC, Sherding RG: *The cat: diseases and clinical management*, New York, 1989, Churchill Livingstone.

21-gauge needle attached to a 3 ml syringe is used; it is difficult to obtain inspissated fluid when a needle of smaller bore is employed. Once the joint is entered, gentle suction is applied until fluid is no longer obtained or blood appears in the syringe.

Once the fluid has been collected, the color, clarity, viscosity, and amount of fluid are noted and recorded. A drop of fluid is used to make a smear for cytological examination, and a portion of the sample is submitted for culture and sensitivity testing. Inoculation of some type of enriched media such as Trypicase-Soy or thioglycollate broth is recommended.[22] Any remaining fluid is placed in a tube containing EDTA anticoagulant and submitted for cell count and biochemical evaluation.

Because the amount of joint fluid obtained is often insufficient for complete analysis, priorities must be established for the analysis to yield the most information. Cytological evaluation and microbiological testing are of utmost importance. When only one or two drops of fluid have been obtained, a small drop of fluid is transferred to a glass slide (without touching the needle to the slide) and a smear made; the needle and syringe are then flushed with enrichment broth to allow culture and sensitivity testing.

Gross Examination

Joint fluid analysis should begin at the very moment that the fluid is withdrawn from the joint. Normal joint fluid is clear (acellular) and is light straw colored or colorless. It has a sticky viscid character because of the presence of hyaluronate and does not clot because of a lack of prothrombin, fibrinogen, factor V, factor VII, and tissue thromboplastin. The viscosity can be estimated by placing a drop of fluid on the fingertip, touching the drop with the pulp of the thumb, and then withdrawing the thumb. Normal fluid will form a 1- to 2-inch-long continuous strand between the apposing digits (Fig. 1-27). Alternatively, viscosity can be estimated by observing a drop of fluid as it falls to the slide that is used to prepare a smear. Only a small amount of fluid is normally present; no more than a few tenths of a milliliter of joint fluid can be collected from most normal joints.

Bloody fluid may be obtained when the arthrocentesis is traumatic; iatrogenic blood is usually incompletely mixed with the joint fluid and is usually bright red or pink. The presence of blood in joint fluid may allow a clot to develop. High numbers of nucleated cells increase joint fluid turbidity; viscosity of joint fluid may decrease because of destruction, dilution, or insufficient production of hyaluronate. Synovitis may result in excessive production of fluid. If joint fluid is discolored or turbid, lacks viscosity, or is excessive in amount, joint

disease is present. Because these abnormalities are characteristic of inflammatory joint disease (Table 1-4), gross evaluation alone can help the veterinarian distinguish between inflammatory and noninflammatory joint disease. Correlation of the gross characteristics of joint fluid with the clinical scenario can help the veterinarian begin to make diagnostic and therapeutic decisions while cytological and microbiological analyses are pending.

Cytological and Microbiological Examinations

Joint fluid analysis should always include microscopic examination of a smear of the synovia. Such examination allows the veterinarian to determine the number and relative proportions of various cell types. It allows the detection of toxic changes in polymorphonuclear cells and may allow the detection of microorganisms. Culture and sensitivity testing should always be performed because it is crucial to differentiate septic from immune-mediated joint disease; such differentiation is not usually possible by gross or cytological examinations alone.

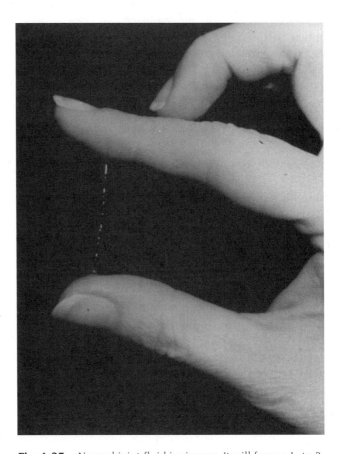

Fig. 1-27   Normal joint fluid is viscous. It will form a 1- to 2-inch strand after a drop has been compressed between opposing digits. Certain inflammatory conditions reduce joint fluid viscosity.

Normal joint fluid contains less than 3000 white blood cells (WBCs)/μl and very few red blood cells. Elevation of WBC count is the hallmark of the inflammatory joint diseases. With as little as 0.5 ml of fluid, it is possible to perform a white and red blood cell count using a hemocytometer counting chamber. The joint fluid is left undiluted or diluted with normal saline solution. Acetic acid in WBC diluting fluid precipitates mucin in joint fluid and therefore should not be used for cell counts.[22] Alternatively, WBC count can be estimated by comparing blood and joint fluid smears. For example, if an average of 10 cells are found per high-power field on the blood smear of a dog having a WBC count of 20,000/μl and there is an average of 20 cells per high-power field on the joint fluid smear, the joint fluid would contain about 40,000 WBCs/μl. With very little practice the veterinarian can accurately determine that the joint fluid WBC count is elevated and can establish the relative proportions of nucleated cells present.

A tremendous variation in WBC count is seen with each of the inflammatory joint disorders, and considerable overlap exists between disorders. Polymorphonuclear cells are the predominant cell type of most inflammatory joint disorders; however, mononuclear cells may predominate in animals having rheumatoid arthritis and plasmacytic-lymphocytic arthritis. The WBC count rarely exceeds 40,000/μl with these diseases, whereas the WBC count may easily surpass this number with SLE, idiopathic immune-mediated arthritis, and septic arthritis.

In addition to culture and sensitivity testing, detecting neutrophils with toxic changes and observing microorganisms on microscopic examination of joint fluid helps the veterinarian distinguish infectious from noninfectious inflammatory joint disease. Unfortunately, culture and sensitivity testing of joint fluid has failed to document the presence of bacteria in known cases of infection, not all infections cause toxic changes in neutrophils, and organisms may not be detected on examination of the smear even if they are present. The veterinarian will have to rely on the clinical scenario and his or her own good judgment when analysis of joint fluid has failed to distinguish between septic and noninfectious inflammatory joint disease (see Chapter 21).

OTHER TESTS AND DIAGNOSTIC PROCEDURES

Historical, physical, radiographic, and joint fluid examinations form the basis for diagnosis and treatment of lameness; however, certain other tests or procedures are occasionally warranted. An understanding of how or why such tests are performed and what the result indicates provides the clinician with an insight concerning the significance of the test in the diagnostic process.

The ideal laboratory test is both sensitive and specific, that is, it has the ability to identify animals with the disease and those without it. Unfortunately, it is usually not possible to combine high sensitivity and high specificity in one test. In addition, the results of serological testing are not absolute values and cutoff points for positive and negative values are based in part on clinical criteria. Individual laboratories may report widely varied results from the same sample. An analysis of laboratories by Healy and Whitehead[14] showed some results to be grossly in error. As such, care must be exercised in interpreting the results of serological testing and pathological examination. The results must be considered within the context established by historical, physical, radiographic, and joint fluid examinations.

Rheumatoid Factor (RhF, RF) Testing

A number of antibodies have been detected in the blood and joint fluid of humans with an erosive or destructive form of arthritis known as rheumatoid arthritis. Collectively, these antibodies have been deemed the rheumatoid factors; their presence suggests that immunological processes may in some way be associated with the pathogenesis of the disease. The exact role that these immunoglobulins play in the pathogenesis of the disease is unknown; they are probably not pathogenic in and of themselves.[8]

An IgM class immunoglobulin is generally considered the rheumatoid factor in dogs. Modified Waller-Rose and latex agglutination tests are most frequently used to detect its presence. There is controversy over what constitutes a positive titer with the Waller-Rose test. Bennett and Kirkham[7] suggest that the test is positive with titers of 1:40 or greater; others have considered a titer as low as 1:8 to be positive.[10,20]

Rheumatoid factor has been detected in dogs having septic arthritis and SLE. In addition, it has been detected in apparently healthy dogs and in dogs with nonarticular diseases. Of 141 apparently healthy dogs, 57 had detectable rheumatoid factor using the Waller-Rose test.[7] A titer of 1:20 was found in 14 of these dogs and 3 had a titer of 1:40. In the same report, 11.7% of dogs with diseases other than polyarthritis had significant levels of rheumatoid factor; 6.4% of dogs having degenerative joint disease had a titer of 1:40.

It would be imprudent to make a diagnosis of rheumatoid arthritis or to eliminate it from the list of differential diagnoses solely on the basis of a positive or negative RF test. The rheumatoid factor test is only one of several criteria used to make a diagnosis of rheumatoid arthritis (see Chapter 21). In one report,[4] only 22 (73%) of 30 dogs with rheumatoid arthritis had a positive titer and 6 of the dogs had tested negative on one or more occasions. Thus it is reasonable to repeat the test in dogs having negative or insignificant titers when the clinical and radiographic features of the disease suggest that rheumatoid arthritis is the diagnosis. In human patients, rheumatoid factors have been measured to monitor the response to therapy. If this is to be done, samples should be collected at regular intervals then frozen and analyzed by the same laboratory at the same time.[8]

Antinuclear Antibody (ANA) Testing

A variety of autoantibodies have been detected in the serum of humans having SLE.[15,16] The presence of autoantibodies suggests that immunological processes play a role in the pathogenesis of this disease. The presence of antinuclear antibodies is one the criteria used to make the diagnosis of SLE (see Chapter 21).

ANAs are detected in a variety of ways; no method of detection is ideal.[1] Indirect immunofluorescence testing (FANA) is considered the most reliable.[1,6] Detection of neutrophils and other white blood cells that have phagocytized nuclear material in vitro, so-called LE cells, is another means of determining the presence of antinuclear antibodies. Unfortunately, the LE cell test can be difficult to interpret because of confusion of nondiagnostic nucleophagocytic cells with true LE cells. The test is laborious, and reliability depends on the experience and diligence of the technician performing the test.[9] In addition, the LE cell test is considered insensitive; formation of LE cells seems to depend on the concentration of antibody; many human hospitals require a high-positive FANA as a prerequisite to performing the LE cell test.[1,6,9]

The indirect immunofluorescence test is considered a sensitive indicator of SLE. There is some controversy over what constitutes a significant titer. Titers of 1:20 or greater were considered significant by Grindem and Johnson.[9] Bennett[6] suggests that a titer of 1:32 or greater is abnormal. Halliwell[11,12] found that it is not unusual for normal dogs and dogs having other diseases to have titers of 1:40 or less. Positive FANA titers have been detected in dogs with autoimmune skin disease, rheumatoid arthritis, and bacterial endocarditis. Positive titers have been documented in dogs receiving hydralazine.[3]

The definitive diagnosis of SLE is based on other criteria in addition to the presence of ANA (see Chapter 21). Some think that diagnosis of "suspected" SLE may be justified even when ANA has not been detected. Halliwell[11,12] reported 267 cases of *suspected* canine SLE; only 31 had an ANA titer of 1:40 or greater and 146 cases were completely negative. Even though a positive titer does not necessarily mean that the animal has SLE, most authorities believe the definitive diagnosis rests on detection of ANA at appreciable levels.[5,11] Bennett[5] described 13 cases of *definite* SLE in dogs; all had a positive ANA titer. Since the criteria established for SLE in humans have been used as a model for the disease in dogs and cats, emphasizing the importance of detecting antinuclear antibodies would seem reasonable. More than 80% of human patients with SLE have a positive ANA titer.[15,21]

Borrelia Burgdorferi (Lyme Disease) Testing

Exposure to the spirochete *Borrelia burgdorferi* causes an antibody response that can be documented with indirect immunofluorescent antibody testing.[2,18,19] The organism causes Lyme disease, a systemic illness that often has articular manifestations (see Chapter 21).

A positive titer to *B. burgdorferi* is important in the diagnosis of Lyme disease because the causative spirochete is difficult to culture or otherwise identify in dogs with suspected borreliosis.[17] Unfortunately, many apparently normal dogs in one endemic area had positive titers as well; although the geometric mean titer in affected dogs was found to be significantly higher than that found in clinically normal dogs, there is considerable overlap in titers.[17]

Because the clinical signs of Lyme disease are varied, nonspecific, and similar to those seen with other inflammatory joint disorders, the significance of a positive titer to *B. burgdorferi* must be carefully considered. Dogs with nonerosive immune-mediated arthropathies living in areas where *B. burgdorferi* is endemic could easily be misdiagnosed as having Lyme disease. Confusion over what constitutes a positive titer as well as public and commercial pressures generated by an enormous amount of publicity have probably adversely influenced the diagnostic process and increased the likelihood of overdiagnosis.

Synovial Membrane Examinations

Microbiological and pathological examinations of the synovial membrane have value in the diagnosis of joint disease. Although many histopathological abnormalities are nonspecific, an experienced pathologist can provide the clinician with valuable information. Histopathological examination is especially valuable in diagnosis of neoplasia and may help confirm or deny the clinical diagnosis of noninflammatory or inflammatory joint disease (see Chapter 21). When coupled with microbiological examination, synovial membrane analysis may help differentiate infectious arthritis from other inflammatory disorders.

Synovial membrane analysis may be warranted when the cause of joint disease remains undetermined or when symptomatic treatment has proven ineffective. Histopathological and microbiological examinations of the synovial membrane should be performed anytime exploration of a joint has failed to uncover the cause of lameness or when an apparent cause has been found but the membrane appears uncharacteristically thick, hyperemic, or discolored. Rupture of the cranial cruciate ligament may be the sequela of a number of inflammatory joint diseases. In such cases the synovial membrane usually appears more hyperemic and thickened than a clinician would normally expect with cruciate ligament rupture alone. Failure to examine the synovial membrane might preclude an accurate diagnosis and prognosis and lead to inappropriate and unsuccessful treatment.

Percutaneous needle biopsy of the synovial membrane has been described. Sample size is small, and the large size of some needles limits the use of this technique to larger dogs.[13] Biopsy via surgical arthrotomy has the advantages of allowing complete exploration of the joint, selective sampling of the synovial membrane, and collection of larger samples, and it can be performed on any joint in any size of animal.[13] In addition, treatments such as synovectomy or stabilization procedures can be performed at the same time. Samples of the synovial membrane should include the joint capsule and should be atraumatically harvested. Routine histopathological and microbiological methods are used. Special methods such as immunofluorescence testing have been used.

Miscellaneous

Serological and other testing methods for *Rickettsia* or *Rickettsia*-like organisms and for mycotic infections are indicated when the clinical findings suggest that they may be the cause of lameness (see Chapter 21). Such tests are more likely to be used when the affected animal lives in or has traveled to an area where the organism is endemic.

Measurement of immune complexes and other so-called acute-phase proteins might be of benefit in diagnosis and management of inflammatory joint disorders. There are numerous methods for documenting their presence; however, since the result of such testing is usually nonspecific, these tests are not routinely used in diagnosis or management of joint disease in dogs or cats. Coombs testing is not usually indicated or of diagnostic value in animals with joint disease; it is indicated for use when there is a hemolytic event. The test is sometimes positive in animals with SLE.

REFERENCES

1. Alarcon-Segovia D: Antibodies to nuclear and other intracellular antigens in the connective tissue diseases, *Clin Rheum Dis* 9:161-175, 1983.
2. Anderson JF, and others: Spirochetes in *Ixodes dammini* and mammals from Connecticut, *Am J Trop Med Hyg* 32:818-824, 1983.
3. Balazs T, and others: Hydralazine-induced antinuclear antibodies in beagle dogs, *Toxicol Appl Pharmacol* 57:452-456, 1981.
4. Bennett D: Immune-based erosive inflammatory joint disease of the dog: canine rheumatoid arthritis. 1. Clinical, radiological and laboratory investigations, *J Sm Anim Pract* 28:779-797, 1987.
5. Bennett D: Immune-based non-erosive inflammatory joint disease of the dog. 1. Canine systemic lupus erythematosus, *J Sm Anim Pract* 28:871-889, 1987.
6. Bennett D, Kirkham D: The laboratory identification of serum antinuclear antibody in the dog, *J Comp Pathol* 97:523-539, 1987.
7. Bennett D, Kirkham D: The laboratory identification of serum rheumatoid factor in the dog, *J Comp Pathol* 97:541-550, 1987.
8. Egeland T, Munthe E: Rheumatoid factors, *Clin Rheum Dis* 9:135-160, 1983.
9. Grindem CB, Johnson KH: Systemic lupus erythematosus: literature review and report of 42 new canine cases, *J Am Anim Hosp Assoc* 19:489-503, 1983.
10. Halliwell REW: Autoimmune disease in the dog, *Adv Vet Sci Comp Med* 22:221-263, 1978.
11. Halliwell REW: Skin disease associated with autoimmunity: the nonbullous autoimmune skin diseases, *Compend Contin Educ Pract Vet* 3:156-162, 1981.
12. Halliwell REW: Autoimmune disease in domestic animals, *J Am Vet Med Assoc* 181:1088-1096, 1982.
13. Hardy RM, Wallace LJ: Arthrocentesis and synovial membrane biopsy, *Vet Clin North Am* 4:449-462, 1974.
14. Healy MJR, Whitehead TP: Outlying values in the National Quality Control Scheme, *Ann Clin Biochem* 17:78-81, 1980.
15. Kimberly RP: Lupus erythematosus. In Beary JF, Christian CL, Sculco TP, editors: *Manual of rheumatology and outpatient orthopedic disorders*, Boston, 1981, Little, Brown.
16. Koffler D: The immunology of rheumatoid diseases, *Clin Symp (CIBA)* 31:14, 1979.
17. Kornblatt AN, and others: Arthritis caused by *Borrelia burgdorferi* in dogs, *J Am Vet Med Assoc* 186:960-964, 1985.
18. Magnarelli LA, and others: Parasitism by *Ixodes dammini* (*Acari:Ixodidae*) and antibodies to spirochetes in mammals at Lyme disease foci in Connecticut, USA, *J Med Entomol* 21:52-57, 1984.
19. Magnarelli LA, and others: Borreliosis in dogs from southern Connecticut, *J Am Vet Med Assoc* 186:955-959, 1985.
20. Newton CD, and others: Rheumatoid arthritis in dogs, *J Am Vet Med Assoc* 168:113-121, 1976.
21. Rothfield NF: Systemic lupus erythematosus: clinical and laboratory aspects. In McCarty DJ, editor: *Arthritis and allied conditions*, Philadelphia, 1979, Lea & Febiger.
22. Wilkins RJ: Joint serology. In Bojrab MJ, editor: *Pathophysiology in small animal surgery*, Philadelphia, 1981, Lea & Febiger.

2

Function, Structure, and Healing of the Musculoskeletal System

STEVEN E. WEISBRODE

▶ DEFINITION OF TERMS

articular cartilage Hyaline cartilage of synovial joints. The outer, or articulating, layer is unmineralized. The deepest layer adjacent to the underlying bone is mineralized.

canaliculi Miniscule canals within bone through which the processes of osteocytes extend to one another and to surface osteoblasts.

cement lines Microscopic basophilic lines in bone matrix that are poor in collagen and rich in ground substance and mineral. These lines indicate previous limits of bone resorption and rests in bone formation.

chondrocyte Cell within cartilage matrix. Chondrocytes retain the ability to produce matrix and, under appropriate conditions, can initiate mineralization of cartilage matrix.

collagen Fibrous tissue of the matrix; composed of predominantly type I collagen in bone and type II in hyaline cartilage.

compact bone (cortical bone, osteonal bone, haversian bone) Dense bone of the shafts of long bones and the outer walls of flat bones. In young animals, this bone is compacted (dense) but has not yet undergone remodeling to form osteons.

cutback zone Region in the metaphysis of marked bone resorption on the periosteal surface that tapers the bone from the circumference present at the physis to that of the diaphysis.

diaphysis Shaft or central region of the bone.

endochondral ossification Process by which hyaline cartilage is resorbed and replaced by bone. Bone is deposited on top of mineralized cartilage cores

27

that are created by vascular invasion and chondroclasis of the hyaline cartilage.

endosteum   Osteoblastic (often inactive) lining of the osteons and the cortical bone facing the marrow cavity.

epiphysis   End of the bone; separated from the remainder of the bone by the physis in the growing animal.

ground substance   Amorphous noncollagenous material of bone matrix. Some of the components of ground substance include water, proteoglycans, noncollagenous proteins (including enzymes and paracrine growth factors), pyrophosphates, and lipids.

Haversian canal   See *osteon.*

Howship lacuna   Scalloplike eroded area on a bone surface caused by osteoclastic bone resorption.

intramembranous bone formation   Direct production of bone by osteoblasts derived from metaplasia of osteogenic mesenchymal cells. Intramembranous bone has no cartilaginous precursor.

lacuna   Space in the matrix within which osteocytes and chondrocytes reside. This space in hyaline cartilage is probably a processing artifact. In bone the lacunar space around osteocytes is a true in situ fluid-filled space.

lamellar bone   Bone matrix deposited in an orderly manner so that the collagen fibers form parallel, microscopic layers. All normal bone of the mature skeleton is lamellar.

matrix   Collagen and ground substance of bone. It is bone tissue minus the mineral and cells.

metaphysis   Region of the bone between the physeal plate and the shaft of the bone (diaphysis).

mineral   Hydroxyapatite. Needle-shaped crystals containing predominantly calcium, CO_3, PO_4, OH, and lesser amounts of sodium, magnesium, and iron.

osteoblast   Cell of mesenchymal origin that produces bone (produce and secrete matrix and initiate its mineralization).

osteoclast   Cell of bone marrow origin that resorb bone mineral and matrix. They usually are multinucleated.

osteocyte   Cell within bone that originates from osteoblasts that become surrounded by and embedded in the bone they produce. Osteocytes retain minimum ability to produce bone.

osteoid   Unmineralized bone matrix.

osteon   Completed packet of remodeled compact bone. They are composed of cylinders of concentric lamellae of bone arranged around a central canal containing capillaries, lymphatics, and unmyelinated nerves. Osteons are oriented to the long axis of the bone and usually are perpendicular to the major weight bearing or stress on that bone.

periosteum   Fibrous and osteogenic membrane lining the exterior of the bone.

physis (growth plate, physeal plate)   Zone of hyaline cartilage between the epiphysis and metaphysis in growing animals. Cartilage in growth plate is able to undergo interstitial growth with subsequent endochondral ossification resulting in lengthening of bone.

resting lines   Cement lines with smooth or regular contour that indicate where bone formation ceased.

reversal lines   Cement lines with irregular or scalloped contour that indicate the depth to which osteoclasts resorbed bone.

tidemark   Demarcation line between unmineralized articular cartilage and the underlying mineralized cartilage.

trabecular bone (spongy bone, cancellous bone)   Spicular bone present within the marrow cavity.

Woven bone   Bone matrix deposited in haphazard pattern so that the collagen fibers are somewhat randomly arranged and do not form layers. Woven bone is the initial bone formed in endochondral and intramembranous bone formation and is the initial form of reactive bone in the adult skeleton.

BONE
Function

The most obvious function of bones is to give support to the organism in order to maintain basic form and locomotion. In mammals the skeleton is "internal" compared with the exoskeleton of so-called lower life forms. In addition to providing a framework on which the muscles can act, the bony skeleton offers rigid protection to vital structures such as the brain and spinal cord, as well as protection and a suspension rigging for the viscera of the thoracic and abdominal cavities. Marrow is located within the internal cavities of bone. Although marrow is critically important to life because it produces cells of hematopoietic and immune function, it is not apparent why marrow might need the protection of such sturdy surroundings.

Since the crystal component of bone is so extensive, it is not surprising that bone plays a role in mineral (particularly calcium) homeostasis. Surprisingly, however, the role bone plays in calcium homeostasis *in the normal animal* is rather small and almost passive compared with the ability of the kidneys and intestines. The function of osteocytes and osteoclasts in resorption of bone and release of calcium salts into the interstitial fluid (and eventually into the serum) is discussed later.

Development of the Skeletal System

Except for most of the flat skull bones, the skeleton begins its existence in the form of cartilage, which has to be mineralized, resorbed, and replaced by bone. This process is termed *endochondral ossification.* When the limbs begin to take shape in the fetus, they are composed entirely of hyaline cartilage. This cartilage is able to expand in width and length by both interstitial and appositional growth. Cartilaginous appositional growth occurs by generation of new matrix and cells on the perimeter of the limb by chondroblasts of the perichondrium. Interstitial growth occurs by division of chondrocytes within the cartilage matrix and causes expansion of the limb in all directions in the very early stages of uterine life. Later in the fetal period, interstitial growth in the physis results in directed longitudinal growth of the limb. Because of its fluid content, arrangement of collagen fibers, and lack of mineralization, hyaline cartilage has resilience, or plasticity, that allows interstitial growth not possible in bone. An analogy of interstitial growth is the expansion of clusters of soap bubbles under a stream of water. The dimension of the clusters increases not only because of the enlargement of individual bubbles, but also because of the creation of new bubbles within the mass.

The hyaline cartilage of the developing limbs takes on rudimentary form of their mature counterparts. This probably is genetically programmed rather than caused by physical forces acting on the limb in utero. Endochondral ossification is preceded by formation of a bony collar around the diaphyseal region of the cartilaginous limb. This collar develops by metaplasia of the perichondrium into periosteum. What initiates this metaplasia of perichondrium into periosteum is unknown, but apparently, different genes are now expressed by these cells to produce osteoid matrix and initiate its mineralization. This initial stage of ossification of endochondral bone is, in fact, intramembranous. Simultaneous with the development of the bony collar, chondrocytes in the middiaphysis undergo hypertrophy. Blood vessels from the bony collar invade the cartilage toward the region of hypertrophied chondrocytes and bring with them osteoclast and osteoblast precursors. As the blood vessels from the periosteum range closer to the hypertrophied chondrocytes, the chondrocytes induce mineralization of their surrounding matrix. After matrix mineralization, individual chondrocytes degenerate and die.

The combination of matrix mineralization and death of individual chondrocytes attracts (or triggers?) the invading blood vessels with their osteoclastic cells to penetrate the lacuna, resorb away one side of the mineralized vault, and expose the necrotic chondrocyte debris to the circulation. Technically, the osteoclast resorbing the cartilage would be termed a *chondroclast*. However, no known differences exist between osteoclasts and chondroclasts other than the substrate on which they are acting. This process is complex and is explored further in the discussion of the growth plate.

The invading blood vessels and osteoclasts leave a lattice of mineralized cartilage matrix on which new bone can form. This is the essence of endochondral ossification. A cartilage precursor was resorbed and replaced by bone. The process, however, involves partial resorption

of cartilage with building of bone on top of a "skeleton" of mineralized cartilage matrix rather than complete removal of the preexisting cartilage and deposition of new bone in empty space. The new bone is deposited on the mineralized cartilage spicules by osteoblasts whose precursors were brought into the region with the blood vessels that penetrated from the periosteum. The first spicule of new bone has a central core of mineralized cartilage matrix and is lined on both sides by osteoblasts and a narrow rim of osteoid. After several days, the osteoid becomes fully mineralized, creating a completed trabecula. This region in the middiaphysis of the developing limb is called the *primary center of ossification*. This region expands toward the metaphyses, replacing cartilage for bone as it advances.

At the ends of most bones of the appendicular skeleton, epiphyses are separated from the metaphyses in the growing animal by the physis (Fig. 2-1). The foci of initial endochondral ossification of the epiphyses begin as

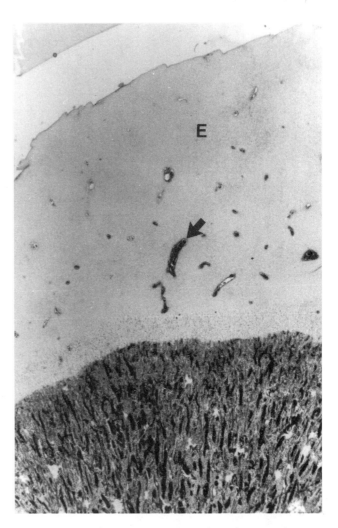

Fig. 2-1 Long bone from a young dog. The metaphysis is completely ossified. The epiphysis (E) has prominent vessels (*arrow*), but no secondary center of ossification has yet occurred.

separate events from the primary ossification of the diaphysis and are called *secondary centers of ossification*. The histogenesis of the process is the same as for the primary ossification center. The onset of secondary ossification centers varies among species, breeds, and bones within the same individual. As the ossification in the epiphyses expands centripetally and the ossification in the diaphysis expands up and down the newly forming marrow cavity, a disk of hyaline cartilage is left between the epiphysis and the metaphysis. This disk is the *physis*, or *growth plate*.

Because the growth plate is composed of cartilage rather than bone, longitudinal growth can continue because of interstitial growth of the hyaline cartilage in the physis. Longitudinal growth is no longer possible by interstitial proliferation in the rigid bony areas of the epiphysis and diaphysis, but the trade-off is that the ends and middle of the bones are capable of supporting the growing animal's weight. Chondrocytes in the physis are arranged into columns, and except for the resting zone, these columns are organized into zones (Fig. 2-2).

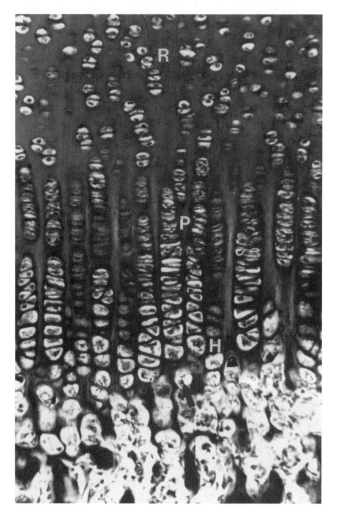

Fig. 2-2 Resting (R), proliferating (P), and hypertrophic (H), chondrocytes form the cellular columns of the physis. The zone of vascular invasion (*arrow*) is closest to the metaphysis.

The zone closest to the epiphysis is the *resting zone*, which is composed of relatively inactive chondrocytes. Chondrocytes in the resting zone are small elliptical cells arranged in clusters surrounded by relatively abundant matrix. In the resting zone the clusters of chondrocytes appear randomly arranged. The zone deep to the resting zone is the *proliferating zone*. Although chondrocytes in mitosis are seen infrequently in the proliferating zone, chondrocytes undergo division here, with production of new cells and matrix. This proliferating zone is largely responsible for extending the length of the bone in the direction of the overlying epiphysis.

The next zone toward the metaphysis is the *hypertrophic zone*, where the chondrocytes and their lacunae enlarge. This enlargement also contributes to longitudinal growth, extending the epiphysis farther from the diaphysis. In the hypertrophic zone the chondrocytes accumulate glycogen; this and swelling, possibly from hypoxia, contribute to the cytoplasmic enlargement. Most of the nutrient supply to the growth plate cartilage comes from the epiphyseal artery, with diffusion of nutrients and oxygen into the metaphyseal end of the plate. Consequently, oxygen tension is least in the hypertrophic zones of the growth plate. With the enlargement of the chondrocytes and their lacunae in the hypertrophic zone, the condensed matrix takes on a ladderlike appearance. The parallel sides of the ladder are the longitudinal cartilaginous septa, and the rungs are the transverse septa. In the distal regions of the hypertrophic zones, mineralization of the longitudinal septum begins.

The initiation of this mineralization is under direct control of the chondrocyte. As in the primary center of ossification in the diaphysis, the conversion of cartilage into bone involves invasion into the cartilage by blood vessels, which bring with them precursors of osteoclasts and osteoblasts. In the center of the growth plate, these vessels are capillary loops derived from branches of the nutrient artery. At the perimeter of the plate, the capillaries are from branches of the metaphyseal arteries. No agreement exists about the precise sequence of events and even the appearance of the cells involved at the *zone of vascular invasion*, also known as the *zone of provisional calcification*. Certainly at this point, the longitudinal septum is fully mineralized, and patchy or no mineralization of the transverse septum occurs. It is also agreed that the last hypertrophied chondrocyte dies, and its transverse septum is penetrated by a blood vessel. Uncertainty surrounds the appearance of the hypertrophied chondrocytes before necrosis. In most specimens the chondrocytes in the hypertrophic zone appear to undergo increasing depletion of glycogen and vacuolar degeneration as they are distanced from the advancing epiphyseal end of the plate and its blood vessels. However, hypertrophied chondrocytes are very sensitive to fixation artifacts, and advanced degenerative changes noted in these cells may be artifacts of preservation.

The invasion and destruction of the transverse septum by blood vessels leave only the mineralized longitudinal cartilage septum as a remnant of the physis (Fig. 2-3). Not all these septa survive; many are resorbed away by osteoclasts (chondroclasts) whose precursors followed the invading capillaries. On the surface of the remaining cartilage cores, osteoid is deposited by osteoblasts that have matured from osteoblast progenitor cells brought with the blood vessels. The deposition of bone matrix (osteoid) on the cartilage core creates the primary trabecula. The sequence of the conversion of cartilage to bone is the same in the physis as in the primary center of ossification; the major difference is that interstitial growth is oriented toward lengthening the bone in the physis. In the epiphyses, there is also a physis between the expanding secondary center of ossification and the remaining epiphyseal cartilage; this is called the *articular-epiphyseal complex.*

The mechanisms that influence the processes of endochondral ossification of the physis plate are com-plex, and the biochemical mediators are not fully under-stood. Investigations center on three major areas: (1) control of proliferation of chondrocytes, (2) control of maturation and mineralization of chondrocytes, and (3) control of vascular invasion. Growth hormone (soma-totropin) has long been known to be needed for longi-tudinal growth. Somatotropin may have a direct effect on the physis plate by inducing chondrocytes to synthe-size insulin-like growth factor 1, a powerful growth stim-ulator. In contrast, the steroid sex hormones of estrogen and testosterone are important in reducing proliferation of chondrocytes and influencing closure of the physis.

With vitamin D deficiency, mineralization and matura-tion of chondrocytes of the physis fail to occur. Some evidence suggests that the vitamin D metabolite $24, 25\text{-}(OH)_2D_3$ has a greater effect on physeal maturation and mineralization than other vitamin D metabolites. Most studies, however, support the concept that all functions of vitamin D are mediated preferentially by its most potent renal metabolite, $1, 25\text{-} (OH)_2D_3$. The effect of vit-amin D on the physis may be indirect, since rickets (widening of the physis because of failure of mineraliza-tion and maturation of chondrocytes from vitamin D deficiency) can be cured in rats by infusing calcium and phosphorus. These observations suggest that the influ-ence of vitamin D and its metabolites on the physis may be secondary to their effect on absorbing calcium and phosphorus from the intestine. When considering the control of mineralization and vascular invasion of the physis, inhibitors of these events may be more signifi-cant than promoters. In physeal cartilage, proteoglycans and pyrophosphates inhibit mineralization, and pro-teases inhibit endothelial cell proliferation and vascular invasion. Therefore, initiation of mineralization and vas-cular invasion probably results from destruction of these inhibitors.

In microscopic and radiographic examination of bone, one can easily forget that the bone is a three-dimensional structure. The mineralized cartilage cores that survive the vascular invasion and chondroclasis at the chondro-osseous junction (interface of cartilage of physis and trabeculae of bone in the metaphysis) are not finger-like projections but, when viewed on edge, are honeycomb-like structures (Fig. 2-4 *A*). The former columns of chondrocytes make up the chambers in the honeycomb, and the walls of the comb are the mineral-ized longitudinal septa. Once this honeycomb is covered with bone (formation of primary trabeculae), modeling of these to secondary and tertiary trabeculae occurs and converts this honeycomb into anastomosing plates of the cancellous bone of the marrow space (Fig. 2-4 *B*).

In the primary trabeculae, both sides are lined by osteoblasts that are depositing bone. Therefore, the sur-faces on the trabecula are moving away from one another, and the trabecula is becoming thicker because of circumferential formation. The primary trabeculae are

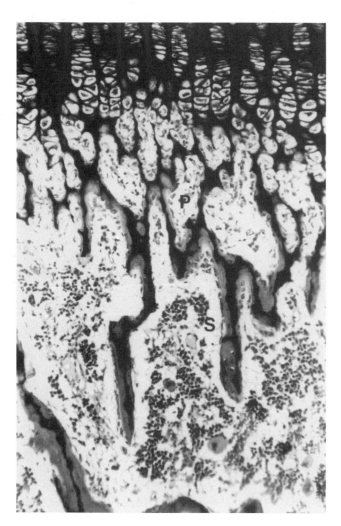

Fig. 2-3 Mineralized cartilage core (*darker matrix*) lined by osteoid (*lighter matrix*) forming primary (P), and secondary (S), trabeculae.

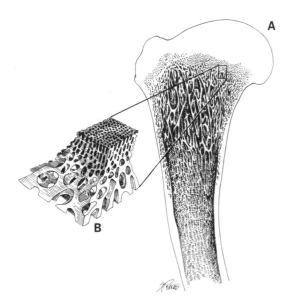

Fig. 2-4 Physis and metaphyseal trabeculae viewed on sagittal section (**A**) and from the epiphysis (**B**). The holes at the top of **B** represent the end of the column of chondrocytes, where the last of the hypertrophic chondrocytes has died and been invaded by vessels. The matrix surrounding the holes represents the mineralized longitudinal cartilaginous septa. The three-dimensional meshwork of trabeculae can be appreciated as interconnecting struts or plates.

more numerous and thinner than secondary trabeculae. Likewise, tertiary trabeculae are fewer and thicker than secondary trabeculae. The transition of primary to secondary to tertiary trabeculae involves the process of modeling.

Modeling is the movement of bone through space and the changing of its shape. Modeling requires formation to occur on one surface and resorption on another. Envision two parallel 1-foot-thick brick walls that are 10 feet apart and continually being added to in length from their proximal ends (primary trabeculae). The goal is to connect these walls gradually at their distal ends into a single centrally placed wall that is 2 feet thick (secondary trabecula). The walls must never have a break. To accomplish this, bricks are removed from the outer surface of each wall and added to the insides of the walls until the inner surfaces meet. Removal of bricks would continue on the outer surfaces until the central single wall is 2 feet thick. In fact, the wall has changed shape and has been moved through space. This is modeling and is accomplished by osteoclastic activity on the "outsides" of opposing trabeculae and formation on the "insides" of opposing trabeculae. By formation on opposing surfaces and resorption on nonopposing surfaces, primary trabeculae may "drift" through space and unite to form a secondary trabecula (see Fig. 2-3).

At the perimeter of the physis, the ends of the cortical bone are formed. In this region the objective is to convert primary trabeculae into compact bone rather than cancellous bone. This is done by compaction. Formation takes place on both sides of a trabecula and continues until there is only a central space left for vessels and nerves. The bone deposited is dense cortical (compact) bone, but it is not deposited in concentric lamellae of osteons. This requires remodeling and osteonization, as discussed later.

Although most bones increase in length by endochondral ossification, all bones increase in width by intramembranous bone formation. The periosteum deposits new bone on the surface of existing bone to widen the cortex (Fig. 2-5). In larger animals, this may be done in multiple layers or laminae at one time and the space filled in between the laminae by compaction, as described previously. To form a cortical wall of appropriate thickness, while formation is taking place on the periosteal surface, resorption is occurring on the endosteal surface. This modeling of cortical bone results in bone drift through space. To appreciate the extent of this movement and drifting, consider the cross-sectional diameter of the thorax of a Great Dane pup and compare it with the diameter in the adult dog. These bones moved through space to attain this difference. Using these ribs in this case as an example, the concept of formation on the outside (periosteum) and resorption on the inside (endosteum) seems at first to be true, but in fact this is the net effect and does not hold true when all surfaces of the bone are considered. With regard to this movement, the rib is considered to have four different surfaces: the periosteum and endosteum of the cortex facing the skin (outer cortex), and a periosteum and endosteum of the cortex facing the pleura (inner cortex). This movement of the growing rib then results from formation on the outer periosteum and the inner endosteum and resorption on the outer endosteum and the inner periosteum.

Remodeling

One of the most remarkable features of the skeletal system is its ability to renew itself. Remodeling is the renewal of bone by activation of resorption followed by formation. In theory the amount of bone replaced is equal to the amount of bone removed so that there is no net difference in bone volume. The advantages of this are that minor damage (microfracture) that has accrued with time can be removed and replaced with new tissue. If microfractures were not "remodeled away," they could increase in size with time and result in structural weakening of the bone.

Primary remodeling of bone is seen most dramatically on microscopic examination of compact bone (cortical

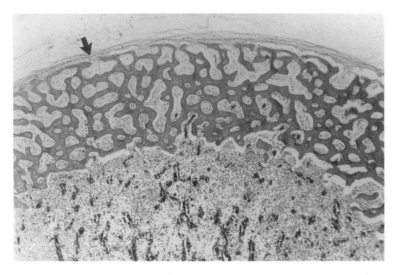

Fig. 2-5 Cross section of the diaphysis of a long bone in a neonatal puppy, with intramembranous bone formation enlarging the cortex from the periosteal surface (*arrow*).

bone) of young animals. As stated previously, compact bone in young animals is formed by compaction (filling in by lamellar bone) between trabeculae at the perimeter of the growth plate and by adding lamellar bone to the width of the bone by the periosteum. This bone is not arranged in osteons. Primary remodeling involves the activation of bone resorption by osteoclasts and the conversion of this nonosteonal compact bone to osteonized compact bone (osteonization). In cortical bone a cluster of osteoclasts acts as a drill bit and bores a longitudinal tunnel in the compact bone. The width and length of the tunnel appear to be genetically programmed. This "drill bit" is referred to as a cutting cone (Fig. 2-6). After the cutting cone, a blood vessel and cells of osteogenic potential mature into osteoblasts. These osteoblasts line the walls of the tunnel and begin to lay down bone in layers. The central canal of the tunnel becomes smaller as the osteoblasts continue to deposit bone. Again, at a genetically programmed stop, the osteoblasts cease depositing bone, and some remain as inactive cells on the bone surface (lining cells). The end product is a tunnel that has been filled in with concentric layers of bone with a central canal for blood vessels and nerves, in other words, an osteon (Fig. 2-7).

In remodeling, resorption precedes formation. In humans the estimated amount of bone formed is about 97% of the amount resorbed. With time there can be a physiological bone loss (osteoporosis) as a result of long-term subtle differences in the balance between amount of bone resorbed and the amount of bone formed during remodeling. The sequence of remodeling is *activation, resorption, and formation* (ARF). The end result of this ARF is a unit of bone referred to as a *basic structural*

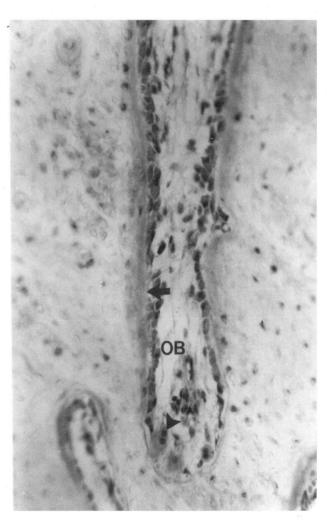

Fig. 2-6 Cutting cone with leading edge of osteoclasts (*arrowhead*) followed by osteoblasts (OB). Beneath the osteoblasts is a layer of osteoid (*arrow*).

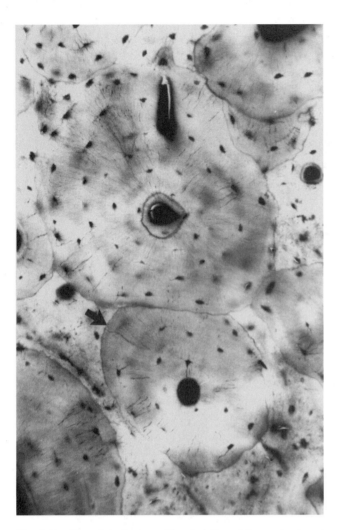

Fig. 2-7 Completed osteon. The dark line at the perimeter of the osteon (*arrow*) is a cement line indicating where resorption had stopped and formation began to reverse the process (reversal line).

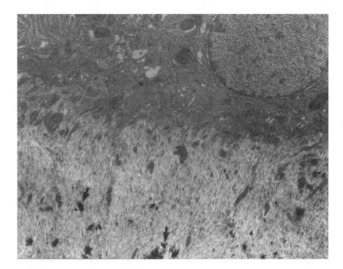

Fig. 2-8 Electron photomicrograph of an osteoblast. The cell has extensive rough endoplasmic reticulum and numerous mitochondria. The Golgi apparatus is not conspicuous in this plane. The adjacent matrix (osteoid) is incompletely mineralized. Initial foci of mineralization are taking place in matrix vesicles (*arrows*).

unit (BSU). In cortical bone the BSU is the osteon. In trabecular bone, no term exists for this unit other than BSU.

Individual Bone Cells and Their Functional Activity

Osteoblasts. Osteoblasts are the cells of mesenchymal origin on the surface of bone. Their function can be divided into four categories: matrix synthesis, matrix mineralization, initiation of resorption, and communication with osteocytes.

Matrix synthesis. Osteoblasts active in the synthesis of matrix are rectangular to columnar cells of relatively high cytoplasmic/nuclear ratio. The prominent cytoplasmic area reflects the abundance of cellular organelles, particularly rough endoplasmic reticulum and Golgi apparatus, required for production and secretion of matrix (Fig. 2-8). The osteoblast is responsible for synthesis of all matrix components. Matrix, which is all the extracellular material in bone other than mineral, can be considered in two major categories: collagen and ground substance (Fig. 2-9).

Collagen is the protein that gives bone its strength rather than hardness and is the major component of bone matrix. When decalcified bone is examined microscopically, the matrix appears as densely packed lamellae of collagen fibers. These fibers in mature bone are arranged in concentric layers in osteons of cortical bone, and parallel the gently curving surfaces of trabeculae in cancellous bone.

In recent years, knowledge of the components of the *ground substance* and their functions has exploded, but for the most part, the ground substance is still poorly understood. Briefly and for the purpose of this text, the ground substance can be divided into three components: proteoglycans, noncollagenous proteins, and lipids. The role of *proteoglycans* in bone is not well understood, but they may act as inhibitors of mineralization. *Noncollagenous proteins* include cytokins, which are capable of influencing activity of other bone cells, and enzymes, which probably play a role in collagen degradation and destruction of inhibitors of mineralization. In addition, noncollagenous proteins act as finding agents for cells, matrix and mineral to each other. *Lipids* are probably associated with fragments of cell membranes extruded into the matrix and probably function in the mineralization process.

Initiation of mineralization. In vitro, mature collagen devoid of cells (e.g., boiled tendon) is able to precipitate

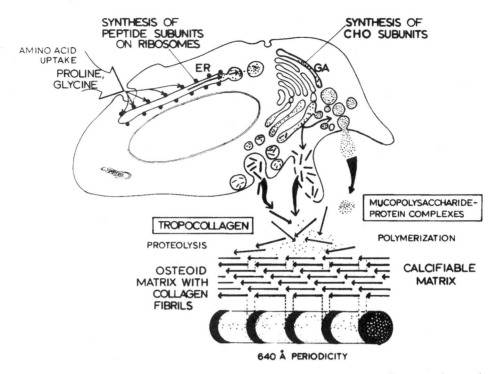

Fig. 2-9   Illustration of an osteoblast synthesizing collagenous (tropocollagen) and noncollagenous (represented as mucopolysaccharides) components in the rough endoplasmic reticulum (ER) and secreting them into the matrix by way of the Golgi apparatus (GA). Note the characteristic layering and gaps between adjacent tropocollagen resulting in a banded collagen fibril. The dark bands in the fibril represent mineral that has been deposited in the gaps.

calcium and phosphorus out of a concentrated solution. In vivo, however, most investigators believe that the initiation of mineralization in bone is under the control of the osteoblast. Small spherical particles of the osteoblast facing the bone-forming surface are pinched off and remain in the unmineralized matrix (osteoid). These spherules are called *matrix vesicles* (see Fig. 2-8). Mineralization is initiated within these matrix vesicles. As described previously for initiation of mineralization of the physis, inhibitors of mineralization may be more important than promoters. The bone fluid in the region of osteoid is suspected to be high enough in calcium and phosphorus to allow spontaneous precipitation. It therefore is not surprising that matrix components can act to inhibit mineralization.

The role of the matrix vesicle is to destroy at least some of these inhibitors and to concentrate precipitated and crystalline calcium and phosphorus in a focus that can overwhelm the remaining inhibitors. The membrane of the matrix vesicle is rich in phosphatase enzymes. One of the substrates of these phosphatases is *inorganic pyrophosphate*. Inorganic pyrophosphates have high-energy phosphate-phosphate bonds and are potent inhibitors of mineralization. They are found in osteoid, as well as cartilage. Once the inorganic pyrophosphates are cleaved by the phosphatase enzymes of the matrix vesicle, not only are their inhibitory effects destroyed, but

the cleaved free phosphorus is made available for incorporation into bone mineral. Lipids of the matrix vesicle are able to bind calcium physically to the surface of the membranes. With free phosphorus in the vicinity of the matrix vesicle, calcium bound to the surface of the vesicle, and inhibitors of mineralization destroyed, the calcium and phosphorus are ready to gain entry into the matrix vesicle. This is accomplished at least partially by phosphatase enzymes, possibly acting as alkaline phosphatase. These enzymes may facilitate calcium and phosphorus transport into the matrix vesicle. Once in the matrix vesicle in sufficient concentration, the calcium and phosphorus, as well as other cations and anions (sodium, magnesium, iron) precipitate out as amorphous mineral. This amorphous mineral stage is short lived, and the mineral crystallizes into the spicule form known as *hydroxyapatite*.

The conversion of the mineral from an amorphous to a crystalline needle-like shape causes a physical rupture of the matrix wall by the spicule. Once the spicule has ruptured the matrix vesicle, it has access to collagen fibers surrounding the matrix vesicle. Although the collagen fibers were unable to initiate the mineralization process (as a result of the presence of inhibitors in the matrix), once the inhibitors are inactivated and a mature crystal contacts a collagen fiber, salts in the form of crystalline hydroxyapatite are precipitated directly out of the bone fluid in the matrix and onto the collagen without matrix vesicles as intermediaries. In other words, once the mineralization process is initiated by matrix vesicles, it can be propagated by collagen fibers. Tropocollagen molecules secreted by osteoblasts arrange themselves in overlapping layers that give type I collagen its typical cross-banded ultrastructural appearance. When the tropocollagen molecules align themselves, they leave a gap or hole between themselves. It is in these gaps that crystals of hydroxyapatite are precipitated (see Fig. 2-9) once mineralization has been initiated by the matrix vesicles.

Initiation of resorption. The osteoclast undoubtedly is the cell most responsible for dissolution of bone mineral and lysis of bone matrix. It was perplexing, therefore, that receptors for hormones that induce osteoclastic bone resorption (e.g., parathyroid hormone [PTH]) were not found on osteoclasts but were present on osteoblasts. The complex sequence of events initiating resorption is not yet fully understood but can be summarized as follows.

Hormones or cytokines that stimulate resorption bind to receptors on the osteoblast. For PTH, this binding to receptors on the plasma membrane causes an increase in intracellular cycle adenosine monophosphate (cAMP). The ultimate effect of this "second messenger" (cAMP) is to phosphorylate specific intracellular proteins. This phosphorylation of specific proteins (a form of "activation") results in the physiological response. The initial structural response of osteoblasts to PTH is a change in shape (Fig. 2-10). *Resting osteoblasts* (also called *lining cells*) form a layer over the bone surface, protecting it from wandering osteoclasts that are hovering above it.

PTH causes osteoblasts to round up and separate from one another. The subsequent gaps that are present between cells allow osteoclasts to gain access to the bone surface. The exposed surface of bone may not be densely mineralized matrix. On many resting bone surfaces, underneath the inactive osteoblasts is a very narrow layer of unmineralized collagen. The purpose of this thin band of connective tissue is unknown, but it may act as a barrier to osteoclasis.

In addition to causing osteoblasts to contract and expose the underlying bone, PTH is thought to cause osteoblasts to release collagenases to destroy this thin, unmineralized layer of collagen. Osteoclasts now can gain access to the fully mineralized bone surface. Besides preparing the surface and "getting out of the way," osteoblasts are likely to produce proteins that are chemotactic for osteoclasts. These chemotactic proteins (*cytokines*) may be released directly into the microenvironment or become deposited into the matrix as noncollagenous proteins.

Communication with osteocytes. During matrix synthesis, osteoblasts send numerous fingerlike cytoplasmic projections into the matrix. Some of these pinch off to become matrix vesicles, and others atrophy and involute when the osteoblast changes from an active osteoblast secreting matrix to a resting osteoblast, or lining cell. Some of these cytoplasmic projections, however, survive and extend through canals in the bone called *canaliculi*. These processes then extend from the lining cells to the osteocytes and from osteocyte to osteocyte. They form gap junctions with each other when they meet in a canaliculus. Since gap junctions are capable of allowing ions and small molecules to travel between cells, the

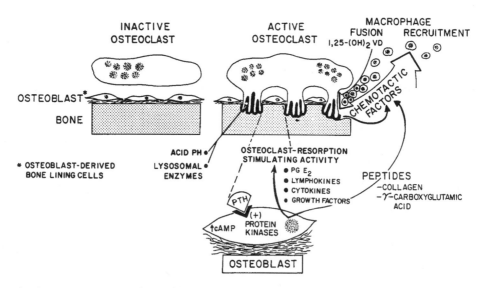

Fig. 2-10   Interaction of osteoblasts and osteoclasts. On the left, osteoblasts form a relatively uniform layer separating the inactive osteoclast from the bone surface. On the right, stimulated osteoblasts have contracted and exposed the bone surface to osteoclasts activated by cytokines released by the osteoblast.

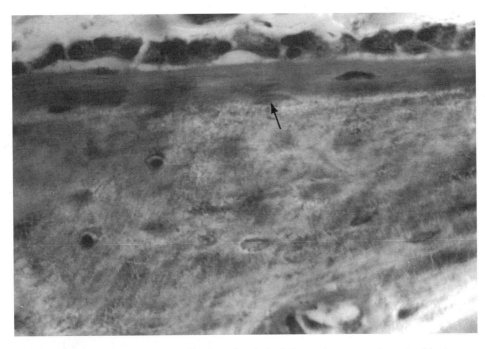

Fig. 2-11 Section of fully mineralized (undecalcified) bone demonstrating osteoblasts on a surface of osteoid. Osteocytes are present within the osteoid layer and within the mineralized matrix. The arrow indicates the line of separation between the osteoid and the mineralized matrix.

osteoblast-osteocyte network means that an extensive amount of bone surface is in indirect contact with the lining cells and eventually the plasma, as discussed next.

Osteocytes. Osteocytes are the cells buried within the bone (Fig. 2-11). The microscopic holes in the bone in which they reside are termed *lacunae*. These cells send out long, thin, cytoplasmic projections that course through the bone in tunnels, or canaliculi (Fig. 2-12). As stated previously, the processes join each other with gap junctions, and this interconnecting network extends between osteocytes and the surface osteoblasts. Osteocytes are osteoblasts that became buried in matrix. Osteocytes deeper in the bone (further from the surface) are older (i.e., buried earlier) than osteocytes closer to the surface. The function of osteocytes is uncertain. It is speculated that they play a role in calcium homeostasis. This certainly makes sense from an anatomical perspective.

Normally, bone surface is thought of as that near the vascular system, for example, the endosteum, periosteum, and central canals of the haversian systems. However, the lacunar and canalicular network of osteocytes is also a surface system, although not in proximity to the vascular system. This surface system of the lacunar and canalicular network is vast, and the solubility of the mineral in the lacunar wall is believed to be greater than for bone mineral in general. It is hypothesized that changes in the metabolic activity of osteocytes could solubilize small amounts of mineral from the lacunar wall. Miniscule fluxes in the deposition and removal of

mineral from these surfaces would have a trivial effect on the structural integrity of the bone but could have marked effects on calcium homeostasis. Mineral released from lacunar or canalicular walls would be transmitted "up" the system to lining cells (inactive osteoblasts), which would pump the calcium into the extracellular fluid. The significance of this "osteocyte-osteoblast pump" is uncertain, and it is probably less important to minute-to-minute calcium homeostasis than the intestine and kidney. However, this pump may

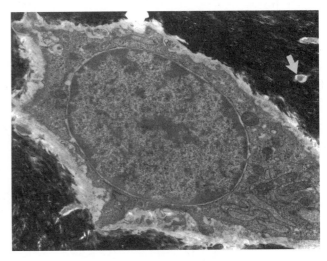

Fig. 2-12 Electron micrograph of an osteocyte. Cellular processes can be seen extending into the bone through channels called canaliculi (*arrow*).

play a role in responding to marked challenges to calcium homeostasis.

Destruction of both matrix and mineral from the lacunar wall has been termed *osteocytic osteolysis*. Osteocytic osteolysis is not a physiological event and probably occurs only with great stresses to calcium homeostasis. Most investigators think that osteocytic osteolysis does not play a significant role in the pathogenesis of bone disease.

Osteoclasts. Osteoclasts are derived from the monocyte-macrophage system under the influence of a variety of agents, including $1,25\text{-}(OH)_2D_3$. Although mature osteoclasts do not have receptors for the vitamin D metabolite, precursors of osteoclasts do have receptors for $1,25\text{-}(OH)_2D_3$, which is required for their genesis. Preosteoclasts are mobile, mononucleated cells that are separated from the bone surface by lining cells. Initiation of resorption has been discussed previously as a function of the osteoblast. Once activated, the preosteoclast fuses with other preosteoclasts, and when it has access to the bone surface, it differentiates further.

The plasma membrane touching the bone surfaces changes into two distinctly different structures (Fig. 2-13). The perimeter of the cell develops a transitional zone that is rich in microfilaments and poor in other organelles. This transitional zone functions to anchor the cell to the bone surface and confine the bone-digesting activity. The central portion of the plasma membrane in contact with the bone surface becomes extremely convoluted and is called a *ruffled*, or *brush, border*. Bone resorption occurs

beneath this ruffled border. Carbonic acid is produced in the cytoplasm of the osteoclast with the aid of the enzyme carbonic anhydrase, and the hydrogen ion is released through the ruffled border by a proton pump (Fig. 2-14). This acidification of the bone surface beneath the osteoclast solubilizes the mineral and by doing so enables enzymes to penetrate the remaining matrix. The enzymes (primarily proteinases rather than collagenases as might be expected) responsible for cleaving the collagen into polypeptides come from the numerous lysosomes in the osteoclast. It is uncertain how much of the matrix degradation products and dissolved salts passes

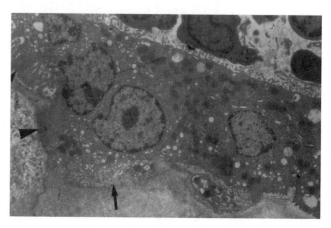

Fig. 2-13   Electron photomicrograph of an osteoclast with portions of the ruffled border (*arrows*) and transitional zone (*arrowhead*) in the plane of section.

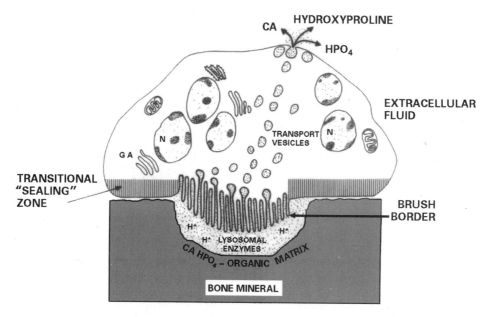

Fig. 2-14   Hydrogen ions from intracellular carbonic acid production are secreted by proton pumps on the surface of the ruffled border into the underlying bone to dissolve mineral. Lysosomal enzymes are secreted to hydrolyze the organic components of the matrix.

through the osteoclast and how much escapes directly to the local environment. The important point is that the resorbed products of both mineral and matrix are released to the extravascular space and ultimately to the intravascular space and are not locally reused for the synthesis of new bone.

Physiological bone resorption associated with remodeling is initiated by osteoblasts, as described previously. In remodeling, after the resorptive phase if over, a formation phase occurs. This association of resorption with formation is called *coupling*. The osteoclast is not thought to play a direct role in coupling. Current theory suggests that growth factors (noncollagenous proteins) deposited in the bone originally during matrix synthesis by osteoblasts are responsible for coupling. A promising candidate for the most important coupling factor is *transforming growth factor β* (TGF-β). TGF-β in vitro is able to inhibit bone resorption and stimulate bone formation. TGF-β apparently exists in the matrix in an inactive form that requires acidification for activation. The osteoclast not only releases TGF-β from the matrix during resorption, but also activates it. As the concentration of TGF-β in the local environment rises, it causes a cessation of resorption and an onset of formation.

Bone resorption in pathological states differs from that described previously for remodeling. Pathological resorption is probably not initiated by osteoblasts but is induced by prostaglandins and cytokines, such as osteoclast activating factor released from inflammatory cells, particularly macrophages. In addition to differences in the means of initiating resorption, the feedback mechanisms that limit the depth of resorption and the coupling of resorption to formation are not present in pathological conditions. Subsequently, clinically significant areas of bone loss may develop with inadequate replacement by new bone in many lesions, particularly those involving neoplasia and inflammation.

Response of Bone to Injury

The matrix and mineral of bone are extracellular and relatively inert. Therefore, changes in the mineral and matrix of bone in response to injury are caused by alterations in the activity of osteoblasts, osteocytes, and osteoclasts. The response of bone cells to injury can result in their atrophy, degeneration, and death, leading to hyperplasia, hypertrophy, or imbalance in the rates and coordination of bone synthesis and resorption. In simple terms, this means that for the matrix and mineral of the skeleton, the response to injury is limited to changing the amount of bone present, changing the shape of the bone present, or changing the rate at which it is replaced (turnover). These responses can be categorized into changes in remodeling, changes in modeling, and focal lytic and productive bone lesions.

Changes in remodeling in response to injury. With regard to changes in remodeling in response to injury, we consider injury in its broadest sense—an insult to the cell. Some injuries are trivial and may be below the threshold of detection by the cell. More serious insults may elicit a response that is within the physiological limits of the cell and therefore is not detected as a clinical problem. Some insults overwhelm the cell and alter its normal activity. An injury that can greatly influence bone remodeling is change in mechanical use. As summarized by Frost, normal mechanical use is necessary to suppress the activation phase of remodeling and stimulate the completion (or formation) phase. In much less precise terms, normal mechanical use suppresses resorption and stimulates formation. Reduced mechanical use then results in net loss of bone (Fig. 2-15). This can take place surprisingly quickly and can be detected experimentally within 72 hours. Such bone loss can be expected in small domestic animals with paralysis and paresis associated with trauma and denervation. The effects of increased mechanical use on remodeling are less clear. The mechanisms by which mechanical use may alter bone cell function are discussed next.

Changes in modeling in response to injury. Modeling is the change of the size, shape, or orientation of bone. It occurs during growth and throughout life as mechanical use of the bone is altered. The observations that a bone can (within limits) alter its structure to accommodate changes in its function have been credited to the German anatomist Julius Wolff (1836-1902) (see references in Frost) and have been termed *Wolff's law*. In practical terms, Wolff's law predicts that the thickness of

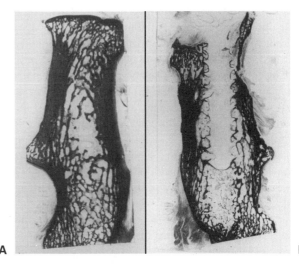

Fig. 2-15 Tibial tarsal bones from an experimental dog. **B,** A stainless steel screw was placed and removed before preparing the section. **A** served as the control. Note the porosity of the cortex and thinning of the trabeculae caused by the stress-shielding (decreased mechanical use) effect of the screw.

cortices and the thickness and orientation of trabeculae change to adapt to the stress placed on the bone. It is not only the trabeculae that are influenced by mechanical forces. In bones, with increased mechanical use, the cortices becomes thicker because of an increase in periosteal bone apposition and inhibition of the normal expansion of the endosteum by resorption. Conversely, decreased mechanical use causes a thinning of the cortex by depressing periosteal apposition and increasing endosteal resorption.

In response to uneven mechanical stress put on a bone, bone forms on the side of compression and resorbs on the side of tension. In a bowed leg, bone forms on the concave or compressed side of the leg and resorbs on the convex or stretched side. These responses of bone to stresses are mediated by osteoblasts and osteoclasts. What tells the bone-forming cells and resorbing cells to act is not precisely known, but electric potentials within bone are thought to play important roles. When bone is placed under strain, the deformation of the collagen produces electric potentials known as *piezoelectric forces* and fluid flows produce streaming potentials. These forces appear to be independent of bone cells and mineral. Electropositive areas of bone tend to undergo resorption, and electronegative areas undergo formation.

Focal lytic and productive lesions of bone

Necrosis. Necrosis means cell death, the result of irreversible cell injury. Necrosis does not take place in the mineral and matrix phases of bone, which are extracellular. The cells that die are the osteoblasts, osteocytes, osteoclasts, and the cells of the marrow. Osteonecrosis can result from a variety of causes, which can be divided into two categories: inflammation and vascular compromise not associated with inflammation.

Necrosis associated with inflammation is common and may be a result of compression of vessels because of pressure buildup from the exudate of the inflammation in the rigid confines of the bone. In addition, necrosis associated with inflammation can be caused by toxins or enzymes released by inflammatory cells or from microorganisms. Bone lysis induced by inflammation (discussed in the following section) also can isolate a fragment of bone from its blood supply, causing its death.

Vascular compromise not associated with inflammation causing ischemic necrosis of bone is usually caused by trauma. Fracture of a bone into multiple fragments may result in one or more of the pieces being avulsed from its blood supply.

Other cases of necrosis of bone not associated with inflammation or overt trauma are presumed to result from vascular compromise and are often grouped as avascular necrosis. Such conditions are seen in the femoral head of small breed dogs. The pathogenesis of this in the dog is not known with certainty but may be secondary to pressure buildup within the joint capsule causing compression of the small veins and arteries that supply the femoral head. Because the precise cause is often difficult to determine, these conditions are often called *idiopathic avascular necrosis.*

The response of bone to necrosis requires an intact blood supply and is greatly altered if the necrosis is associated with inflammation. Following are descriptions of the response of bone to necrosis in which reestablishment of blood supply has been successful and no inflammation occurs. In the acute stages of necrosis, the cells of the bone and marrow are dead but the mineral or matrix is not altered grossly, microscopically, or radiographically. In fact, at this stage the lesion may be clinically silent, and the strength of the bone is not yet altered.

In the subacute stages, at the periphery of the lesion, where the blood supply has been reestablished, a cellular response to the necrosis occurs. In the marrow, early stages of fibrosis may develop. An increase in both bone resorption and formation in the dead bone is likely in response to cytokines from macrophages. The osteoclasts and osteoblasts that accomplish this come, respectively, from the monocyte-macrophage cells and undifferentiated mesenchymal cells from the adjacent viable marrow and bone. The goal of this response is to resorb the dead bone and replace it with normal bone. Although dead bone in the early stages of necrosis is not deficient structurally, with time the bone accumulates microdamage because dead bone is incapable of remodeling.

The formation that takes place in the subacute stages of the necrosis is not limited to replacing dead bone that has been resorbed by osteoclasts. On some dead trabeculae, viable osteoblasts deposit a layer of new woven bone directly on top of the dead bone (Fig. 2-16). Although this sandwich of new bone–dead bone eventually is resorbed, for a time some trabeculae in the lesion are thicker than normal because of this deposition. The purpose of this deposition is uncertain, but it may add strength to the bone while other areas are undergoing resorption. The stimulus for the bone production may be mechanical. During this stage of repair of necrosis of bone, the bone may appear radiodense, possibly because of new bone deposition on top of dead bone and mineralization of the cytoplasm of dead osteocytes.

In the chronic stages of repair of osteonecrosis, the hope is that all the dead bone has been resorbed and replaced with normal bone and that the fibrosis of the marrow also is resorbed. This is unlikely for large lesions, for those in which abnormal weight bearing has occurred during the repair stages, and for those in which inflammation has developed. The femoral head of dogs with idiopathic avascular necrosis often shows extensive resorption of the dead bone and fibrosis of the marrow but little disposition of new bone. The articular carti-

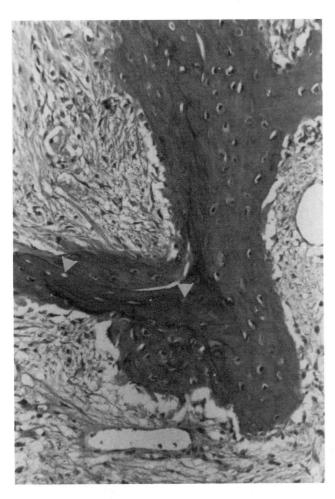

Fig. 2-16 Reactive woven bone with haphazardly arranged osteocytes deposited on a necrotic trabeculus. Note the absence of osteocyte nuclei in many of the lacunae (*arrowheads*).

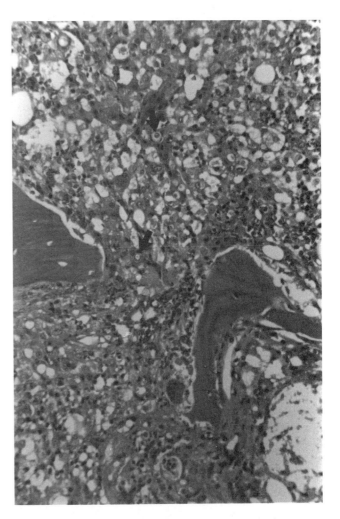

Fig. 2-17 Chronic pyogranulomatous osteomyelitis as a result of B*lastomyces dermatitidis* (*arrows*). Trabeculae of adjacent bone have scalloped surfaces indicating increased resorption, and areas of empty osteocyte lacunae representing necrosis.

lage, no longer supported by the underlying subchondral bone, begins to buckle and fold and eventually collapses into the vacated epiphysis.

Usually, resorption of necrotic bone is limited to osteoclasis on the perimeter of the lesion even if the lesion is very large. This is because marrow capable of giving rise to osteoclasts deep within the zone is dead and because the vascular channels in the bone are thrombosed with necrotic debris, limiting the access of osteoclasts. In large areas of necrosis, especially when portions of cortical bone are involved and inflammation occurs, as with infection, the repair stage may stop. The piece of dead bone that cannot be revascularized or replaced is surrounded by exudate or dense fibrous tissue, and the adjacent viable bone is sclerotic (increased density). The island of dead bone is termed a *sequestrum*, and the sclerotic surrounding bone is called the *involucrum*.

Inflammation. Inflammation of bone is termed *osteitis*. Usually, inflammation also involves the marrow (*osteomyelitis*) and the overlying periosteum (*periostitis*). Osteomyelitis without evidence of periostitis suggests a hematogenous origin of the inflammation.

Periostitis without evidence of osteomyelitis suggests trauma as the source of the inflammation. When diagnosed, however, most cases of osteitis are in advanced stages and involve both the periosteum and the marrow.

Osteomyelitis should be considered to have been caused by an infectious agent until proved otherwise. In small animal practice, these are usually bacteria and fungi. In dogs and cats, bacterial osteomyelitis is usually caused by trauma rather than hematogenous spread. Dogs and cats with sepsis probably have inflammation of their bones, and either the animal dies of the infection before clinical signs of the bone lesions develop or the lesions in the bone remain small and are resolved in response to therapy before they become clinically apparent. The nature of the inflammation varies with the organism; except for *Clostridium species* it is usually suppurative. Fungal osteomyelitis is more common in dogs than cats and the most common causes are *Blastomyces dermatitidis* and *Coccidioides immitis* (Fig. 2-17). In fungal osteomyelitis the exudate is more commonly pyogranulomatous. Cytokines, enzymes, toxins, and pressure from these exudates orchestrate the response of the bone to the infection. The response is mediated by bone cells and results in a mixture of bone lysis, reactive bone formation, and bone necrosis. These lesions in the bone structure can be rapid and extensive, and the physical deformity or weakening of the bone can bring into play mechanical factors that are superimposed on the mediators of inflammation (Fig. 2-18).

As discussed earlier, necrosis of bone in areas of inflammation can result from pressure of the exudate within the rigid confines of the bone that collapses blood vessels, leading to infarction. The central areas of the infarcted bone have no blood supply, and inflammation, which is a vascular-dependent process, cannot progress. Likewise, resorption of the infarcted area cannot take place from the necrotic avascular center that is not in contact with viable marrow elements for replenishment of osteoclastic precursors.

In general, the more extensive the suppuration and aggressive the inflammation, the more bone resorption occurs. If the resorption destroys the cortex and damages the periosteum, there are superimposed attempts of the inflamed bone to deal with repair and form a callus. The bone deposited in these conditions is not the orderly lamellar bone obeying rules of modeling and remodeling, but a rapidly deposited woven bone that is haphazard in arrangement, weak, and poorly mineralized (Fig. 2-19). The results can be an extremely deformed bone. In less aggressive osteomyelitis, the response can be predominantly osteoblastic (Fig. 2-20). Osteomyelitis can become chronic because pockets of bacteria may become sequestered in areas of necrotic or inflamed bone and be relatively inaccessible to antibiotics. The exudates from these pockets track in dependent fashion along paths of least resistance. Fistulas from the tracks may break out in the skin and appear as pus draining from ulcerations that ultimately connect with pockets of osteomyelitis.

Trauma. Trauma greater than a trivial insult but not capable of breaking the bone usually results in elevation of the periosteum because of edema and hemorrhage. The periosteum is programmed to proliferate and produce new bone when irritated. Thus, trauma to a bone surface may result in *exostoses* nodular to fusiform bony protuberances from the surface of the bone. Usually, little bone resorption is associated with such periosteal trauma. Except for the pain associated with the original trauma, these exostoses are usually incidental findings unless they compress vessels or nerves or compromise joint movement.

Fracture. When a bone is fractured, substantial damage to adjacent soft tissue may occur. This includes extensive hemorrhage and variable laceration and crushing of muscle. It is now being recognized that the hematoma that forms around the broken ends of the bone is not an inert clot but a miraculous soup of chemical mediators that stimulates the formation of bony callus to bridge the break and provide temporary

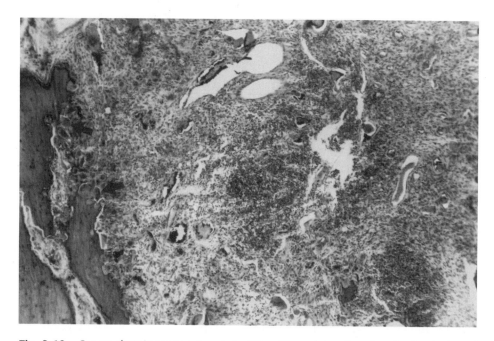

Fig. 2-18 Severe chronic suppurative periostitis with pockets of exudate in the thickened periosteum. The subjacent bone surface is being excavated by numerous osteoclasts (*arrows*).

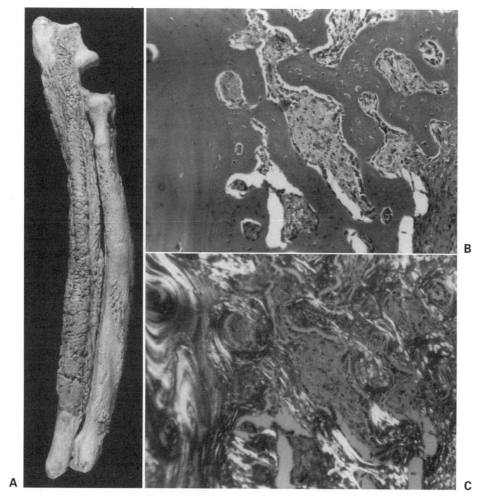

Fig. 2-19   **A**, Radius and ulna from a patient with hypertrophic pulmonary osteopathy (HPO). The surface of the bones is irregular and cobblestone-like because of reactive periosteal bone formation. The pathogenesis of HPO is not understood completely, but hyperperfusion of the periosteum occurs with minimal cellular infiltrates. The reactive bone may result from the hyperperfusion. HPO is usually associated with pulmonary lesions, which may cause the hyperperfusion by irritation of the vagus nerve as it traverses the thorax. Vagotomy reduces the hyperperfusion and allows for some amelioration of the bone lesion. **B** and **C,** Reactive periosteal new bone formation in response to adjacent inflammation and lysis visualized by routine bright-field light microscopy (**A**) and with polarized light (**B**). There is orderly arrangement of both lamellae and osteocytes in the underlying normal compact bone. The projections of reactive woven bone typically radiate perpendicularly from the bone surface and have enlarged and irregularly spaced osteocytes, with lamellae oriented in varying planes.

stability. Coagulation can activate complement to bring in inflammatory cells, particularly macrophages, which can release interleukins to stimulate prostaglandin synthesis and release. Platelets in the clot are rich in growth factors such as transforming growth factor beta, platelet-derived growth factor, and epidermal growth factor. The damaged soft tissue and bone also release "factors" into the clot that stimulate mitosis and differentiation of mesenchymal cells. In addition to acting as a sump for growth factors, the clot plays a physical role. Fibrin in

the clot acts as a temporary support lattice for invading mesenchymal cells and blood vessels. During the first 24 to 48 hours after the fracture occurs there is no stability or production of new bone.

Within a day or two of the fracture, mesenchymal cells of the endosteum and cambium layer of the periosteum begin to proliferate and invade into and onto the clot (Fig. 2-21*A*). The stimulus for these cells to proliferate is probably a combination of growth factors in the clot released from the damaged bone and soft tissue and an

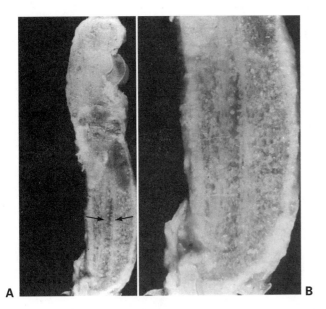

Fig. 2-20 Chronic low-grade osteomyelitis of a metatarsal bone of a cat. **A,** Opposing arrows delineate the approximate original periosteal surface. **B,** On closer view the original cortex has undergone extensive resorption and in some areas is indistinct. The periosteal reactive bone has remodeled so that it is oriented parallel with the bone surface. The porosity of the cortex in this case is probably caused by a combination of bone lysis as a result of inflammation and stress shielding from the excessive collar of reactive bone.

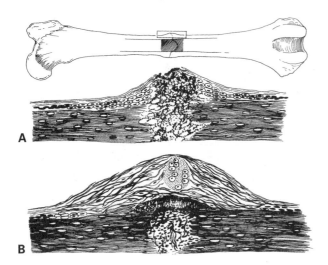

Fig. 2-21 Fracture repair in a stable fracture but without rigid fixation. The views are from a region indicated in the box in the bone at the top and include one cortex and the overlying periosteum. **A,** Within 24 to 48 hours, the swelling consists of hemorrhage, edema, and hypertrophy and hyperplasia of osteogenic cells in the periosteum. **B,** By 2 weeks, a primary callus is formed by woven bone produced by the osteogenic cells of the periosteum that invaded into the clot. In the thickest portion of the callus, hyaline cartilage may form, which can subsequently undergo endochondral ossification.

intrinsic programmed response of endosteum and periosteum to proliferate when physically lifted or disrupted. This response is most intense in the periosteal and endosteal surfaces that have been directly damaged (but are still viable) and dissipates farther from the fracture site. This gradation of response eventually gives the callus a fusiform appearance, which is greatest over the fracture and tapers toward the more normal distant endosteal and periosteal surfaces.

The mesenchymal cells that migrate into and onto the clot are pluripotential and can differentiate into fibroblasts, osteoblasts, and chondroblasts. Along with these mesenchymal cells, blood vessels invade the clot. These vessels may come from the marrow, periosteum, or adjacent soft tissue (e.g., muscle), and the stimulus for their proliferation and invasion is probably angiogenic growth factors in the clot. The soft tissue contribution is probably important; fractures heal poorly when overlying soft tissue is removed traumatically or iatrogenically.

In addition to the invading individual mesenchymal cells, buds of osteogenic tissue begin to protrude into and around the clot. These buds arise from the periosteum and endosteum and maintain contact with them. As the buds become more extensive and thicker and the invading mesenchymal cells begin to differentiate and produce matrix, the primary callus begins to take shape. The portion of the callus derived from the periosteum is called the *external callus*, and that from the endosteum is called the *internal callus*. The earliest mineralized osseous matrix in the callus is present by 1 week, and a radiographic "shadow" is present by 2 weeks. Between 1 and 2 weeks the external callus is able to bridge the fracture gap with woven bone (Figs. 2-21*B* and 2-22). As the osseous portions of the callus increase, the clot portion becomes smaller as the cells and fibrin are phagocytosed and removed.

Ideally, the pluripotential cells invading the clot all differentiate into osteoblasts and rapidly produce woven bone of repair. Unfortunately, this requires ideal conditions of compression and adequate oxygen supply. When the supply of oxygen to the callus is low, more cartilage tends to form. Some hyaline cartilage in the callus is normal. In most "normal" fractures, cartilage usually is present in the periphery of the thickest portion of the callus. This location may reflect a lower oxygen tension in the callus in this region. Hyaline cartilage in a callus eventually is able to undergo mineralization and subsequent endochondral ossification, as described previously for the growth plate. The disadvantage of excessive cartilage in the callus is the reduction in rigidity and therefore stability for the fracture site until endochondral ossification of the cartilage in the callus is complete. Compression that is not so great as to cause necrosis promotes osseous differentiation in the mesenchymal

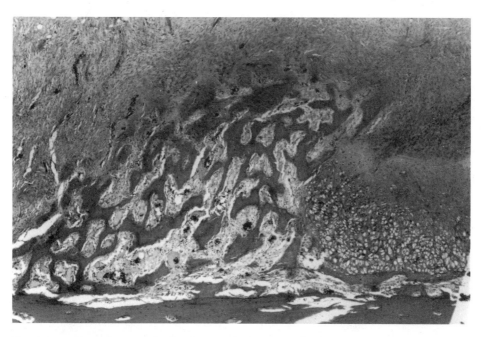

Fig. 2-22   Photomicrograph of a portion of a fracture callus at 4 weeks with changes similar to those in Fig. 2-21, B. The external callus is not yet complete and consists of proliferative fibrous and osseous tissue from the periosteum, and a central area of the callus (*right*) with hyaline cartilage.

cells of the callus. Tension on the callus encourages the mesenchymal cells to differentiate into fibroblasts.

Dense mature fibrous tissue (scar tissue) and inflammation are the enemies of normal fracture healing. Fibrous tissue in the callus is undesirable for two major reasons. Excess fibrous tissue makes the callus "rubbery" and without sufficient rigidity for the fracture ends to heal. In addition, in contrast to hyaline cartilage, fibrous tissue does not normally have a matrix that undergoes mineralization. Therefore, fibrous tissue that is formed cannot be converted to bone. Turnover of fibrous tissue is very slow, and a marked buildup of fibrous tissue between the bone ends may result in a nonunion and require surgical intervention.

In a stable fracture with adequate blood supply, there should be a complete bony callus by 6 weeks (Fig. 2-23). At this time the gap between the fracture ends may appear radiographically to be wider because of resorption of the dead bone at the fracture site. These dead edges may extend back several millimeters from the fracture line and result from vascular compromise at the time of the break. After 6 weeks the callus should begin compaction and remodeling. Compaction is the same concept as described previously for development of cortical bone. Osteoblasts on both sides of the trabeculae of woven bone in the callus deposit bone and "fill in" the space between the trabeculae to convert trabecular bone into compact bone. This compaction is composed

of lamellar bone and takes place more slowly than the deposition of the woven bone of the initial trabeculae. Again, as in the developing skeleton, this compact bone is deposited in lamellae, but as yet no true haversian canals exist. The haversian canals are formed when remodeling takes place. Cutting cones of osteoclasts drill through the compact bone of the callus, and the long drill holes are filled in with concentric lamellae and produce a typical osteon. Complete remodeling of the callus may take years.

In addition to remodeling of the callus, modeling occurs in that the callus becomes flatter and more

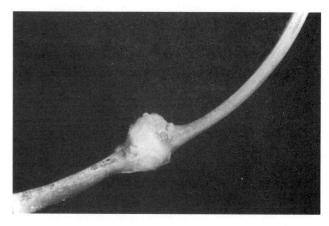

Fig. 2-23   Complete bony callus on rib.

fusiform, with trabeculae oriented to the long axis of the bone over time. The size of the callus and therefore the distortion of the bone depend on stability. The less stable the fracture, the larger is the callus. A large callus may not only create a cosmetic problem but could be in a location to interfere with locomotion by impinging on muscle, nerves, or adjacent bones. The clinical value of limiting the motion of a fracture is not only to reduce the size of the callus, but also to reduce tension on the bone ends and avoid compromise of blood flow (and therefore oxygen) to the callus in order to keep fibrous tissue and cartilage formation to a minimum.

A large part of this textbook deals with surgically stabilizing a fracture to facilitate its repair. The goal of many of these procedures is to provide absolute stability at the fracture site by means of wires, plates, screws, pins, or other implants. Properly applied, these techniques help keep callus formation to a minimum. The means by which the fracture heals depends on the size of the gap between the fracture ends. If stabilization is not achieved, callus formation occurs to varying degrees (the greater the instability, the greater the callus), as described previously. When surgery has been successful in achieving complete stability, the ends of the fracture can be in contact with each other or have a small gap between them.

Direct or contact healing of an anatomically reduced and rigidly stabilized fracture is done directly by remodeling. No temporary osseous tissue is deposited because no space exists for it to be deposited into. Cutting cones, as in the cutting cones of normal remodeling, drill holes across the fracture site, and subsequently a new osteon forms and is one of the new bony cables that connect the broken ends. In contact healing the "gap" is so small that osteoclasts of the cutting cones can "jump" the gap and continue the drilling on the other side of the fracture. Likewise, during the formation phase, osteoblasts are able to bridge directly over the fracture (Fig. 2-24). The remodeling rate in contact healing is greater than in normal bone. Probably because of chemotactic and physical factors, the activation rate of remodeling is increased. This increased activation means that more cutting cones are started. The rate of resorption and formation in each new osteon, however, is not different from normal.

The ends of most surgically reduced fractures are not in direct contact but are separated from one another by a small gap. If the gap is less than 1 mm, lamellar bone is directly deposited into the gap (appositional formation of compact bone). This deposition begins after the second week and progresses at a rate of 1 to 2 μ per day. The orientation of this new bone, however, is perpendicular to the axis of the bone in the ends of the fracture. Although this repair bone is of excellent quality, because

its collagen fibers are perpendicular to the normal axis of the bone, a structural weakness occurs at the repair site (Fig. 2-25). Not until remodeling through this repair tissue has occurred can osteonal bone with orientation compatible with the adjacent bone be achieved.

In gaps larger than 1 mm, the gap is initially filled with a coarse woven bone with prominent vascular spaces. Within several weeks the vascular spaces begin to fill in with concentric layers of lamellar bone. The result then of the unremodeled repair is a mixture of lamellar bone and woven bone. The orientation of the woven bone is

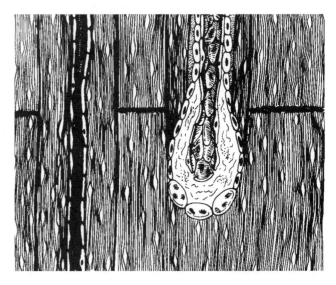

Fig. 2-24 Direct or contact healing. The fracture line is represented by a vertical line. In the lower portion of the illustration, a cutting cone is crossing the fracture and subsequently filling in with bone. At the upper portion, a completed osteon is present that has crossed the fracture.

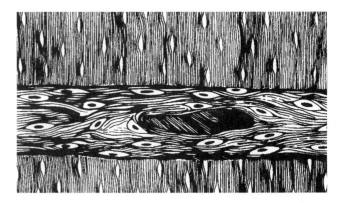

Fig. 2-25 A small gap healing. The gap has been filled with lamellar bone deposited in a plane perpendicular (vertical in the illustration) to the fracture ends.

somewhat random, but in general it is oriented perpendicularly to the long axis of the bone (Fig. 2-26). Remodeling of the repair bone is required to create osteonal bone in the gap with orientation parallel with the long axis of the bone.

To achieve complete stabilization of a fracture, it may be necessary to apply rigid implants to the bone, such as metal plates and screws. These plates may shield the bone from stress and create a localized disuse atrophy. The mechanisms of disuse atrophy (bone loss caused by decreased mechanical use) are discussed in the preceding section. Use of plates of an inappropriately large size can lead to marked stress shielding and pronounced atrophy of the bone. Such bone, even with a plate attached, may be predisposed to fracture.

CARTILAGE

This discussion is restricted to hyaline cartilage of synovial joints and physes. Articular cartilage provides a lubricated, low-friction surface that can withstand and disseminate the mechanical forces of movement and weight bearing to underlying structures. Physeal cartilage provides a "plastic" environment within which interstitial growth is possible with eventual conversion to bone (endochondral ossification).

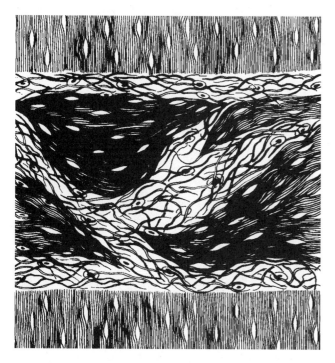

Fig. 2-26 A fracture healing with a large gap. The gap is filled with fibro-osseous tissue and lamellar bone generally perpendicular to the fracture ends.

Structure and Function

Articular cartilage. Articular cartilage is easy to define in the adult animal. It is the hyaline cartilage at the end of the bones that is not mineralized. In the growing animal, the unmineralized cartilage at the end of the bones consists of an outer layer of articular cartilage and a deeper layer of epiphyseal cartilage. The epiphyseal cartilage is the cartilage that has yet to undergo endochondral ossification to become the bony epiphysis. After the neonatal stages, no blood vessels exist in the articular cartilage; only the epiphyseal cartilage has blood vessels.

The cells within hyaline cartilage are called *chondrocytes*. When hyaline cartilage is routinely preserved for microscopic examination, the chondrocytes appear to be in lacunae. If special fixatives are used to prevent loss of proteoglycans, no space is present between the chondrocyte and the adjacent matrix. It is now thought that lacunae around chondrocytes in hyaline cartilage are probably shrinkage artifacts. In comparison, the lacunae around osteocytes in bone appear to be true spaces. Another difference between the "housing" of osteocytes and chondrocytes is no canaliculi are present in cartilage. The lack of canaliculi probably reflects the ability of molecules to diffuse through the watery gel of the chondroid matrix compared with the rigid, water-poor matrix of bone.

Articular cartilage is organized into three layers (Fig. 2-27). The surface layer is called the *superficial layer*. Chondrocytes and collagen fibers in this layer are oriented parallel with the joint surface. The layer deep to the surface layer is the *transitional layer*. In this layer, chondrocytes and collagen fibers are arranged obliquely to the surface. The deepest layer is the *radial layer*, in which the chondrocytes and collagen fibers are arranged perpendicular to the joint surface. The arrangement described for articular chondrocytes and collagen is overlapping arcades, with the arch of the arcade being at the surface and the parallel walls being the radial layers. This architecture enables the fibers parallel with the surface to withstand the shearing forces on articular cartilage and the fibers perpendicular with the surface to withstand the compressive forces.

In growing animals, beneath the radial layer is the epiphyseal cartilage. At the junction of the epiphyseal cartilage and epiphyseal bone is a zone of endochondral ossification (in other words, the "physis" of the epiphysis). The zone, including the articular cartilage and the subjacent epiphyseal cartilage with its zone of endochondral ossification, has been called the *articular-epiphyseal complex*. In the adult, when expansion and growth of the epiphysis are complete, a thin rim of mineralized epiphyseal cartilage remains beneath the

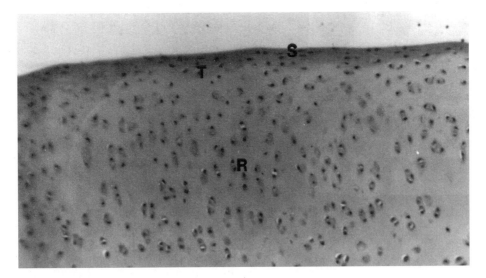

Fig. 2-27 Articular cartilage with surface (S), transitional (T), and radial (R) layers.

articular cartilage. The junction between the mineralized layer of epiphyseal cartilage and the unmineralized articular cartilage is called the *tidemark* (Fig. 2-28). This differs from the metaphyseal growth plate, which at maturity is completely removed and replaced by bone. There is no advantage to the body to retain a disk of cartilage in the metaphysis of a fully grown bone, even if the cartilage is mineralized. The advantage of retaining the layer of mineralized cartilage beneath the articular cartilage is that it acts as a transition zone between the overlying unmineralized articular cartilage and the underlying mineralized bone of the epiphysis (called the *subchondral plate*).

The matrix of articular cartilage is greatly different from that of bone. The most essential differences are the water content, the size and concentration of proteoglycans, and the collagen type. Articular cartilage consists of 75% water. This water is bound loosely in the matrix similar to a gel. The binding is caused mostly by the proteoglycans. Proteoglycans are complex protein-polysaccharide molecules. They have a protein core from which protrude branches of sugars known as *glycosaminoglycans*. Major glycosaminoglycans of proteoglycans include karatan sulfate and chondroitin sulfate. The physical appearance of the proteoglycan with protein core and protruding branches of glycosaminoglycans has been likened to a bottle brush. Proteoglycans are rarely present as single molecules in articular cartilage but are bound to hyaluronic acid (which itself is a glycosaminoglycan but not one that is part of the proteoglycan molecule) and called *proteoglycan aggregates*. These proteoglycan aggregates are very large macromolecules with very strong electronegativity. The electronegativity causes these macromolecules to repel one another and trap water. The combination of the physical structure of the proteoglycan aggregates, the trapping of

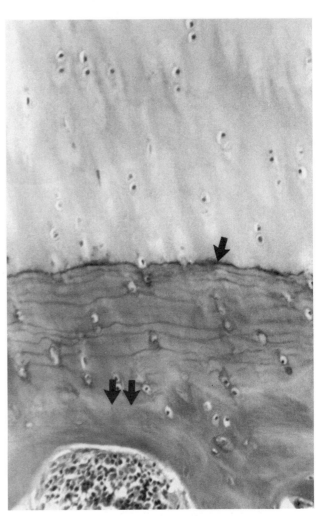

Fig. 2-28 Tidemark (*single arrow*) between the overlying unmineralized articular cartilage and mineralized cartilage. Multiple past tidemarks are within the mineralized cartilage, indicating periods of previous temporary growth arrest. The subchondral bone is beneath the mineralized cartilage (*double arrows*).

water, and the electronegative forces keeping the aggregates away from each other gives articular cartilage its resilience and resistance to compressive forces.

The collagen of articular cartilage is type II rather than type I collagen of bone. The differences between these collagen types are well understood biochemically, but the biological significance of these differences is poorly understood.

Synovial joints are encased by a joint capsule. The outer layer of the capsule if fibrous and continuous with the periosteum. The inner layer is called the *synovial membrane*. The surface of the synovial membrane has an incomplete lining of synovial cells. These cells are admixed with a loose collagen matrix. The synovial cells are responsible for producing and secreting synovial fluid, which is necessary for nourishment of the avascular hyaline cartilage and lubrication of the synovial membrane. In addition to production of synovial fluid, synoviocytes have the ability to become phagocytic (type A cells) and fibroblastic (type B cells).

The mechanism of joint lubrication is not completely understood. Simply stated, there are two types of lubrication: boundary and weeping. *Boundary lubrication* is provided by coating a surface with mucins produced by the synovial membrane. These mucins are primarily hyaluronic acid and glycoproteins. Boundary lubrication is most important on the non-weight-bearing surfaces or the surfaces bearing only light loads. *Weeping lubrication* is provided by a thin film of water and proteoglycans that is squeezed out of the cartilage under pressure of weight bearing. As the load is reduced, the water and proteoglycans are taken back into the cartilage matrix. This in-and-out movement not only provides lubrication, but also facilitates entry of nutrients and exit of metabolic by-products into and out of the cartilage.

The structure and function of hyaline cartilage of the growth plate have been discussed earlier.

Responses of Hyaline Cartilage to Injury

The response of adult hyaline cartilage to injury is restricted by its avascularity and limited ability to proliferate. There are four categories of responses to injury of hyaline cartilage: (1) degeneration and necrosis, which can lead to erosion and ulceration if it is articular cartilage; (2) hyperplasia of chondrocytes with production of new matrix (a very limited capacity in adult cartilage); (3) modeling of cartilage; and (4) persistence, or retention of cartilage that should have undergone endochondral ossification.

Degeneration and necrosis of cartilage. Degeneration and necrosis of hyaline cartilage is very common and may even be considered a normal change with advanced age. Central to cartilage degeneration and necrosis is the loss of proteoglycans from the matrix.

Loss of proteoglycans results in failure of normal binding of water. The failure to bind water normally results in inadequate lubrication of weight-bearing surfaces and reduced ability of the cartilage to withstand compression. Loss of proteoglycans in response to injury creates cartilage even more susceptible to injury, and a vicious cycle is established. The reduction of cartilage proteoglycans in response to injury is the result of the net changes in proteoglycan synthesis and breakdown. Factors that influence proteoglycan synthesis and breakdown can come from the chondrocytes themselves, the synovium, and subchondral bone.

Trauma to chondrocytes causes reduction in their synthesis of proteoglycans and secretion of proteases capable of destroying proteoglycans. Trauma to the synovium can trigger synovial cells to release prostaglandins, which inhibit proteoglycan synthesis by chondrocytes. In addition, traumatized synovial cells can secrete interleukins that stimulate chondrocytes to produce proteoglycan-degrading proteases. Hyaluronidase can be secreted by injured synovial cells and cause secondary damage to chondrocytes by destroying hyaluronic acid on synovial and articular surfaces, thus reducing boundary lubrication.

When synovium is inflamed, not only do synovial cells release prostaglandins, interleukins, and hyaluronidase, but inflammatory cells in the exudate can produce these agents, as well as lytic enzymes and collagenases ,which may directly digest cartilage matrix and cells. In cases of chronic fibrinous or lymphoplasmacytic arthritis, pannus can contribute to the destruction of articular cartilage. Pannus is discussed in the following section on hyperplasia.

Loss of proteoglycans and proper water binding by cartilage results in reduced ability to withstand normal compressive and shearing forces. This process begins the cartilage on an unrelenting path toward degenerative joint disease. The initial structural change of this abnormal water binding is, almost paradoxically, an increase in water content of the cartilage. This makes the cartilage softer to the touch and has been termed *chondromalacia*. The biochemical mechanism of this increase in water is not certain. What is certain is the water is not complexed properly with proteoglycans and detracts rather than adds to the ability of the cartilage to withstand use. The chondromalacic cartilage loses the top two layers (the surface layer and transitional layer) to wear. The cartilage at this time has less water content and the remaining radial collagen fibers become condensed because they are not being "held apart" by the effects of the proteoglycan-water interaction. These condensed radial fibers can now be seen grossly as a frayed surface resembling a shag rug. This change is called *fibrillation* (Fig. 2-29). Wearing down of the fibrillated cartilage is known as *erosion*. Eventually the cartilage may wear down to the subchondral bone,

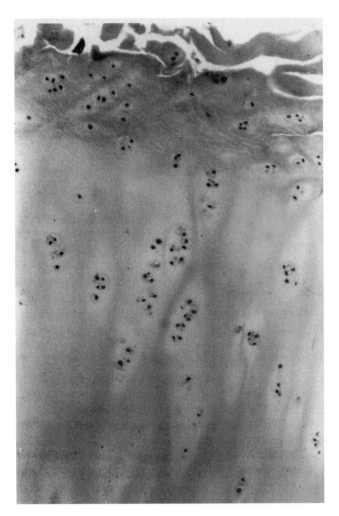

Fig. 2-29   Fibrillated articular cartilage with fraying of surface, hypocellularity from death of chondrocytes, and hyperplasia (chondrone formation) of residual chondrocytes.

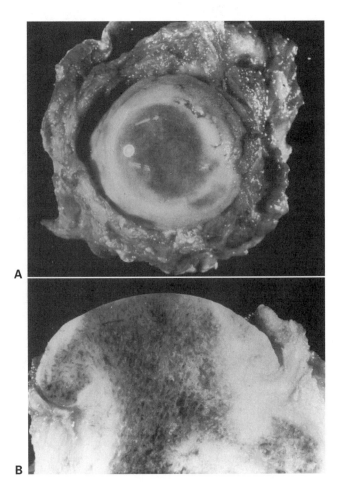

Fig. 2-30   **A,** Surface, and **B,** cross section of ulcerated and eburnated femoral head. The central darkened area has complete loss of articular cartilage. The dark appearance is caused by blood and hematopoiesis in the marrow cavity.

at which point it can be called an *ulcer*. The underlying bone can become polished smooth by wear (Fig. 2-30). This polishing and compensatory thickening of the bone as a result of increased mechanical use results in a dense white surface that is ivorylike and has been called *eburnated bone.*

Because of its location and function, consequences of degeneration and necrosis of cartilage of the physis differ greatly from degeneration and necrosis of articular cartilage. These consequences depend on the age of the animal and the location of the lesion within the plate. Lesions of the resting and proliferating zones of the plate may cause premature closure (Fig. 2-31). Lesions at the zones of hypertrophy and mineralization may cause a disruption of endochondral ossification and result in a separation of the cartilage from the underlying secondary trabeculae. Since the proliferating cells are not affected, the chondrocyte columns accumulate, leading to a thickened plate. Lesions in a plate that is almost

ready to close have minimal effects on the structure and integrity of the bone, since endochondral ossification and the influence of the plate on bone modeling are slight at this time. Damage to a plate of a rapidly growing animal could result in marked asymmetrical growth of the bone and therefore skeletal deformity if the lesion is located at either side of the plate. If the lesion is central or diffuse, there could be stunting of the bone and a structural weakness at the metaphysis, where the continuity of the metaphysis is disrupted because of lack of endochondral ossification.

Hyperplasia of cartilage and synovium. Chondrocytes proliferating in response to injury form clusters known as *chondrones.* The matrix around chondrones is rich in newly synthesized proteoglycans. Chondrocytes in adult articular cartilage have limited ability to proliferate and produce new matrix, and there is little evidence that chondrocyte proliferation is beneficial in healing cartilage.

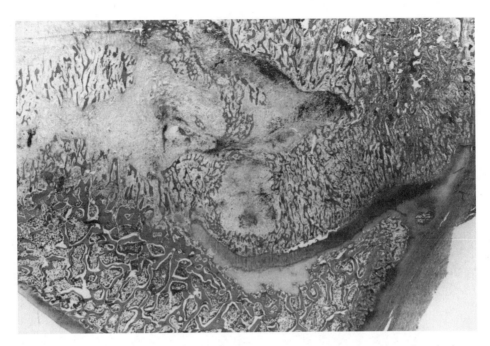

Fig. 2-31   Physis of distal ulna that has focally closed and been replaced by trabecular bone and adjacent fibrosis. The pathogenesis in this case was uncertain but suspected to result from local ischemia secondary to trauma.

Although adult articular hyaline cartilage has limited ability to proliferate, the same is not true for tissue of chondrogenic potential in the adult. Examples of this are the perichondrium and the attachment site of the joint capsule with bone. Irritation of these sites either by trauma or inflammation typically leads to marked proliferation of pluripotential mesenchymal cells with differentiation into both cartilage and bone. Proliferations that begin as cartilage usually undergo endochondral ossification. These proliferations are called *osteophytes* and may become quite large and impinge on the joint space. Osteophytes around the intervertebral joints may impinge on the foramina of the spinal roots and cause pain and sensory or locomotor defects. Osteophytes that begin at the insertion of the joint capsule do so on the synovial side of the insertion, and the osteophytes may break loose from the synovium and become free in the synovial space, where they are called "joint mice."

Synovial tissue has marked ability to proliferate. Grossly, synovium is usually an inconspicuous soft membrane on the inner surface of the joint capsule. In response to trauma, sterile inflammation (often immune mediated), and infection, synovium proliferates to form a shag rug–like surface with villouslike projections that may extend a centimeter from the surface (Fig. 2-32). This proliferation consists of type A and B synovial cells, as well as subsynovial fibrous stroma. If the initiating injury is inflammatory, the stroma is infiltrated with inflammatory cells, usually lymphocytes and plasma cells. Even if the exudate in the joint space is suppura-tive, few neutrophils remain in the synovium. Most neutrophils rapidly migrate out of vessels, through the synovial stoma, and pass out into the synovial fluid.

In chronic inflammatory lesions of the synovium, especially in erosive immune-mediated arthritis (e.g., rheumatoid-like) and fibrinous arthritis, the synovium along with granulation tissue may grow onto the surface of the cartilage or actually invade under the cartilage. This proliferative synovial tissue is called *pannus* (Fig. 2-33). Pannus is destructive to cartilage in several ways. When pannus grows over the cartilage, it prevents diffusion of nutrients into the cartilage. Probably of greater importance is the ability of cells in the pannus to secrete collagenases and prostaglandins, which directly and indirectly cause breakdown of the cartilage. In addition, pannus contains macrophages capable of resorption of cartilage and underlying bone.

In its early stages, synovial hyperplasia probably has good intentions of increasing the amount of snyovial fluid and lubricants to help the joint respond to injury. Likewise, inflammation of the synovium in response to infectious agents may be helpful and necessary for the joint to destroy the invading microorganism. In the extreme, however, both these processes have a deleterious effect on the cartilage.

Modeling of cartilage. In response to abnormal mechanical use, which could be secondary to trauma, inflammation, or developmental abnormalities, articular cartilage is able to change its contour to match the modeling

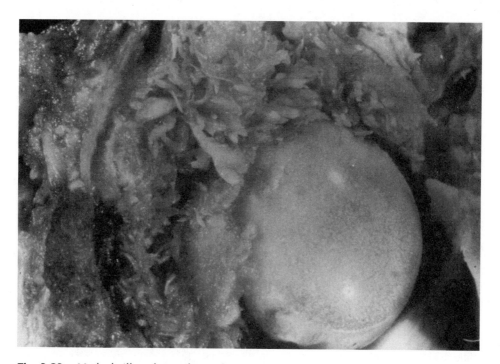

Fig. 2-32 Marked villous hyperplasia of synovium in the coxofemoral joint with ulceration of the femoral head.

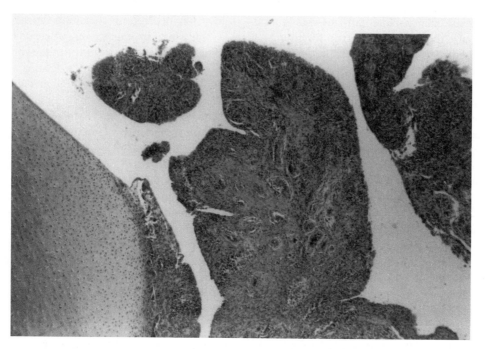

Fig. 2-33 Marked hyperplasia and inflammation of the synovium with early attachment and growth of the synovium onto the cartilage surface (pannus).

changes in the underlying bone. The mechanism of this process is poorly understood because it is very slow but must involve both removal and production of new cartilage (Fig. 2-34). This appears to contradict well-accepted observations that cartilage has minimal ability to proliferate. These differences cannot be reconciled except with the factor of time. If the modeling changes in the bone are slowly progressive, the cartilage appears to have time to adapt. If the changes are rapid, the cartilage cannot adapt, and the result is abnormal wear on

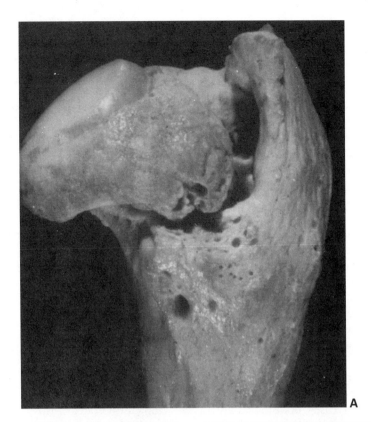

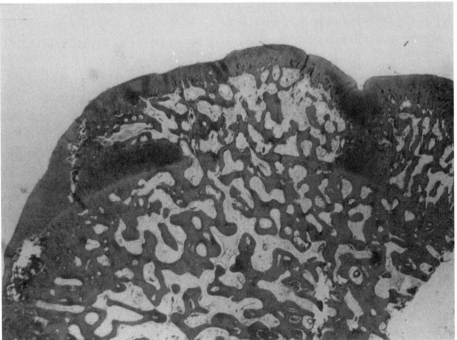

Fig. 2-34 **A,** Marked flattening and modeling of the femoral head. Much of the periarticular hard tissue probably was produced by the periosteum at the site of insertion of the joint capsule. **B,** Another case of marked modeling of the epiphysis. Here the modeling is caused by proliferation of the articular cartilage with subsequent endochondral ossification. The original contour of the subchondral bone is still mostly intact.

the cartilage, leading to degeneration and necrosis rather than modeling.

Persistence. This refers to persistence of growth cartilage either at the articular-epiphyseal complex or at the metaphyseal growth plate. This is a common lesion in veterinary medicine and may have a variety of causes. It most often occurs as a multifocal temporary failure of endochondral ossification called *osteochondrosis*. Osteochondrosis is a condition of rapidly growing animals. It is a major problem in horses, pigs, and poultry but also affects cattle and sheep. It is a significant clinical problem in larger breed dogs. The condition is virtually unheard of in the cat probably because of the ratio of body weight to rate of growth for the cat. The cause of osteochondrosis is not known. Some believe that is it normal to have multifocal temporary delays in endochondral ossification in rapidly growing animals and that only in the exceptional cases do these minor foci become clinical lesions. The cause has been studied most in swine and horses, but these findings may not be relevant to the dog. Excess caloric intake and excess dietary calcium have been incriminated in the dog, but these findings do not appear to explain many clinical cases.

In the dog, most clinical cases of osteochondrosis involve the articular epiphyseal cartilage, predominantly of the proximal humerus. Resulting from the failure of endochondral ossification, the growth cartilage of the articular epiphyseal cartilage does not become resorbed and replaced by bone. The growth cartilage appears as an irregular projection of cartilage into the bony epiphysis and radiographically appears as a lucency (Fig. 2-35). Likely because of a combination of mechanical forces

and inadequate diffusion of nutrients, the deeper layers of the persistent cartilage undergo degeneration and necrosis. This leads to a fissure within the cartilage that, again probably because of mechanical forces, can dissect into the articular cartilage and create a flap of cartilage. These flap lesions are known as *osteochondritis dissecans*. This flap may tear loose from the cartilage and become a "joint mouse."

Healing of Articular Cartilage Defects

Small defects that do not penetrate the tidemark may remain static for years. Even though articular cartilage can proliferate and the matrix can "flow" into adjacent defects, these properties are very limited and most small defects do not heal. Larger defects that do not extend through the tidemark not only do not heal, but because of loss of normal contour and proteoglycans, also cause degeneration and necrosis that can progress to degenerative joint disease.

Defects through the tidemark have the advantage of stimulating fibrovascular ingrowth into the cartilage from the underlying bone. This fibrovascular repair tissue is able to create fibrocartilage within the defect. The long-term effect of this fibrocartilage has not been adequately studied under controlled conditions.

HEALING OF MUSCLE AND TENDON

Muscle is able to heal by regeneration or by scar (reactive fibrosis). The occurrence of these depends on the type and extent of the injury. Injuries that preserve the basal lamina (basement membrane) allow for muscle

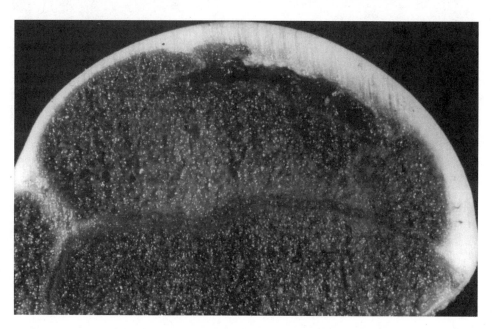

Fig. 2-35 Humeral head with osteochondrosis characterized by thickening of the cartilage because of failure of endochondral ossification. Beneath the thickened cartilage is an area devoid of bone because of a combination of necrosis and failure of bone formation.

regeneration. Injuries that destroy the basal lamina heal by fibrosis. Noninvasive and nonlytic injuries to muscle, such as moderate localized ischemic and pressure injuries and toxic and metabolic myopathies, are able to heal by regeneration. Extensive lacerations and inflammation of muscle are more likely to heal by fibrosis.

Muscle regeneration occurs by proliferation of satellite cells. Mature muscle nuclei themselves are not capable of division. Satellite cells are inconspicuous cells that live within the basal lamina but outside the myofiber. With injury, these cells are stimulated to proliferate and "invade" into the myofiber. Once the degenerate and necrotic myofilaments are removed by phagocytes, the cytoplasm of the proliferating satellite cells is able to fuse together, resulting in a syncytium of nuclei, organized myofilaments, and sarcoplasm (Fig. 2-36). This process is able to reform muscle indistinguishable from the original.

If the basal lamina is damaged, fibroblasts from the endomysium are able to gain access to the injured myofiber. After the necrotic debris is removed by phago-cytosis, fibroblasts divide and produce collagen to replace the lost muscle.

Tendons consist of dense, parallel arranged fibrous tissue with a characteristic wave pattern known as *kinking*. If tendon tissue is abnormally stretched but not ruptured, the collagen fibers may lose their normal kinking, and the tendon may not recoil to normal length. Mature tenocytes (the fibrous cell of the tendon) have essentially no ability to divide, and therefore, regeneration of tendon is not possible. If tendon tissue is ruptured, it can be removed by phagocytosis by macrophages. If the injury extends to the peritenon, fibroblasts can invade the tendon and produce scar tissue to replace the damaged tendon. This scar tissue, as with most scar tissue, initially contains myofibroblasts, which are fibroblasts rich in contractile intracellular filaments. As the scar tissue matures, these filaments enable the scar tissue to contract. With time, fewer of the fibroblasts in the lesion have this extent of contractile filaments. The scar tissue formed may eventually develop a kink pattern, but it is out of synchrony with the original pattern. In addition, the collagen of the repair may have a greater extent of type III collagen than the original tendon, which is essentially only type I collagen. These factors make the repair tissue less strong than the original tendon. Repair tissue from the peritenon may cause fibrous adhesions of the tendon to the adjacent soft tissue, reducing the glide of the tendon.

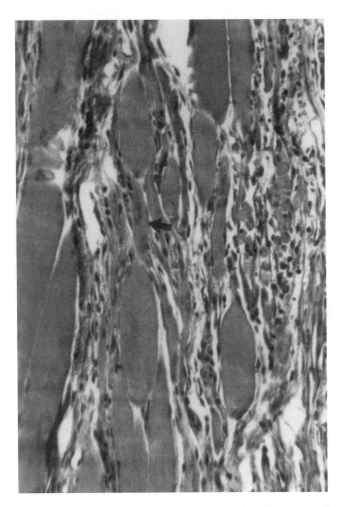

Fig. 2-36 Reaction of muscle in a region of crush injury and necrosis. The multinucleated elongated cells (*arrow*) are reactive myoblasts attempting to form new myofibers.

SUGGESTED READINGS

Frost HM: The biology of fracture healing: an overview for clinicians. Part I, *Clin Orthop* 248:283-293, 1989.

Frost HM: The biology of fracture healing: an overview for clinicians. Part II, *Clin Orthop* 248:294, 1989.

Frost HM: Skeletal structural adaptations to mechanical usage (SATMU). 1. Redefining Wolff's law: the bone modeling problem, *Anat Rec* 226:403-413, 1990.

Frost HM: Skeletal structural adaptations to mechanical usage (SATMU). 2. Redefining Wolff's law: the remodeling problem, *Anat Rec* 226:414-422, 1990.

Hamerman D: The biology of osteoarthritis, *N Engl J Med* 320(20): 1322-1330, 1989.

Hughes PF, Fitzgerald RH Jr: *Musculoskeletal infections*, Chicago, 1986, Year Book.

Hulth A: Current concepts of fracture healing, *Clin Orthop* 249: 265-284, 1989.

Mankin HJ: The reaction of articular cartilage to injury and osteoarthritis (part 1), *N Engl J Med* 291(24):1285-1292, 1974.

Mankin HJ: The reaction of articular cartilage to injury and osteoarthritis (part 2), *N Engl J Med* 291(25):1335-1340, 1974.

Marks SC, Popoff SN: Bone cell biology: the regulation of development, structure and function in the skeleton, *Am J Anat* 183:1-44, 1988.

Mayne R: Cartilage collagens: what is their function, and are they involved in articular disease? *Arthritis Rheum* 32(3):241-246, 1989.

Mohan S, Baylink DJ: Bone growth factors, *Clin Orthop Rel Res* 263:30-48, 1991.

Vaes G: Cellular biology and biochemical mechanism of bone resorption: a review of recent developments on the formation, activation and mode of action of osteoclasts, *Clin Orthop* 231:239-271, 1988.

3

Practical Biomechanics

Donald A. Hulse
William Hyman

MECHANICAL CONCEPTS AND TERMINOLOGY

Biomechanical analysis relies on the proper understanding and use of concepts and terms adopted from physics and engineering. These concepts and terms describe how materials and structures behave when they are subjected to steady or time-varying external loads. A knowledge of basic mechanical principles is helpful in understanding the normal body response to the environment. Additionally, knowledge of mechanical principles leads to a better understanding of injury mechanisms of the musculoskeletal system and a better understanding of the prevention and treatment of orthopedic injuries. Familiarity with mechanical terms and concepts used to define the responses of the musculoskeletal system to physiological and nonphysiological forces is the cornerstone to understanding applied orthopedic biomechanics. This section discusses definitions and accompanying diagrams that explain mechanical terms frequently used in descriptions of the musculoskeletal system.

Forces and Moments

The nature of the loads to which a system is subjected is described in terms of the forces and moments that act on the system. Forces act in a straight line and tend to cause the system to move in the direction of the force. Forces are considered positive if they are pulling on a system, and negative if they are pushing on the system. To describe a force properly, it is necessary to know its magnitude and direction. Frequently used terms in biomechanics are discussed next.

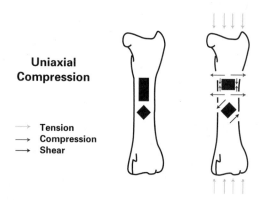

Uniaxial Compression

→ Tension
→ Compression
→ Shear

Fig. 3-1 Generation of tension, compression, and shear stresses associated with an axially applied compressive load. Note the change in relationship between the sides of the diamond box. Shear stress is produced at an oblique angle to the longitudinal axis of the bone.

From Hulse D: *Biomechanics of fracture fixation failure*, Philadelphia, 1991, Saunders.

Uniaxial force. A force applied in one direction and distributed evenly over the surface of the loaded structure is a uniaxial force. It can be tension or compression and is expressed in units of kilograms (kg) or newtons (Fig. 3-1).

Ground reaction force. This is a force exerted in response to the foot contacting the ground. It is equal to but in the opposite direction of the force generated by foot contact. In general, this force is referred to in terms of the *vertical ground reaction force* (VGRF), which designates the vertical axial force exerted by the ground (Fig. 3-2). VGRF is measured in newtons or kilograms.

Moments. Moments arise when forces act a distance from some point of interest. A moment is equal to the magnitude of the force times the perpendicular distance from the point of interest to the line of action of the force (Fig. 3-3). This perpendicular distance is called the *moment arm*. Moments tend to cause the object to which they are applied to rotate about some axis. In reference to cylindrical objects, such as most bones, some moments give rise primarily to bending deformations whereas others give rise primarily to twisting. Twisting moments also are called *torques*.

Deformation. When a force or moment is applied to a fixed object, the object changes shape. This change in shape can be elongation, shortening, bending, or twisting and is referred to as *deformation*. A graph (force/deformation curve) can be constructed, with the vertical axis representing the amount of force and the horizontal axis the amount of deformation (Fig. 3-4). A force/deformation curve is representative of the *structural* properties of an object.

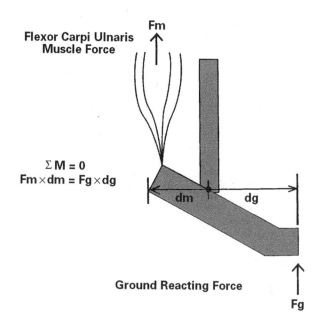

Flexor Carpi Ulnaris Muscle Force Fm

$$\Sigma M = 0$$
$$Fm \times dm = Fg \times dg$$

dm   dg

Ground Reacting Force

Fg

Fig. 3-2 Balance of moments generated about the carpal joint. The ground reaction force (FG) acts about the moment arm (*dg*), causing a cranial bending moment (FG × *dg*). To maintain normal posture, this moment must be balanced by a moment generated from contraction of the flexor carpi ulnaris (F*m* × *dm*).

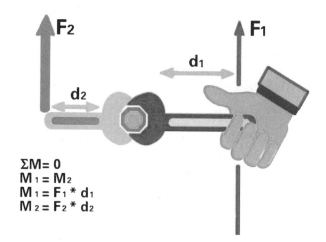

F_2 F_1 d_1 d_2

$$\Sigma M = 0$$
$$M_1 = M_2$$
$$M_1 = F_1 * d_1$$
$$M_2 = F_2 * d_2$$

Fig. 3-3 Opposite moments acting about the nut in the center of the two wrenches. A moment is equal to the magnitude of the force (F_1 and F_2) times the perpendicular distance from the point of interest (nut) to the line of action of the force (d_1 and d_2). The sum of the moments must equal zero for equilibrium.

Stress and Strain

Although forces and moments are useful in describing the external loads acting on an object, these terms are not sufficiently descriptive in many cases, especially when considering the nature of the loads that are being carried within a material. Additional concepts and terminology are needed to describe the deformation that an object undergoes when forces and moments act on it.

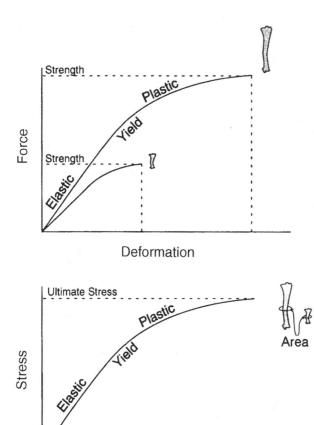

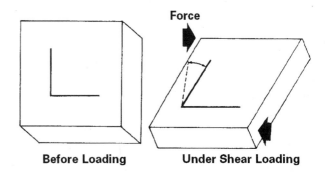

Fig. 3-4 A force/deformation curve representing structural properties and a stress/strain curve representing material properties of bone. The elastic region, yield point, and plastic region of each curve are shown. The stiffness is represented by the slope of the force/deformation curve in the elastic region. The modulus is the slope of the stress/strain curve in the elastic region.

Stress. The concept of stress is used to describe local force intensity either on the surface of a material or on a plane inside the material. Internal stress is important because it gives rise to internal deformations that can affect physiological function. Excessive internal stress can also lead directly to fracture of the material. Stress represents the amount of force exerted on a specific surface area or cross-sectional area of an object. It is defined as *normal* stress if the applied force is perpendicular to the surface and as *shear* stress if the applied force is oblique or parallel to the surface of the object. The level of stress is determined by dividing the total force applied to an area by the calculated surface area at that point. Stress is measured in newtons per square millimeter (mm²). It should be noted that for an interior point in a material, the values of the normal and shear stresses depend not only on the point of interest, but also on the plane of interest. Therefore, internal stresses must always be specified with respect to a particular plane of interest.

Strain. Any material that is subjected to external forces and moments develops internal stresses, which in turn are associated with internal deformations. Internal deformations are described in terms of strain. Axial strain is the local deformation of a finite area of an object. It is defined as *normal* strain if the change in shape of the area is elongation or shortening. To determine normal strain, the original length of the area of interest is calculated and then divided by the calculated change in length of the area after the load is applied (Fig. 3-5). Strain is defined as *shear* strain if the change in shape is a deflection of the area in question. To determine shear strain, two lines that intersect to form a 90-degree angle in the plane of interest are chosen as a point of reference. Shear strain is a measure of the change in angle between these two lines, which were originally perpendicular to each other (Fig. 3-6). A graph

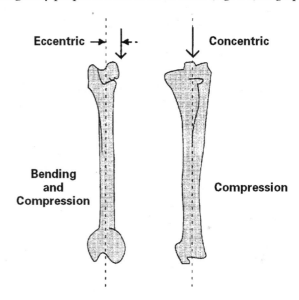

Fig. 3-5 Eccentric or concentric loading of bony columns. If the joint load application is not in line with the column of bone (femur), a bending moment is produced. If the joint load is in line with the center of the bony column, an axial load is produced.

Fig. 3-6 When a structure is loaded in shear, lines originally at right angles on a plane surface within the structure change their orientation, and the angle becomes obtuse or acute. This angular deformation indicates shear strain.

Modified from Frankel and Burstein, 1970.

(stress/strain curve) can be constructed, with the vertical axis representing the amount of stress and the horizontal axis the amount of strain. A stress/strain curve is representative of the material properties of an object.

Material Properties

Stress/strain curve. The mechanical behavior of a material generally is characterized by the relationship between stress and strain that exists in the material. Stress/strain rather than load/deformation is used because a stress/strain curve is independent of the size of the test specimen, whereas a load/deformation curve is dependent on the size of the specimen. In a typical stress/strain diagram, an initial elastic region exists over which the strain returns to zero if the stress is removed (Fig. 3-7). For orthopedic implants (e.g., stainless steel) this portion of the curve is linear, and their behavior is described as *linearly elastic*. The slope of the linear portion is an important material property because it is a measure of the stiffness of the material (this should be distinguished from the stiffness of the structure, which is discussed later). The slope typically is called the *elastic modulus* or *Young's modulus*. Materials such as stainless steel continue to deform linearly until they reach a point, called the *yield point*, at which the material begins to permanently deform; that is, when the load is removed, the strain does not return to zero. This portion of the curve is called the *plastic region*. Materials that undergo large plastic strains are called *ductile*, whereas others undergo little or no plastic strain and are referred to as *brittle*. As the load continues to increase, the material eventually fails. The stress at which failure occurs is

called the *ultimate stress*. The ultimate stress of steel is usually considered to be independent of the rate of loading. However, the ultimate stress of bone has been determined to depend somewhat on the rate of loading; a higher ultimate stress is reached for rapidly applied loads.

Viscoelastic properties. For many materials the stress/strain relationship is essentially independent of the rate at which load is applied or the time over which the load is maintained. The behavior of other materials, such as bone, does depend on time. Such materials are described as being viscoelastic. If the axial loading experiment previously described is performed on a viscoelastic material, some additional behaviors are noted. If the load is maintained for some time, the material continues to deform. This continued deformation is called *creep*. In addition, if the material is stretched out to a given amount of deformation (strain), the force required to maintain that strain decreases with time. This is called *stress relaxation*.

Fatigue. Another important time-dependent behavior is fatigue. Fatigue failure occurs with repeated loading even though the load is not sufficient to cause failure from a single application. Fatigue is very important in designing systems such as implants, which are subjected to repeated loads. Fatigue behavior generally is described in terms of an *S/N* curve; where the stress to failure, *S*, is plotted against the number of cycles to failure, *N* (Fig. 3-8). As shown, usually this is done on a log scale to accommodate a large variation in *N*. The failure

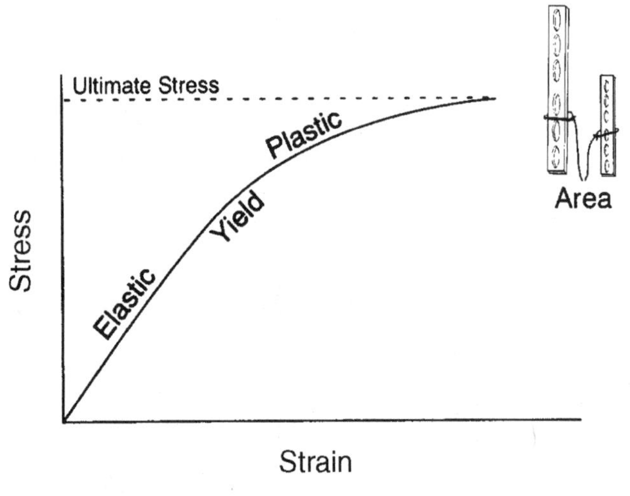

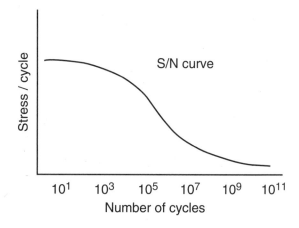

Fig. 3-7 Stress/strain curve for a large plate and a small plate. The two plates are normalized by dividing by cross-sectional area. The ultimate stress and modulus are shown by this curve and represent the material properties of each plate.

From Hulse D: *Biomechanics of fracture fixation failure*, Philadelphia, 1991, Saunders.

Fig. 3-8 An S/N curve. The curve depicts the relationship between the allowable stress, number of cycles, and stress/cycle. In the left-hand part of the curve, high stress/cycle lowers the number of cycles necessary to cause failure. The right-hand part of the curve represents failure that occurs at low stress/cycle and high numbers of cycles.

From Hulse D: *Biomechanics of fracture fixation failure*, Philadelphia, 1991, Saunders.

point for a given material is referred to as the *allowable stress*. For most structural materials, as the number of cycles required is increased, the allowable stress decreases. Fatigue failure is characterized as a succession of small cracks, which propagate throughout the material until the remaining area cannot support even a single load application. The material then undergoes ductile failure on the next load cycle. This behavior can be seen during visual metallurgical analysis of failed structures. Some materials have a stress below which fatigue failure does not occur. This value is called the *fatigue strength*. Since orthopedic implants must support repeated loading, they must be designed so that the maximum stress is below the fatigue strength or so that the number of cycles that can be sustained is very large.

Structural Properties

Force/deformation curve. The structural behavior of an object depends on the properties of the material from which the object is made, as well as the geometry of the object. As an example of structural properties, consider the difference in the tensile strength and stiffness of a tibia from a poodle and a tibia from a Great Dane (see Fig. 3-4). Assuming each bone has identical organic and inorganic composition, as the bones are subjected to increasing tensile loads, they deform until failure occurs. The larger bone from the Great Dane is expected to deform less at a given load and ultimately fail at a larger load than the smaller bone from the poodle. The ultimate load at fracture and stiffness of each bone can be determined through examination of the force/deformation curve. Initially, each bone reacts to a given force in a linear manner; that is, the deformation is directly related to the amount of force. This section of the curve is called the *elastic region* because when the force is removed, the bone returns to its original shape. The lower end of the elastic region most likely represents the range of in vivo physiological loading. Beyond some point the force causes permanent change in shape such that the deformation in the bone remains when the force is removed. In materials such as stainless steel, this point is well defined and is called the *yield point*. The upper limits of the elastic region and the yield point probably represent levels of force where significant damage to the microstructure of bone occurs. The section of the curve from the yield point to where the bone catastrophically breaks is called the *plastic region*, and the point of failure is the *ultimate load* or *ultimate strength*.

Structural stiffness. The structural stiffness of each bone is given by the slope of the force/deformation curve within the elastic region. As may be appreciated from examining the differences in stiffness and ultimate strength of the two tibias, structural properties depend not only on the material composition of each bone, but also on the dimensions of each bone. Important geometric dimensions are the cross-sectional area (amount of bone mass), distribution of bone about the neutral axis (shape of the bone), and the length of the bone.

The importance of the geometric dimensions of a whole bone in determining its structural properties can be seen by examining the parameters that influence structural strength and stiffness. Structural strength and stiffness are directly related to the modulus and moment of inertia and are inversely related to the applied force and cubic length. The *modulus* is representative of the material composition of the bone (collagen, mineral, etc.), and the *moment of inertia* represents the effect of cross-sectional shape on resistance to bending and twisting. Since strength and stiffness of bone increase as the moment of inertia increases, knowledge of those factors that influence the value of the moment of inertia is helpful. The most important factor in the determination of the moment of inertia is the radius of the structure in question. The moment of inertia increases exponentially (4th power) as the radius of the structure increases. This means that the strength and stiffness of a bone are direct functions of the fourth-power radius of that bone. The large radii of the metaphysis and epiphysis at the ends of each long bone explain how the porous and relatively weak cancellous bone of these areas can have adequate structural strength to withstand physiologic loading.

Another important use of the concept of moment of inertia is seen in fracture healing. Nature increases the radius of a healing diaphyseal fracture by deposition of periosteal callus around the external surface of the bone. By doing so, the moment of inertia of the healing bone is increased, which allows for adequate structural strength before remodeling callus into dense cortical bone.

Normal Forces and Moments of the Skeletal System

Long bones are subjected to physiological and nonphysiological forces. Nonphysiological forces occur in unusual situations, are transmitted to bone directly, and may easily exceed the ultimate strength of bone, giving rise to a fracture. An example is the force exerted to the leg by a blow from an automobile. In this situation the local inertial force is very large and is directed perpendicular to the bone surface. As discussed later, rapid local bending occurs, which gives rise to local shear and tensile stresses. The magnitude these two stresses derive as a result of the high inertial force can easily exceed the normal strength of bone and cause a fracture. Physiological forces are generated by weight bearing, muscle contraction, and associated physical activity. They are transmitted to the bone through the joint surfaces and muscle contraction. Physiological forces act along straight lines, which can be parallel or at an angle to the axis of bone. They result in tension or compression and can give rise to torsional and bending moments. Physiological forces do not usually exceed the ultimate strength of bone and are not responsible for bone fractures except in unusual cases.

The physiological force of weight bearing occurs as the foot makes contact with the ground. Simultaneously, the ground responds with an equal but opposite reaction, the ground reaction force. The magnitude of the ground reaction force varies proportionately with body acceleration and the distribution of body weight carried by the foot at impact. In addition to magnitude, the time over which the foot is in contact with the ground can be important in determining the effect of the force. Therefore, rapid loading can have a different effect than the same force applied slowly. In dogs, during slow walking, the ground reaction force can equal 30% of the body weight with each forelimb and 20% of the body weight with each rear limb. However, as a result of acceleration effects, the ground reaction force may increase to more than five times body weight at a fast trot, at a run, or when landing from a jump.

The ground reaction force causes axial compression, bending moments, and torsional moments in the bone. These moments must be balanced by muscle contraction to control motion and maintain equilibrium. For example, when the front foot strikes the ground, a ground reaction force (primarily vertical) is produced. The perpendicular distance from the line of action of the ground reaction force to the carpal joint is the *moment arm*. The product of the ground reaction force and the moment arm is the bending moment, which causes the foot to rotate cranially about the carpal joint. The moment of the ground reaction force acting at the carpal joint is balanced by muscle contraction to maintain equilibrium. Because of relatively short moment arms (lever arms), muscles must exert considerable force to maintain equilibrium. For example, if the ground reaction force in a large dog equals 30 kg and the perpendicular distance from the vertical line of action of the ground reaction force to the radiocarpal joint (moment arm) equals 6 cm, the bending moment tending to cause cranial rotation of the joint is 180 kg-cm. If the moment arm of the ulnaris lateralis muscle (distance from the accessory carpal bone to the radiocarpal joint) equals 2 cm, the muscle needs to contract with a force of 90 kg to balance the moment of the ground reaction forces (see Fig. 3-2). Although the sum of the moments (in this case the ground reaction force balanced by the contraction of the ulnaris lateralis muscle) is zero at equilibrium, there remains a net force, which is transmitted to the long bones via the joint surface. Although this is an oversimplified model, it demonstrates how very large loads are created and transmitted to the bones through the joints.

The sum of the physiological forces is transmitted to the bones and causes axial compression, axial tension, bending moments, and torsional moments on the column of bone (for simplicity, bending moments and torsional moments are referred to as *bending* or *torsion* the rest of this chapter). The percentage of the joint load transmitted as axial compression or bending is determined by the point and direction of force application at the articular surface relative to the column of bone, the normal curvature of the bone, and limb position. If the force is applied eccentric (off center) to the bony column, both compression and bending occur; a force applied concentric (in line) with the bony column produces compression. Bones loaded more eccentrically therefore are subject to greater bending than bones loaded more concentrically. A second factor that determines the amount of bending versus axial compressive force is the normal curvature of the bone. The radius and distal tibia are loaded through a joint surface that is more in line with the longitudinal axis of the bony column and are subject to compressive loading. However, the normal curvature of these bones does result in significant bending. In fact, in vivo strain analysis shows that 85% to 89% of the predominant internal stress in most bones is derived from bending. The only long bone tested to date that is loaded primarily in compression is the equine metacarpus.

Torsion arises from the twisting of the body when the foot is firmly planted on the ground. Muscle forces also contribute significantly to torsion, since their points of attachment are peripheral to the axis of rotation of the bone and their line of axis is at an angle to the axis. The axis of rotation of the bone generally corresponds to the center of the marrow cavity. As such, muscle contraction occurs with a moment arm (lever arm) that is the distance from the center of the marrow cavity to the point of muscle attachment onto the cortical surface. The force of muscle contraction results in a torsional moment (force × moment arm) that causes rotation of the bony column. This is most significant when the line of muscle force is perpendicular to the longitudinal axis of the bone, as with the iliopsoas muscle and external rotators of the proximal femur. Torsional moments that are not resisted when a proximal femoral fracture is present result in healing with increased anteversion.

Stresses and Strains of Normal Bones

When axial forces and moments are applied to any structure, it deforms from its original shape, and internal stresses and internal strains are produced. The four primary physiological forces are (1) axial compression, (2) axial tension, (3) bending, and (4) torsion. Each of these alone or in combination results in a complex pattern of internal stresses and strains within the bone. When a fracture occurs, these internal stresses and strains affect the fracture line interface. It is important to understand the generation of internal stresses and strains so they can be neutralized with internal or external stabilizing devices.

Stresses arising from compression. When the joint force is evenly distributed over the articular surface and in line (concentric) with the column of bone, axial compression of the bone occurs. The resulting internal stresses and strains are (1) compression stress parallel to the column of bone, which causes shortening; (2) strain perpendicular to the column of bone, which causes expansion; and (3) shear stress oblique to the column of bone, which causes shortening and lateral displacement (see Fig. 3-1). Clinically, the perpendicular strain from axial compression is not important because significant expansion of the bone is unlikely. However, the compressive and shear stresses are significant in that they cause collapse of a comminuted or oblique fracture if not resisted.

Stresses arising from tension. Axial tension is the direct result of muscle contraction at a point of insertion. The resulting internal tensile stress must be resisted by orthopedic implants to prevent significant gapping of the fracture surface. Axial tension from muscle contraction is the only physiological force of significance in certain fracture types. Examples are fractures of the greater trochanter, the olecranon, and the tibial crest. These injuries are best treated with the tension band principle, which applies pins and wire or bone plates and screws to resist internal tensile stress.

Stresses arising from bending. When a significant component of the joint force is transmitted eccentric to the column of bone or when the bone has significant curvature (radius), bending of the bone occurs. When a structure such as bone undergoes bending, internal tensile stress is produced on the convex surface of the bone, and internal compressive stress is produced on the concave surface of the bone (Fig. 3-9). As a result, bone on the tensile side undergoes stretching, and bone on the compression side undergoes shortening. The magnitude of these compression and tension stresses increases as the distance from the center of the marrow cavity (neutral axis) increases. Proceeding from the concave surface toward the convex surface, the *neutral axi* is the point within the structure where compressive stress ends and tensile stress begins. The maximum tensile stress is present at the periosteal surface on the convex surface of the bone, and maximum compressive stress is present on the concave surface of the bone. The surface of bone experiencing tension is referred to as the *tension surface*, whereas while the surface experiencing primary compressive stress is referred to as the *com-*

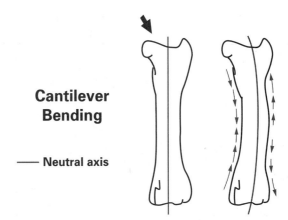

Fig. 3-9 Physiological bending. Note the compression stress on the concave surface and tensile stress on the convex surface. Maximum stress is present at the periosteal surface that is the greatest distance from the neutral axis. This point represents a point of zero stress because the stresses are changing from compression to tension.

From Hulse D: *Biomechanics of fracture fixation failure*, Philadelphia, 1991, Saunders.

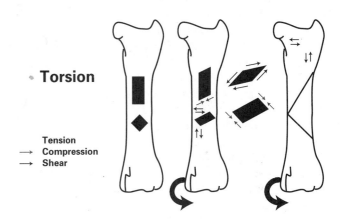

Fig. 3-10 Tensile, compressive, and shear stresses associated with a torsional force.

pression surface. Because tensile stress pulls apart fracture surfaces, it is important to know the tension surface of each long bone so that stress may be resisted and fracture surface widening prevented. The tension surface of the femur is the craniolateral surface, the craniolateral surface in the tibia, the craniolateral surface of the humerus, the cranial surface of the radius, and the caudal surface of the ulna.

Stresses arising from torsion. Torsion causes internal shear stress perpendicular to the long axis of bone. The result is rotational deformation and lateral displacement of the fracture surface. Torsion also causes internal tensile and compressive stress oblique to the longitudinal axis of the bone (Fig. 3-10). Clinically, internal shear stress arising from rotational instability can cause a delay union or nonunion of a transverse fracture if not controlled. Internal tensile stress must be resisted to prevent gapping of an oblique or spiral fracture.

Although is it convenient to address each of these physiological forces and subsequent internal stresses individually, clinically the bones experience combined compression, tension, bending, and torsional loading. An appreciation of the normal and shear stresses and strains generated by physiological forces coupled with the knowledge of an implant's ability to resist these stresses is important for optimum fracture management.

Structure and Composition of Bone

Bone is a mineralized connective tissue whose function is to provide structural support, protect vital internal organs, and facilitate body movement. It is composed of bone cells, mineral elements, organic matrix, and water. The mineral elements consist mostly of calcium and phosphate in the form of small hydroxyapatite crystals embedded in collagen fibers. These mineral crystals are strongest when placed under compression and therefore function primarily to resist internal compressive stress arising from physiological loads. The organic matrix is 5% gelatinous ground substance and 95% collagen fibers. The gelatinous ground substance is made of polysaccharides in the form of complex molecules called *proteoglycans*. The proteoglycans function as a cementing substance that surrounds each osteon to bind the layers of mineralized collagen fibers. The collagen fibers are oriented parallel to the longitudinal axis of the bone. They are strongest in tension and as such, function primarily to resist internal tensile stress arising from physiological loads. The microscopic architecture of the bone composite is such that the collagen, minerals, and proteoglycans functioning together as a unit are more resistant to internal shear, tensile, and compressive stress than each separate component alone. As such, the hydroxyapatite crystals embedded within the collagen fibers and surrounded by proteoglycans are ideally constructed to provide the necessary supportive and protective roles for the body.

Microscopically, cortical and cancellous bone are made of layers of mineralized collagen fibers embedded in the gelatinous ground substance. The layers of mineral and fiber are arranged as lamellar sheets and have three different orientations that make up the bone structure (Fig. 3-11): (1) circumferential lamellae, which encircle the outer bone surface; (2) osteon or haversian lamellae, which are the basic building structure of cortical bone; and (3) interstitial lamellae, which fill the spaces between the osteon lamellae. The osteon is the most abundant of the three lamellar organizations and is made of sheets of mineralized collagen fibers organized around a central haversian canal. The haversian channel contains blood

vessels and nerves, which serve as the nutrient supply and information network for bone cells. Along the surface of each layer (lamella) of collagen fibers within the osteon are small cavities called *lacunae*. Each lacuna houses an osteocyte, whose function is to maintain metabolic homeostasis. Surrounding individual osteons is a thin layer of proteoglycan ground substance called the *cement line*, which serves to encase each osteon. Although collagen fibers weave between the layers of lamellae within a single osteon, they do not cross the cement line to interconnect with other osteons. The lack of mineralized collagen fibers throughout the cement line renders it the weakest link in bone structure; this site is often the point of fracture initiation and propagation.

Macroscopically, bone is divided into two distinct types, cortical bone and cancellous bone. Although both types of bone have a lamellar structure made of the organic and inorganic substances described previously, the density and thickness of each bone type vary in accordance with functional demand. Cortical bone is mostly fabricated of osteons, but its porosity may vary from 5% to 30%. It is thicker and is more compact in the diaphyseal region of each long bone corresponding to the area of smallest cross-sectional diameter. Examples are the distal third of the tibial and humeral diaphysis. At the end of each long bone, the cortical bone becomes less compact and forms a thin outer shell covering the cancellous bone. Cancellous bone is made of lamellae whose orientation and density also vary depending on functional demand. Cancellous bone is more dense in the epiphyseal and metaphyseal regions of long bones, where there is a relatively small cross-sectional diameter of bone and a high load per unit area. Examples are the femoral head and humeral condyles. Cancellous bone is more porous in areas with a greater cross-sectional diameter of cancellous bone and low load per unit area. Examples are the cranioproximal humeral metaphysis and the cranioproximal tibial metaphysis.

Biomechanically, the strength and stiffness of bone are the properties that give it the ability to withstand the functional demands of normal physiological loading. At a fundamental, structure-free level where the properties of individual osteons are compared, all bone has the same properties. At this level, mechanical properties depend on the relative proportions of the organic and inorganic phases. However, most biomechanical studies into the properties of bone are reported in terms of a specified unit area of cortical and cancellous bone (material property) or as the whole bone (structural property).

As a material, cortical bone has a tensile strength of 100 to 200 megapascals (MPa) and a tensile modulus of 10 to 20 (GPa). Cancellous bone exhibits a tensile strength of 10 to 20 MPa and a tensile modulus of 0.2 to 0.5 GPa. Cortical bone undergoes approximately 1 to 3% strain before failure, and cancellous bone undergoes 5%

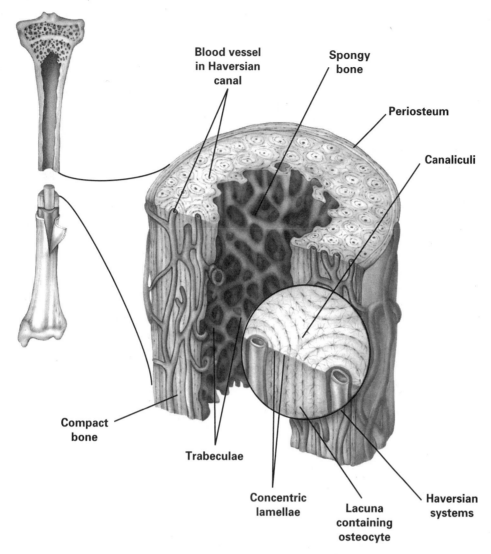

Blood vessel
in Haversian
canal

Spongy
bone

Periosteum

Canaliculi

Compact
bone

Trabeculae

Concentric
lamellae

Lacuna
containing
osteocyte

Haversian
systems

Fig. 3-11 Fine structure of bone schematically illustrated in a section of the shaft of a long bone depicted without inner marrow. The osteons, or haversian systems, are apparent as the structural units of bone. In the center of the osteons are the haversian canals, which form the main branches of the circulatory network in bone. Each osteon is bounded by a cement line. One osteon is shown extending from the bone.

From Thibodeau G: *The human body in health and disease*, St Louis, 1992, Mosby.

to 7% strain before failure. To determine structural properties, whole bones are loaded in direct compression, tension, bending, and torsion. The ultimate force the whole bone can withstand without failure depends on the composition of the organic and inorganic phases of the cortical and cancellous bone, degree of porosity, and the geometric shape of the bone. Under compressive or tensile loads, the cross-sectional area of the bone is the only important geometric feature; in this case a bone with more mass (greater cross-sectional area) withstands a greater force. When a whole bone experiences bending loads and torsional loads, not only is the mass of

bone important, but also the distribution of the bone mass (shape of bone). The distribution of the bone about the neutral axis determines the moment of inertia, which is an important geometric feature in determining strength and stiffness. The moment of inertia is a function of the fourth-power radius of the whole bone. Therefore the amount of bone, its material property, and its distribution (shape) are all important in determining the structural strength and stiffness of a whole bone.

Bone is viscoelastic and anisotropic. Cortical and cancellous bone being viscoelastic means that their mechanical properties depend on the rate of loading. Bone that is loaded very rapidly exhibits an increase in strength and stiffness compared with bone that is loaded slowly. This property of bone protects the animal from experiencing fractures during strenuous physiological activity, such as that associated with rapid impacts (e.g., jumping, falling). Because the strength and stiffness of bone increase with rapid loading, the energy absorbed by bone (as represented by the area underneath the force/deformation curve) also increases. If the load exceeds the ultimate strength of bone, a fracture occurs and the stored energy is released to the soft tissues. Therefore, with high-velocity injuries, energy dissipation can cause significant soft tissue injury. Bone is anisotropic, which means that the strength and stiffness depend on the direction of loading. In general, bone is strongest if loaded along its longitudinal axis and weakest if a load is applied perpendicular to its longitudinal axis.

Mechanism of Bone Failure

The various loading modes to which bones are subjected (compression, bending, torsion) lead to specific fracture patterns. Since bone is weakest when subjected to shear stress or tensile stress, failure occurs within the zones of high shear and tensile stress. Bones subject to compressive loads generally fail oblique to the longitudinal axis corresponding to the plane of maximum internal shear stress. Bending loads initiate a transverse fracture corresponding to the high internal tensile stress on the convex surface of the bone. A small fragment may occur on the compression surface of the bone initiated at the zone of high internal shear stress. If compression and bending occur at the same time, the internal shear stress is accentuated on the concave surface, resulting in a larger "butterfly" fragment or comminution of the concave surface. Torsional loads create internal shear stress parallel to the column of bone and can initiate a fracture at the point of maximum shear stress. The fracture is then propagated in a spiral fashion around the circumference of the bone corresponding to the zone of maximum internal tensile stress. Clinically, fractures may be simple low-energy fractures in which the failure force can be deduced, or more often, the fracture pattern is more complex because of combinations of loads.

BIOMATERIALS

Various metals are used in manufacturing implants for fracture fixation devices. Examples are the iron-based alloys (stainless steels), cobalt-based alloys (e.g., Vitallium), and titanium-based alloys. The specifications for a variety of these alloys have been codified by the American Society for Testing and Materials (ASTM) and, for stainless steel, by the American Iron and Steel Institute (AISI). Before an alloy can be used for internal fracture stabilization, several requirements must be satisfied. Among

these are a suitable combination of properties to permit fabrication of properly sized and shaped implants, suitable mechanical properties relative to allowable sizes for implantation, and compatibility in vivo. Another factor that plays a significant role in veterinary orthopedics is the cost of the implant. Although the titanium-based and cobalt-based alloys enjoy a degree of popularity in human orthopedics, economics favors the use of the stainless steel alloys almost exclusively in veterinary orthopedics. As such, this discussion is limited to fabrication principles and mechanical properties of stainless steel.

Alloy fabrication begins with the extraction of metal ores from mineral deposits. In the case of stainless steels, the base element is iron with other elements, such as chromium, nickel, and molybdenum, added during fabrication. There are four basic types of stainless steels, and two of these, martensitic and austenitic stainless steels, are frequently used in orthopedics. The martensitic steels are very hard and tough and thus are favored for the manufacturing of surgical instruments. The superior corrosion resistance of austenitic alloys, such as 316L stainless steel, has led to their dominance in implant fabrication. The designation 316L comes from the AISI. This alloy is equivalent to the special-quality stainless steel for surgical implants designated by the ASTM specifications for F138 and F139 alloys. The composition of austenitic 316L stainless steel is iron (62% to 62%), chromium (17% to 20%), nickel (13% to 16%), and molybdenum (2% to 3%). Carbon is limited to less than 0.03%, and the remainder of ingredients consists of small amounts of other elements.

Each element has a specific purpose in the total composition of the alloy. Nickel is added to stabilize the alloy in the more corrosion-resistant austenitic microstructure. Molybdenum controls corrosion of stainless steel but can only be used in small amounts because it greatly hardens the alloy, making it difficult to work with. Chromium is added to form a stable chromium oxide surface layer, which helps to prevent corrosion. Carbon is important in some stainless steel applications because it forms carbide precipitates, which render the surface very hard. This is advantageous in manufacturing surgical instruments such as osteotomes or carbide tip needle holders. However, excess carbon is a disadvantage in the fabrication of surgical implants because of rapid corrosion of the carbide precipitates in vivo. To prevent formation of carbide precipitates and subsequent corrosion, the carbon content of surgical implants must be very low. The L designation in 316L stainless steels denotes low carbon levels (less than 0.03%) and should be present in the name placed on stainless steel alloys used as surgical implants. The letters VM as part of an alloy name on some surgical implants designate a remelting of the alloy in a vacuum to further remove impurities, which, if present, can accelerate corrosion or lower the mechanical properties. Standardized designations such as 316L or VM should not be confused with proprietary material names used by some manufacturers.

The properties of stainless steels not only are sensitive to chemical composition, but are also sensitive to the manufacturing process. Formation of 316L stainless steel is accomplished by combining the appropriate elements and melting them together under suitable conditions into cast bars or rods. However, cast structures are relatively weak and must undergo further processing to make pins or bone plates with suitable mechanical strength and stiffness. Further refinement of mechanical properties of the cast alloy is accomplished by forging. Forging in this context is similar to the art of the blacksmith; the metal is heated and hammered into shape. However, in the manufacture of surgical implants, forging consists of gradually shaping the implant through compression in dies.

After forging, the implant is cold-worked to elongate the grain structure into fibrous shapes parallel to the long axis of the implant and expected deforming forces. This microstructure provides optimum strength to prevent breakage of the implant. However, as cold working increases the strength, it also increases the stiffness, which reduces the work required for breakage (area beneath the stress/strain curve). Therefore, excessive cold working can result in premature failure of the implant when subject to the cyclical stress of in vivo loading. Also, if the implant becomes too stiff after cold working, the ability to contour the implant at surgery is lessened.

Since a degree of ductility is optimum to prevent brittle failure of an implant exposed to in vivo cyclical loading and allow contouring of the implant at surgery, each implant can be further refined by heating. To attain the desired strength and stiffness, stainless steel can be made more ductile by heating (annealing) in special ovens. The degree of ductility can be varied to attain properties desired for each implant. For example, 316L cerclage wire is more ductile than bone plates, which in turn are more ductile than Steinmann or Kirschner pins.

After the desired mechanical properties are attained, the implant undergoes passivation through acid treatment. This process converts surface elements such as chromium into oxides, producing a surface layer that gives superior surface characteristics and provides corrosion resistance. It is important not to damage the surface of an implant during surgery in order to preserve the oxide layer. For example, care must be taken when contouring a bone plate to use appropriate bending pliers, which prevents unnecessary scratching of the plate surface. Scratching of the surface can remove the oxide layer, permitting corrosion and stress concentration that can lead to failure. The ultimate tensile strength of surgical stainless steel is set at minimum of 70,000 psi and at maximum cold working, 125,000 psi. The yield strength ranges from 25,000 to 100,000 psi depending on the degree of cold working. The maximum strain is 40% with minimum cold working and 12% with maximum cold working.

The mechanical characteristics of implants discussed previously are generally determined under low-cycle or static conditions. However, orthopedic implants must remain in service for months or years and are subject to time-dependent mechanical properties. One time-dependent mechanical property of importance in orthopedics is fatigue. *Fatigue* refers to failure of an implant that occurs as a result of repeated stress at levels below that required to cause breakage from a single load (ultimate stress). Generally, the greater the peak stress produced with a given cycle of loading, the fewer are the cycles needed to break the implant. The relationship between the peak stress and number of cycles to failure is represented by the *S/N* curve (see Fig. 3-8). This curve demonstrates the need for adherence to principles of application of implants to facilitate load sharing between the implant and bone during the healing period. In the left-hand section of the curve, the allowable stress (point of implant failure) is reached with a low number of cycles and high loading. This can be seen clinically in patients when an implant must span a section of fragmented bone that cannot be reconstructed so as to offer bony support under loading. Examples are a buttress plate or an external skeletal fixator that must support a highly fragmented injury (Fig. 3-12). Also, the allowable stress may be

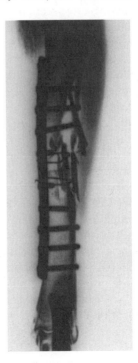

Fig. 3-12 Craniocaudal radiograph of a dog undergoing bone plate osteosynthesis for a comminuted tibial fracture. In this case, initial load sharing occurs between the implant and bone, resulting in high stresses on the implant.

From Hulse D. *Biomechanics of fracture fixation failure*, Philadelphia, 1991, Saunders.

reached with a low number of loading cycles when high physiological loads result from the patient falling or jumping on the leg postoperatively. In the right-hand section of the curve, the allowable stress is such that failure occurs with low loads but an excessive number of loading cycles. This is observed clinically when the patient's activity is not limited after surgery or when delayed union occurs and the implant must remain functional beyond a reasonable amount of time.

Function of Implants in Osteosynthesis and Mechanisms of Failure

Intramedullary pins. The biomechanical advantage of an intramedullary pin is resistance to applied bending loads. In contrast to other implants (bone plates, external fixators), the pin is equally resistant to bending loads applied from any direction. This is caused by the circular nature of intramedullary pins. The bending support afforded by intramedullary pins depends on load sharing between the bone and pin, the working length of the pin, and the size of the pin. Several biomechanical disadvantages to intramedullary pins exist, including poor resistance to axial or rotational loads and lack of fixation (interlocking) with the bone. The only resistance to rotation or axial loads given by an intramedullary pin is the friction generated between the pin and the bone. The actual contact of the pin and bone is not substantial because of the varying cross-sectional diameter of the marrow cavity, limiting the degree of friction created between the two surfaces. Also, the contact between the pin and cancellous bone in the epiphysis varies with the amount of cancellous bone present and the accuracy of pin placement. Therefore the friction created between the pin and cancellous bone also varies. In general, the friction generated between the pin and bone is not sufficient to prevent rotational movement or axial collapse of a fracture. This same concept applies to the stability of an intramedullary Steinmann pin within the bone, that is, the factors that prevent premature pin migration. Again, only the friction created between the pin and bone prevents premature pin migration. If the fracture is unstable because of an unrealistic expectation of implant performance, the stress at the pin-bone interface exceeds the frictional stability between the pin and bone and may cause premature pin migration.

Intramedullary pins can fail by breakage, plastic deformation (bending), or premature loosening. Plastic deformation and breakage are not common and occur when physiological loads exceed the yield point or ultimate strength of the pin. Factors that contribute to plastic deformation or breakage of an intramedullary pin are points of stress concentration, a pin too small in diameter, and lack of postoperative restraint. Stress concentration occurs with an abrupt change in cross-sectional di-

ameter along the shaft of the pin. This occurs with the threaded trocar Steinmann pin at the junction of the smooth and threaded sections of the pin shaft. In addition to the point of stress concentration, the smaller shaft diameter of the threaded section reduces the moment of inertia and therefore ultimate strength in this section of the pin. When the threaded point of the pin is seated securely in bone, a cyclical cantilever bending stress is concentrated at the thread/smooth shaft junction during physiological loading. The result can be plastic deformation or breakage of the pin at the point of stress concentration (Fig. 3-13). Plastic deformation or breakage of a pin can also occur if the original pin diameter is too small. This is particularly true if the patient's activity is not restricted postoperatively.

Although mechanical failure of an intramedullary pin is possible, the more common mode of failure is premature loosening. Premature loosening is caused by bone resorption at the pin-bone interface and occurs because of excessive local strains between the pin and endosteal surface of the bone. Clinically excessive local strains are the result of poor decision making preoperatively, poor surgical technique, or poor patient restraint postoperatively. An example is the use of a single pin to provide rotational and axial support in a fractured long bone. The only resistance to rotation or axial stress provided by an intramedullary pin is the friction generated between the

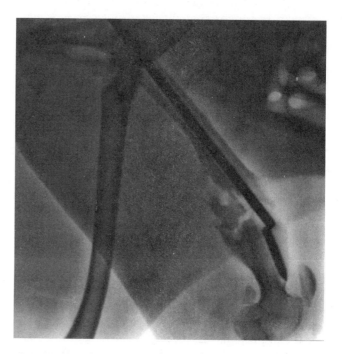

Fig. 3-13 Lateral radiograph showing breakage of a threaded Steinmann pin at the junction of its smooth shaft and threaded shaft.

From Hulse D: *Biomechanics of fracture fixation failure*, Philadelphia, 1991, Saunders.

pin and endosteal surface of the bone. Within the bone, the actual contact between the pin and endosteum is not substantial because of the varying cross-sectional diameter of the marrow cavity. This limits the contact and therefore the degree of friction created between the surface of the pin and the cortical bone. In general, the friction generated between the pin and bone (endosteum and cancellous) is not sufficient to prevent movement of the fracture. Movement of the fracture causes local stresses at the pin-bone interface that exceed the frictional hold between the pin and bone. The result is micromotion and excessive local strains incompatible with bone tissue survival. Osteoclastic resorption of bone enlarges the original drill hole, reducing local strain but loosening the pin. Once the pin is loose, it may migrate or simply remain in the marrow cavity (Fig. 3-14). If the pin migrates from the marrow cavity, all fracture stability is lost and further osteosynthesis is needed. If the pin is loose and remains in the marrow cavity, it may provide some bending support and, depending on biological factors, union may occur.

Cerclage wire. Cerclage is the use of heavy-gauge orthopedic wire to supplement other fixation devices in the stabilization of fracture surfaces. Indications for cerclage wire include long oblique fractures, spiral fractures, and comminuted fractures. Cerclage wire may be used to adapt fracture surfaces or used as an ancillary stabilizer in creating friction between fracture surfaces. To function as an ancillary stabilizer, the fracture surface should be 2.5 to 3 times the diameter of the marrow cavity in the area of placement. If the fracture surface is too short in length, it becomes difficult to place the needed minimum of two cerclage wires across the fracture surface. Consequently, only one wire is placed, which acts as a fulcrum to concentrate stress and produce high local strains.

Additionally, for cerclage wire to function as an ancillary stabilizer, there should be no more than two fragments when viewed in any transverse plane. If more than two fragments are present, cerclage wire may be used only to adapt or hold the fragments in their anatomical location. An analogy to the use of cerclage wire for adaptation is the use of metal rings to hold slats in a wooden barrel. As can be perceived, collapse occurs if one slat (bone fragment) is loosened. The most common cause of cerclage wire failure is inappropriate use of the wire as a stabilizer when the comminution of the fracture is such that the wire should be used only for adaptation. An example is shown in Fig. 3-15, where an attempt was made to stabilize a comminuted fracture with an intramedullary pin and cerclage wire. As discussed previously, an intramedullary pin offers little support against axial collapse of a fracture. Also, the comminution is such that cerclage wire cannot serve as a stabilizer

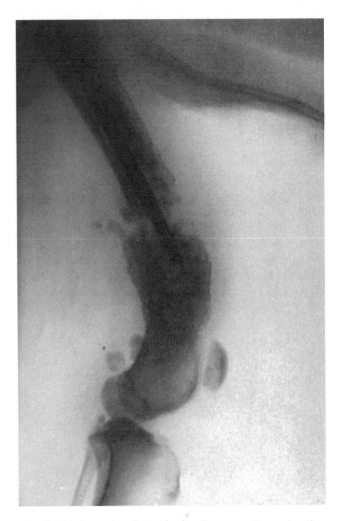

Fig. 3-14 Lateral radiograph showing premature migration of an intramedullary pin.

From Hulse D: *Biomechanics of fracture fixation failure*, Philadelphia, 1991, Saunders.

in preventing collapse of the bone fragments. As with the wooden barrel, when one fragment loosens, the entire structure collapses.

Hemicerclage wire is the use of orthopedic wire to assist in rotational and bending support with transverse fractures. Only the cruciate hemicerclage wire pattern is recommended, since it has been shown to be superior to other hemicerclage wire patterns. The wire should be placed on the tension side of the bone to give rotational as well as bending support. Hemicerclage is recommended only with transverse fractures or oblique fractures that have been bayoneted to prevent axial collapse.

External skeletal fixation. Strength and stiffness of the fixator-bone composite is determined by various factors, including frame configuration, pin number, pin size, pin placement, bar placement, fracture configuration,

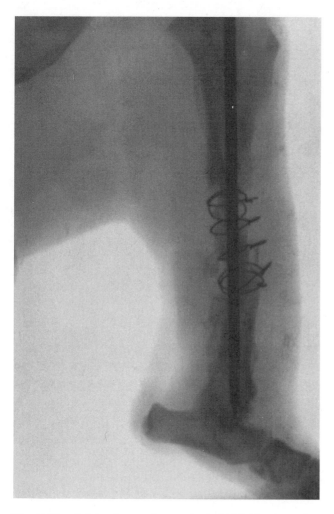

Fig. 3-15 Axial collapse of comminuted tibial fracture after attempted stabilization with an intermedullary pin and cerclage wire.

and material from which the fixator is made. In general, the greater the size and number of bars connecting the pin assembly, the greater is the strength and stiffness of the fixator. In addition, since bones are subject to bending in two planes (mediolateral and craniocaudal), biplanar fixators are more effective in resisting physiological bending loads than are fixators with connecting bars in the same plane.

Static strength evaluation of different external fixator configurations shows type Ia, type Ib, type II, and type III external fixators to be successively stronger in resisting bending, axial compression, and torsion. The greater the number of pins per fragment, the greater is the stiffness and surface area over which to distribute stress at the pin-bone interface. This is true up to four pins per fragment. Beyond this number, the amount of stiffness increase is negligible. Studies also indicate that pin diameter has an effect on stiffness and stress at the pin-bone interface. An increase in pin diameter exponentially in-

creases the stiffness of the pin, since stiffness is directly related to the fourth power of the radius (increasing the diameter by 2 mm increases the stiffness by a factor of 16).

The placement of the pins relative to the fracture also affects the stiffness of the pin-bone composite. Stiffness in bending is inversely related to length (stiffness = modulus × moment of inertia/length). Therefore the greater the length over which the force is distributed, the longer is the working length and the more flexible the structure. This concept relates to the position of the pins relative to the fracture. One pin should be placed 2 cm proximal to the fracture and one placed 2 cm distal to the fracture. The closer these pins are placed on either side of the fracture, the shorter the distance between connecting clamps on the external bar; therefore, the shorter the length of the bar sustaining the load and the greater the stiffness of the fixator. The proximal and distal pins are placed in their respective metaphyses while remaining pins are spaced evenly in the proximal and distal fragments.

The concept of working length also applies to the position of the fixation bar. The shorter the distance from the external fixator clamp to the point of cortical entrance by the pin, the shorter is the pin length. Therefore the external fixation bar must be placed as close to the bone as is possible without the clamps or bar impinging on the skin surface.

Another important factor that affects the stiffness of the external fixator bone composite is the fracture configuration. If the fixator and bone share the load during healing, less load is carried by the fixator. For example, if the fracture is comminuted, the entire load must be carried by the fixator until healing has progressed sufficiently to produce bone contact with callus that has enough mechanical strength to share the weight-bearing forces. As the callus becomes more mature, the bone is able to carry more of the physiological load, thus reducing the stress on the fixator and pin-bone interface. If the fracture is transverse, the fixator and bone share the load initially, reducing the stress at the pin-bone interface (this is particularly true if compression is applied to the bone by prestressing the fixation pins). Pin implantation is done with a low-speed power drill.

In a study comparing low-speed insertion with hand chuck insertion, acute pullout force was less with the hand chuck insertion. In chronic pullout tests, both methods of insertion were comparable in force required to extract the pins. Considerable emphasis has been placed on pin design with the rekindled interest in external fixators. Numerous studies have been conducted with the goal of modifying pin design to increase pin-bone interface stability. One investigation studied the strength and holding power of smooth pins and a one cortex threaded pin (Ellis pin). The Ellis pin had similar bending strength to smooth pins but was seven times more resistant than smooth pins to pullout 8 weeks after insertion. Although the Ellis pin has a mechanically weak junction at the threaded and smooth shafts, when properly inserted, this juncture lies within the marrow cavity and is protected from cyclical stress. A recent experimental study compared the acute and chronic pullout strengths of smooth pins, Ellis pins, and Turner Hip pins. The Turner Hip pin is a threaded pin with "rolled-on threads" similar to a bone screw. This study showed that Ellis and Turner Hip pins had similar pullout strengths, but both were superior to the pullout strength of smooth pins. A recent clinical study compared the use of threaded pins (Turner Hip pins) and smooth pins in clinical patients. Limb use, patient comfort, and stability at the pin-bone interface were increased when threaded pins were used alone or in combination with smooth pins.

The most common mode of external fixation failure is premature loosening of fixation pins (Fig. 3-16). If loosening occurs before biological callus stabilization of fracture surfaces, fracture mobility and loosened pins can cause patient discomfort. Also, once a fixation pin has loosened, associated inflammation predisposes the pin-tract to infection. If this occurs, inflammation is intensified and patient discomfort becomes more evident. In turn, patient discomfort leads to limb disuse, fracture disease, and prolonged bone healing. The cause of premature loosening is bone resorption at the fixation pin-bone interface. This may be the result of one or two factors acting alone or in combination: local bone damage and micromotion at the fixation pin-bone interface.

Local bone damage results from the production of microfractures or excessive heat production during insertion of fixation pins. Local microfractures are associated with the use of dull fixation pins and occur when the torque produced with pin insertion exceeds the shear strength of bone. Thermal heat necrosis of local bone

can occur with the use of dull fixation pins or drilling with too many revolutions per minute (rpm) during insertion. In either situation, the friction generated between the pin and bone produces enough heat to cause local bone damage. Damaged bone as a result of microfractures or thermal necrosis undergoes osteoclastic resorption, which in turn enlarges the drill hole and loosens the fixation pin.

Osteoclastic bone resorption at the fixation pin bone interface is also induced by micromotion or excessive local stress. Micromotion causes local strains at the fixation pin-bone interface, which, if too high, exceed those compatible with bone tissue survival. Osteoclasts then resorb bone to enlarge the space between the fixation pin and bone. This action relieves high local strains, but the enlarged drill hole leads to a loosened fixation pin. Once the pin is loose, physiological loads produce more micromotion at the fixation pin-bone interface. The result is a cycle of high local strain, osteoclastic resorption of bone, enlarged drill hole, and more pin loosening. Excessive stress can occur when the pin must transfer high loads to the bone. This stress can exceed the ultimate strength of bone, causing local microfractures that lead to bone resorption.

Micromotion and local stress at the pin-bone interface are directly related to stiffness of the fixator-bone composite and pin design. Therefore the common clinical cause of external skeletal fixation failure is inappropriate choice of fixator type and pin design. A clinical example is the use of a four-pin, type I external fixator frame used for fixation of a severe gunshot injury of the tibia in an adult dog. In this case, biological factors, such as age and soft tissue injury, dictate a prolonged healing time. Mechanically, the fixator must function as a buttress because the fragmentation precludes load sharing between the bone and external fixator. These biological and mechanical factors predict that high stress levels will be present at the fixation pin-bone interface for an extended time. If the appropriate fixation pin design and the factors that influence fixator stiffness are not considered, premature loosening of the fixation pin is likely.

Bone plates and screws. Bone plates function with the bone to form a bone plate-fractured bone composite after implantation. Bone plates function differently depending on whether compression of the fracture surfaces is achieved and on the method used to apply compression to the fracture surface. If compression, and therefore fracture fragment contact, is achieved, the plate functions as a compression plate or a neutralization plate. A compression plate osteosynthesis is designated as one in which compression of the fracture surface is achieved through application of the plate to the bone. An example is application of a Dynamic Compression Plate to a transverse fracture. Proper eccentric placement of

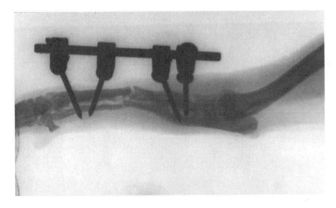

Fig. 3-16 Lateral radiograph showing premature loosening of external fixation pins in the radius of a dog.

From Hulse D: *Biomechanics of fracture fixation failure*, Philadelphia, 1991, Saunders.

the drill holes achieves compression of the fracture surface when the screws are tightened. In a neutralization osteosynthesis, lag screws are used to compress fracture lines and the plate used to support and neutralize the forces acting on the reconstructed cylinder of bone. An example is the use of lag screws and a bone plate to stabilize an oblique fracture. A bone plate serves as a buttress when it serves to maintain axial alignment. Examples are when the fragmentation of the diaphysis is such that compression between the fragments is not possible or when an articular fragment must be held in alignment during healing.

The stiffness of the bone plate–bone composite is important in maintaining the interfragmentary strain at a level compatible with bone union. Stiffness is directly proportional to the modulus of the bone-implant composite and can only approach that of intact bone if compression is achieved through a compression plate or neutralization plate. Compression preloads the fracture surface to maintain contact between the surfaces under dynamic load. As long as the preload exceeds the physiological tensile stress attempting to separate the fracture, stability and stiffness are maintained. Compression also creates friction between the fracture surfaces, which will maintain stability as long as the friction exceeds the shear stress from physiological loading. If no compression of the fracture surfaces is achieved, the stiffness of the bone-plate composite is equal to that of the plate alone and is considerably less than that of intact bone.

In addition to compression, an appropriate length of plate must be applied. Stiffness is also directly related to the moment of inertia of the plate-bone composite. Since the moment of inertia depends on the fourth-power radius, maintaining the effective radius of the bone-plate composite is important. This is accomplished surgically by reconstructing the transcortex so that the plate functions as a compression or neutralization plate. If the plate functions as a buttress plate (i.e., the transcortex is not compressed), the radius of the bone-late composite is that of the bone plate alone. Consequently, the moment of inertia is smaller, which reduces the stiffness of the bone-plate composite (Figs. 3-17 and 3-18). Stiffness of the bone-plate composite is inversely proportional to the working length of fixation. The *working length* refers to the distance between the innermost screws on either side of the fracture plane. The greater the distance between the innermost screws, the longer is the working length and the less stiff the plate-bone composite. An example of a short working length is a transverse fracture in which the screws on each side of the fracture line are in place. A longer working length is present if the length of multiple fracture lines prevents placement of screws in the center of the plate.

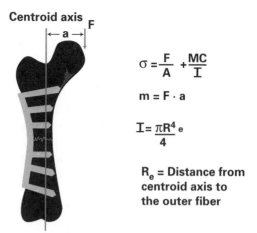

Fig. 3-17 Bone plate osteosynthesis of a femoral fracture. In this case the transcortex was reconstructed. σ, Allowable stress; F, axial force; A, cross-sectional area; M, applied bending moment; C, radius; I, moment of inertia. Because the transcortex is intact, the applied moment is small and the moment of inertia large. As such, it is unlikely that the allowable stress of the bone plate will be reached.

From Hulse D: *Biomechanics of fracture fixation failure*, Philadelphia, 1991, Saunders.

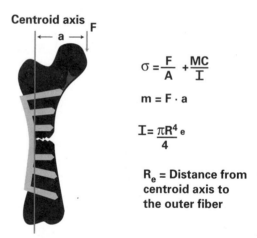

Fig. 3-18 Bone plate osteosynthesis of the femur in which the transcortex was not reconstructed. In this case the moment arm is larger than in Fig. 3-17, which increases the applied bending moment. Also, the effective radius of the structure is reduced, which decreases the moment of inertia of the bone-plate composite. Physiological loads may approach the allowable stress of the bone plate.

From Hulse D: *Biomechanics of fracture fixation failure*, Philadelphia, 1991, Saunders.

Bone plates and screws fail by plate or screw breakage, bending of the plate or screw, screw loosening, or screw pullout. For breakage or bending to occur, the ultimate allowable strength or allowable yield strength (static or fatigue) must be exceeded. This occurs more often in bone plates when the transcortex of the long bone is not reconstructed. In this situation the applied moment increases while the moment of inertia of the bone-plate composite decreases. These factors, coupled with excessive loading cycles from lack of postoperative restraint, may lead to premature bending or breakage of the plate as defined by the *S/N* curve. Screws can also bend or break when the allowable yield strength or ultimate strength is exceeded. Clinically, this can occur when the screw is subject to greater-than-expected loads, as when the surgeon inadvertently chooses a screw with too small a diameter or when excessive loads on the screw result from poor surgical technique. An example of the latter is poor bone-plate contouring leading to a loss of frictional hold between the cortex and plate. In this case the applied axial load is carried by the screws and shear breakage of the screw heads may occur.

Screw loosening occurs from bone resorption at the screw-bone interface. Bone resorption ensues when microdamage of the bone occurs during screw insertion or when excessive stress is present at the screw-bone interface. Bone resorption also follows excessive micromotion at the screw-bone interface. Damage to the bone occurs when unsharpened instruments are used to prepare the drill hole for screw insertion. An example is the use of a dull drill bit, which may cause excessive torque. If the torque exceeds the shear strength of bone, microfractures of the cortex occur. The damaged bone is then resorbed, enlarging the original drill hole and loosening the screw. Loosening can also result when local strains at the screw-bone interface are too high. Local strain is related to screw design and stiffness; therefore, too small a screw or the wrong type of screw design can result in micromotion and bone resorption.

Screw pullout occurs infrequently and is related to screw design, bone strength, and applied tensile forces parallel to the screw shaft. Physiological bending gives rise to such tensile forces when the plate is on the tension surface of the bone. If excessive, the tensile stresses can exceed the shear strength of bone interposed between the screw threads. When this occurs, the bone fractures adjacent to the screw threads, and the screw pulls out of the cortex (Fig 3-19).

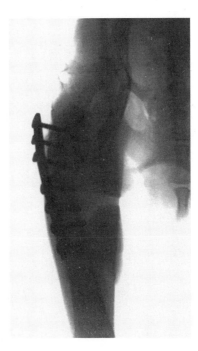

Fig. 3-19 Craniocaudal radiograph of a dog showing proximal stress screw pullout after bone plate osteosynthesis. In this case the plate did not extend proximal enough to the fracture relative to the length of the proximal femur. The tensile stress from the physiological bending moment exceeded the screw's holding ability, resulting in pullout.

From Hulse D: *Biomechanics of fracture fixation failure*, Philadelphia, 1991, Saunders.

SUGGESTED READINGS

Carter DR, Spengler DM: Biomechanics of fractures. In Sumner-Smith G, editor: *Bone in clinical orthopedics*, Philadelphia, 1982, Saunders.

Nordin M, Frankel V: *Biomechanics of the musculoskeletal system,* ed 2, Philadelphia, 1989, Lea & Febiger

Perren S: Primary bone healing. In Bojrab MJ, editor: *Pathophysiology in small animal surgery*, Philadelphia, 1981, Lea & Febiger.

Perren S, Rahn BA: Biomechanics of fracture healing. 1. Historical review and mechanical aspects of internal fixation, *Orthop Surv* 2:108, 1978.

Radin EL: *Practical biomechanics for the orthopedic surgeon*, New York, 1979, John Wiley & Sons.

Rahn BA: Bone healing: histologic and physiologic concepts. In Sumner-Smith G, editor: *Bone in clinical orthopedics*, Philadelphia, 1982, Saunders.

4

Slings, Padded Bandages, Splinted Bandages, and Casts

TODD A. TOBIAS

GOALS OF BANDAGING

The primary goal of support bandaging is to facilitate healing by immobilizing an injured part of the body. Different injuries require different degrees of immobility. In general, the more rigid the bandage, the more expensive are the materials and the greater the potential for complication. Secondarily, bandages can limit limb swelling and provide protection, medication, absorption, and debridement for open wounds.

Success with bandaging starts with an appropriate candidate. All injuries do not lend themselves to treatment with bandages. The decision to perform surgery, apply a bandage, or do nothing must be made on a case-to-case basis. The most common indications for bandaging are addressed later; however, a comprehensive discussion on the management of orthopedic injuries is not within the scope of this chapter. The second ingredient for success is an appropriate choice of bandage. It is important to realize that no single support bandage exists for any given injury. Numerous approaches can and have been used successfully for similar injuries. Third, once an appropriate bandage is chosen, a successful outcome cannot be expected without adequate application and monitoring. Proper application depends on an understanding of basic principles and a mastery of bandaging technique. Although specific instructions are detailed later, consistent success is only achieved with practice and experience with a variety of cases.

Finally, veterinarians must always remember that bandages need protection not only from the environment, but from the patients themselves. Even a perfectly applied bandage, used for an appropriate injury, can significantly exacerbate the original problem if soiled, wetted, or damaged by the patient or environment. As a result, enthusiasm for the use of a support bandage must always be tempered by the potential for complication.

DEFINITIONS

Slings, padded bandages, splinted bandages, and casts are defined as external support devices, which, in the order listed, can increasingly immobilize a body part, usually an extremity. The function of these devices is determined by the method of application and the materials used in their construction. The term *external coaptation* is usually reserved for splinted bandages or casts, which in some instances can provide adequate stability for injured ligaments or fractures. For purposes of simplicity, the terms *external support device* and *bandage* are considered synonymous and inclusive for all slings, padded bandages, splinted bandages, and casts.

Slings

Slings provide minimal stability and are usually designed only to prevent weight bearing or maintain a protective orientation for the limb. Slings are often constructed solely of elastic adhesive tape. Because no underlying padding exists, and because adhesive tapes are strong and have limited pliability, slings must be applied and monitored carefully so that pressure-induced sores are prevented or detected early.

Padded Bandages

Padded bandages provide more stability than slings but generally are not considered adequate for injured ligaments or fractures. They are most often applied as an aid for soft tissue injury. Besides providing minimal support, they can limit the degree of limb swelling and provide protection, gentle debridement, and absorbency for open wounds.

Splinted Bandages

Splinted bandages are constructed similarly to padded bandages but have an associated splint for added rigidity. In addition to the advantages provided by padded bandages, the splinted variety provides adequate stability to permit healing of some ligament injuries and fractures. This type of bandage is also used to protect surgically repaired connective tissue injuries and openly reduced but tenuously repaired fractures.

Casts

Casts provide the greatest stability of all external support devices. Stability is afforded by a rigid outer layer constructed of casting material. Casts provide adequate stability for some ligament injuries or fractures and can protect fragile repairs of connective tissue or bone. However, the usefulness of casts is severely diminished in injuries associated with severe soft tissue swelling or open wounds.

Bandage Layers

The different layers of material are as important to a bandage's function as the techniques with which they are applied. It is important to identify and characterize the layers because of their significance to a bandage's characteristics and because of their functional synonymy between bandages of differing types (Fig. 4-1). Homology with previous descriptions of bandage component layers is maintained where applicable.[16]

The *contact layer* lies closest to the skin and is often a protective material such as tube stockinette, orthopedic felt, or material designed specifically for wound coverage. The "stirrups," usually made from adhesive tape, are included in the contact layer and prevent distal slippage of the bandage. The *padding layer* is usually made of cotton cast padding or roll cotton and is applied in some bandages to distance a less pliable layer (ie., cast or splint material) from the contact layer and limb. The padding provides some support, when tightly compacted, but also provides absorbency. The *compressive layer*, made from conforming roll gauze, is applied with circumferential tension to compact the padding and, with splinted bandages, to bind a splint firmly to the limb. Care must be taken to place this layer evenly and without excessive tension, or venous and lymphatic obstruction with limb swelling

may occur. The *splint layer* does not completely encircle the limb and is made of moldable or nonmoldable rigid material such as aluminum rod, thermally sensitive plastic, plaster, fiberglass, and metal or plastic "spoon" splints. This layer provides the predominant support in splinted bandages and is bound to the layers beneath with additional conforming gauze. The *outer layer*, although porous, is usually somewhat more water resistant than the underlying cotton layers and is frequently made of an elastic fabric with adhesive properties. It is the sole layer in most slings and the most external layer in support and splinted bandages, where it prevents layers underneath from fraying and protects them from dirt and moisture. The *cast layer* is used only with casts and is made from a stiff material such as fiberglass or plaster. It is applied circumferentially and provides the sole stability for these support devices (Fig. 4-1).

BIOMECHANICS

Bandages immobilize limbs by providing resistance to distracting forces. The degree of immobilization has three major determinants: the stiffness of the stiffest layer, the intimacy of this layer to the limb bones, and the relative position of the unstable injury within the bandage.

Bandage Layer Stiffness

The stiffness of a bandage layer is determined by its inherent material properties and the thickness, geometry, and compression used in its application. Stiffness is a measure of resistance to bending. The effects of material properties and thickness on resistance to bending are relatively intuitive: the less pliable and thicker the material, the stiffer the layer. Geometry is also important, especially for splinted bandages. Most layers are applied circumferentially, providing them with ringed cross-sectional geometry, which is extremely resistant to bending forces (Fig. 4-2, *A*). The splint layer, however, can be fashioned in a variety of ways. Most simply, fiberglass or plaster tape can be layered evenly to produce a rectangular cross-sectional shape, which weakly resists bending forces (Fig. 4-2, *B*). Alternately, the material can be molded with a spine or arch so that the cross-sectional geometry approximates a partial ring and provides higher resistance to bending forces (Fig. 4-2, *C* and *D*).

Compression is also an important determinant of stiffness, especially for layers constructed of low-density materials such as roll cotton. The large amount of air in cotton allows free movement between the fibers, making it a very pliable material in a noncompressed state. However, when placed under compression, air is forced out, the cotton fibers are more tightly packed, and the entire layer is much more resistant to bending. In this

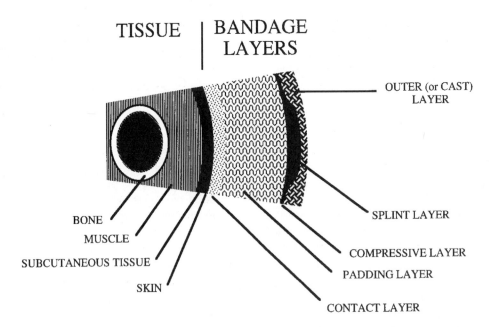

Fig. 4-1 Important bandage and tissue layers to consider when applying an external support device to a limb.

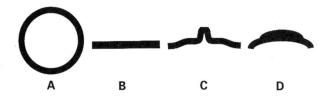

Fig. 4-2 Cross-sectional geometry of the bandage layers. **A,** Ring is typical of most bandage layers because of their circumferential application. **B,** Thin rectangle is typical of taped splintage that is layered. **C,** Splintage molded with a spine. **D,** Splintage molded with an arch.

compressed state, although the chemical nature of the material is unaltered, the mechanical properties are changed dramatically.

The stiffest layer is the primary determinant of the entire bandage's stiffness. When applied correctly, the padding layer, splint layer, and cast layer are the stiffest layers of the padded bandage, splinted bandage, and cast, respectively.

Intimacy of Stiffest Layer to the Limb Bones

To be effective, the stiffest layer of the bandage must be intimately coupled with the bones proximal and distal to the injury. Proximity and compression are the most important determinants of this coupling. Proximity is determined by properties of both the bandage and the limb. The degree of compression is determined by the tension applied to the compressive layer.

With regard to a bandage's construction, it is important to ensure that the stiffest layer is not excessively distant from the limb. This concept of proximity is easily applied to splinted bandages and casts. An excessively thick contact or padding layer distances the splint or cast layer from the limb, resulting in poor stability (Fig. 4-3). However, the relationship between proximity and bandage stability is more difficult with padded bandages. Although thicker padding distances the outer and compressive layers from the limb, these layers are not the stiffest layers in the bandage. The padding layer itself provides the most support in a padded bandage. Therefore, the concept of proximity suggests that increasing padding layer thickness should have no effect on bandage stability, since the padding layer usually contacts the limb directly, and proximity between the layer and the limb does not change. In reality, the thickness of the padding layer has a dramatic effect on the stability provided by a padded bandage. The thicker the padding layer, the less effectively applied compression can compact the material located most axially, or closest to the limb. Therefore, bandages with excessively thick padding layers provide less stability because the compacted and stiff outer sublayer of the padding is distanced from the limb by a less compacted and more pliable inner sublayer (Fig. 4-4).

Properties of the limb also greatly affect these concepts of bandage-to-bone coupling. Coupling is enhanced if the distance between the bandage and the affected bones is minimized. All interposed tissue, including skin, subcutaneous fat, and muscle, naturally distances the

TISSUE | BANDAGE LAYERS

A

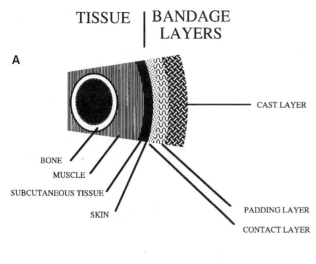

CAST LAYER

BONE
MUSCLE
SUBCUTANEOUS TISSUE
SKIN

PADDING LAYER
CONTACT LAYER

B

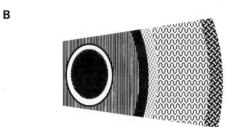

Fig. 4-3 Cross section of a cast applied to a limb. **A,** Good stability provided by a cast applied with a thin padding layer, allowing close proximity between the cast layer and limb (traditional cast). **B,** Poorer stability provided by a cast applied with a thick padding layer, distancing the cast layer from the limb (soft padded cast).

TISSUE | BANDAGE LAYERS

BONE
MUSCLE
SUBCUTANEOUS TISSUE
SKIN

PADDING LAYER
CONTACT LAYER
COMPRESSIVE LAYER
OUTER LAYER

Fig. 4-4 Cross section of an excessively thick padded bandage. Only the outer sublayer of padding, closest to the compressive layer, has been compacted adequately. The axially located sublayer is less compacted, contributing to instability.

bandage from the bone and decreases stability. The thicker the interposed tissue, the greater is the distance and the poorer the stability. These concepts must be remembered, especially in extremely obese or edematous limbs, where the subcutaneous tissues are excessively thick. Most importantly, however, these concepts affect the stability achieved when bandaging the proximal limbs. The bones distal to the elbow and stifle are easily palpated because of the absence of large muscle masses in these regions. Alternately, the humerus and femur are poorly palpated because they are encased, circumferentially, in thick musculature. Stability is enhanced with bandages of the distal limbs because less interposed muscle results in closer proximity between the bones and bandage. Conversely, when attempting to stabilize the brachium or thigh, surrounding large muscles limit proximity and interfere with bandage-bone coupling.

Compression, afforded by the compressive layer, is an important determinant of stability. The higher the compression, the more intimate the coupling is between the stiffest layer and the affected bones. Specifically, stability is enhanced by compacting the padding layer, approximating the stiffest layer to the affected bones, and increasing the friction between all bandage layers and the limb. Although a degree of compression is critical, too much can cause a tourniquet-like effect, leading to vascular stasis and limb swelling. Caution and experience are needed to ensure that adequate compression is applied without obstructing venous and lymphatic drainage.

Position of Unstable Area within the Bandage

The position of an unstable area within a bandage is analogous to the position of a fracture relative to a plate or pin. Stability is achieved only when there is adequate purchase of the stabilizing implant, proximal and distal to the injury. Usually, this means that stability is best when the implant is centered over the unstable area. Similarly, *an unstable area should be centered within a bandage so that purchase is obtained on the limb proximal and distal to the injury* (Fig. 4-5).

The issue of centering the unstable area relative to the bandage is addressed by the familiar guideline requiring immobilization of the joints proximal and distal to the injury. However, this concept of centering may also help explain why stability can be achieved without necessarily incorporating the adjacent joints, as long as adequate purchase is obtained.[14]

The inability to center a bandage adequately over injuries of the humerus or femur also limits the stability that bandages can provide to these bones. As a result, this concept of centering further justifies the longstanding

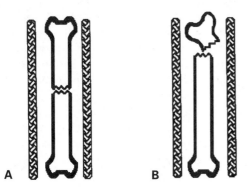

Fig. 4-5 Bandage applied to a fractured limb. **A,** Midshaft fracture is centered within a bandage, affording adequate purchase and good stability. Reduction is maintained. **B,** Proximal shaft fracture is located near the end of a bandage, affording *inadequate* purchase and poor stability. *Loss* of reduction occurs.

conviction that bandages usually provide inadequate stability for fractures involving bones of the proximal limbs.

Biomechanical Limitations of External Support

Even if the principles of bandaging are understood and applied correctly, the injured area may still be subjected to distracting forces. This is because an appropriately stiff bandage, with good bandage-to-limb intimacy and centered suitably over the injury, still does *not* provide rigid stability. Support bandages are eventually limited by the biomechanical characteristics of interposed soft tissue.[14] Additionally, because of their cylindrical construction, support bandages have difficulty neutralizing forces that are specifically transmitted along the longitudinal axis of the bone.

Bending forces, which are transmitted primarily perpendicular to the longitudinal axis of the bone, are usually neutralized quite well with appropriately applied splinted bandages and casts. However, torsional, compressive, and tensional forces, which are transmitted parallel to the longitudinal axis, are less completely neutralized. Torsional forces may be adequately neutralized in most cases, as long as an appropriate bandage with good stiffness, intimacy, and position is applied to a fracture with some inherent stability.[2] However, patients with fractures susceptible to compressive or tensional forces, including oblique and comminuted fractures or avulsion fractures, should be considered poor candidates for external support. Incomplete or minimally displaced transverse fractures of the radius/ulna or tibia/fibula, with partially intact periosteal sleeves, are naturally resistant to compressive, tensional, and rotational forces and

are the most appropriate fractures for primary therapy with external support.

INDICATIONS FOR EXTERNAL SUPPORT

Numerous indications exist for the use of support bandages. The most common involve accidental or iatrogenic trauma to an extremity, which in turn causes soft tissue injury, ligament injury with joint instability, and/or fracture. *In general, rigid stability is rarely achieved with external support, and moderate stability is only achieved for bones and joints **distal to the elbow** in the thoracic limb and **distal to the stifle** in the pelvic limb.* For this reason, external support is usually reserved to treat distal limb injuries that require only limited stability.

Anatomically, it is extremely difficult to provide even limited stability to injuries of the proximal limbs. Because of the normally angled carriage of the brachium and thigh and because of the broad skin folds located in the axillary and inguinal regions, it is usually very difficult to apply bandages well proximal of the elbow or knee. If the patient is ambulatory, a full-limb bandage often sags somewhat, causing the most proximal edge to move distally. The additional weight of the bandage along with sagging can produce a fulcrum, often at the level of the injury. This can reduce stability and potentially exacerbate the injury itself. For this reason and others, indications to use support bandages with proximal limb injures are very limited.

Fractures or luxations of the proximal limbs, including the elbow, stifle, shoulder, hip, humerus, femur, and pelvis, are extremely difficult to immobilize. Therefore, the goals of external support for injuries in these areas are necessarily limited to minimizing gross movement, preventing weight bearing, or maintaining the limb in a specific orientation. Closed fractures or luxations in quiet animals can often be managed without bandaging temporarily until definitive therapy can be administered. If the fracture is open or the animal is in excessive pain, support bandaging may be indicted. The spica splint is the best method of immobilizing the proximal aspect of the thoracic or pelvic limb because the torso is incorporated within the splint (see Fig. 4-24). However, the spica splint does *not* usually afford adequate stability to allow primary healing of ligament derangements or fractures of the humerus and femur. Slings (Velpeau, carpal flexion, pelvic, Ehmer) that prevent weight bearing but do not significantly immobilize the limb are helpful in some patients. All animals with proximal limb injuries should be confined to a cage with good footing and kept as quiet as possible.

One must remember that the potential benefits provided by external support are sometimes overshadowed by the potential complications. With injuries of the proximal limbs, a therapeutic decision to offer no support is often superior to a bandage that is unlikely to fulfill its purpose and liable to exacerbate the original injury.

Open Wounds and Surgical Incisions

Open wounds, primary or delayed wound closures, exiting drains, and surgical incisions are the most common indications for bandages. Padded and splinted bandages are appropriate devices for these injuries and perform various beneficial functions, including maintaining cleanliness, preventing desiccation, protecting from further injury and self-mutilation, supplying padding over bony protuberances as with decubital ulcers, limiting excessive motion, affording patient comfort, facilitating drainage by supplying absorbency, providing gentle debridement, retaining topical medication, and minimizing soft tissue swelling and edema. Padded and splinted bandages can be used with adherent, nonadherent semiocclusive, and nonadherent occlusive wound dressings. The specific indications for these dressings are addressed elsewhere.[12,15,16]

Restraint

In addition to protecting wounds, bandages are frequently used as restraint devices to prevent self-mutilation, abrasion, excessive scratching or licking, and catheter occlusion. Paretic animals with spinal cord or peripheral nerve disease often knuckle and abrade the dorsal aspect of their distal limbs during ambulation. Similarly, some animals with sensory deficits and anesthetized distal limbs, as with brachial plexus injury, may continually lick and chew at the affected paw, leading to self-mutilation and loss of limb. Padded bandages or "spoon"-splinted bandages are often used in these neurologically affected animals to prevent self-induced injury.

Many other indications exist for the use of bandages as restraint devices. Pelvic limb hobbles are effective restraints for animals that have a tendency to scratch injuriously with their pelvic limbs. Body splints are useful for pelvic or perineal wounds, such as perianal fistulas, to prevent licking or chewing. A Schroeder-Thomas splint can be very effective in patients with positionally occluded catheters by maintaining traction and limiting flexion of the elbow or stifle.

Connective Tissue Injury: Ligaments, Tendons, and Joint Capsule

Indications for splinted bandages or casts include acute, moderate to severe (second-degree to third-degree) ligament sprains of the carpus, tarsus, or phalangeal joints with associated swelling, pain, subluxation, luxation, or palpable instability. Whether handled conservatively or surgically, splinting or casting should be provided to protect the healing ligament and joint capsule for 3 to 5 weeks.[6] Ligament or joint capsule injuries resulting in laxity of the elbow or stifle are more difficult to stabilize with external support. A special type of splinted bandage, the spica splint, can be used for treating these injuries in some cases. Spica splints are difficult to apply effectively, especially for pelvic limbs in male dogs when the penis must be avoided. Additionally, they are usually quite restricting of the animal's ability to ambulate and are occasionally poorly tolerated.

Ligament or joint capsule injuries resulting in laxity of the shoulder or hip are special cases for which a sling or spica splint can often provide adequate stability for the most frequently seen problems. The specific indications are discussed later under postoperative repairs and under descriptions of specific bandages.

Musculotendinous strains occasionally benefit from external support. Acute, mild to moderate (first-degree to second-degree) strains are usually managed successfully with forced rest or confinement. Severe (third-degree) strains involving complete rupture of the muscle-tendon unit often require primary surgical repair.[6] External support and confinement are critical components of effective therapy and are discussed under postoperative repairs.

Fractures

Fractures distal to the elbow in the thoracic limb and distal to the stifle in the pelvic limb are potential indications for stabilization with support bandages. The surgeon must distinguish fractures amenable to stabilization with splinted bandages or casts from fractures that need more rigid stability, as with internal or external fixation. When assessing whether a fracture can be appropriately managed with external support, the surgeon should ask the following questions:

1. Can the fracture be adequately reduced in a closed fashion?
2. Does the fracture have enough inherent stability so that fragment reduction can be maintained with support bandaging alone?
3. Can the fragments be held in reduction long enough, with support bandaging, to permit healing?

If the answer to all three questions is unequivocally "yes," external support devices such as splinted bandages and casts are likely to be successful. If the answer to any of the three questions is "no," external support should not be attempted as the primary method of repair.

Can the fracture be adequately reduced in a closed fashion? First and most importantly, the fragments must be easily palpable. Usually, this is only possible distal to the elbow and stifle, where the surrounding soft tissues, especially muscle, are relatively scant. Profound soft tissue swelling also prevents adequate palpation of the fragments, even in the distal limbs. Second, the fracture should be fresh. With chronicity, as early as 5 days in a young animal, muscular contracture, fibrosis, and callus formation can make reduction extremely difficult, especially in a significantly displaced or overriding fracture.

Does the fracture have enough inherent stability so that fragment reduction can be maintained with support bandaging alone? Once reduced, the support bandage must be capable of maintaining reduction. For this to occur, the fracture must have some inherent stability, since support bandages do not provide rigid fixation. When assessing whether a fracture has inherent stability, four factors should be addressed.

1. *The fracture type should be simple or two piece.* Comminuted fractures are rarely stable and are usually inappropriate choices for support bandaging.
2. *The fracture should be transverse rather than oblique.* Since compressive forces are poorly neutralized with support bandages, the fracture configuration must be resistant to this distracting force. Transverse fractures resist displacement when placed under compression, unlike oblique fractures, which tend to override. Exceptions to this rule are torsionally induced long, spiral fractures with partially intact periosteal sleeves. Often, these fractures have some stability when placed in torsion opposite to that which caused the fracture.
3. *The fracture fragments should not be greatly displaced.* With minor displacement, often a portion of the periosteal sleeve remains intact, which in turn provides some stability when the fracture is subjected to bending forces opposite to those that caused the injury (Fig. 4-6, *A* to *C*). Even a two-piece transverse fracture has little inherent stability if significant displacement or overriding causes complete loss of an intact periosteal sleeve (Fig. 4-6, *D*).
4. *The fracture must be carefully but forcibly manipulated to detect for instability.* This is usually performed with the patient sedated or anesthetized. Although radiographs can provide clues, inherent stability is best demonstrated with careful palpation.

Can the fragments be held in reduction long enough, with support bandaging, to permit healing? If the fracture is reducible and if external support is

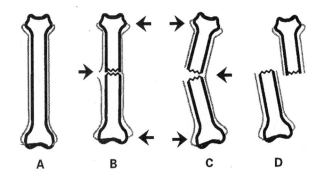

Fig. 4-6 The importance of a partially intact periosteal sleeve to fracture stability. **A,** Intact bone and periosteal sleeve. **B,** Fractured bone with an intact periosteum on one side only. Note how the periosteum provides stability and prevents *overreduction* when forces *opposite* to those that created the fracture are applied. **C,** Fractured bone with an intact periosteum on one side only. Note how reduction is lost, and the fracture "breaks open" when forces similar to those that created the fracture are applied. **D,** Complete loss of the periosteal sleeve leading to an unstable fracture with significant displacement.

capable of maintaining reduction, the splinted bandage or cast must still be maintained, reasonably undisturbed, until the fracture heals. External supports are difficult to maintain for more than 3 weeks without change. For this reason, quick bony union in about 3 to 5 weeks helps to ensure success. As a result, young animals that heal quickly are probably the best candidates for support bandaging as the sole method of repair. Additionally, open wounds often preclude the use of splinted bandages or casts as the primary modes of stabilization because of the need for frequent bandage changes. Windows can be cut into casts over open wounds to permit daily care. However, these windows structurally weaken the cast and must be replaced after wound treatment to prevent soft tissue swelling into the fenestration.

Considering all these restrictions, it becomes clear that only selected fracture types lend themselves to sole repair with support bandaging. Fractures typical of this category are partial, incomplete, or greenstick fractures of the radius/ulna or tibia/fibula. Minimally displaced radial physeal fractures and fractures of the radius without ulnar fracture are also good candidates, since partially intact periosteal sleeves usually provide some inherent stability. Homologous decision making holds for the tibia/fibula. Similarly, metacarpal/metatarsal fractures with intact bones spanning or "splinting" the fractured ones usually have significant inherent stability and are managed successfully with external support alone.

· · ·

The rules and examples just stated are intended to be general guidelines designed to achieve optimal success with support bandaging. Certainly, comminuted largely displaced chronic fractures in older animals have been successfully treated with external support alone. However, the previous guidelines, although conservative, provide optimal success in the management of fractures treated solely with closed reduction and external support.

Perioperative Protection for Connective Tissue and Fracture Repair

Preoperative immobilization of a fracture or luxation is an attractive indication for padded or splinted bandages. The potential benefits include minimizing continued soft tissue injury, limiting progressive swelling and edema, protecting associated cutaneous wounds, and diminishing the pain associated with instability. As already described, these goals are best achieved with injuries distal to the elbow and stifle.

Postoperative immobilization of a fracture or luxation is often an invaluable ingredient toward final success. Ideally, surgical repair of ligament, tendon, joint capsule, or bone should be secure enough to allow freedom of movement in the postoperative period. Freedom of movement is beneficial because it *prevents* complications associated with immobilization. Complications leading to loss in range of motion and poor limb use include muscular, tendinous, and periarticular fibrosis; cartilage degeneration; ligamentous laxity; and osteoporosis.[1] However, freedom of movement must be restricted with orthopedic repairs, which are tenuous because of the nature or complexity of the injury. In these cases, attempted limb use or minor accidental trauma (e.g., fall) may be sufficient to disrupt the primary repair. External support can be an invaluable aid toward protecting the repair until healing provides adequate strength to withstand minor trauma or the normal forces of limb use.

Specific indications for protection of orthopedic repairs distal to the elbow and stifle

Fractures. Fractures involving small fragments are frequently difficult to reduce and stabilize. Typically these fractures are highly comminuted or involve small bones and joints of the distal limb, such as the malleolus, carpus, tarsus, metacarpus/metatarsus, and phalanges. Nonreducible small fragments often prevent anatomical reconstruction and lead to a weaker bone implant construct. Reducible small fragments often require small implants, which may have inadequate strength or purchase compared with the forces applied during ambulation. When anatomical reduction is impossible and implant purchase or strength is questionable, external support can be used adjunctively to help assure a successful outcome.

Arthrodesis. Similar concerns of implant purchase and strength exist with arthrodeses of the distal limb. Partial arthodesis or panarthrodesis of the carpal, tarsal, or phalangeal joints often requires the use of small implants, with limited purchase in biomechanically disadvantaged positions.[11] In these patients, it is often wise to protect the surgical repair until limited primary healing occurs.

Ligament, tendon, and joint capsule injury. For repairs of joint capsule, ligament, or tendon, the factors limiting a repair's durability include suture material strength, suture pattern, and the substance of the soft tissues themselves. Ligaments and tendons, with parallel collagen bundles, heal slowly and hold suture poorly.[9,13] Additionally, the small size of the structures demand use of fine, relatively weak suture material, even in large-breed animals subjecting their limbs to tremendous forces. Common connective tissue injuries in which these concerns about repair are relevant include traumatically ruptured or sheared carpal/tarsal/phalangeal collateral ligaments, ruptured common calcaneal tendons, and lacerated flexor tendons. Because of the prolonged healing and inherent weakness of repair, these connective tissue injuries often require external support despite primary surgical reconstruction.

Specific indications for protection of orthopedic repairs of the elbow, stifle, brachium, and thigh.

Difficulties associated with bandaging the brachium and thigh severely limit the stability that can be provided to these areas. As a result, goals related to bandaging proximal limb injuries must be less ambitious than those related to the distal limb. Instead of providing significant stability, bandages of the proximal limb are usually designed to prevent weight bearing or constrain the limb to a particular orientation.

Fractures. Indications for postoperative support of the proximal extremities are naturally similar to those of the distal limbs. Highly comminuted fractures of the humerus, femur, scapula, or pelvis and fractures involving small fragments are difficult to reduce and stabilize. Common examples of proximal limb fractures typically involving small pieces include humeral or femoral condylar fractures, supraglenoid tubercular avulsions, and scapular neck fractures. As stated previously, issues concerning anatomical reduction, implant purchase, and implant strength must be considered when determining whether external support is indicated.

Arthrodesis. Arthrodeses of the shoulder, elbow, and stifle are difficult to perform and carry the same concerns as arthrodeses in the distal joints. The use of small implants with limited purchase in biomechanically disadvantaged positions indicates postoperative protection with external support.

Ligament, tendon, and joint capsule injury. As mentioned earlier, the determinants of stability after surgical repair of ligament, tendon, or joint capsule injury include the strength and character of the connective tissue, the strength of the suture material, and the suture pattern. Examples of connective tissue repairs that may require protective external support include collateral ligament rupture or shear injury of the elbow and stifle, medial capsulotomy when approaching the medial coronoid, rupture of the straight patellar tendon, and traumatic luxation of the elbow, stifle, shoulder, or hip.

Shoulder luxation. The appropriate bandage for a shoulder luxation depends on whether the humeral head luxates medially or laterally. With medial instability, the external support should force the humeral head laterally to protect the medially located injury or repair. The Velpeau sling, which orients the distal humerus medially and the humeral head laterally, is the appropriate bandage for medial shoulder luxation. With lateral instability, the humeral head should be forced medially or kept in a neutral position; this is best accomplished with a spica splint (see specific bandages for more detailed discussions).

Hip luxation. Open or closed reductions of the hip often require bandaging to maintain the femoral head within the acetabulum. Craniodorsal luxations of the hip are clinically the most common. In these, internal rotation and abduction of the hip are the most important joint orientations to maintain. The modified Ehmer sling is a tried and tested bandage that maintains these orientations effectively when applied correctly. Caudoventral luxation, with tearing of the ventral joint capsule, is the next most frequently directed luxation. Once the hip is reduced, abduction can force the femoral head ventrally, causing reluxation. This coxofemoral abduction can be effectively prevented with tarsal or stifle hobbles (see specific bandages for more detailed discussions).

Stifle surgery. Many surgeons typically apply padded bandages postoperatively in patients with cruciate repair or patellar luxation. The goal behind this practice is to provide support and limit swelling in the early postoperative period. However, swelling is usually minimal with these surgeries, and the support provided is limited because of the difficulty of achieving purchase on the distal femur. Therefore, I do not routinely apply postoperative bandages for these patients.

Summary

The type of external support used postoperatively depends on the degree of stability required. Splinted bandages or casts are most appropriate for tenuously repaired fractures, arthrodeses, or ligament/tendon injuries of the distal limb requiring significant added support. The spica splint is for similar indications in the proximal limb. If stability of the repair is adequate, short of withstanding the forces of weight bearing, a less-restrictive sling might be more appropriate, more comfortable, and less expensive.

It is important to remember that traditional padded bandages, splinted bandages, or casts are usually inappropriate support devices for proximal limb injuries. Only the spica splint and the various thoracic and pelvic limb slings should be reserved as external supports for limb injuries proximal to and including the elbow and stifle.

BANDAGE COMPLICATIONS

Unfortunately, complications associated with bandaging are extremely common. Measures to prevent bandage-related complications must address the most frequent etiologies: poor bandage application, poor bandage care, and joint immobilization. Efforts to minimize the potentially devastating effects of bandage complications require familiarity with their most common signs so that careful monitoring can then lead to early, aggressive treatment.

The most common complications are discussed next and include joint stiffness or laxity, limb swelling, cutaneous erosions and ulcers, and bandage loosening.

Joint Stiffness

Joint stiffness is a common complication associated with bandaging and can be expected in any joint bandaged for more than a couple of days. The degree of joint stiffness is determined by the degree of soft tissue injury and the duration of immobilization. The more severe the injury and longer the immobilization, the more extensive and restrictive are the adhesions which limit range of motion.

Varying degrees of disability are caused by bandages, which cause joints to be frozen in partial to full extension. Bandages contribute to this complication in two ways. First, they limit the normal range of motion for all incorporated joints. This immobilization, in combination with soft tissue injury, leads to varying degrees of periarticular fibrosis. Fibrosis can adhere joint capsule, muscle, tendon, and bone, which limits the normal sliding between these structures and causes reduced range of motion. Second, bandages tend to straighten limbs because the compressive layer tends to extend all incorporated joints. Acting together, these two processes can cause a joint to be stiffened in extension long after the bandage is removed. A severe form of this problem is termed *fracture disease* which, besides joint stiffness, includes periarticular and musculotendinous fibrosis, cartilaginous degeneration, muscular atrophy, and osteoporosis.[1]

The severity of the disability is also related to the nature of the joint involved. The degree of normal joint motion during ambulation is a very important factor related to disability because a reduced range of motion in some joints is better tolerated than in others. For example, the carpus and tarsus, even if ankylosed in extension, cause little to no gait disturbance, since compensation can occur more proximally in the limb. The stifle, however, if fixed in extension, may cause severe gait abnormalities, including complete disuse of the limb.

One of the most disabling forms of fracture disease is called *quadriceps contracture*. This syndrome is most often seen in young growing dogs with severe orthopedic injury to the femur and thigh.[4] The stifle and tarsus become fixed in full extension, and the animal often has little to no use of the limb. At this stage, the prognosis for returning normal function to the affected limb is guarded to poor. Rigid fracture fixation and early ambulation are the most effective methods for prevention. For this reason and others, femoral fractures are rarely treated with prolonged external coaptation.

Joint Laxity

Prolonged immobilization can contribute to joint laxity.[17] Clinically, this complication is most frequently seen in the carpus in young growing dogs, which occasionally demonstrate mild to severe carpal hyperextension after protracted immobilization. Treatment includes controlled exercise on soft surfaces providing sure footing, such as grass. The prognosis is usually good, with patients showing improvement in 2 to 6 weeks. It is important to note that prolonged immobilization is contraindicated for treatment of *carpal laxity syndrome* in young large-breed dogs because of the likelihood of exacerbating the associated carpal hyperextension.

Limb Swelling

Limb swelling is most often caused by applying a bandage too tightly. However, a bandage, initially applied appropriately, can become too tight when a limb later swells from ensuing infection or previous surgical trauma. When too tight, the bandage acts as a tourniquet, which then variably compresses and occludes the vascular elements in the limb. With increasing compression, the first to be occluded are the lymphatics and veins. Venous and lymphatic congestion leads to increased interstitial fluid accumulation and a progressively worsening interstitial edema distal to the obstruction. Interstitial edema increases the diffusion distance for oxygen and contributes to tissue ischemia. When compressive pressures equal or exceed systolic arterial pressure, the arterial blood supply can be slowed or stopped. When this occurs, irreversible tissue ischemia, resulting in necrosis, can occur within 2 to 3 hours.

Cutaneous Erosions and Ulcers

Cutaneous injury is an extremely common complication associated with bandages, especially casts and slings, which normally provide little to no padding between the cast or adhesive outer layers and the skin. Underlying skin can be injured with exposure to excessive pressure, frequent abrasion, or constant wetness. Excessive pressure, caused by bandages that are placed too tightly, can occlude dermal veins and arterioles, resulting in dermal ischemia and necrosis. Motion of the limb within and around the bandage can cause physical abrasion, especially over bony protuberances and at the bandage's proximal and distal ends. Constant wetness caused by immersion or repeated moistening of the bandage can weaken the skin's natural defense mechanisms.[5] Overgrowth of pathogenic bacteria can cause pyoderma and maceration.

Bony protuberances typically involved with cutaneous injury include the accessory carpal bone, lateral epicondyle of the elbow, olecranon, patella, tibial malleolus, and calcaneus. In these areas, overlying skin is especially susceptible to injury because the underlying bone is poorly cushioned with subcutaneous tissue. Special attention to bony protuberances when bandaging is often appropriate, especially when applying casts that have minimal padding.

Similarly, skin underlying the proximal and distal edges of a bandage is often subjected to abrasion, especially the axillary and inguinal skin folds and dorsal surface of the toes. Trauma to the skin is exacerbated if a bandage is constructed with its proximal or distal edges ending at the level of a joint. Periarticular skin is particularly vulnerable to abrasion by the bandage's edge because of joint motion during ambulation. Careful construction and additional padding at the most proximal and distal aspects of a bandage can prevent this injury.

Bandage-associated dermal injury can be extremely serious. Once the skin has been breached with pathogenic bacteria, infection can dissect along muscular, tendinous, and fascial planes. A necrotizing cellulitis or fasciitis can propagate through considerable tissue underneath a bandage before overt signs of infection are noticed. Without aggressive early therapy, in the form of surgical debridement and parenteral antibiotics, these invasive infections can lead to limb loss.

Bandage Loosening

Even if applied appropriately, a bandage can loosen significantly with time. Most often, limb swelling at the time of bandage application subsides, leaving a bandage that is in effect, too large. Additionally, the materials used to construct the bandage can stretch, especially in animals that are insufficiently exercise restricted.

Bandage looseness causes instability of the injured area, leading to delayed or incomplete healing and continued soft tissue injury. Looseness also permits increased motion of the limb within the bandage, which contributes to cutaneous abrasion, as described previously.

Prevention of Complications

Effective prevention of the common bandage complications requires clinical experience, sound judgment, good bandaging skills, and meticulous bandage care. Joint stiffness is often an unavoidable complication with prolonged bandaging. However, clinicians can best prevent disabling joint stiffness and fracture disease by reserving the use of support bandages for appropriate injuries. For example, bandaging techniques should rarely be used as the primary mode of stabilization for fractures of the proximal limb. *When used for humeral or femoral fractures, bandages alone are likely to exacerbate the instability, contribute to soft tissue injury, and maintain the elbow or stifle in near-full extension.* For the hind limb, quadriceps contracture, a disabling form of fracture disease, may become a likely sequela regardless of the fracture's fate.

Appropriate bandaging skills can also be used to limit the disabling effects of joint stiffness. As mentioned, a bandage tends to straighten the incorporated limb. However, with the limb held in partial flexion, a cast can be applied or splintage material molded to maintain the limb in a functional position. As a result, when the cast or bandage is removed, although range of motion is decreased, compensation and disability are minimized. Finally, since joint stiffness is related to the duration of immobilization, reductions in range of motion can be minimized by maintaining the bandage only as long as necessary.

Carpal hyperextension can be minimized with careful positioning of the carpus when applying a cast or molding a splint. Maintaining 10-15 degrees of flexion and 10-15 degrees of medial deviation (varus) at the carpus can lessen this manifestation of joint laxity frequently seen after forelimb bandage removal in young, large breed dogs.

Limb swelling is difficult to prevent in some cases, even for skilled bandagers. Clinical experience is invaluable in determining the degree of tension when applying the bandage's compressive layer so that adequate stability is obtained without contributing to vascular occlusion. Helpful guidelines to prevent swelling include using an appropriately thick padding layer and applying uniform tension to the compressive layer. Uneven compression along the limb can cause vascular occlusion,

diminishing venous/lymphatic drainage and contributing to swelling.

Prevention of cutaneous injury requires severe exercise restriction and protective measures to keep the bandage clean and dry. These measures limit motion-related abrasion and help maintain the health of underlying skin. Extra padding or a thicker contact layer can help, particularly around bony protuberances and at the proximal and distal edges of the bandage. This is especially true with casts, which have little padding themselves and are often used for extended periods without removal.

Bandage loosening is an unavoidable problem in limbs that are very swollen at the time of bandage application. These animals should be reevaluated every few days until the swelling subsides and the bandage can be replaced. Exercise restriction helps limit the loosening that occurs via stretching of the bandage materials themselves.

BANDAGE CARE

Meticulous bandage care, although difficult, is essential to achieve successful results with immobilization. The main obstacles are the patients themselves and the owners, who provide most of the nursing care and must be educated and sensitized to the early signs of problems. Important components of bandage care include enforcing exercise restriction, maintaining the support device clean and dry, and monitoring carefully for signs of limb swelling or infection. A sensible plan for reevaluation and bandage replacement must also be scheduled.

Restricting Exercise

One of the most important but most-difficult-to-enforce elements of bandage care is strict patient rest. Exercise restriction improves the chances of success because it preserves the bandage's integrity, helps ensure adequate stability, and minimizes the incidence of motion-related cutaneous sores. As mentioned, the materials of most external supports, although durable, are not designed to withstand the wear and tear of constant exercise. Enforced rest prolongs the effective life of any bandage. Second, even a well-applied splinted bandage or cast does not provide rigid stability. Enforced rest minimizes the instability created by excessive movement or weight bearing. Third, exercise can exacerbate epidermal abrasion from limb motion within or around the bandage. Cutaneous trauma is most often seen around joints, overlying bony protuberances, and underlying the proximal and distal edges of the bandage.

The degree of exercise restriction depends on the dog, the bandage, and the underlying problem. In most cases the animal should be restricted to a cage, kennel, or small room, effectively isolated from other animals and small children. A rough or textured surface, such as a rug, should be provided for sure footing. Running, jumping, and playing are prohibited, and exercise outside must be limited to leashed walks only. Extremely hyperactive patients may need tranquilization for the first few weeks, until they adapt to the new restricted exercise regime.

Maintaining the Bandage Clean and Dry

Unprotected bandages often become excessively soiled or wetted and require changing. Cotton, an extremely absorbent material, is usually the major component of the contact and padding layers in most bandages. Fecal matter, urine, or water can easily be absorbed into these layers and remain in constant contact with the underlying skin or open wounds. If wetness or excrement is allowed prolonged contact with skin, breakdown of the normal defense mechanisms may allow entry of pathogenic bacteria, leading to pyoderma and maceration.[17] Wet bandages also allow environmental bacteria, traveling with the moisture, access to underlying wounds. Consequently, a sterile contact layer should be considered contaminated if the overlying bandage becomes wet. Wetness is usually caused by the bandage's contact with surface water or urine. However, an occlusive covering, such as a plastic bag, prevents the escape of moisture normally evaporating from the skin. Humidity can increase, resulting in significant moisture deposition within the bandage.

Bandages should have an absorbent nonocclusive or "breathable" protective covering at all times. Tube stockinette or a cotton sock can be used for this purpose. When the animal is taken outside, a plastic bag and second stocking are placed over the bandage. The second stocking protects the thin underlying bag from tearing, while the bag keeps moisture from contacting the bandage. Alternately, thick tear-resistant plastic, such as from an intravenous fluid bag, can be placed over the bandage as a waterproof covering (Fig. 4-7).[7] On returning inside, the outer stocking and bag or heavy plastic are removed. Elevating the water and food bowls may help keep bandages clean and dry, especially for dogs that tend to slobber, overturn, or step into their food. Once a bandage becomes wet, a clinician must decide whether to replace it. Most bandages or casts slightly or superficially damp will dry without a problem; however, once soaking wet, a bandage or cast must be changed.

Monitoring for Swelling or Infection

Clients or caretakers must be sensitized to the signs of swelling or infection. With most support bandages, digits three and four are left protruding from the most distal aspect of the bandage. Caretakers should be instructed

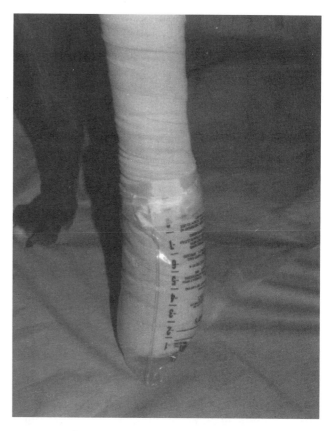

Fig. 4-7   Tear-resistant plastic boot fashioned out of a used intravenous infusion bag provides protection from dirt and moisture on walks outside.

to visualize and palpate these digits at least twice per day. The claws should remain close to one another, and the interdigital areas should palpate warm and dry. Signs that a bandage is too tight include swollen digits with claws that have spread from one another, interdigital areas moistened from the weeping of serum, cyanotic nail beds, and cool interdigital temperatures.

Caretakers must also anticipate the formation or worsening of preexisting wounds underneath a bandage. Signs of an uncontrolled infection under the bandage include discoloration of the outer layer from seepage of underlying exudate and malodor detected from the distal or proximal aspects of the support. Complaints of recent licking or chewing at the bandage in an animal previously tolerant of the restraint may indicate a complication as well. Any sign of discomfort, excessive tightness, or uncontrolled infection demands immediate investigation and usually bandage removal.

Reevaluating and Replacing the Bandage

Scheduled reevaluations for bandage examination and replacement are important components of bandage care. The frequency of reevaluation depends on numerous factors and must be tailored to the individual patient and client. Important factors include the presence of open wounds, stability required to heal the injury, patient age, limb swelling at time of bandage application, and owner compliance. All bandages should be checked daily by the caretakers and at least every 2 weeks by a veterinarian.

Presence of open wounds. Open wounds, before the formation of a granulation bed, are usually quite exudative. Adherent dressings and daily bandage changes are indicated to provide gentle debridement and encourage drainage. Once a healthy granulation bed covers the wound, the exudation usually subsides dramatically. At this time, a nonadherent dressing and twice-weekly bandage changes are continued until the bed completely contracts and epithelializes.

Stability required to heal the injury. The stability required by the injury strongly influences the frequency of bandage replacement. An unstable injury should be disturbed as infrequently as possible. Ideally, a fracture should not be destabilized by bandage removal until healing is complete. Premature destabilization with motion at the fracture site can lead to loss of reduction. Frequent destabilization can also delay revascularization of the fragments, slow the healing callus, and contribute to delayed union or nonunion. Similarly, repeated destabilization of an area with ligamentous instability can reinjure and stretch the healing scar tissue, leading to permanent laxity. For this reason, unstable fractures and ligament injuries should not have bandages removed more frequently than every 2 weeks, unless signs of complication are observed.

Patient age. Puppies under 9 months of age are prone to bandage-related complications. Young animals in a period of rapid development may outgrow a bandage quickly, especially large-breed dogs that have tremendous potential for growth. Also, the rambunctious nature of puppies predisposes them to motion-related complications, such as bandage wear and cutaneous injury. Long-term tranquilization may be indicated in severely hyperactive patients until they adapt to the forced exercise restriction. Because of their rapid growth and frenetic nature, puppies should be reevaluated for bandage replacement every 1 to 2 weeks.

Limb swelling at time of bandage application. Bandages placed on excessively swollen limbs are predisposed to loosening as the swelling abates within the first few days after application. As discussed, loose bandages provide less support and are more likely to create cutaneous abrasions. Therefore, bandages placed on swollen limbs should be reevaluated every 2 to 3 days to ensure that adequate compression and stability are maintained.

Owner compliance. The veterinarian's confidence in the owner's ability to detect bandage-related complications should influence the reevaluation schedule. Fastidious owners who maintain strict exercise restriction and provide meticulous care generally can follow a more liberal schedule with infrequent reevaluations. Alternately, when dealing with less trustworthy owners, a more regimented reevaluation schedule should require frequent monitoring by the veterinarian.

BANDAGE REMOVAL

The incidence of bandage complications increases the longer a bandage is maintained. Therefore, bandages should be removed as soon as the indications for their original application are resolved.

Bandages covering open wounds, primary wound closures, or incisions are usually removed after the wound bed epithelializes or the incision heals. Prolonged bandaging for these problems is only indicated when self-mutilation is anticipated or wounds are located over bony protuberances, as with healed decubitus ulcers.

Ligament injuries and tenuously repaired fractures should generally be protected with support bandages at least 3 to 4 weeks. Stability and bony union should be assessed with careful palpation and radiography. If healing has progressed adequately and the bandages are permanently removed, exercise restriction should still be enforced an additional 2 to 4 weeks.

Fractures repaired solely with external coaptation generally remain bandaged for 4 to 8 weeks. Intrinsically stable fractures in younger patients caused by minor trauma require shorter bandaging times than extremely unstable fractures in older patients that have suffered severe trauma. Bandage changes should be performed as infrequently as possible to prevent loss of reduction and minimize reinjury to the healing callus. As mentioned, adequate healing is assessed by palpation and radiography. Exercise restriction should be continued for 2 to 4 weeks after bandage removal.

Bandage removal is often followed by reapplication with a less rigid support. For example, casts can be replaced with splinted bandages, which then can be replaced with padded bandages. This stepwise reduction in bandage rigidity permits a controlled reduction in stability and affords continued protection of the limb while gradually permitting greater forces to be transmitted through the injured site. With this technique, more rapid healing and greater mobility can be achieved while minimizing the chances of catastrophic reinjury.

BANDAGE APPLICATION
Contact Layer

The contact layer includes components of the bandage that are always in direct contact with the skin. These include wound dressings, limb stocking,* orthopedic felt,[†] and adhesive tape[‡] "stirrups." The indications for adherent, nonadherent, semiocclusive, or occlusive wound dressings are beyond the scope of this chapter and are described elsewhere.[12,15]

Limb stocking is thin, tubed, socklike material often placed underneath casts or splinted bandages. Appropriately wide stocking material, usually 1 to 3 inches, is cut 50% longer than the length of the limb. The material is stretched proximally and distally by two assistants (see Fig. 4-25, A) so that it conforms closely to the contours of the limb without wrinkling. Limb stocking provides some protection to underlying skin without significantly distancing the cast or splint layer from the limb.

Orthopedic felt is thick synthetic feltlike material into which holes are usually cut to make doughnut-shaped pads (see Fig. 4-25, B). The material is positioned to encircle bony prominences without covering them. This helps protect these susceptible areas from injury without significantly diminishing the intimacy between the bandage and limb.

Stirrups are adhesive strips of tape, usually 1/2 to 1 inch wide, that are used to help prevent distal slippage of the bandage. The strips are applied laterally and medially or cranially and caudally to the distal aspect of the limb, avoiding open wounds and the dewclaws (see Fig. 4-18). They should be applied with firm pressure over dry hair to ensure adequate adhesion. These strips should extend distally past the claws for at least 10 cm and are adhered to each other or to a tongue depressor. Once the padding and compressive layers are applied, the stirrups are separated from each other distally. They are wrapped proximally under tension, twisted 180 degrees, and adhered to the underlying compressive layer. These ends can be further affixed with one or two circumferential strips of adhesive tape, if desired.

Padding Layer

The padding layer, composed of cotton cast padding[§] or roll cotton, protects the limb from the overlying layers and provides absorbency for exudative injuries. The limb is maintained in a functional position, and the padding layer is wrapped evenly, distally to proximally as snugly as possible; generally, the padding material tears before it can be applied too tightly. The material is applied circumferentially with 50 to 75% overlap wrapping cranially to caudally around the medial aspect of the limb and caudally to cranially around the lateral aspect, as shown in Fig. 4-19, A. Spiraling the material in this direc-

tion helps minimize external rotation (supination), a tendency most frequently seen when bandaging the forelimb. At the anticipated level of the bandage's proximal edge, the material is torn, and the next layer is again started from the distal aspect. This is repeated until the desired thickness of padding is achieved. The diameter of the cylindrical bandage should remain uniform. Distally, only the central two digits should be left protruding (see Fig. 4-20), however, the entire paw can be incorporated when wounds involve the digits or pads. Proximally, the bandage edge is positioned from the midshaft to proximal one-third of the radius/tibia (half limb) or midshaft to proximal one-third of the humerus/femur (full limb), *not* at the level of a joint. Having a bandage edge at the level of a joint can predispose the underlying skin to abrasion (see Bandage Complications). The shoulder and hip can be abducted and extended to stretch the axillary and inguinal skin folds, providing easier application proximally for full-limb bandages. Often, the most proximal and distal aspects of the bandage have the thinnest layers of padding; extra layers should be added to protect these locations, which are predisposed to injury (see Figs. 4-19, C, and 4-25, D).

The final thickness of padding depends on the nature and purpose of the bandage. Casts usually have a very thin padding layer to minimize the distance between the cast layer and limb (see Fig. 4-3). Usually, only one or two layers of padding are used, with a thickness no greater than 0.5 cm. Padded bandages (modified Robert Jones bandage) and splinted bandages generally have 1.5 to 2 cm of cotton padding. Without splintage, this thickness of cotton provides minimal stability, even after compaction with the compressive layer. The classical Robert Jones bandage is much thicker, with 4 to 8 cm of cotton padding. The added padding provides increased stability and absorbency. It is important to remember that padding layers that become too thick resist compaction axially and diminish the stability provided (see Fig. 4-4 and Biomechanics).

Compressive Layer

The compressive layer is composed of conforming roll gauze,* which is applied with circumferential tension to compact the underlying padding. With splinted bandages, the compressive layer is also used to bind the splint firmly to the limb. As with the padding, this layer is applied distally to proximally with about 50% overlap and in a direction which minimizes external rotation (supination) of the distal limb. The limb should be cupped with one hand and the material applied snugly with the other (see Fig. 4-19, D). The material is applied until the desired compression is achieved and all irregularities and constricting bands

*Tube Stockinette, Balfour Health Care, Rockwood, Tenn.
[†]Orthopedic Felt, Smith & Nephew Richards, Inc., Memphis.
[‡]Durapore, 3M Medical-Surgical Division, St. Paul, Minn.
[§]Specialist Cast Padding, Johnson & Johnson, New Brunswick, NJ; Webrill II, The Kendall Co., Boston.

*Conform, The Kendall Co., Mansfield, Mass; Flexicon, CoNco Medical Co., Bridgeport, Conn.

are eliminated from the surface. Proximally, this layer should be advanced only to within 1.5 to 2 cm of the padding layer's edge to ensure that the skin is never contacted directly by this restrictive nonelastic material.

The degree of tension applied to the compressive layer depends on the thickness of the padding, nature of the injury, and purpose of the bandage. If the bandage is designed to provide stability or limit swelling, the compressive layer is applied more firmly than for a bandage used only as a wound covering. In a classical Robert Jones bandage, with 4 to 8 cm of padding, the compressive layer is usually applied as tightly as possible to provide adequate support. However, this degree of tension would cause limb swelling in most padded and splinted bandages, with only 1.5 to 2 cm of padding. In these bandages the tension needed to provide stability without causing venous/lymphatic obstruction and limb swelling is difficult to define. Subjectively, the compressive layer, once applied, should deform only temporarily when indented firmly with a finger. If the layer is nondepressible or if the depression remains after indentation, the material may be too tight or too loose, respectively. If swelling occurs, early detection is the most important determinant for preventing injury.

Splint Layer

Splints are constructed of moldable or nonmoldable material and provide the predominant stability for splinted bandages. Moldable splints include plaster-,* fiberglass-,† and resin-impregnated‡ tapes; aluminum rod;§ and thermally sensitive plastic.ǁ Nonmoldable or prefabricated splints include metal or plastic "spoon" splints.¶ The splint layer is incorporated after the compressive layer is applied. Moldable splintage is usually contoured on the lateral aspect of the limb, whereas spoon splints are usually applied caudally. Both types of splintage are bound to the bandage with additional layers of conforming gauze. The additional gauze is applied with similar tension and direction to that used for the underlying compressive layer. Splint material should extend from the distal aspect of the bandage to a point proximally, 1.5 to 2 cm short of the bandage's edge.

Aluminum rod (⅛, ³⁄₁₆, or ⅜ inch) should be contoured to the lateral aspect of the padded bandage so that it maintains the limb in a functional position (see Fig. 4-22

and 4-32.) The rod should form a continuous loop contacting the proximal, distal, craniolateral, and caudolateral aspects of the bandage. The ends of the rod are overlapped and taped together with nonelastic adhesive tape. This taped junction is the weakest part of the loop and should not be positioned at the level of a joint or unstable injury.

Plaster-, fiberglass-, and resin-impregnated tapes are versatile materials that can be layered and molded to produce custom splints. At least three layers of tape should be used to obtain desired stiffness. The material can also be molded with a spine or arch to provide additional resistance to bending (see Fig. 4-2). These impregnated tapes are also used to construct casts. Once removed, one or both halves of a cast can be reused as a custom splint or bivalved cast (see Bandage Removal and Miscellaneous Casts).

Thermally sensitive plastic is a versatile material gaining popularity with veterinarians that can be used effectively for custom splints. An appropriately sized piece is cut from a plastic sheet and heated with warm water or hot air. At the appropriate temperature, the material is easily molded and becomes tacky, so partially overlapping flaps can be adhered together (Fig. 4-8). Binding the plastic to the bandage while still in a moldable state ensures that the material is contoured perfectly to the limb (Fig. 4-9, *A*). To provide optimal stability, this material should be fashioned so that it encircles the limb more than 180 degrees (Fig. 4-9, *B*).

Spoon splints are prefabricated in many different sizes out of plastic or aluminum (Fig. 4-10). These splints are used to provide stability and protect injuries *distal to the elbow* in the forelimb and *distal to the tarsus* in the hind limb. Unlike the other splint materials, they are placed on the caudal aspect of the bandage, extend distal to the

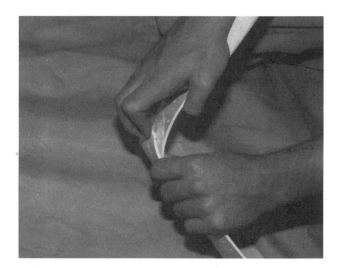

Fig. 4-8 Thermally sensitive plastic can be fashioned so that overlapping flaps are adhered to one another at the appropriate temperature.

---

*Specialist Plaster Bandage, Johnson & Johnson, New Brunswick, NJ.
†Vetcast Plus, 3M Animal Care Products, St. Paul, Minn; CaraGlas Xtra, Carapace, Tulsa.
‡CutterCast Casting Tape, Cutter Biomedical, Pompton Plains, NJ.
§Splint Rods, Osteo-Technology International, Inc., Timonium, Md.
ǁOrthoplast II, Johnson & Johnson, New Brunswick, NJ; CaraForm Veterinary Thermoplastic, Carapace, Tulsa.
¶Mason Meta Splint, Osteo-Technology International, Inc., Timonium, Md.

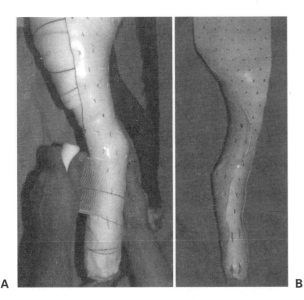

Fig. 4-9 Thermally sensitive plastic, cut from a flat sheet or roll, can be custom-contoured to the limb at the appropriate temperature. **A,** Binding the plastic to the bandage while still in a moldable state ensures the material is contoured perfectly to the limb. **B,** Plastic should encircle the limb more than 180 degrees to provide optimal stability.

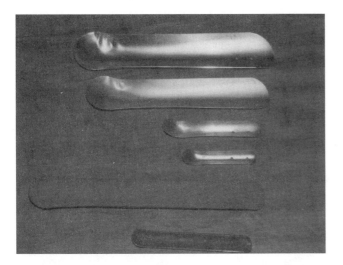

Fig. 4-10 Prefabricated "spoon" splints are made in many sizes out of aluminum or plastic.

paw, and contact the ground during weight bearing. Proximally, they should not extend above the olecranon on the forelimb or the calcaneus on the hind limb. They often must be cut with a hacksaw or heavy shears to obtain the proper length. With injuries proximal to the paw, the padded bandage underlying a spoon splint may be applied with the middle digits exposed. If the digits or pads are involved, the entire paw is usually incorporated within the bandage. In this case, care must be taken to ensure that the compressive layer and additional conforming gauze binding the splint to the bandage are not

applied too tightly, since the digits cannot be examined for evidence of swelling.

Outer Layer

The outer layer is usually applied using a nonocclusive elastic fabric with adhesive properties.* This layer is applied circumferentially over the compressive layer and acts to protect all underlying layers from wear, dirt, and moisture. The tape is applied distally to proximally with 50% or less overlap and should cover the underlying layers without contacting the skin. Moderate tension is used during application; however, the tension should be significantly less than that used for the compressive layer. Usually, only one layer of the taped fabric is needed.

After the outer layer is applied, the padding and compressive layers are still exposed at the distal aspect of most bandages. In these cases, small strips of the elastic fabric can be fashioned to protect this part of the bandage, which may be subjected to dirt and moisture during weight bearing (Fig. 4-11).

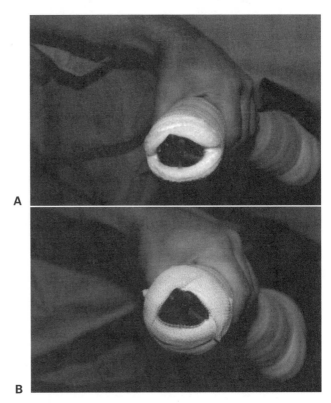

Fig. 4-11 Distal end of a padded or splinted bandage. **A,** Often, padding is exposed distally after application of the outer layer. This padding is easily soiled or wetted. **B,** Padding is protected by small strips of elastic adhesive tape.

---

*Elastikon, Johnson & Johnson, Arlington, Texas; Vetrap, 3M Animal Care Products, St. Paul, Minn.

The strength and limited pliability of outer-layer material increase the likelihood of pressure or abrasion-related cutaneous injury when they are applied in direct contact with the skin. For this reason, slings which are constructed solely of outer-layer material are prone to bandage-related complications. Complications can be prevented by protecting the limb with underlying padding or by incorporating pleats wherever the elastic tape encircles the limb (see Fig. 4-15 and Thoracic Limb Slings).

Cast Layer

The cast layer is applied with a taped fabric impregnated with plaster, fiberglass, or water-activated polyurethane resin.[8] Plaster, the traditional casting material, is strong and inexpensive but has lost favor among veterinarians because of various disadvantages relative to other materials. First, plaster's heaviness tends to make casts unwieldy, especially for cats and small dogs. Also, plaster tends to chip on impact and limits radiographic quality because of its radiopacity. Plaster also weakens once wet and dries very slowly. The newer materials, including the fiberglass and resin-impregnated tapes, are lightweight, strong, impact resistant, and radiolucent. These materials do not lose strength when wet and are more easily dried.[8] The major disadvantage of these newer materials is their higher cost.

The cast layer is applied circumferentially over thin layers of stockinette and padding. Using gloves, one immerses the roll of casting tape in cool to lukewarm water. After saturation, one allows the excess water to drip from the material without squeezing the roll. The tape is applied distal to proximal wrapping cranially to caudally around the medial aspect of the limb and caudally to cranially around the lateral aspect, as shown in Fig. 4-25, E. Spiraling the material in this direction helps minimize external rotation (supination), a tendency most frequently seen when casting the forelimb. Starting distally, one applies the material snugly with even tension while holding the roll close to the limb. Constricting bands and finger indentations are avoided. One should allow the rolled material to follow its own path when crossing over angled joints, such as the elbow, tarsus, or stifle. Portions of cast padding initially exposed are covered when the casting tape courses back over the area. The cast layer should end 1.5 to 2 cm below the proximal extent of the padding. Subsequent layers should be applied before the first hardens, although no more than two or three layers are necessary. Once the cast layer hardens, underlying stockinette and stirrups are reflected over the ends of the cast and held in place with additional casting material or elastic tape. Many clinicians tend to leave the thickness of the cast layer too thin at the proximal and distal ends. These locations are predisposed to wear during weight bearing and should be reinforced with two or three extra layers of casting material.

One must ensure that the cast's distal end is positioned at the level of the second phalanx for digits three and four. If the cast is positioned too far distally, it impedes walking and undergoes excessive wear during weight bearing. If positioned too proximally, the metacarpo(tarso)phalangeal joints extend during weight bearing, leading to contact between the edge of the cast and digits. This can cause serious cutaneous injury to the dorsal aspects of the middle digits, usually at the level of the first phalanx. As mentioned, the proximal end of the cast should be positioned from midshaft to proximal one-third of the radius/tibia (half-limb cast) or midshaft to proximal one-third of the humerus/femur (full-limb cast), *not* at the level of a joint.

Cast removal is best performed with a circular oscillating saw.* These instruments cut through casting material very efficiently but are less likely than other saws to cause injury if contact with the skin is made. Motion of the saw blade on the surface of the cast material should be directed inward, to an appropriate depth, then outward (Fig. 4-12). This inward and outward motion is repeated, connecting the individual cuts until a full-thickness continuous groove is formed. The saw should

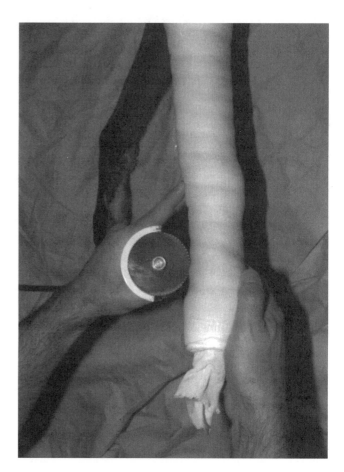

Fig. 4-12   Cast removal with a circular oscillating saw.

*M-PACT Cast Cutter, Cast Removal Systems, Eudora, Kan.

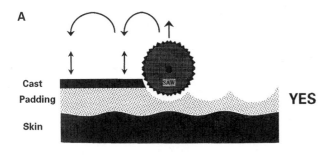

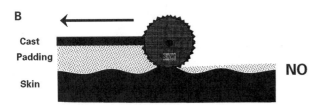

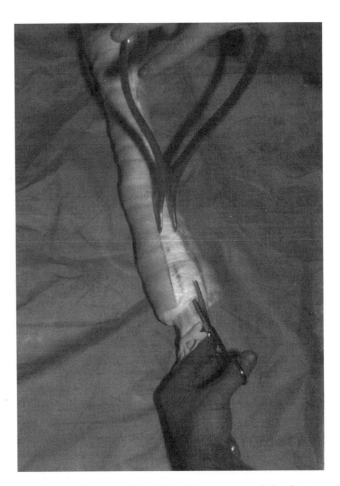

Fig. 4-13 Motion of an oscillating circular saw blade when removing a cast. **A,** Blade should be moved inward and outward so that individual cuts are connected to form a full-thickness continuous groove. **B,** Dragging the saw through the casting material predisposes the skin to injury if contact with the blade occurs.

Fig. 4-14 Cast spreaders widen the groove made by the saw and permit cutting of underlying bandage layers.

not be dragged through the casting material because injury to the skin is likely if contact with the blade occurs (Fig. 4-13).

Cast removal is easiest after two full-thickness grooves are created approximately 180 degrees apart from each other. Cast spreaders are used to separate the halves and scissors to cut the underlying bandage layers (Fig. 4-14). If the cast is going to be saved and reused as a splint or bivalved cast, it should be cut into medial and lateral halves by positioning the two grooves on the cast's cranial and caudal aspects. One or both halves can be reapplied if a splint or bivalved cast is indicated (see Bandage Removal and Miscellaneous Casts).

Bandage Material Width

When applying cast padding, conforming gauze, or casting material, one often has a choice among various widths of material (2, 3, and 4 inch). The wider the roll, the more material is applied with each encircling wrap and the fewer the rolls needed to achieve an appropriate thickness of material. However, wider tapes make it more difficult to maintain the limb in a functional position because the material does not course as evenly over partially flexed joints. As a result, wider rolls tend to straighten underlying joints more than narrower rolls, which can be wrapped more anatomically along limb contours.

Generally, the smaller and thinner the limb, the narrower is the roll of material. As a rule of thumb, bandages

for cats and small dogs are best applied with 2-inch-wide material. Three-inch material is used for midsized dogs (25 to 50 pounds), and 4-inch material is reserved for only the largest breeds.

THORACIC LIMB SLINGS

Slings are general-purpose bandages designed to prevent weight bearing or maintain a protective orientation for the limb. Slings usually afford significant mobility to the incorporated limb and should therefore be reserved for injuries requiring minimal stability.

It is important to remember that slings are prone to bandage-related complications. Elastic fabric is often adhered directly onto the skin, since slings are usually constructed with little to no padding. Skin underlying the tape can be irritated directly by the adhesive or by excessive pressure from material wrapped too tightly. These complications may be prevented by applying a protective layer of padding and conforming gauze underneath the elastic tape wherever it must encircle the limb. Pressure-related cutaneous injury can also be minimized by incorporating pleats in the elastic tape. Pleats can separate with tension, providing more "give" than tape that is applied circumferentially. In this way, pleats act as safety valves if excessive tension is used during sling application or if the incorporated limb swells significantly after application (Fig. 4-15).

Carpal Flexion Sling

The carpal flexion sling prevents weight bearing but provides free mobility to the proximal limb. The carpus is partially or fully flexed and taped into position with elastic adhesive tape (Fig. 4-16). The tape is applied circumferentially around the dorsal aspect of the paw and distal radius, with little to no tension. Swelling of the paw can occur if the tape is applied too tightly or if the carpus is forced into maximum flexion. Cast padding and conforming gauze underneath the tape help prevent skin irritation caused by direct contact with the adhesive, but slippage is more common.

Indications for the carpal flexion sling include stable forelimb injuries that would benefit from temporary protection from weight-bearing forces. Typically, this includes postoperative protection of repaired forelimb fractures or luxations. The carpal flexion sling is also used to protect repairs of the accessory carpal bone or flexor tendons, which can be subjected to disruptive forces when the carpus extends.

Velpeau Sling

The Velpeau sling prevents weight bearing and provides some stability to the proximal limb. Two or three layers of padding are placed circumferentially around the torso and limb while it is held partially flexed and adducted against the ventrolateral chest. The layers should be wrapped in front of and behind the contralateral brachium to prevent cranial slippage of the incorporated

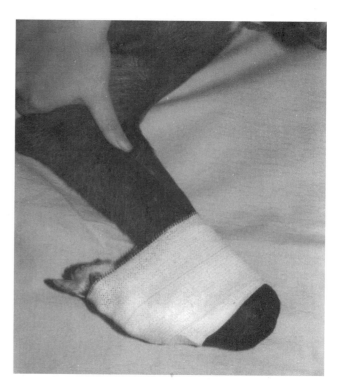

Fig. 4-16 Carpal flexion sling. Tape is applied with minimal tension around the dorsal aspect of the paw and distal radius.

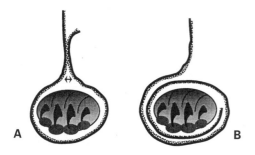

Fig. 4-15 Attaching elastic adhesive tape to the limb when applying a sling. **A,** Pleats can be formed by attaching adhesive surfaces to one another when placing tape around the limb. These pleats can separate if excessive tension is applied to the tape or if the limb subsequently swells. **B,** Adhesive tape that encircles the limb will *not* unwrap if tension becomes excessive. As a result, this technique is more likely to cause pressure sores or necrosis of the skin.

limb (Fig. 4-17). A compressive layer with moderate tension and an outer layer are then placed in a similar manner. Forced flexion of the incorporated carpus should be avoided to prevent swelling of the paw. Caution must also be used when applying material around the chest because excessive tension can compromise respiration.

The Velpeau sling can occasionally be used as the primary mode of therapy for proximal limb connective tissue injuries and fractures. Bicipital bursitis and traumatically induced medial shoulder luxation can be rested effectively with this sling. Sufficient stability can also be provided for minimally displaced, intrinsically stable fractures of the scapula and humerus. Most often the Velpeau sling is used adjunctively to protect tenuous repair of a fractured scapula or humerus or to protect repair of medial shoulder luxation. By adducting the distal limb, the sling forces the humeral head laterally within the joint, thereby reducing stresses to any imbrication or tendon transfer performed on the medial aspect. For lateral shoulder luxation, a spica splint should be used as primary or adjunctive therapy.

THORACIC LIMB PADDED AND SPLINTED BANDAGES
Padded Bandage

The padded bandage (modified Robert Jones) is a general-purpose application with numerous indications for injuries *distal to the elbow*. Padded bandages are constructed with contact, padding, compressive, and outer layers and permit weight bearing but provide minimal stability. For injuries distal to the carpus, the proximal end of the bandage should extend up to the middle or proximal one-third of the radius (half limb). For injuries to the carpus or antebrachium, the bandage should extend up to the middle or proximal one-third of the humerus (full limb). Proximally, the bandage should *not* end at the level of a joint (i.e., carpus or elbow). Distally, the digital pads and claws of digits three and four should protrude from the end of the bandage.

Application. The specific techniques used to apply the various bandage layers are described earlier in this chapter. In brief, the stirrups are applied firmly to the hair on the lateral and medial aspects of the distal limb. Distally, the ends of the stirrups are adhered to each other or to a tongue depressor so that they extend at least 10 cm distal to the digits (Fig. 4-18). Using cast

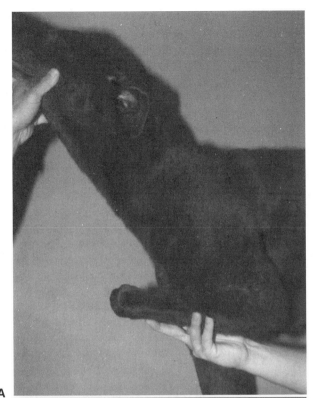

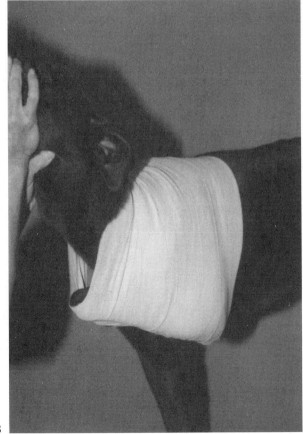

Fig. 4-17 Velpeau sling. **A,** Limb held partially flexed and adducted against the ventrolateral chest. **B,** Cast padding, conforming gauze, and elastic tape hold the limb in place.

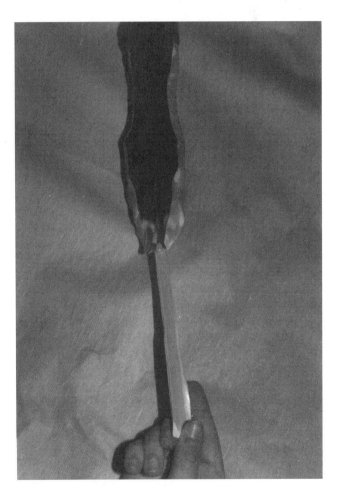

Fig. 4-18 Stirrups are applied firmly to the hair on lateral and medial aspects of the distal limb; wounds and dewclaws are avoided. Stirrups should extend approximately 10 cm distal to the paw, adhered to each other or to a tongue depressor.

padding or roll cotton, the padding layer is applied distally to proximally with about 50% overlap wrapping cranially to caudally around the medial aspect of the limb and caudally to cranially around the lateral aspect, to minimize external rotation (supination). (See Fig. 4-19, *A*.) The padding is continued up to the anticipated proximal end of the bandage and torn. Additional layers are applied in a similar manner until the appropriate thickness is obtained. Usually, 1.5 to 2 cm of cotton cast padding (five to seven layers) is adequate (Fig. 4-19, *B*). Two or three additional layers of padding are applied to the most proximal and distal ends of the bandage to provide added protection in these locations (Fig. 4-19, *C*). With the limb cupped in one hand, conforming gauze is applied evenly and snugly with the other, (Fig. 4-19, *D*). The conforming gauze should be spiraled proximally

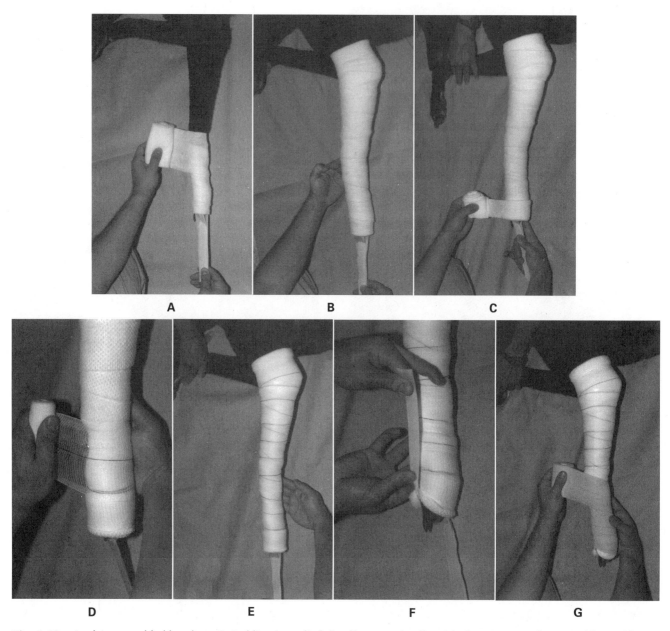

Fig. 4-19 Applying a padded bandage. **A,** Padding is applied distally to proximally, with about 50% overlap. **B,** Additional layers of cast padding are applied until a thickness of 1.5 to 2 cm is achieved. **C,** Two or three additional layers of padding are added to the proximal and distal edges to protect the underlying skin in these injury-prone areas. **D,** Limb is cupped in one hand, and conforming gauze is applied with the other. **E,** Two or three layers of conforming gauze are applied, extending to within 1.5 to 2 cm of the padding's proximal edge. Conforming gauze should not contact the skin. **F,** Stirrups are reflected up and over the padding and compressive layers. Moderate tension when reflecting the stirrups helps prevent distal slippage. **G,** Outer layer is applied with elastic adhesive tape extending no further proximally than the conforming gauze. The adhesive tape should not contact the skin.

in the same direction as the underlying padding. Two or three layers of conforming gauze are usually adequate. The compressive layer should compact all but the most proximal 1.5 to 2.0 cm of padding; direct contact with the skin should be avoided (Fig. 4-19, *E*). The stirrups are separated, reflected proximally with tension, and held in place with a circumferential loop of adhesive tape (Fig. 4-19, *F*). Finally, elastic tape is applied to protect the underlying layers (Fig. 4-19, *G*). Direct contact between the outer layer and skin should be avoided.

Padded bandages are applied so that digits three and four protrude from the distal end to facilitate examination (Fig. 4-20). However, injuries to the digits or pads may require the entire paw be incorporated within the bandage (Fig. 4-21). In this case, special care is taken to ensure that the compressive layer is *not* applied too tightly, since the digits cannot be examined for signs of swelling.

Indications. Padded bandages are used primarily or adjunctively for the treatment of relatively superficial injuries that do not need significant additional stability (see Indications for External Support). The most common examples include open wounds, primary or delayed wound closures, and surgical incisions. The specific benefits of these bandages have been discussed in detail.

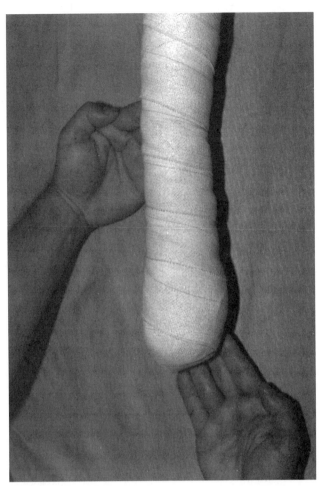

Fig. 4-21 With injuries to the pads or digits, the entire paw can be incorporated within the bandage.

Most importantly, they can minimize swelling of traumatized limbs, absorb exudate, and protect, debride, and medicate underlying wounds.

Robert Jones Bandage

The Robert Jones bandage (R-J bandage) is a variation of the padded bandage with a much thicker padding layer. As with padded bandages, the R-J bandage is constructed with contact, padding, compressive, and outer layers and is indicated for injuries *distal to the elbow*. The proximal aspect of the R-J bandage usually extends as high up on the limb as possible (full limb). The R-J bandage provides more stability than a padded bandage because of its added thickness; however, its extremely bulky size is unwieldy and restricts ambulation.

Application. Application of the R-J bandage is performed similar to that of the padded bandage except for the padding and compressive layers. Much thicker padding (4 to 8 cm) is applied using rolled cotton instead of

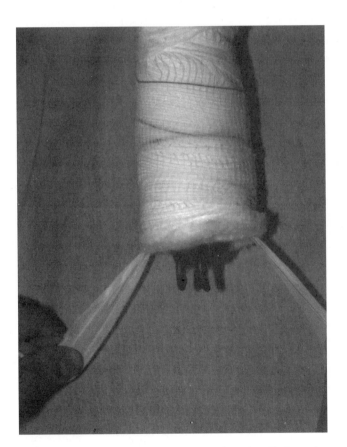

Fig. 4-20 Digits three and four protruding distally from the end of a support bandage.

cast padding. Usually, three to five layers of cotton roll are wrapped as snugly as possible to achieve the desired thickness. The compressive layer is then applied, as tightly as possible, with conforming gauze. The thicker padding and tightly applied compressive layer afford increased stability without contributing to vascular occlusion. The stirrups and outer layer are fashioned identical to the padded bandage.

Indications. The major advantages of the R-J bandage include its increased stability over padded bandages and its tremendous absorbent capacity. However, if the padding layer becomes too thick or the compressive layer is not applied tightly enough, stability is diminished because axially located cotton adjacent to the limb is not adequately compacted (see Biomechanics). Additionally, the bandage's bulk, which limits mobility and requires a significant investment in bandaging material, makes repeated application impractical. Therefore, the R-J bandage is usually used as a temporary "field dressing" for fractures or wounds distal to the elbow until definitive repair, splinting, or casting can be performed.

Splinted Bandage

The splinted bandage is a support bandage for injuries *distal to the elbow* that permits weight bearing and provides moderate stability. The bandage is constructed with contact, padding, compressive, splint, and outer layers. For injuries distal to the carpus, the proximal aspect of the bandage should extend up to the middle or proximal one-third of the radius (half limb). For injuries to the carpus or antebrachium, the bandage should extend up to the middle or proximal one-third of the humerus (full limb). The proximal aspect of the bandage should *not* end at the level of a joint (i.e., carpus or elbow), and only the pads and claws of digits three and four should protrude distally.

Application. The specific techniques used to apply the bandage layers are described earlier in this chapter. In brief, the first three layers, including the stirrups and padding and compressive layers, are applied identical to those of the padded bandage, as described earlier. Moldable splintage, such as a metal rod (⅛, ³⁄₁₆ or ¼ inch), thermally sensitive plastic, or casting tape, is then contoured to the bandage's lateral aspect. At the carpus, 10-15 degrees of flexion and 10-15 degrees of medial deviation (varus) may be incorporated into the splint to minimize the carpal hyperextension often seen after bandage removal (See Bandage Complications). A functional position for the elbow joint should also be maintained with full-limb splints (Fig. 22, *A*). The splint layer is then applied laterally, superficial to the compressive layer, and is bound to the bandage with additional layers of con-

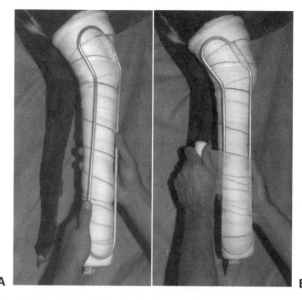

Fig. 4-22 Splinted bandage, thoracic limb. **A,** Aluminum rod splint has been contoured to the limb's lateral aspect. A functional angle for the elbow has been maintained. **B,** Splint layer is incorporated into the bandage with additional layers of conforming gauze.

forming gauze (Fig. 4-22, *B*). These additional layers of conforming gauze should be applied evenly, spiraling in the same direction and with similar tension to that of the underlying compressive layer. The stirrups are then reflected, and the outer layer is applied routinely.

Spoon splints are a special form of splintage material that are prefabricated out of plastic or aluminum. They are best used to protect injuries distal to midshaft radius. Unlike the other splint materials, they are placed on the bandage's caudal aspect and extend distally, past the paw, to contact the ground during weight bearing. Proximally, they should not extend past the olecranon. If needed, the splints can be hacksawed or cut with heavy shears to the appropriate length. With a radial, carpal, or metacarpal injury, the padded bandage underlying a spoon splint may be applied with digits three and four protruding (Fig. 4-23, *A*). If the digits or pads are injured, the entire paw is often incorporated (Fig. 4-23, *B*). In this case, care must be taken that the compressive layer is not applied too tightly, since the digits cannot be examined for evidence of swelling.

Indications. Splinted bandages are usually used primarily or adjunctively for the treatment of injuries that require significant additional stability (see Indications for External Support). The most common examples include luxations, fractures, and postoperative protection of tenuous orthopedic repairs. For open wounds, splinted bandages provide all the benefits of padded bandages and increased stability.

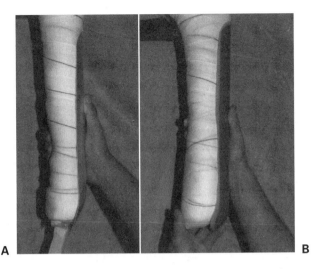

Fig. 4-23 Spoon splint, thoracic limb. **A,** Spoon splint is applied to the caudal aspect of a padded bandage, with digits three and four protruding distally. **B,** Spoon splint is applied to the caudal aspect of a padded bandage that incorporates the entire paw.

Spica Splint

The spica splint is a special form of splinted bandage for injuries of the proximal limb, including the elbow, humerus, shoulder, and scapula. It permits weight bearing and limited ambulation and provides moderate stability. The bandage is constructed with contact, padding, compressive, splint, and outer layers. Stability to the proximal limb is afforded because the bandage and splint span the entire limb and incorporate the thorax (Fig. 4-24). As with the other padded and splinted bandages, only the pads and claws of digits three and four should protrude from the bandage distally.

Application. The specific techniques used to apply the bandage layers are described earlier in this chapter. In brief, the stirrups and padding, compressive, and splint layers are applied similar to those of the splinted bandage except that the entire limb and thorax are incorporated. The padding layer is applied as high proximally on the limb as possible and is then continued circumferentially around the thorax, cranial and caudal to the contralateral limb. Conforming gauze is applied similarly, using caution to extend no closer than 1.5 to 2 cm from the padding's edge. Care must also be used when applying tension to material wrapped around the thorax. Respiration can be compromised if the conforming gauze or outer layer material is applied too tightly. This is especially true in patients with preexisting thoracic trauma, such as hemothorax, pneumothorax, or pulmonary contusion. Moldable splintage is then contoured to the lateral aspect of the limb and thorax, maintaining a functional position for the elbow and shoulder (Fig. 4-24). To provide optimal

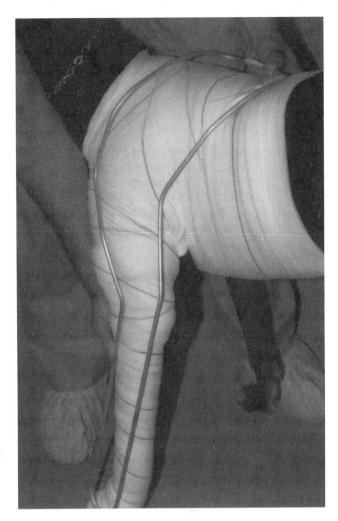

Fig. 4-24 Spica splint, thoracic limb. The bandage incorporates the entire limb and thorax. A functional position has been maintained for the carpus, elbow, and shoulder.

stability, the splint material should extend from the most distal aspect of the bandage to at least the dorsal midline of the thorax. The splint layer is then bound to the bandage with additional layers of conforming gauze. The additional conforming gauze should be applied evenly, with similar tension to that of the underlying compressive layer. The stirrups are then reflected, and the outer layer is applied.

Indications. Spica splints are used primarily or adjunctively for the treatment of injuries to the elbow, humerus, shoulder, and scapula that require additional stability (see Indications for External Support). The most common indications include elbow luxation; lateral shoulder luxation; and minimally displaced, intrinsically stable fractures of the humerus or scapula. Additionally, spica splints are often used to protect tenuous orthopedic repair of these associated bones and joints postoperatively. The spica splint is not a frequently applied bandage, even though indications for its use are common. The increased bandaging material required to incorporate the chest makes this splint relatively expensive to apply. Also, the splint's bulkiness and significant restriction of the elbow and shoulder severely limit patient ambulation.

THORACIC LIMB CASTS

The cast is a support bandage for injuries distal to the elbow that permits weight bearing and provides near-rigid stability. The cast is constructed with contact, padding, and cast layers. For injuries distal to the carpus, the cast's proximal aspect should extend up to the middle or proximal one-third of the radius (half cast or half-limb cast). For injuries to the carpus or antebrachium, the cast should extend up to the middle or proximal one-third of the humerus (full cast or full-limb cast). The proximal aspect of the cast should *not* end at the level of a joint (i.e., carpus or elbow), and only the pads and claws of digits three and four should protrude distally.

Application

Cast application is usually performed with the patient anesthetized to permit reduction of the fracture/luxation and prevent motion of the limb while the cast layer hardens. For injuries with instability along the medial aspect of the limb, the patient should be positioned in lateral recumbency with the affected limb down. In this position the injured area tends *not* to "break open," valgus deformity is minimized, and reduction is maintained more easily. Rolling the patient dorsally a small amount helps when applying the cast as far proximally as possible. Alternately, for injuries with instability along the limb's lateral aspect, the patient is positioned in lateral recumbency with the affected limb up.

The specific techniques used to apply the bandage layers are described earlier in this chapter. In brief, the stirrups are applied firmly to the hair on the medial and lateral aspects of the distal limb. Appropriately sized tube stockinette (usually 1 to 3 inches wide) is cut 50% longer than the limb and is stretched proximally and distally by two assistants so that the material conforms to the contours of the limb without wrinkling (Fig. 4-25, *A*). "Doughnuts" may be fashioned out of cast padding or orthopedic felt by cutting circular holes in small pieces of the material. These doughnuts are then centered over bony protuberances, such as the olecranon or lateral epicondyle of the humerus, so that the prominences themselves are encircled but not covered with material (Fig. 4-25, *B*). Cast padding is then applied distally to proximally with 50% overlap, using no more than one or two layers (Fig. 4-25, *C*). However, two to three additional layers of padding may be applied to the most proximal and distal extents of the bandage to provide additional protection for the skin in these injury-prone locations (Fig. 4-25, *D*).

The limb is held in reduction by assistants and the casting material applied over the padding layer. A functional position for the elbow should be maintained for full-limb casts. At the carpus, 10-15 degrees of flexion and 10-15 degrees of medial deviation (varus) may be incorporated into the cast to minimize the carpal hyperextension often seen after cast removal (See Bandage Complications). The bandager should wear gloves to protect hands from the fiberglass, resin, or plaster. Starting distally and working proximally, one applies the material snugly and circumferentially, with about 50% overlap. The casting tape is wrapped cranially to caudally around the medial aspect of the limb and caudally to cranially around the lateral aspect to minimize external rotation (supination); see Fig. 4-25, *E*. Using even tension, one should allow the casting material to follow its own path when crossing over angular portions of the limb. When the layer approaches within 1.5 to 2 cm of the proximal extent of the padding, it is cut and the next layer is started distally. Two or three layers of casting material are usually sufficient. Creases, wrinkles, and finger indentations should be avoided during application. The cast's proximal and distal ends are subjected to the most wear and should be reinforced with two or three extra layers of casting material. Once the cast layer hardens, the stockinette and stirrups are reflected over the ends of the cast and are held in place with additional casting material or elastic tape (Fig. 4-25, *F* and *G*).

Indications

Casts are used primarily or adjunctively for the treatment of injuries that require significant additional stability (see Indications for External Support). The most common indications include luxations, fractures, and postoperative protection of tenuous orthopedic repairs. Contraindications for casts include severely swollen limbs and injuries associated with open wounds. Casts placed on severely swollen limbs are often loose within days as the swelling abates. Once loose, casts provide minimal stability and may contribute to motion-related epidermal abrasion. Injured limbs with open wounds are also poor choices for stabilization with casts. Although windows can be cut over open wounds to allow daily care, these openings structurally weaken the cast and must be replaced after wound treatment to prevent underlying soft tissue from swelling into the fenestration.

PELVIC LIMB SLINGS

General comments pertaining to the indications, construction techniques, and potential dangers of slings are addressed earlier (see Thoracic Limb Slings).

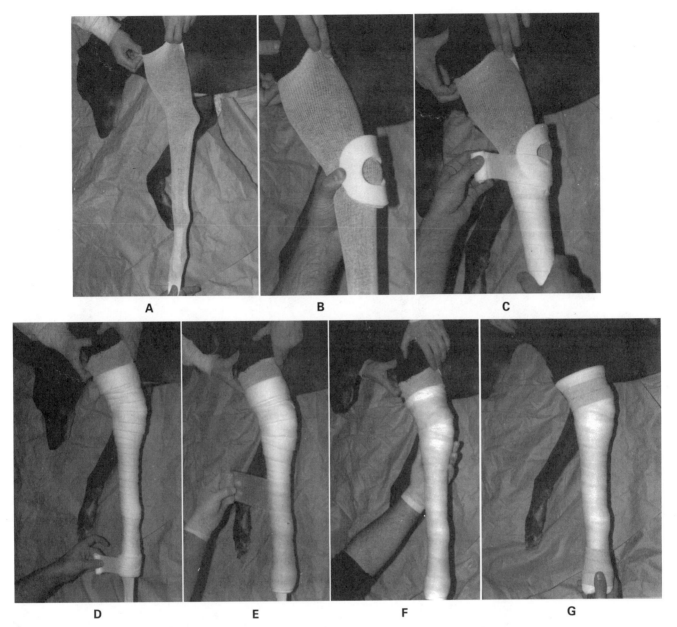

Fig. 4-25   Cast, thoracic limb. **A,** Tube stockinette is stretched proximally and distally by two assistants so that the material conforms to the contours of the limb without wrinkling. **B,** "Doughnuts," fashioned out of cast padding or orthopedic felt, are applied to encircle bony protuberances such as the olecranon. **C,** One or two layers of cast padding are applied and hold the orthopedic felt in place. **D,** Two or three additional layers of padding are added to the most proximal and distal edges of the bandage. This helps protect the underlying skin in these injury-prone areas. **E,** Using gloves, one applies two or three layers of casting material snugly over the padding. The material is applied distally to proximally, with 50% overlap. One allows the roll to follow its own path when crossing over angular portions of the limb; all exposed padding eventually becomes covered. **F,** Proximal and distal ends of the cast are reinforced with two or three extra layers of casting material. The tube stockinette and stirrups are reflected over the ends of the cast and held in place with additional casting material or elastic tape. **G,** Completed cast.

Ehmer Sling

Application. The *classical Ehmer sling* prevents weight bearing of the pelvic limb by maintaining the tarsus and stifle in partial flexion. Elastic adhesive tape is carefully pleated around the metatarsus with the material directed proximally and the adhesive surface laterally (Fig. 4-26, *A*). The stifle and tarsus are flexed, and the material is directed proximally and medial to the thigh (Fig. 4-26, *B*). The material is brought over the thigh, as proximally as possible, and is directed distally over the limb's lateral aspect back toward the pleat (Fig. 4-26, *C*). This circumferential loop is continued plantar to the metatarsus and medial to the limb (Fig. 4-26, *D*). After the material is brought over the thigh again, it is directed caudodistally, medial to the tarsus (Fig. 4-26, *E*). The material is twisted 180 degrees and directed laterally, along the plantar aspect of the metatarsus at the level of the initial pleat (Fig. 4-26, *F*). The roll is then directed cranioproximally medial to the thigh and again twisted 180 degrees (Fig. 4-26, *G* and *H*). This figure-eight application is continued for one or two complete revolutions.

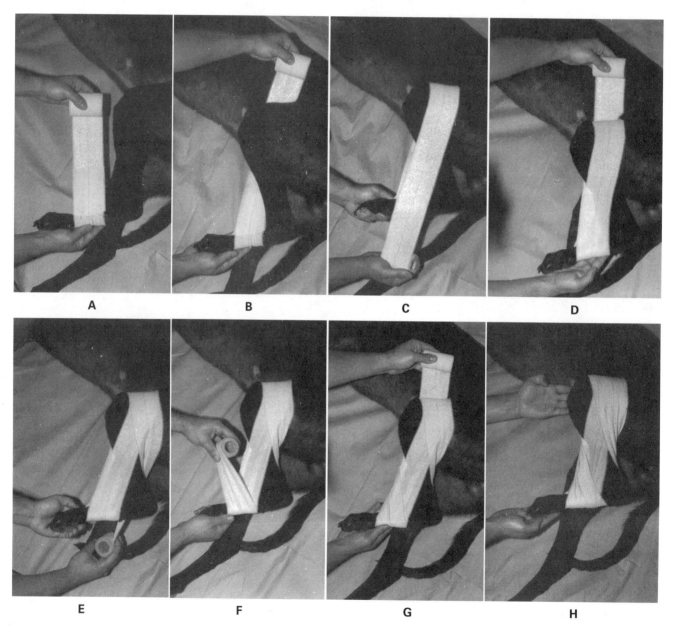

Fig. 4-26 Ehmer sling. **A,** Elastic adhesive tape is pleated around the metatarsus so that the material is directed proximally and the adhesive surface laterally. **B,** Stifle and tarsus are flexed, and the material is directed proximally and medial to the thigh. **C,** Material is brought over the thigh, as proximally as possible, and is directed distally over the limb's lateral aspect back toward the pleat. **D,** Material is continued plantar to the metatarsus and medial to the limb. **E,** Coming over the thigh, it is now directed caudodistally, medial to the tarsus. **F,** Material is twisted 180 degrees and directed laterally, along the plantar aspect of the metatarsus at the level of the initial pleat. **G,** Tape is then directed cranioproximally medial to the thigh and again twisted 180 degrees. This figure-eight application is continued for one or two complete revolutions. **H,** Completed classical Ehmer sling.

The *modified Ehmer sling*, as with the classical version, prevents weight bearing of the pelvic limb but also maintains the hip joint flexed, abducted, and internally rotated. The bandage is applied similar to the classical version except that an additional revolution of tape is applied. After the material is brought caudodistally, medial to the tarsus, and twisted, it is directed over the plantar aspect of the calcaneus, tarsus, and proximal metatarsus (Fig. 4-27, *A*). The material is then directed cranioproximally with significant tension and is incorporated into a caudal abdominal belly band constructed of elastic adhe-

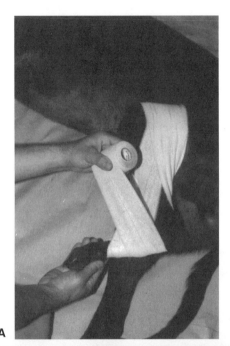

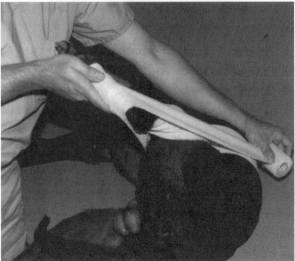

A

B

Fig. 4-27   Modified Ehmer sling. **A,** After a classical Ehmer is applied, a final revolution is directed over the plantar aspect of the calcaneus, tarsus, and proximal metatarsus. **B,** Material is then directed cranioproximally with significant tension and is incorporated into a caudal abdominal belly band. Additional strips, connecting metatarsus to torso, may be needed to support the limb as desired.

sive tape (Fig. 4-27, *B*). Additional strips, connecting metatarsus to torso, may be needed to support the limb as desired.

With both versions of the Ehmer sling, the band crossing over the proximal aspect of the thigh has a tendency to slip forward over the stifle, causing the bandage to unwrap. This often occurs in long-haired dogs, with the tape adhering to long mobile hair rather than firmly attaching to the limb. Looping around the thigh as proximally as possible and clipping or shaving the upper limb help prevent this problem.

Finally, protection in the form of cast padding and conforming gauze is often placed around the tarsus, metatarsus, and distal tibia to prevent sores caused by the irritation or excessive pressure from elastic tape.

Indications. Traditionally, the Ehmer sling is used to maintain the femoral head within the acetabulum after open or closed reduction of a craniodorsal coxofemoral luxation. However, the classical Ehmer does not cross the hip joint and cannot effectively restrict the hip's orientation or mobility. Alternately, the modified Ehmer, by suspending the metatarsus from the torso, forces the hip into flexion, abduction, and internal rotation, which are the optimal orientations to maintain reduction after a craniodorsal luxation.

Pelvic Limb Sling

Application. The pelvic limb sling (Robinson sling) prevents weight bearing by maintaining the tarsus, stifle, and hip in partial flexion.[10] Two- to three-inch elastic or nonelastic adhesive tape is unrolled to an amount at least equal to the distance from the lumbar dorsal midline to the affected limb's metatarsus. The proximal end of the tape is held at the level of the dorsal midline, and the roll is directed distally, positioning the tape medial to the limb with the adhesive surface directed laterally (Fig. 4-28, *A*). The tape is wrapped around the plantar aspect of the metatarsus and then attached to itself proximally, forming a pleat (Fig. 4-28, *B*). The material is further unrolled, doubling back on itself to the dorsal midline, attaching adhesive surface to adhesive surface (Fig. 4-28, *C*). The paw is raised 5 to 8 cm off the ground by drawing the doubled material up proximally and incorporating it into a caudal abdominal belly band made of elastic adhesive tape (Fig. 4-28, *D*). The pleat and doubled material can be further secured to the limb with additional encircling strips of tape. Additionally, the metatarsus can be cushioned from the pleat with a thin underlying layer of padding and conforming gauze.

Indications. Most often the pelvic limb sling is used adjunctively to protect tenuous fracture repair of the tibia or femur or repair of stifle luxation. The sling is an attractive alternative to support bandages if minimal stability is

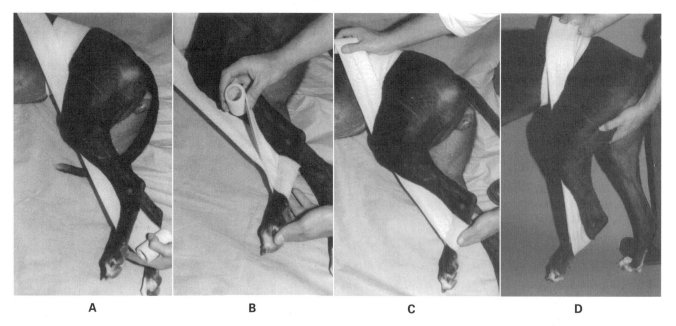

A   B   C   D

Fig. 4-28 Pelvic limb sling. **A,** Two- or 3-inch elastic or nonelastic adhesive tape is unrolled with the free end held at the level of the dorsal lumbar midline and the roll at the metatarsus. Tape is positioned medial to the limb with the adhesive surface directed laterally. **B,** Tape is wrapped around the plantar aspect of the metatarsus and then attached to itself proximally, forming a pleat. **C,** Material is further unrolled, doubling back on itself to the dorsal midline, attaching adhesive surface to adhesive surface. **D,** Doubled material is drawn up proximally, raising the paw 5 to 8 cm off the ground. It is then incorporated into a caudal abdominal belly band. The pleat and doubled material can be further secured to the limb with additional strips of tape.

needed. By maintaining the paw only inches off the ground, the sling protects the affected limb from the normal forces of weight bearing while maintaining a functional position and allowing significant freedom of movement.

90-Degree–90-Degree Flexion Sling

Application. The 90-degree–90-degree flexion sling is a variation of the classical Ehmer and prevents weight bearing of the pelvic limb by maintaining both the tarsus and stifle in approximately 90 degrees of flexion.[3] With the tarsus and stifle flexed to 90 degrees, elastic adhesive tape is simply wrapped circumferentially around the thigh and metatarsus (Fig. 4-29). This differs from the Ehmer sling, where the material is then passed distally around the caudomedial aspect of the tarsus in a figure-eight fashion. Additional tape can be applied circumferentially at the level of the distal tibia to help prevent slippage of the proximal and distal loops.

Indications. The 90-degree–90-degree flexion sling has been described as a prophylactic maneuver to prevent quadriceps contracture after complicated femoral fracture repair in young dogs.[3] Patients at high risk for quadriceps contracture are defined as immature patients (especially under 6 months) with considerable fracture comminution and soft tissue injury. It is recommended that the sling be maintained for no longer than 10 days.

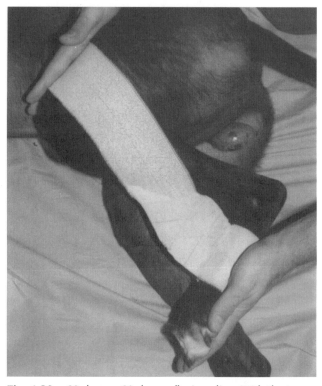

Fig. 4-29 90-degree–90-degree flexion sling. With the tarsus and stifle flexed to 90 degrees, elastic adhesive tape is wrapped circumferentially around the thigh and metatarsus. Additional tape can be applied circumferentially at the level of the distal tibia to help prevent slippage of the proximal and distal loops.

Hobbles

Application. Hobbles are designed to permit weight bearing but prevent abduction of the pelvic limbs. Elastic tape is applied circumferentially around the hind limbs, taking care to maintain a between-limb distance similar to that of the standing position. When applying tape to each limb, it is better to form pleats than to apply the tape circumferentially (see Bandage Application). Cast padding and conforming gauze can be applied underneath the elastic tape, if desired. Additional tape placed around the pleats on the medial aspect of both limbs can help prevent premature pleat separation and distal slippage. *Tarsal hobbles* are positioned just proximal or just distal to the tarsi, at the level of the distal tibia or midmetatarsus (Fig. 4-30). *Stifle hobbles* are positioned just proximal to the patellae, at the level of the distal femur (Fig. 4-31). An additional strip of tape coursing over the pelvic dorsum and connecting the lateralmost aspects of the stifle hobbles is often necessary to prevent distal slippage.[8]

Indications. Indications for hobbles include caudoventral coxofemoral luxation, pelvic trauma, and pelvic limb restraint. Caudoventral coxofemoral luxation must be handled differently than the more typical craniodorsal luxation. Although craniodorsal luxation is usually associated with diffuse capsular tears, caudoventral luxation is often associated with focal tearing of only the ventral joint capsule. Dorsocranially, the capsule is usually intact and provides excellent intraarticular stability once reduction is achieved. However, severe abduction of the hip forces the femoral head ventrally, toward the area of weakened capsule. Hobbles can very effectively limit this severe abduction and prevent reluxation. Patients with multiple pelvic injuries often have difficulty maintaining the hind limbs adducted. When walking, pelvic limbs can suddenly abduct, especially on slippery floors, causing the animal to fall and further injure itself. Hobbles are useful in providing support to patients with this tendency. Finally, hobbles can be used as a restraint device for animals that injuriously scratch themselves with the pelvic limbs. Bandages, wounds, incisions, or pruritic skin can be protected from self-induced trauma with these restraint devices.

Tarsal and stifle hobbles perform similar functions; however, each has its own unique advantages. Some patients recovering from caudoventral coxofemoral luxation can still manage to abduct the hip at the level of the

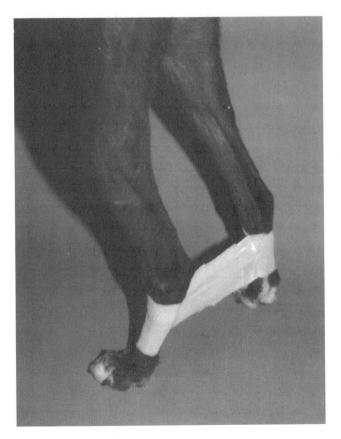

Fig. 4-30 Tarsal hobbles.

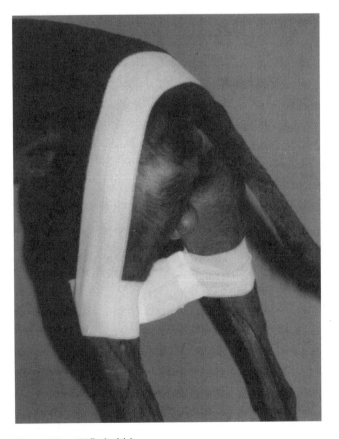

Fig. 4-31 Stifle hobbles.

stifles, despite tarsal hobbling. Stifle hobbles are more effective at preventing reluxation in these patients. Additionally, stifle hobbles can usually be maintained longer, especially in female dogs, who tend to soil tarsal hobbles with their caudally directed urine stream. Alternately, tarsal hobbles are more useful when providing restraint for excessive scratching, since greater control of the distal limb is achieved.

PELVIC LIMB PADDED BANDAGES, SPLINTED BANDAGES, AND CASTS

The indications and methods of application for padded bandages, splinted bandages, and casts of the pelvic limb are analogous to those of the thoracic limb (see Thoracic Limb Padded and Splinted Bandages and Thoracic Limb Casts). These bandages are appropriate for injuries *distal to the stifle* and permit weight bearing with varying degrees of stability. For injuries distal to the tarsus, the proximal aspect of the bandage should extend up to the middle or proximal one-third of the tibia (half limb). For injuries to the tarsus or crus, the bandage should extend up to the middle or proximal one-third of the femur (full limb). The proximal aspect of the bandage should *not* end at the level of a joint (i.e., tarsus or stifle), and only the pads and claws of digits three and four should protrude distally.

Application of Spoon Splints in Pelvic Limb Splinted Bandages

Spoon splints are a special form of splintage that are prefabricated out of plastic or aluminum. They are best used to protect injuries of the distal limb as far proximally as the tarsometatarsal joint. Unlike the other splint materials, they are placed on the caudal aspect of the bandage and extend distally past the paw to contact the ground during weight bearing. Proximally, they should not extend past the calcaneus. If needed, the splints can be hacksawed or cut with heavy shears to the appropriate length. With a metatarsal injury, the bandaging underlying a spoon splint may be applied with digits three and four exposed (see Fig. 4-23, *A*). If the digits or pads are involved, the entire paw is often incorporated (see Fig. 4-23, *B*). In this case, care must be taken that the compressive layer and additional conforming gauze binding the splint to the bandage are not applied too tightly, since the digits cannot be examined for evidence of swelling.

Specific Cautions Relative to the Pelvic Limb

Disabling stiffness with joint extension is a more frequent complication in the pelvic limb than the thoracic limb after prolonged bandaging. Bandages that apply compression to any degree tend to straighten joints and extend limbs (see Bandage Complications—Joint Stiffness). In the forelimb the carpus is fully extended during normal weight bearing. Therefore, stiffness or reduced flexion in this joint does *not* cause a significant gait disturbance. Alternately, the tarsus and stifle of the hind limb are partially flexed during weight bearing. Inability to flex these joints interferes with the normal swing phase during ambulation and can cause significant gait disturbance. When bandaging the pelvic limb, care should be used to maintain a functional position. This is especially true with the splinted bandage and cast, which are often applied for prolonged periods and can be custom-contoured to maintain the tarsus and stifle in partial flexion (Fig. 4-32).

Pelvic Limb Spica Splint

Pelvic limb spica splints deserve special mention because the pelvic anatomy makes them more difficult to apply

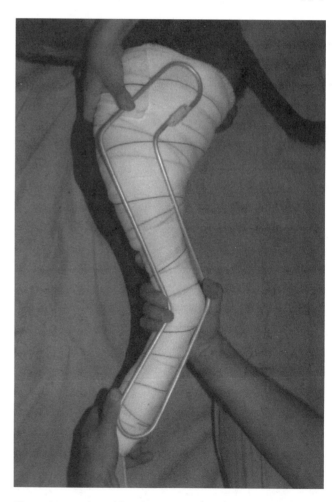

Fig. 4-32 Splinted bandage, pelvic limb. The aluminum rod splint has been contoured to the limb's lateral aspect. Functional angles for the tarsus and stifle have been maintained.

and maintain. As with the thoracic limb, the spica splint incorporates the entire limb and associated torso. Incorporating the pelvis predisposes the bandage to soiling because of the proximity of urinary and gastrointestinal excrements. This is a problem especially in males, in whom encircling bandage material often overlies the prepuce and becomes soiled during urination. In debilitated male patients, closed-system urinary catheterization can be instituted so that urine is diverted away from overlying bandage material. Otherwise, the splintage must be directed cranially, at its most proximal extent, and incorporated in an abdominal wrap positioned just cranial to the prepuce. Stability is somewhat diminished with this configuration because of the greater distance between the limb and incorporated torso.

Incorporating the pelvis also predisposes the scrotum to injury. When applying bandage material ventrally, care must be taken to avoid excessive compression, which can lead to swelling or abrasion of the scrotal sac.

MISCELLANEOUS SPLINTED BANDAGES
Schroeder-Thomas Splint

The Schroeder-Thomas splint (S-T splint) provides stability by suspending the limb within a rigid custom-contoured frame. This splint is appropriate for injuries *distal to the elbow and stifle*. The biomechanical function of the S-T splint is similar to that of a crutch. The limb is protected from weight-bearing forces, which are instead transmitted up the rigid frame and into the torso at the axillary or inguinal region.

Application. The splint is constructed from aluminum rod, sized appropriately so that it can withstand weight-bearing forces without bending. The diameter of the brachium or thigh is estimated proximally at the level of the axillary or inguinal region. A circle with slightly larger diameter than the limb is formed by wrapping the rod 1½ revolutions around the appropriate stage of a pyramidal cylinder* (Fig. 4-33). The whole ring is angled 45 degrees (Fig. 4-34, *A*) and then padded with cast padding, conforming gauze, and elastic tape. The ring's distal aspect is directed medially as the limb is placed through (Fig. 4-34, *B*). The ring is advanced snugly into the axillary or inguinal region and the frame contoured while maintaining the limb in a functional position. The frame's distal aspect should extend past the paw only 2 to 5 cm. First, tape is applied connecting the paw to the distal aspect of the frame. Encircling material, such as cotton padding, roll cotton, or combine roll is then applied at appropriate locations to suspend the limb

*Osteo-Technology International, Inc., Timonium, Md.

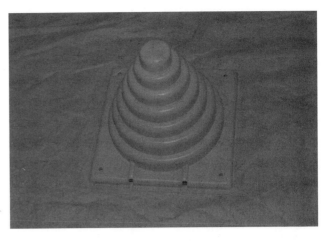

Fig. 4-33 Mold of pyramidal cylinder used in construction of a Schroeder-Thomas splint.

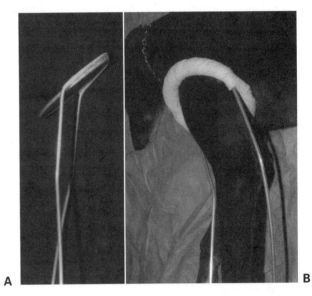

Fig. 4-34 Schroeder-Thomas splint. **A,** Ring is angled 45 degrees. **B,** Ring is padded with cast padding, conforming gauze, and elastic tape. With the distal aspect of the ring directed medially, it is advanced snugly into the axilla. The remainder of the frame can then be contoured to the limb.

within the frame (Fig. 4-35). The goal is to provide stability and traction while maintaining a functional position for the limb.

Indications. Indications for the S-T splint are similar to those for other splinted bandages (see Indications for External Support). Fractures, luxations, and orthopedic repairs distal to the elbow and stifle, requiring a limited amount of additional stability, are the most common indications. The splint also works well for restraint purposes. By effectively resisting limb flexion, the S-T splint can be extremely helpful when placing catheters in fractious

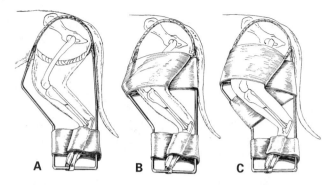

Fig. 4-35 Application of a Schroeder-Thomas splint for a midshaft tibial fracture. **A,** Cotton padding, roll cotton, or combine roll is used to sling the metatarsus and provide distal traction to the limb. **B,** Similar bandaging is added proximally to pull the femur forward and apply traction to the tibia. **C,** Proximal sling is continued distally to provide medial support for the tibia.

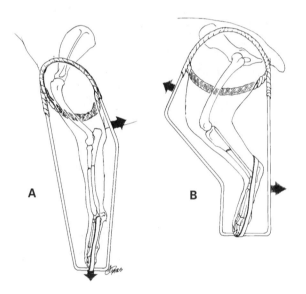

Fig. 4-36 Direction of tractional forces to employ when applying a Schroeder-Thomas splint for temporary stabilization of injuries to the distal limb. **A,** Thoracic limb, radial-ulnar fracture. **B,** Pelvic limb, tibial-fibular fracture.

animals or in maintaining patency for positionally occluded catheters. *The S-T splint should never be used for proximal limb injuries, such as humeral or femoral fractures.* With these injuries, the medial aspect of the ring can act as a fulcrum, contributing to instability and soft tissue injury.

The framed construction affords the S-T splint unique advantages. Suspending the limb within an encircling external framework permits one to apply tractional forces along the long axis of bones (Fig. 4-36). This may be beneficial, temporarily, with overriding fractures when muscular contracture is a significant concern. Additionally, the framed structure's crutchlike function

can completely protect the distal limb from compressive forces during weight bearing. The ability to provide traction and eliminate compressive forces affords the S-T splint distinct benefits over other bandages.

Despite these advantages and the numerous potential indications, the S-T splint is used infrequently by most veterinarians. Unfortunately, the S-T splint is difficult to apply correctly and, if misused or misapplied, can result in disastrous complications, including nonunion, malunion, or fracture disease. Use of the S-T splint is especially dangerous in the hind limb, where it tends to cause excessive straightening when applied incorrectly. Severe concurrent injury to the femur or thigh can predispose such a patient to quadriceps contracture (see Bandage Complications). As a result, most veterinarians prefer to use other bandages that are more easily applied and serve similar functions.

Body Splint

The body splint is used as a restraint device to prevent self-induced trauma to the caudal body. When applied unilaterally or bilaterally, the body splint severely limits lateral flexion of the head, neck, and torso. In this way, it effectively discourages patients from licking or chewing at wounds or incisions in the pelvic or perineal region. The splint is especially useful in patients in whom the Elizabethan collar restraint is not tolerated or is contraindicated.

Application. Body stockinette is applied in sweater-like fashion, extending from the neck to the cranial aspect of the thigh. Splints constructed out of wood or aluminum rod are fabricated to a length equal to the distance between the angle of the mandible and last rib. The splints are padded with cast padding, conforming gauze, and elastic tape and then protected with 2-inch stockinette (Fig. 4-37). The splints are attached to the torso, unilaterally or bilaterally, with 2- or 3-inch elastic tape applied circumferentially around the neck and caudal thorax. The body sweater is reflected over the ends of the splints and is secured with adhesive tape (Fig. 4-38).

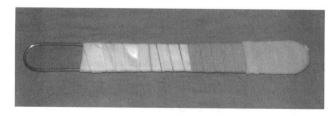

Fig. 4-37 Constructing side bars for the body splint. The aluminum rod splints are padded with cast padding, conforming gauze, and elastic tape. They are then protected with 2-inch stockinette.

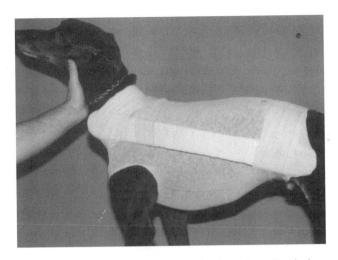

Fig. 4-38 Completed body splint with unilateral side bar. The splint is attached to the torso with 2- or 3-inch elastic tape, applied circumferentially around the neck and caudal thorax. The body sweater is reflected over the ends of the splint and secured with adhesive tape.

A unilateral splint is usually adequate for a unilateral lesion. In this case the splint is applied on the same side as the lesion for optimal restraint. Cast padding and conforming gauze can be placed around the neck and thorax, underneath the splints, to protect underlying wounds or to limit mobility of the neck more severely. Care must always be taken to ensure that the elastic tape or conforming gauze is not applied too tightly around the neck or thorax, compromising respiration.

MISCELLANEOUS CASTS
Soft Padded Cast and Bivalved Cast

A soft padded cast affords intermediary stability between a splinted bandage and a traditional cast. It is constructed by substituting elastic adhesive tape (outer layer) with casting material in the application of a padded bandage (see Thoracic Limb Padded and Splinted Bandages). Because of its thicker padding layer, the soft padded cast combines the key advantages of the padded bandage with those of the cast. The thicker padding provides protection and absorbency for underlying wounds while the cast layer enhances stability. As with the padded bandage, the soft padded cast can be used as a half-limb or full-limb application.

Indications. Specific indications for soft padded casts include tenuously repaired orthopedic injuries requiring significant protection postoperatively. These bandages are especially useful in situations when anticipated swelling contraindicates the use of a traditional cast. Other indications include injuries that require more stability than a splinted bandage affords but have accompanying open wounds that preclude the use of a tradition-

al cast. In these cases the soft padded cast lends itself readily to *bivalving*, in which the cast layer is cut into two halves and reused. After the two halves are carefully separated from the underlying layers, the padding and compressive layers are removed. The wounds are treated, padding and conforming gauze reapplied, and the two halves of the cast layer replaced and secured with circumferential adhesive tape. This device is called a *bivalved cast* (see Bandage Application—Cast Layer).

Walking Bar Cast

Aluminum rod, contoured into a U shape, can be applied to a cast's distal aspect so that the metal contacts the ground and protects the cast during weight bearing. The aluminum U, or walking bar, is positioned with the distal aspect 2 to 3 cm distal to the paw. It is attached to the cast with encircling adhesive tape.[10] The walking bar is used to prevent excessive wear to the distal aspect of a cast in patients who are allowed to ambulate on a hard surface.

The walking bar is also indicated to prevent or protect digital sores. These wounds occur especially in patients with casts that do not extend to the second phalanx of digits three and four.[8] In these patients, digital extension during weight bearing can cause repeated contact with the cast material, resulting in cutaneous injury along the dorsal aspect of the digits (see Bandage Application—Cast Layer).

REFERENCES

1. Anderson GI: Fracture disease and related contractures, *Vet Clin North Am* 21:845-858, 1991.
2. Arnoczky SP, Blass CE, McCoy L: *External coaptation and bandaging*, Philadelphia, 1985, Saunders.
3. Aron DN, Crowe DT: The 90-90 flexion splint for prevention of stifle joint stiffness with femoral fracture repairs, *J Am Anim Hosp Assoc* 23:447-454, 1986.
4. Bardet JF: Quadriceps contracture and fracture disease, *Vet Clin North Am* 17:957-973, 1987.
5. Bellah JR: Intertriginous dermatitis. In Bojrab MJ, editor: *Disease mechanisms in small animal surgery*, Philadelphia, 1993, Lea & Febiger.
6. Brinker WO, Piermattei DL, Flo GL: *Handbook of small animal orthopedics and fracture treatment*, Philadelphia, 1990, Saunders.
7. Clarke KM: Personal communication, 1994.
8. DeCamp CE: External coaptation. In Slatter, D, editor: *Textbook of small animal surgery*, Philadelphia, 1993, Saunders.
9. Killingsworth CR: Repair of injured peripheral nerves, tendons, and muscles. In Harari J, editor: *Surgical complications and wound healing in the small animal practice*, Philadelphia, 1993, Saunders.
10. Knecht CD, and others: *Fundamental techniques in veterinary surgery*, Philadelphia, 1981, Saunders.
11. Lesser AS: Arthrodesis. In Slatter D, editor: *Textbook of small animal surgery*, Philadelphia, 1993, Saunders.
12. Lozier SM: Topical wound therapy. In Harari J, editor: *Surgical complications and wound healing in the small animal practice*, Philadelphia, 1993, Saunders.

13. Peacock EE, VanWinkle W: *Wound repair*, Philadelphia, 1984, Saunders.

14. Smith GK: Biomechanics pertinent to fracture etiology, reduction, and fixation. In Newton CD, Nunamaker DM, editors: *Textbook of small animal orthopaedics*, Philadelphia, 1985, Lippincott.

15. Swaim SF: Bandages and topical agents, *Vet Clin North Am* 20:47-65, 1990.

16. Swaim SF, Wilhalf D: The physics, physiology, and chemistry of bandaging open wounds, *Compend Cont Educ* 7:146-157, 1985.

17. Tomlinson J: Complications of fractures repaired with casts and splints, *Vet Clin North Am* 21:734-744, 1991.

5

Principles of Fracture Repair

MARVIN L. OLMSTEAD
ERICK L. EGGER
ANN L. JOHNSON
LARRY J. WALLACE

One organization, more than any other, has influenced the art and science of veterinary orthopedics around the world.[1,2] This group, which originated in Switzerland to study orthopedics in humans, is known as AO International, and the veterinary branch of the organization is AO-Vet. The letters AO stand for the German phrase *Arbeitsgemeinschaft für Osteosynthesefragen*. In North America this organization is the Association for the Study of Internal Fixation (ASIF). Sometimes the two names are combined to become AO/ASIF. A very early working relationship between veterinary and human orthopedic surgeons developed in 1943, when Knoll, Willenegger (human orthopedic surgeons), and Jenney (a veterinary orthopedic surgeon) successfully treated a dog's fractured femur with surgical implantation of an intramedullary nail.[1] The AO/ASIF orthopedic goals of early limb motion and normal bone healing are well suited to the veterinary patient, since bed rest is not an option open to the veterinary orthopedic surgeon. Basic and clinical research by members of the AO/ASIF group is the foundation for many principles related in this chapter. Educational programs sponsored by this group have contributed to the orthopedic expertise of veterinarians worldwide.

Even the simplest fractures can be extremely difficult to repair successfully if the veterinary surgeon does not adhere to the principles of fracture repair. The objective of treating a patient's fracture is not only to have the bone heal, but also to have the body part where the fractured bone is located function as near normal as possible. For every fracture, more than one method of fixation exists that will give an acceptable result. The choice of fracture fixation method for a given patient is based on several factors. The surgeon must have a thorough understanding of the principles of application of each repair technique. Each method has advantages and disadvantages that must be considered when selecting the best technique for the individual patient and fracture. Other factors include the type and location of the fracture; the patient's age, size, and activity levels; the potential for owner compliance; the loads acting on the fracture site; the owner's economic situation; and the surgeon's capabilities. All these elements must be carefully weighed when choosing the method of fixation that will provide the patient with the greatest potential for successful fracture repair while being exposed to the least risk.

REFERENCES

1. Brinker WO, Hohn RB, and Prieur WD, editors: *Manual of internal fixation in small animals*, Berlin, 1984, Springer-Verlag.
2. Müller ME, Allgöwer M, Schneider R, and Willenegger H, editors: *Manual of internal fixation*, ed 3, Berlin, 1991, Springer-Verlag.

SECTION A   Primary and Auxiliary Implants and Techniques

Marvin L. Olmstead
Erick L. Egger

The veterinary orthopedist can choose from many different implants and techniques for fracture stabilization or repair. The implants and techniques available include intramedullary pins, external fixators, orthopedic wire, bone screws, bone plates and screws, casts, and splints. (The use of casts and splints is discussed in Chapter 4.) Except for bone plates, which are always used for primary repair, these implants and techniques can have either primary or auxiliary function in fracture stabilization. When an implant or technique functions as the *primary* repair method, it is expected to stabilize the fractured bone and to withstand or neutralize most or all of the loads generated at the fracture site during normal weight bearing and muscle contraction. It may do this by itself or with the assistance of auxiliary fixation. Implants with an *auxiliary* role in fracture repair are used to withstand or neutralize specific loads in a limited portion of the fracture site. They are always combined with a primary implant and alone cannot withstand weight-bearing or muscle-generated loads. The role of a given implant or technique depends on the fracture configuration and how other implants or techniques have been employed in the repair. Some fractures are repaired with only one of the previously mentioned implants or techniques, whereas others may need a combination of implants or techniques to be effectively stabilized.

It is usually not acceptable to combine casts and splints with internal fixation devices. For example, if a transverse fracture of the tibia is primarily repaired with an intramedullary pin and is found to be rotationally unstable, applying a cast to the limb is not an acceptable means of neutralizing the rotational forces. The application of the cast negates the benefits of performing internal fixation on this fracture. Early limb motion and controlled weight bearing are both compromised when the cast is applied. It is also impossible to check the surgical incision. The presence of the cast increases the moisture in the microenvironment around the incision. This may lead to complications with wound healing and infection. It is necessary to reevaluate a limb with a cast more frequently than a limb that has had internal fixation. A limb is also at a greater risk of developing complications such as pressure sores and fracture disease because of the cast. In some situations, however, the negative aspects of combining a cast or splint with internal fixation are outweighed by the benefits of combining them. These generally involve situations when implants that can withstand the loads generated during walking are not available. A good example is when intramedullary pins are used to stabilize a fractured metatarsus or metacarpus in a large dog. The bone is too small to accept an implant that can overcome weight-bearing loads, and a cast or splint must be used to protect the fixation from being overloaded.

Properly applying a technique(s) greatly increases the chances a fracture will heal successfully and the bone will be able to resume normal function. The principles of application of various orthopedic implants and techniques that aid in fracture stabilization and healing are covered in the remainder of this chapter.

ORTHOPEDIC WIRE

Orthopedic wire may be used as a primary means of fixation in some flat bone fractures, such as in the mandible and maxilla, but it never provides secure enough fixation to be used as primary fixation of long bone fractures. Wire is used as either a cerclage or a hemicerclage wire to secure bone fragments in anatomical or near-anatomical position. Cerclage wire is passed completely around the diameter of the bone, whereas hemicerclage wires pass through holes that have been drilled into the bone on either side of the fracture line (Fig. 5-1).

Orthopedic wire is made of 316L stainless steel, as are the other orthopedic implants typically used in veterinary medicine. Because of the way orthopedic wire is manufactured, it is more ductile (malleable) than an intramedullary pin of the same size. The most common wire sizes used in veterinary medicine are 22 gauge (0.025 inch, 0.635 mm), 20 gauge (0.032 inch, 0.812 mm), and 18 gauge (0.04 inch, 1.02 mm). Twenty-gauge wire is used in most medium-sized dogs, whereas the 18 gauge is reserved for large dogs and the 22 gauge is best applied to small dogs and cats.

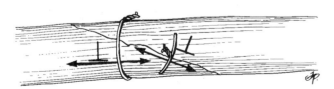

Fig. 5-1 Cerclage wire completely encompasses the outside diameter of a bone. It is oriented 90° to the long axis of the bone to give it the smallest possible diameter. This reduces the risk of the wire becoming loose as the animal loads the bone. A hemicerclage wire passes through 2 holes drilled in the bone's cortex. This wire is best oriented perpendicular to the fracture line. This provides compressive load to the fracture surface.

At one time, many incorrectly believed that applying orthopedic wire so it encircled the bone would significantly disrupt the blood supply of the healing fracture. It is now known that the failures after orthopedic wire was used as part of the fracture stabilization usually resulted from a violation of the principles of wire application. Properly placed and adequately tightened wire(s) should not be detrimental to fracture healing.

Passing Wire Around or Through the Bone

It is critical when passing the wire to maintain as much soft tissue attachment to the bone as possible. The soft tissues provide the blood supply to the bone during the early phases of bone healing. The wire may be passed around the bone through a special wire-passing instrument. The tip of the wire passer is kept tightly against the bone's surface while it is being worked around the bone. Once the tip is exposed on the other side of the bone, the wire is passed through the hollow center of the instrument and the passer withdrawn. The wire is left in place, passed around the bone. In another method for passing the wire, the surgeon carefully passes a large forceps around the bone. The forceps can be used to grasp the wire's end and pull the wire around the bone's circumference. Care must be taken when using either of these instruments to ensure that no nerves or vessels are trapped or traumatized by the wire and that the wire is positioned as close to the bone as possible (Fig. 5-2).

To pass a wire that will be used as a hemicerclage, two holes slightly larger than the wire to be used are drilled in the bone's cortex. These holes may be located in opposite cortices of the same fragment if the intent is to trap another bone fragment, or they may be located in two separate fragments (Fig. 5-3). If the holes are to be placed in separate fragments, it is best to hold the fragments in a reduced position with a bone clamp while the holes are being drilled. This will properly align the holes relative to the proper anatomical relationship of the two fragments. The loads created while the wire is being tightened will pull the fragments out of alignment if the holes in the bone segments are not aligned properly. The surgeon should be able to pass the wire through the holes in the bone while the fragments are reduced.

Wire Tightening

There are two methods for securing wires once they have been applied: (1) creating a locking loop of wire or (2) twisting the two ends of the wire around each other until the wire is secured. Several wire tighteners are available to create either the locking loop or the twist in the wire's two ends.

The instrumentation for the locking loop is designed to create a loop that secures maximum tension in the

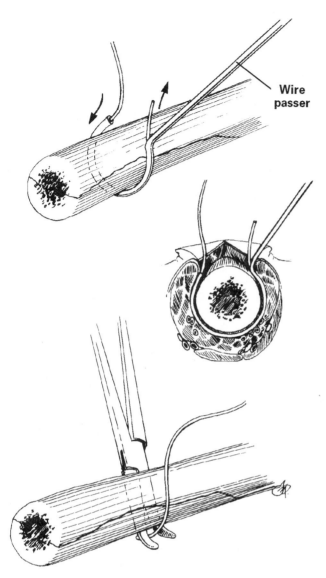

Fig. 5-2 Wire may be passed around the bone with the use of either a cannulated wire passer or a curved forceps. Both instruments should be kept close to the bone while they are being positioned to accept the wire, so important structures such as vessels and nerves are not encompassed by the wire. Wire should also be passed in a manner that disrupts minimal amounts of blood supply to the bone.

wire. The wire for the locking loop system has an "eye" twisted into one end of it, whereas the other end is straight. The straight end of the wire is passed around the bone, usually via the wire passer, and through the wire's eye. The wire's straight end is then passed through the wire tightener and the hole in the tightening handle. The handle is turned until the wire is tight around the bone. The wire is bent by pulling the strand coming out of the instrument away from the eye. Once the wire is bent, the tension on the wire is released by turning the tightening handle in the direction opposite the one used to tighten the wire. This exposes enough

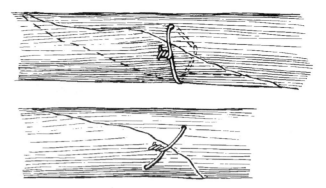

Fig. 5-3 Hemicerclage wire may be passed through holes in the same bone segment or through holes in the opposing bone fragments. Holes are placed in the same segment when the intent is for the wire to trap a long spike of bone from the opposing fragment. In such cases the wire is placed 90° to the bone's long axis to minimize the potential arch the wire can move through. When the wire is placed in the opposing bone fragments, it should be placed perpendicular to the fracture line to maximize compressive loads.

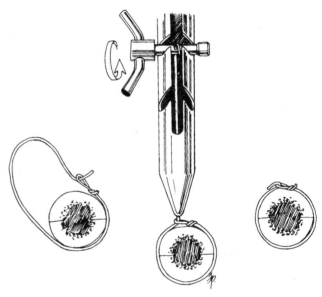

Fig. 5-4 The looped wire has an "eye" at the end through which the straight part of the wire is passed after the wire is placed around the bone. The wire tightener is used to create the smallest diameter, tightest fitting cerclage possible. The wire passing through the eye is bent over to lock the wire in position and cut off 5 to 8 mm from the bend.

wire to allow a section of the wire to be pushed toward the bone. This creates a locked loop of wire. The wire of the locked loop is cut 5 to 8 mm from the eye (Fig. 5-4).

The second method of securing the wire entails twisting the strands of the wire around themselves until the wire is secure. Several instruments are available to aid the surgeon in tightening the wire. Although specially designed wire-tightening instruments are available to do the job, I have found that an old pair of needle drivers with holes drilled perpendicular to the flat surface of the tips makes an excellent wire twister. The holes in the tips should be slightly larger than the largest wire that would ever be used. Once the strands of wire have been passed around the bone, they are bent 90 degrees approximately 2 to 3 cm above the bone. The free ends of the wire are then passed through the holes in the jaws of the needle driver, and the needle driver is clamped shut. Tension is applied to the wire during the twisting process by pulling up on the needle driver (Fig. 5-5). It is important to keep the tension even on each side of the wire. Otherwise, one strand of wire wraps around the second strand, creating a "barber pole" effect (Fig. 5-6). The wire position must be maintained at 90 degrees to the bone's long axis. The wire tends to rotate in the direction of the twist. If the wire is allowed to rotate, a wire loop is created that is larger than the bone's diameter (Fig. 5-7). This allows the wire to loosen during limb motion. Wire rotation can be prevented by placing the jaws of a large forceps loosely on either side of the wire. The jaws are used to block rotation of the wire during tightening, thus maintaining the wire's proper orientation (Fig. 5-8). When the wire twists begin to get close to the bone, the forcep can be removed. Tension while twisting is maintained by pulling on the needle drivers while holding the bone fragments still. When the wire's

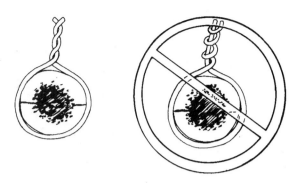

Fig. 5-6 The applied tension must be even in each side of the wire being twisted for the strands to properly interlock. When uneven tension is applied one strand of the wire remains straight while the other strand is wrapped around it. No interlocking of the wire strands occurs when this happens.

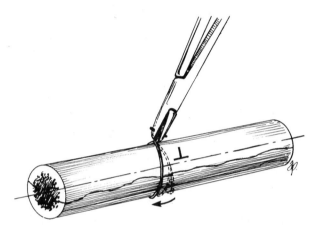

Fig. 5-7 If the wire loop around the bone is able to rotate while the ends are being twisted together, a loop with a diameter larger than the diameter of the bone results. This loop has the potential of moving when the bone is loaded and could cause fixation failure or interfere with revascularization of the bone.

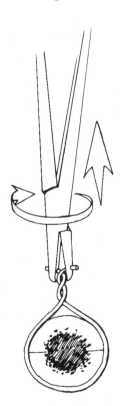

Fig. 5-5 Needle drivers with holes drilled in the tips are effective wire tighteners. The two free ends of the wire are placed through the holes in the drivers. The wire strands are twisted together by rotating the needle drivers while applying tension away from the bone on the wire and the drivers.

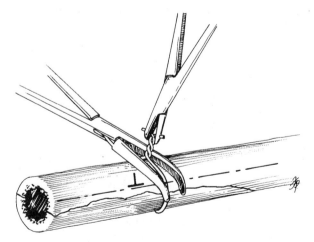

Fig. 5-8 The jaws of a forceps loosely aligned on either side of the wire can be used to keep the wire loop around the bone from rotating while the wire is being twisted. This technique helps keep the loop of the cerclage wire oriented 90° to the bone's long axis.

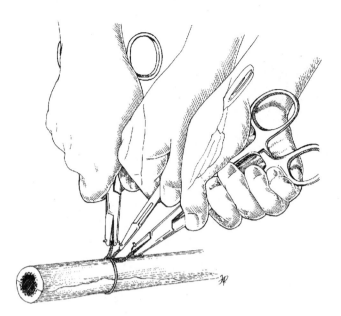

Fig. 5-9 Tension is applied while twisting the wire until the twisted portion of the wire tightly engages the bone's surface. The surgeon's hand and wrist continue the twisting motion in the same direction **without** applying tension to the wire. This causes the wire to lie flat on the bone's surface.

twisted part begins to engage the bone, tension is no longer applied and the surgeon's hand and wrist are allowed to move in the same direction as the twist (Fig. 5-9). This causes the wire to lie flush against the bone and helps maintain the tension in the wire better than bending the wire over. The wire is cut, leaving four to six twists intact.

When each wire is secured into place, the surgeon should check for tightness by pushing on the wire with a hemostat's tip. If any motion in the wire is detected, it should be replaced. When the fracture is completely stabilized, the limb should be put through a full range of motion and all wires again checked for tightness with the hemostat. Since a loose wire does more harm to the process of bone healing than no wire at all, any motion in the wire is unacceptable.

Numbers of Wires

If cerclage wires are to be effective in stabilizing fracture segments, the fracture line should be at least twice the bone's diameter. If the fracture line is shorter than this, the wires will cause fragment slippage. Cerclage wires should not be used on short oblique or transverse fractures (Fig. 5-10).

A single cerclage wire should never be used alone to stabilize a complete fracture. Fracture fragments pivot around a single point of fixation but are fixed in place by two points of fixation (Fig. 5-11). Thus the minimum

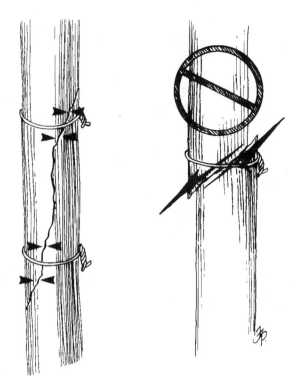

Fig. 5-10 To use cerclage wires in fracture stabilization the length of the fracture line should be at least 2 times the diameter of the bone and a minimum of two wires should be used. If the fracture line is shorter than 2 times the diameter of the bone, shear loads are created that cause the fragments to shift out of alignment.

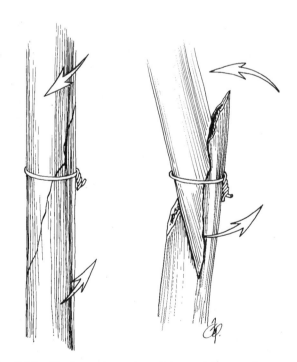

Fig. 5-11 Single cerclage wire used to stabilize two bone segments fails because the segments can rotate on the single point of fixation. A minimum of two wires should be used that are at least 1 cm from fracture ends and 1 cm apart.

number of wires that should be used to stabilize a complete fracture is two. The only time a single cerclage wire may be used is to prevent a fissure fracture(s) from becoming complete. If more than one cerclage wire is to be used, they should be placed at least 1 cm apart. The cerclage wire should also be placed at least 1 cm away from the end of the fracture line.

Preventing Wire Slippage

Because most bones are wider at the metaphysis than at the diaphysis, cerclage wires sometimes tend to slip toward the middle of the bone. Two methods exist to prevent slippage. A small intramedullary pin may be placed through the bone so that its tip just penetrates the opposite cortex. The end of the pin protruding from the near cortex is bent over to prevent pin migration. The pin is placed just distal or proximal to the cerclage wire, depending on which direction the wire would slide. Another method to prevent sliding is by putting a very small notch in the bone. The wire will slip into the notch, preventing further slipping. It is best to keep this notch as shallow as possible because the notch acts as a stress concentrator and could result in fracturing of the bone when weight-bearing forces are applied to the limb.

Hemicerclage Wiring

Hemicerclage wires act as sutures holding bone fragments together. To insert a hemicerclage wire, a hole slightly larger than the size of the wire is drilled through both cortices of one bone fragment or through a single cortex in two separate fragments. When the hole passes through two cortices of one fragment, the wire is used to trap a fragment in place, and the wire should be positioned at 90 degrees to the bone's long axis (see Fig. 5-3). If the wire is placed at a different angle than 90 degrees to the long axis of the bone, the wire may loosen. When the wire is placed 90 degrees to the long axis of the bone, it has the smallest circumference. A larger circumference allows the wire to move through an arc. When the wire is used as a suture to fix two bone segments together incorporating both segments, the wire should be placed 90 degrees to the fracture line (see Fig. 5-3). The loads generated when the wire is placed perpendicular to the fracture line and tightened are compressive. A wire that is not 90 degrees to the fracture line produces shear forces along the fracture line.

Figure-Eight Skewer Pin

The figure-eight skewer pin is a technique that combines a small intramedullary pin and orthopedic wire. Because the intramedullary pin is more rigid than wire, the frag-

ments will not shift when this technique is employed. A small intramedullary pin (Kirschner wire) is driven from one fragment to the other. The pin's tip is allowed to protrude 2 or 3 mm beyond the outer cortex of the far fragment. An orthopedic wire is positioned in a figure-eight pattern around the pin as it enters and exits the bone. The portions of the wire with the free strands should not pass underneath the continuous part of the wire that crosses the bone surface. If the free strand of wire is underneath the wire's continuous part, the continuous part will be elevated when tension is applied on the free strands during the tightening process (Fig. 5-12). The figure-eight wire is tightened as previously described for cerclage wires. Even tension must be maintained on the wire during the tightening process so that the knot ends up halfway between the entrance and exit points of the pin.

The small intramedullary pin is bent 90 degrees at its insertion site. To bend this intramedullary pin, it is best to move the hand chuck 8 to 12 cm away from the insertion point. The hand chuck is hand-tightened around the pin, and the pin is pushed toward the bone. Because of

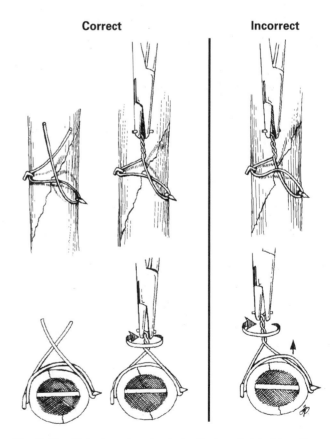

Fig. 5-12 If the free strands of wire that are twisted together are under the continuous portion of the wire, the continuous portion of the wire is elevated off the bones surface when tension is applied to the free strands during twisting. The free strands should be above the continuous strand which should be flush with the bone's surface.

the long length of exposed pin and the pin's flexibility, a sharp bend of the intramedullary pin is produced at the point the pin enters the bone. The pin is cut off, leaving 4 to 6 mm of pin exposed at the insertion site. The pins are bent to prevent their migration during the convalescent period. The pin cannot migrate forward because of the bend and will not migrate backward because it will be covered with normal tissue and fibrous tissue that develops during fracture healing. Tight application of the figure-eight wire also helps trap the pin by creating friction where the wire contacts the pin.

Figure-eight skewer pins may be placed at either 90 degrees to the fracture line or perpendicular to the bone's long axis. A decision is made at surgery as to which placement is the best to prevent slippage of the fragments during weight bearing.

Tension Band Wiring

Tension band wiring is used to stabilize avulsion fractures (Fig. 5-13). The tension band wire counters the tension created during locomotion in a tendon or ligament that is attached to a bone fragment. If these loads are not countered, they cause distraction at the fracture site. Since they are countered by the tension band, the loads are converted into dynamic (cyclic) compression at the fracture site (Fig. 5-14). Because wire does not easily stretch under tension loads, it acts as a direct counter to the distraction forces created by locomotion.

To create the tension band effect, one or two relatively small intramedullary pins are used to secure the fracture fragments in place and act as an anchor for the tension band wire. The use of two pins is more rotationally stable than a single pin, but some bone fragments are too small to insert two intramedullary pins. If two pins are used, they should be separated by at least 1.0 to 1.5 cm at their insertion point. They should be driven perpendicular to the fracture line and should not penetrate the far cortex of bone in the main fragment. These two pins are bent at 90 degrees using the same technique described for bending the figure-eight skewer pin.

A hole is drilled in the main bone fragment perpendicular to the long axis of the bone, which is slightly larger than the size of the wire used for the tension band. Keeping it taut, the wire is passed through the hole in the bone and placed in figure-eight fashion around the two pins. The wire should be straight and not arched between the hole in the bone and the pin. As the wire makes sharp bends at these two points, its length is fixed. The wire is tightened as previously described.

In some instances it may not be possible to have the wire lie flush against the bone because of the bone's conformation, such as the concave surface of the caudal ulna. The surgeon should ensure the wire is taut after the tightening procedure.

One technique allows both sides of the figure-eight wire to be twisted. This is accomplished by creating a twisting loop in the continuous strand of wire. This

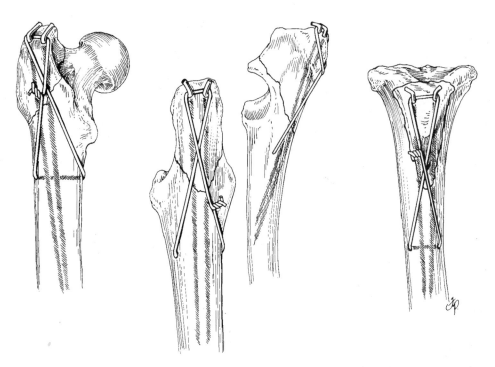

Fig. 5-13   Fractures or osteotomies of bone segments that are the origin or insertion point for muscles, tendons or ligaments are stabilized with a tension band wiring technique.

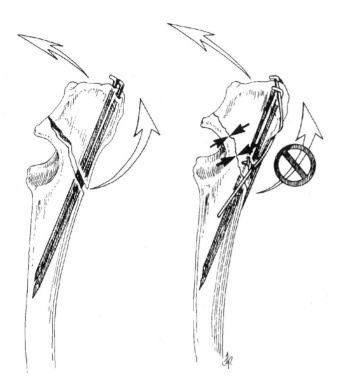

Fig. 5-14 Two intramedullary pins provide rotational stability, axial alignment of the bone fragment and an anchor site for the orthopedic wire. The wire provides the tension band effect by directly countering tension loads applied to the bone by muscle pull or weight bearing. If tension loads are not countered the fracture lines will be distracted. Countering tension loads creates compression loads along the fracture line.

allows the wire to be twisted in the part of the figure eight opposite the portion created by twisting the two free strands together (Fig. 5-15). The idea is that this will provide even tension in both sides of the figure-eight wire. Although the theory is sound, I have found that this technique provides no practical benefit over the technique with only one side of the wires twisted, as described earlier.

INTRAMEDULLARY PINS

Intramedullary pins are the most frequently used primary means of fracture stabilization in veterinary medicine. The most common pin used in repair of veterinary fractures is the round Steinmann pin, which measures 9 to 12 inches in length and 1/16 to 1/4 inch in diameter. Small round pins known as Kirschner wires are available with diameters of 0.035, 0.045, and 0.062 inch. The size of pin selected for a given fracture depends on the size of the intramedullary cavity, the bone in which the pin is to be inserted, and the type of fracture.

Intramedullary pins come with a point at one end or at both ends. The available points are the chisel point, the trocar point, or the threaded trocar point (Fig. 5-16). The trocar point has a better cutting action than the chisel point. The chisel point is less likely to penetrate the bone cortex. As an intramedullary pin for long bone fracture stabilization, the threaded trocar point has no

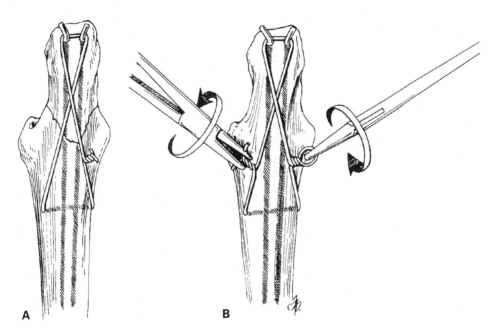

A   B

Fig. 5-15 Two commonly used techniques for applying the tension band wire exist. **A,** In the first technique the wire is passed through the hole in the bone and brought in a straight line around the anchor pin. The wire is pulled tight as it is bent around the pin, locking it in place. The wire is bent around the second pin and the free ends are twisted together. **B,** The second method is to create a loop in the side where the wire is continuous. This loop can be twisted as the free strands of the wire are twisted, tightening both sides of the figure eight evenly.

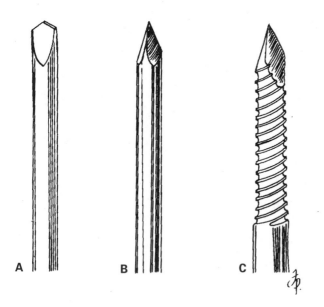

Fig. 5-16   Intramedullary pins have three different tips available: **A,** the chisel point **B,** the trocar point, and **C,** the threaded trocar point. These tips may be at one or both ends of the pins.

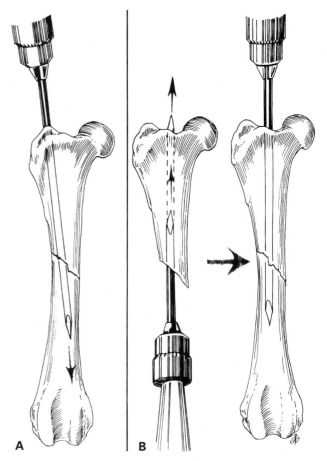

Fig. 5-17   **A,** Intramedullary pins driven in a normograde fashion are started at one end of the bone and driven to the other without changing directions. **B,** When a pin is driven retrograde, the pin is introduced at the fracture site and driven out one end of the bone. The fracture is reduced and the pin is driven to other end of the bone, thus the pin changes direction of advancement during the procedure.

advantage over a smooth point. In fact, there may be a disadvantage in that the pin is weakest at the thread/pin shaft junction, which often ends up being close to a fracture line.

Pin Insertion

Pins may be inserted in either a closed or an open fashion. With closed insertion the fracture site is not approached surgically. A surgical approach to the fracture site is made in an open reduction. Pins are also inserted either retrograde or normograde (also referred to as orthograde) (Fig. 5-17). The retrograde insertion means that the pin is driven in one direction, then the direction of insertion is reversed. To achieve this, the pin must start at the fracture site and be driven out one end of the bone. Once the fracture is reduced, the pin is driven into the opposite fragment. A pin driven normograde always goes in the same direction starting at one end of the bone and driving toward the other end without changing directions.

Normograde pinning can be done with either the closed or the open method of pinning, whereas retrograde pinning can only be accomplished in open-fracture fixation. Closed pinning should be reserved for two-piece fractures that are minimally displaced. With closed pinning the fragments are aligned by palpation while the pin is driven through the medullary cavity of the first fragment and into the medullary cavity of the second fragment. If post-insertion radiographs show the

fracture fragments not to be aligned properly or the pin inserted in an improper place, the fracture repair must be redone. It is generally easier for most surgeons to make a small surgical incision over a fracture site and visualize reduction of the fracture while the pin is inserted.

To insert pins into the bone, the pin is placed in either a hand chuck or a power driver with a chuck attachment. No matter which method is used, a sharp cutting edge on the pin is essential to reduce trauma to the bone and to ensure proper pin position. If a hand chuck is used, the orthopedist's wrist and forearm should move as a unit while the hand chuck is being rotated back and forth (Fig. 5-18). Driving the pin in this manner creates the least amount of wobble at the insertion site and forms a hole in the bone that is approximately the same size as the pin. If a power driver is used to insert the pin, the pin can be driven with no wobble because the driver can easily be held in a fixed position. To prevent thermal necrosis of the bone during insertion, the pin should not turn at extremely high revolutions, and excess force should not be used to advance the pin. Just enough pressure is applied to allow the pin to cut its own path in the bone.

Pin Position, Size, and Number

The angle of pin insertion influences its course through the bone. Generally the angle of insertion of most pins is parallel or almost parallel to the bone's long axis. If the angle of insertion is too large relative to the bone's long axis, the pin may traverse one cortex and penetrate through the opposite cortex without crossing the fracture line. If the insertion point is close to the bone's edge, as with the tibia, it is sometimes necessary to start a pin at a large angle to obtain adequate pin purchase in the bone. However, once the pin has purchased the bone, the angle of insertion is decreased until it parallels the bone's long axis (Fig. 5-19). If the pin is flexible, it

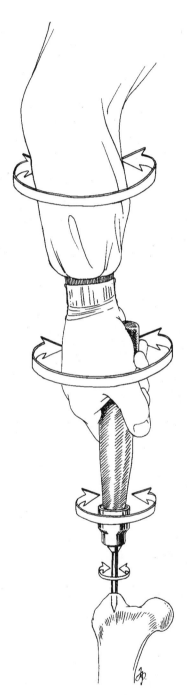

Fig. 5-18 When driving a pin there should be as little wobble as possible at the point where the pin enters the bone. To achieve this the surgeon's wrist and forearm should rotate as a unit in a back and forth motion.

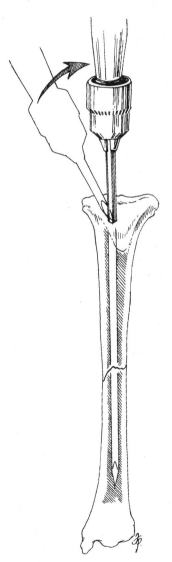

Fig. 5-19 When a pin is inserted close to the bone's edge, such as the proper tibial insertion site, it may be necessary to start the pin at a large angle relative to the long axis of the bone. When the point of the pin has adequately purchased the bone, the angle of insertion can be decreased until the pin is aligned properly with the intramedullary canal.

may bounce off the bone's endosteal surface, bending as it traverses the medullary cavity. The smaller the pin, the more flexible it is. The pin's tendency to bend gives it more endosteal contact points, which may aid in fragment stabilization. A stiff pin tends to straighten the bone fragments along the pin's axis and eliminate the bone's natural curve.

Pins that traverse the bone's length are usually inserted until they are embedded in cancellous bone. A pin should not be exposed at either end of the bone if this allows the pin to damage joint surfaces or interfere with joint function. The distance a pin has been inserted is checked in each case by several different methods. Aligning a pin of the same length with the inserted one and checking its position relative to the bone's ends indicates the inserted pin's position. Putting the joints at either end of the bone through a full range of motion while feeling for the pin scraping on the joint's surface or interfering with joint motion is another method. The final determination of pin position is made from at least two different postoperative radiographic views of the bone. If the pin is found to be improperly positioned or inadequate in any way on the postoperative radiograph, the patient should be taken back to surgery and the pin position corrected.

Once the pin has been inserted, it is cut off as close to its exit point from the bone as possible. An appropriate-sized pin cutter is used to accomplish this. If the pin has been driven through the skin, the blades of the cutter are placed around the pin. The skin and underlying fascia and muscle are pushed as far as possible toward the bone with the cutter. The pin is cut off and the skin pulled over the cut end. This is done at the end of the surgical procedure and before taking postoperative radiographs.

The size of pin chosen for primary fracture fixation depends on the number of pins inserted, the fracture configuration, the type(s) of auxiliary fixation used, and the bone involved. If a single pin is to be used for primary bone fixation, it must be of sufficient size to be able to withstand the loads generated at the fracture site during weight bearing. In some fractures it may be desirable to choose a pin that is the same size as the diameter of the bone at its isthmus. These fractures are generally short oblique fractures or transverse fractures with interdigitating spikes in either the humerus or the femur. When the pin fills the medullary cavity at the isthmus, the risk of segments in these fracture types shifting with weight bearing is minimal (Fig. 5-20). Pins of this size, when placed in the tibia or radius, tend to straighten the bone's natural curve more than is acceptable. For fractures of the radius and tibia, a pin approximately two-thirds the diameter of the medullary cavity at its isthmus is chosen. This size of pin is also more appropriate for more complex fractures of the humerus and femur. When

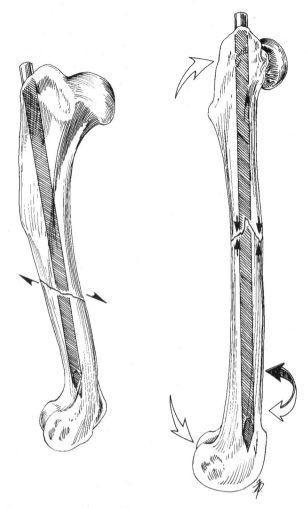

Fig. 5-20 In short oblique fractures a pin that fills the intramedullary canal prevents slippage of the bone segments when shear loads are applied. Transverse fractures with interdigitation are stabilized because the pin resists bending forces and provides axial alignment. The configuration of the fracture negates rotational and compressive loads.

the fracture is more complex, auxiliary fixation such as orthopedic wire and external fixators are added to this fixation. Thus the intramedullary pin is not expected to negate all the loads generated along the fracture line during weight bearing.

In the humerus and femur, it is possible to stack two or more pins in the medullary cavity. When stacked pins are used, their combined diameter should be approximately the same as the bone's endosteal diameter. Multiple pins tend to provide more rotational stability to the fracture than a single pin because more contact or fixation points exist between the pin and the bone. They also create less interference with endosteal blood supply than a single pin with the same diameter as the combined diameters of the stacked pins (Fig. 5-21). Most

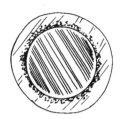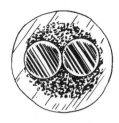

Fig. 5-21   Single pin with the same diameter as the combined diameter of two stacked pins leaves less open intramedullary canal and thus less space for endosteal blood supply.

often, only two pins are used for the stacked-pin technique because each additional pin is more difficult to insert. However, if the surgeon finds that the two pins do not provide the desired stability, adding more pins to the stack is an option. The stacked-pin technique accommodates better for the natural curvature of long bones than a single pin because the pins do not have to be inserted to the same depth in the bone (Fig. 5-22). Stacked pinning is not recommended for the tibia or radius because of the configuration of these two bones.

Pins may be stacked in either a normograde or a retrograde manner. In the humerus and femur, normograde-driven pins are inserted proximally at either the greater tubercle or the greater trochanter. The appropriate-sized pins are chosen based on comparison with the radiographic endosteal diameter and the surgically exposed true endosteal diameter. One of the pins is driven until fully seated in the most distal fragment. While the exposed portion of the seated pin is pulled out of the way by a surgical assistant, the second pin is seated. Retrograde pins are driven from the fracture site proximally in both the humerus and the femur. When driving the pins retrograde, both pins are simultaneously pushed by hand into the proximal cancellous bone. One pin is removed from the medullary canal and the other driven proximally through the greater tubercle or trochanteric fossa. The hand chuck is fixed to the pin's proximally exposed portion, and the pin is withdrawn until its distal end is level with the fracture line. The second pin is reinserted and driven proximally. It is withdrawn to the fracture line as the first pin was. The fracture is reduced and the pins seated in the distal fragments as described for the normograde technique.

Pins and Weight-Bearing Loads

Intramedullary pins help maintain axial alignment of the bone and resist bending loads. Pins alone usually cannot resist shear or rotational loads. If the fracture is transverse, compression loads are not a factor with the use of intramedullary pins. The two bone fragments have full

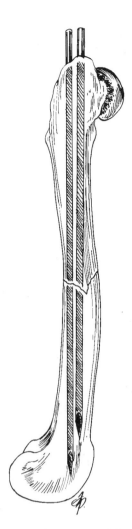

Fig. 5-22   Because the pins used for stacked pinning are smaller than a single pin used to stabilize the same fracture would be, the stacked pins can be inserted to different depths in the bone. When the bone curves as the femur does, at least one pin can be secured in a greater amount of bone at the distal end.

contact along the fracture line, and the fracture line is perpendicular to the compressive load's orientation. However, if the fracture is a long oblique or comminuted, compressive forces cause the fracture to collapse if only a pin is used (Fig. 5-23).

Often, one or more auxiliary methods of fixation are combined with the use of intramedullary pins to overcome the loads generated by weight bearing. Orthopedic wire and external fixators are among the most common auxiliary fixation used with intramedullary pins. In some instances the stacking of pins in the medullary cavity helps diminish the effects of rotational forces on the fracture line. Also, if the fracture fragments interdigitate well, rotational forces and shear forces may be negated.

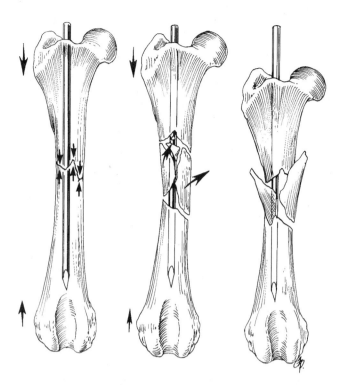

Fig. 5-23 A single pin is adequate to stabilize a transverse fracture with interdigitation because the fracture configuration controls those loads the pin is unable to. A comminuted fracture can not be adequately stabilized with a single intramedullary pin alone. The fracture collapses causing displacement of the fragments and shortening of the bone.

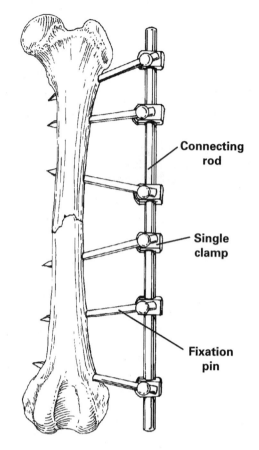

Fig. 5-24 Components of an external fixation apparatus identified on a single-connecting-bar type I configuration.

EXTERNAL SKELETAL FIXATION

External skeletal fixation consists of percutaneously introduced fixation pins that penetrate the bone cortices internally and are connected by linking components to form an external frame (Fig. 5-24). These components can be assembled in different configurations, each of which possesses unique mechanical and postoperative management attributes. External fixation can provide stable fixation of bone fragments with minimal additional damage to soft tissues and osseous vascularity while avoiding the need for implants in the fracture site or immobilization of adjacent joints. Consequently, it is particularly useful in complex fractures with vascular compromise or arthrodesis that require prolonged fixation. In addition, the low initial cost investment and wide spectrum of indications make the fixator particularly useful for veterinarians in the general practice setting.

History and Development

Parkhill[44] and Lambotte independently developed the first external fixators similar to modern devices around the turn of this century. In the 1930s, Hoffman and Stader, among others, developed the designs that are still the basis of many devices in use today.[28] Ehmer[22] modified the Roger Anderson splint specifically for veterinary use in the late 1940s and had it manufactured by the Kirschner Company. During World War II, external skeletal fixation splints were often incorrectly applied to human casualties under battle conditions. Significant complications were first critically reported in 1944,[45] and consequently, external fixator use declined in the United States for many years. During the last two decades, improvements in fixator design and application technique in both human[28] and veterinary orthopedics[4,10,16,20] have resulted in significantly fewer complications and increased fixator use.

Circular fixators were developed by Ilizarov in the 1940s and have been used extensively in Eastern Europe.[28] However, they have only recently been introduced to North America. Circular (ring) fixators use small-diameter, flexible Kirschner wires instead of rigid fixation pins.[33] These wires are driven through the bone fragments at perpendicular angles and attached under tension to rigid rings. The rings are connected together with adjustable longitudinal rods (Fig. 5-25). The device

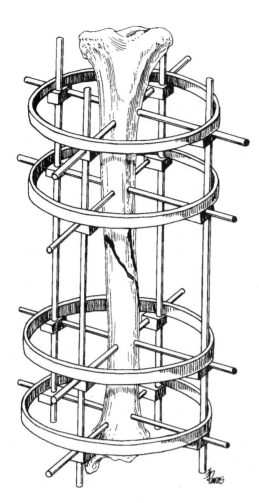

Fig. 5-25 Circular (Ilizarov ring) fixator.

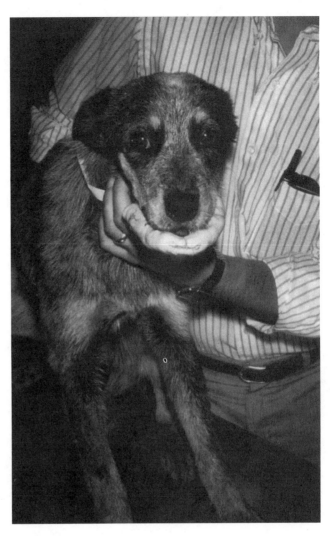

Fig. 5-26 Acrylic pin external fixator applied to mandibular fracture.

was originally designed for fracture fixation, but its complex application probably limits its use for this purpose. Circular fixators most likely have more potential use for progressive limb lengthening and deformity correction in the treatment of premature physeal closures. Reports of veterinary application are beginning to appear in the literature,[36,37,48] and one device designed for veterinary application is commercially available.*

Acrylic pin splints are external fixators in which the connecting clamps and rods are replaced by acrylic columns. They are particularly useful for mandibular fractures and transarticular application because the acrylic connecting columns are easily contoured to the shape of the body (Fig. 5-26).

Biomechanics

Any form of fixation must control disruptive forces at the fracture to be successful. The forces that act at any

*Jorgensen Laboratories, Inc., 1450 N. Van Buren Ave., Loveland, CO 80538.

given fracture depend on the fracture location and pattern. *Bending* is a force that must be controlled in nearly all fractures and can occur in all planes around the longitudinal axis. Experimental work has suggested that bending in the craniocaudal plane is the most significant with walking.[6] External fixators control bending well, particularly in the plane perpendicular to the fixation pins. *Axial compression* results from muscle pull and weight bearing. With oblique or comminuted fracture patterns, axial compression results in fracture collapse or overriding unless adequately controlled. With simple more transverse fractures, axial compression results in fracture impaction and increased fracture stability. The external fixator's ability to control axial compression depends greatly on the device's configuration. *Torsion* is the force that results in rotation if not controlled. Whereas long oblique fractures tend to resist torsion, comminuted or transverse fractures tend to be unstable in torsion. Fixators are relatively good at controlling torsion. *Tension* is the force applied by a muscle or ligament to a bony avulsion fracture and results in distraction of the fracture unless adequately controlled. Since tension tends to be applied to small avulsion fragments that limit fixation pin purchase, external fixation is a poor choice for controlling this disruptive force.

Once the disruptive forces acting at a fracture are determined, a configuration of external fixation can usually be designed or modified to control the force(s) consistent with anatomical and wound management.

Biomechanics of fixator configuration. The simplest configurations of external fixation use fixation pins that pass through only one side of the limb and both bone cortices and are called *half-pins*. The pins are connected on one side of the limb to form a type I (half-pin) splint. Type I configurations can be used on the humerus or femur to avoid interfering with the body wall. They can also be positioned to avoid soft tissue injuries on the lower limbs. The original Kirschner-Ehmer apparatus copied the Anderson splint[1] in using double connecting clamps and an additional bar to connect individual half-pin splints in each fragment (Fig. 5-27). This avoided the need for linear fixation pin alignment and allowed significant adjustment of fracture reduction after fixation application. However, clinical experience and biomechanical testing has shown that this double-clamp type I configuration does not provide adequate resistance to weight-bearing loads because of inherent weakness in the double clamp.[11,16] Consequently, its routine use for fracture treatment is not recommended, and its usefulness is limited to rapidly healing situations such as corrective osteotomies.

With proper application techniques, all the fixation pins can be attached to a single connecting bar (see Fig. 5-24). This type I single-connecting-bar configuration provides adequate resistance to bending forces for treating most relatively stable simple fractures in smaller animals.[11,16] Furthermore, this configuration is lighter and requires less expensive equipment. For larger animals or less stable fractures that must be treated with a type I configuration, a second connecting bar can be added to the same fixation pins, creating a double-connecting-bar design (Fig. 5-28). This nearly doubles the splint's resistance to compressive forces by converting the resulting bending force seen by a single connecting bar into compressive force on the inner bar and tensile force on the outer bar.[17] Two half-pin splints can be oriented parallel and at 60 to 90 degrees of axial rotation to each other. The two splints can be linked to form a triangular cross section. The resulting biplanar type I configuration (Fig. 5-29) is more resistant to craniocaudal bending forces than even full-pin uniplanar splints.[18] More importantly, the biplanar type can be applied to very proximal or distal fractures because fixation pins can be inserted from two planes.

Full pins pass through both sides of the limb and the bone. The pins can be connected to form a type II (full-pin) splint (Fig. 5-30). Type II configurations are very

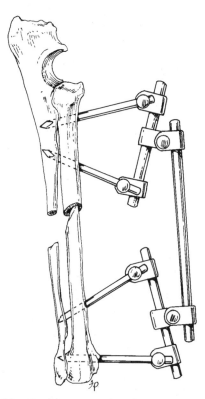

Fig. 5-27 Double-connecting-clamp type I configuration.

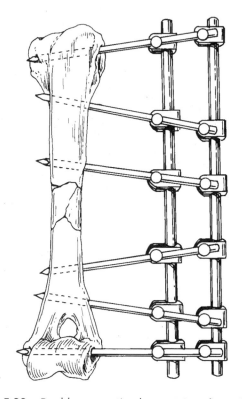

Fig. 5-28 Double-connecting-bar type I configuration.

resistant to compressive forces.[11,16] Therefore, they can be used on relatively unstable fractures. However, to avoid interference with the body wall, they are generally limited to use below the elbow or the stifle. Since it may be difficult to obtain perfect alignment of all full pins for attachment to connecting bars on both sides of the limb, many surgeons prefer to modify the type II splint by only using one full pin in each fragment, with additional half-pins inserted from one or both bars for adequate stability (Fig. 5-31). This not only greatly simplifies application, but also increases the number of fixation pins that can be used with the same number of clamps.

Combining a type I and type II splint forms a type III (trilateral) configuration (Fig. 5-32), which is the most rigid of currently used designs, approximately 10 times as resistant to axial compression as type I splints.[16] Consequently, type III splints are used for highly unstable or infected fractures, nonunions, and arthrodeses when the need for prolonged rigid fixation is anticipated.[23]

External fixators are most often used as the primary fracture fixation. Alternately, an external fixator may be successfully used in conjunction with an intramedullary pin,[24] which controls bending forces while the fixator controls torsional loads. Often the fixator can then be removed in 4 to 6 weeks once early callus formation occurs. To increase the montague's bending strength and

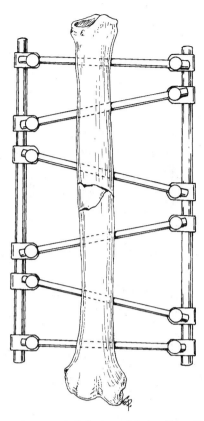

Fig. 5-30   Type II (full-pin or bilateral) configuration.

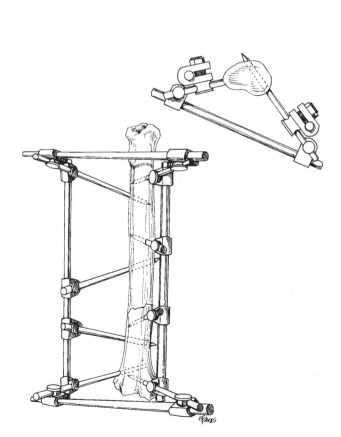

Fig. 5-29   Biplanar type I configuration.

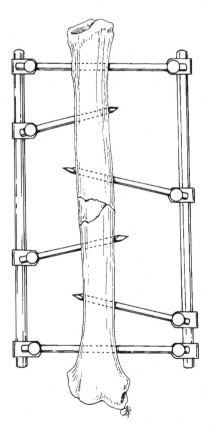

Fig. 5-31   Modified type II configuration, in which only two fixation pins are applied as full pins, making application easier.

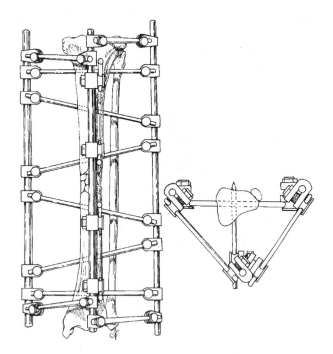

Fig. 5-32 Type III (trilateral) configuration.

further reduce the incidence of postoperative complications, the proximal end of the type I fixator can be "tied in" to the proximal end of an appropriately sized intramedullary pin using an additional connecting bar and double connecting clamps (Fig. 5-33).[5]

Circular fixators possess somewhat unique biomechanical attributes. Because the stiffness of fixation is directly related to the tension of the Kirschner wires that penetrate the bone, and because tension is increased as frame loading increases, frame stiffness is greater with larger loads.[33] Consequently, some motion occurs at the fracture site with relatively low loads, but increasing the loads results in a minimal increase in fracture motion. This technique is one means of obtaining controlled axial motion, which is currently being popularized as "dynamization."[30]

Effect of fixator arrangement on biomechanics. The number of pins placed in each fragment affects the fixator's stiffness. Although the exact effect of pin number depends on various factors, including fixator configuration and pin diameter, mechanical studies on a type II fixator found that increasing from two to three pins per fragment resulted in a 66% increase in axial stiffness, and increasing to four pins per fragment resulted in an additional 33% increase.[9] Using more than four pins per fragment had relatively little effect on stiffness. More importantly for longevity of fixation, increasing the number of pins avoids overloading the bone surrounding each pin.[12] Overloading causes microfractures of the bone, and the subsequent resorption results in premature pin loosening (Fig. 5-34). Consequently, in our practice we

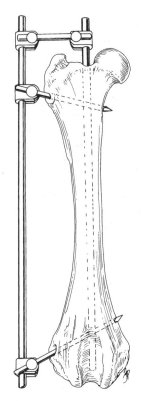

Fig. 5-33 Intramedullary pin "tied in" to a type I fixator configuration to increase strength and preclude premature fixator loosening.

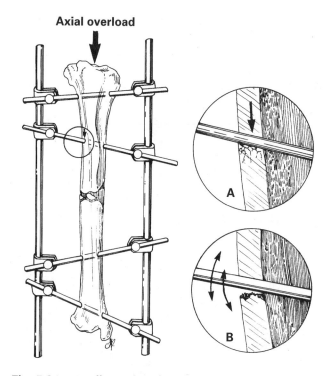

Fig. 5-34 **A,** Effects of inadequate pin number with weight bearing are overload and microfracturing of the bone. **B,** Subsequent resorption of dead bone results in a loose pin.

use a minimum of three and preferably four pins on each side of a fracture. The fixation pins are best spread over the length of the fractured bone to distribute the disruptive forces and maintain maximum fixator strength.[12]

The fixation pins' diameter is determined based on the bone's diameter. If the pin diameter is too small, the pins are too flexible and allow excessive motion with potential loss of fracture reduction. If the pin diameter is too large, the bone is weakened and pin hole fracture may result.[12] We generally select a pin diameter of about 20% of the bone diameter.

If all nonthreaded fixation pins are used, at least two pins in each fragment should be placed at a divergent angle to each other to maintain a mechanical grip on the bone. An angle of 30 to 40 degrees between the outermost pins placed in each fragment has been suggested as offering the best compromise between pin strength and bone grip.[9] The balance of the pins in the frame can be angled or perpendicular as most convenient. If threaded fixation pins are used, they can be perpendicularly oriented to the bone. This makes pin placement easier, allows placement of more pins in a shorter length without resulting in interference, and shortens the pin's effective length (from bone to clamp), which makes the overall frame stiffer.

As the frame is constructed, the positioning of the connecting bar must be considered. Some distance must be provided between the skin and the bar to allow for swelling and callus formation without encroachment of skin on the clamps. However, increasing this distance significantly reduces the frame's stiffness and strength. A good compromise appears to be about 2 to 3 cm for a medium-sized dog.[3] Obviously, this distance should be scaled to the patient's size and the device's location.

Traditionally, nonthreaded fixation pins were used with fixators.[22] One Steinmann pin or double-pointed Kirschner wire (for very small patients) could be cut in half to make two fixation pins. Much recent research has investigated the use of threaded fixation pins. Both clinically and experimentally, threaded pins offer a much better grip on the bone[4,7] and increase stiffness of the fixator[9] compared with nonthreaded pins. Although partially threaded (thread is cut into the pin shaft) Steinmann pins provide greater resistance to pin pullout,[4] the stress collector effect at the threaded/nonthreaded junction has often been the location of pin bending or breakage. One solution is the Ellis pin,* which is threaded only a short distance (about three times the pin's diameter) from the tip so the pin threads only into the far cortex, thus protecting the weak stress collector in the medullary canal (Fig. 5-35).[7] Alternately, pin designs with a positive thread profile, in which the inner thread diameter is that of the nonthreaded shaft

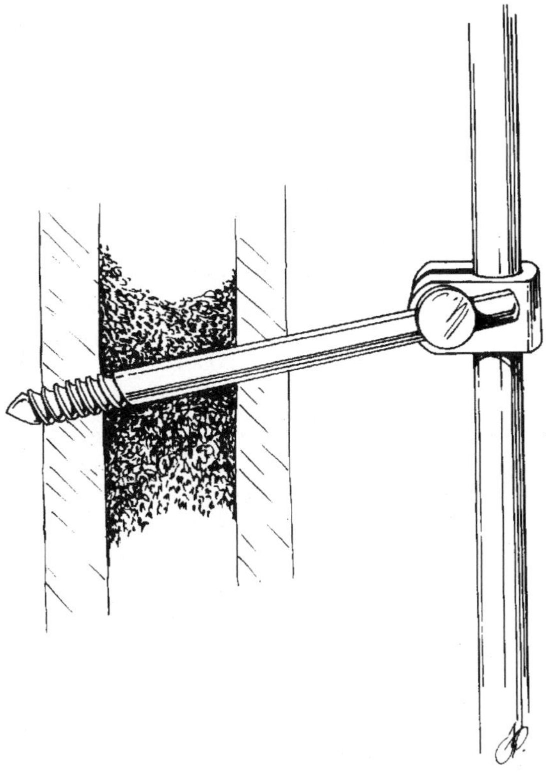

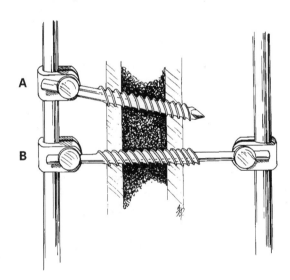

Fig. 5-35   Ellis pin, with its short threaded portion, places the stress riser junction within the protected medullary canal.

Fig. 5-36   Raised half-thread (**A**) and full-thread (**B**) pin designs offer enhanced bone holding and maximum bending strength.

and the outer thread diameter is greater (Fig. 5-36), have recently become available in sizes for veterinary application.* Clinical experience has suggested using a combination of nonthreaded and threaded pins to minimize the postoperative complications of pin loosening and pin

---

*Kirschner Medical Orthopaedic Division, 10 W. Aylesbury Rd., Timonium, MD 21093.

*Gauthier Medical, Inc., 3105 N.W. 22nd St., Rochester, MN 55901; and IMEX Veterinary, Inc., 1227 Market St., Longview, TX 75604.

tract drainage while maintaining fixation pin strength at a reasonable cost.[4]

Fracture Healing

The pathway of fracture healing depends on the character of the fracture and the rigidity of fracture fixation. Generally a fracture treated with a relatively flexible fixator that allows some interfragmentary motion heals with more periosteal callus proliferation. One group of investigators found that 1 mm of induced axial micromotion improved the healing of ovine tibial osteotomies.[25] This concept is also endorsed by the users of the circular fixators that allow some motion of the fracture with weight bearing but stiffen with more loading to prevent deleterious excessive motion.[33] Conversely, a well-reduced fracture stabilized with very rigid fixation often heals with direct crossing of the fracture by osteons and very little periosteal callus formation. Many studies have shown this pattern of healing results in faster return of strength.[38,52,53]

No "best" method of fracture healing exists for all fractures. Fortunately, the ease with which the rigidity of external skeletal fixation can be adjusted allows the clinician to manipulate the mechanical environment that directs this healing process. The current trend in human orthopedics appears to be toward some degree of interfragmentary motion or loading.[30] One such strategy (called destabilization[19,21] or dynamization) involves modification of an initially rigid frame to allow axial compressive loading of the fracture with physiological weight bearing once early healing occurs.[11] This should enhance hypertrophy and remodeling of the fracture while providing protection from excessive stress, which might impede healing or cause refracture. This concept is most useful in unstable fractures that initially require a relatively rigid configuration of fixation to maintain reduction. Our experimental studies have indicated that about 6 weeks after surgery is the optimum time for dynamization of fractures in dogs.[19,21] This can be achieved by removing the connecting bars and pins from one side of a type II or type III splint or by removing alternate fixation pins of a type I splint.

Current External Fixator Devices

Kirschner apparatus. In North America the Kirschner apparatus* is the most frequently used veterinary fixator. It is based on the Anderson splint, which was designed in 1934 for treatment of distal extremity fractures in humans.[1] In 1946, Ehmer modified the size and material of the design slightly, had it manufactured by the Kirschner machine shop, and introduced it as the

Kirschner-Ehmer splint.[22] Over the years the fixator evolved into the Kirschner apparatus, a device that is currently reproduced in four sizes. Three of the sizes are useful for small animal application (Fig. 5-37). The small device is used on cats and small dogs weighing less than 20 to 25 pounds and depending on bone size. The medium-sized device is used on most medium and large dogs. The large device is based on Kirschner's human tibial frame, which employs large, threaded fixation pins and can be useful on giant breed dogs.

The "heart" of the Kirschner apparatus is the single connecting clamp used to affix the fixation pins to the connecting rods. The single connecting clamp consists of a U piece (through which the connecting rod passes), bolt (through which the fixation pin passes), and nut (Fig. 5-38). All nuts, bolts, and the U of the small and medium clamps are made of stainless steel, whereas the U of the large clamps is anodized aluminum. Tightening the nut compresses the fixation pin to the U and squeezes it around the connecting rod, thus locking both simultaneously. This design allows the use of fixation pins the same diameter as or smaller than the hole in the bolt (3/64 inch for small, 1/8 inch for medium, 3/16 inch for large). Consequently, a variety of fixation pin diameters can be used with just two or three sizes of clamps.

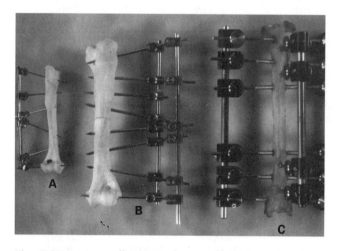

Fig. 5-37 (**A**) Small, (**B**) medium, and (**C**) large Kirschner apparatus.

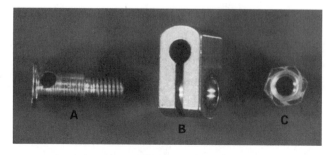

Fig. 5-38 Components of Kirschner apparatus with single connecting clamp. **A**, bolt; **B**, U piece; **C**, nut.

---

*Kirschner Medical Orthopaedic Division, 10 W. Aylesbury Rd., Timonium, MD 21093.

Selection of fixation pin diameter is determined by the patient's size (generally a pin diameter of about 20% of the bone diameter is recommended). For example, in fixing a tibial fracture of a 30-pound dog, ³⁄₃₂ inch fixation pins through medium clamps might be appropriate. However, the U design requires a specific connection rod diameter for each clamp size (⅛ inch for small, ³⁄₁₆ inch for medium, ⁷⁄₁₆ inch for large). Stainless steel connecting clamps are quite durable and can routinely be reused multiple times.

Double connecting clamps are used to attach two connecting rods. Using two double connecting clamps together allows universal adjustment of fixator alignment. They are therefore employed in construction of fixator configurations that allow manipulation of reduction after the entire device is placed. However, double connecting clamps are relatively expensive and heavy, and their mechanical stability is limited.[16] Consequently, their use is generally avoided or limited to rapidly healing, stable situations.

The small and medium Kirschner connecting rods are made of standard stainless steel stock, whereas the large rods are aluminum. Steinmann pins can be used as connecting rods, but this is actually more expensive, since the process of grinding trocar tips on the pins is a major part of their cost.

Acrylic pin splints. The first reports of acrylic pin splints used very long orthopedic screws as fixation pins.[41] The screws were inserted in the bones leaving the heads extended externally, where they were connected with dental acrylic. Commercial kits have been developed for acrylic pin splints in human orthopedics because of their ability to provide maximum support of difficult fractures and ease of application with minimum cost.[28] Use of these human devices for small animal fracture treatment has been reported,[29] but their size and expense have limited widespread application. Recently, a commercial system (APEF*) specifically designed for veterinary use has been developed (Fig. 5-39). The medium kit contains all material needed for construction of fixators comparable in size and strength to the medium Kirschner apparatus. The small kit contains similar materials for fixators and is comparable to the small Kirschner.

Homemade acrylic pin splints are similarly constructed using methylmethacrylate, which is available as hoof repair or dental molding acrylic.† The acrylic can be poured into molds made of thin-walled tubing or hand-molded around the pins once the acrylic cures to dough stage. Mechanical testing suggests a column diameter of ¾ inch provides superior fixation stability to a medium Kirschner apparatus.[51]

*Gauthier Medical, Inc., 3105 N.W. 22nd St., Rochester, MN 55901.
†Jorgensen Laboratories, Inc., 1450 N. Van Buren Ave., Loveland, CO 80538

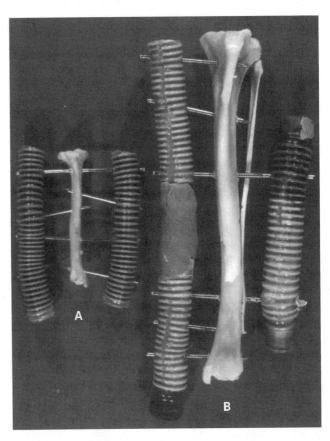

Fig. 5-39   Acrylic Pin External Fixation (APEF) kit creates fixators comparable to small (**A**) or medium (**B**) Kirschner frames.

Application of External Fixation

External skeletal fixation is easy to apply, but close adherence to several principles improves results and reduces the incidence of postoperative problems.

Although the bulk of the external fixation is outside the body, the fixation pin bone interface is usually the limiting factor in determining the longevity and stability of fixation. Consequently, the insertion of these pins must be done under the same aseptic conditions as would be used in placing any other orthopedic implant.

One of the most important advantages of external skeletal fixation is that it can be applied with little additional damage to vascularity and thus to the healing process. Closed reduction of the fracture minimizes such damage. Therefore, some clinicians prefer this approach.[35] However, closed reduction may not provide adequate fracture reduction or alignment, particularly with complex fractures or fractures located proximal to the elbow or stifle joint. Delayed union, nonunion, or malunion can result.[35] Consequently, we generally prefer a limited open approach to achieve better overall fracture alignment and reduction. A limited open approach also allows the placement of autogenous cancellous bone graft into fracture defects. Using either open or closed reduction, the standard guideline for minimal acceptable reduction is at least 50% cortical contact on the *worst* of two orthotopic (craniocaudal and mediolateral) radiographic projections.

As noted by Coombs,[14] "External fixation is only as effective as the pin contact with bone." Since premature loosening of fixation pins is the most common cause of postoperative problems, and even fixation failure,[4,26] attention to pin application is essential.

The method of pin insertion is important. In the past, hand chuck placement has been advocated to avoid thermal necrosis of bone from frictional heat.[4,10,39] However, wobbling with a hand chuck can result in oversized pin holes and pin loosening. Furthermore, hand placement in cortical bone is difficult work, often resulting in less than the optimum number of pins being used. Consequently, direct power insertion is preferred. Research has shown that direct slow-speed (150 rpm or less) power drill placement does not result in significant temperature elevation or premature pin loosening in canine diaphyseal bone.[20] However, excess pressure and high speed must be avoided. Predrilling the pin hole with a slightly smaller twist bit (about 90% pin diameter) is an accepted technique in human orthopedics[26] and should be considered in dense bone such as the olecranon.[4] Also, recent research has demonstrated that predrilling a slightly undersized pilot hole before pin insertion results in "radial preload" of the surrounding bone that, in turn, results in less pin loosening with cyclical pin loading, as occurs with unstable fractures.[32]

Before any pins are placed, the fracture should be approximately reduced so excessive skin tension does not develop against the pins when final reduction is achieved. When pins are inserted, they should be placed through small, separate skin incisions. This decreases the tendency for soft tissues to wrap up around the rotating pin and subsequent skin necrosis. The pins should not be placed through the approach incisions because this makes closure very difficult. When possible, the fixation pins should not penetrate large muscle masses and are of extensive soft tissue motion, since this is a common cause of poor postoperative limb use and pin tract drainage. The pins should be placed through the bone's widest diameter to provide the most strength and avoid cracking the bone. When applying a half-pin splint, the pins need to be driven so the tip completely penetrates the far cortex. The triangular shape of the pin tip tends to make incompletely penetrating pins back out and loosen.

In certain oblique and comminuted fractures, interfragmentary fixation such as lag screws and cerclage wires can be used to achieve better reduction. However, the manipulation required to apply these devices may damage vascularity and slow healing. In addition, rigid interfragmentary devices should not be used with a flexible frame configuration because they have a stress-concentrating effect.[27] This may actually cause further fragmentation of the fracture. We prefer to use divergent Kirschner wires. These wires can be applied with minimal additional soft tissue damage, and they provide adequate stabilization without the stress-concentrating effect.

General Procedure for Fixator Application

The general procedure for application of an external fixator follows.

1. Fracture is approximately reduced by either closed manipulation or through a limited open approach, minimizing soft tissue damage.
2. The most proximal and distal fixation pins are driven through small skin incisions into the two fragments at appropriate angles (Fig. 5-40, *A*).
3. Connecting clamps and a connecting bar are slid onto the end pins, with the anticipated number of "open" clamps in the middle of the bar (Fig. 5-40, *B*).
4. The fracture is reduced. With an open approach, bone clamps can be used to facilitate manipulation and to maintain reduction. In selected comminuted or oblique fractures, interfragmentary fixation may be employed to hold fragments in place.
5. The connecting bar is positioned far enough from the body to allow for swelling and callus formation without encroachment of the skin on the clamps, and the end clamps are tightened (Fig. 5-40, *C*).
6. If a more rigid configuration is required, a second connecting bar can be "stacked" on top of the first to create a double connecting bar, type I (half-pin) splint. Distal to the elbow or stifle, the second bar can be added to the opposite end of full pins to form a type II configuration.
7. The remaining fixation pins are driven through the open clamps at appropriate angles, usually alternating sides of the fracture (Fig. 5-40, *D*).
8. The clamps are tightened as each pin is placed, and fracture reduction is rechecked.
9. Excessive fixation pin length is removed with a pin cutter (Fig. 5-40, *E*).

Technique for Acrylic Pin Splint Application

An acrylic pin fixator is often applied with a two-stage technique.

Stage I (sterile)

1. Fixation pins, usually a combination of threaded pins for optimum bone-pin integrity and nonthreaded pins for economy, are inserted in the bone fragments (Fig. 5-41, *A*).

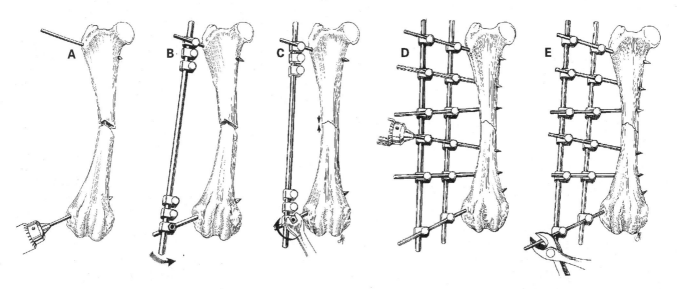

Fig. 5-40 Application of a type I Kirschner apparatus. **A,** End fixation pins are inserted into each fragment. **B,** Connecting bar with the appropriate number of clamps is loosely applied to the pins. **C,** Fracture is reduced, and the end clamps are tightened. **D,** Fixation pins are driven through the open clamps and the small skin incisions into the bone. **E,** After tightening each clamp, excess fixation pin length is removed.

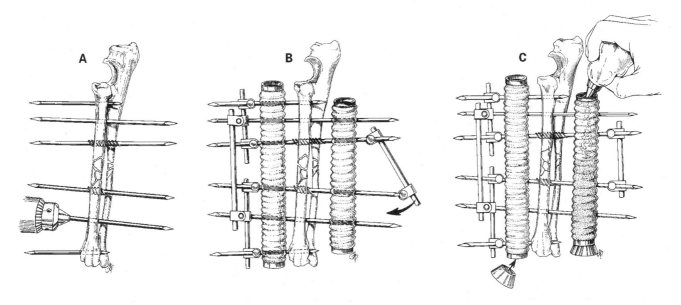

Fig. 5-41 Two-stage application of an acrylic pin external fixator. **A,** Fixation pins are implanted in the bone fragments. **B,** Acrylic column molding tubes are "impaled" on the ends of the tubes and positioned about ½ to 1 inch from the skin parallel to the bone. Temporary alignment is added to the end of the pins outside the molding tubes. **C,** Fracture is reduced and the alignment frame locked. Approach incisions are closed. Fracture reduction may be radiographically confirmed if closed reduction was performed. Acrylic is mixed and poured into molding tubes. After the acrylic cures, the temporary alignment frame is removed and excess pin length cut off.

2. The acrylic column molding tubes are "impaled" on the pin ends and the tubes positioned parallel to the limb about ½ to 1 inch from the skin (Fig. 5-41, *B*).
3. A temporary alignment frame consisting of mechanical clamps and rods is constructed on the ends of the pins outside the tubes (Fig. 5-41, *B*).
4. The fracture is reduced by either closed manipulation or a limited open approach, and the temporary frame is locked. The surgical incision is closed, and any open wounds are bandaged. Radiological evaluation may be used at this time to confirm adequate fracture reduction (Fig. 5-41, *C*).

Stage II (nonsterile)

5. The most dependent end of each molding tube is plugged.
6. The acrylic is then mixed and poured into the open end of each tube (Fig. 5-41, *C*).
7. The acrylic is allowed to cure (6 to 10 minutes), and the temporary alignment frame and excess pin length are removed (Fig. 5-41, *C*).

Postoperative Management of External Fixation

Hospital care. After surgery, distal long bone fractures are routinely placed in a compressive (Robert Jones) bandage to protect the incision and minimize swelling. Any open wounds or incisions are covered with a sterile nonadherent dressing, and roll cotton or cast padding is packed around the pins and under connecting bars. Additional cotton or padding is rolled on the leg from the toes to above the injury. The padding is then compressed with elastic gauze and fixed with tape (Fig. 5-42). In most cases this bandage is removed after 2 to 5 days. With open fractures or with severe soft tissue injury, the wound is often debrided, lavaged, and rebandaged every 2 to 3 days until it is covered with granulation tissue. Because of the stability the fixator provides, such frequent bandage changes can be performed without traumatizing early vascular proliferation and callus formation. When the compressive bandage is no longer necessary, it is replaced with a gauze and tape cover that envelops the fixator's connecting clamps and bars (Fig. 5-43). This cover protects the animal and the owner from the sharp ends of the fixation pins and decreases the incidence of entangling the apparatus on fixed objects. The cover should be applied so it does not contact the skin but allows air circulation around the skin-pin interface.

The use of antibiotic treatment with external fixation is still somewhat controversial.[45] A broad-spectrum antibiotic is indicated for contaminated open or infected fractures until a culture and sensitivity can direct more specific therapy. Furthermore, because of the soft tissue trauma attending even most closed fractures, we tend to use a broad-spectrum antibiotic for 4 to 7 days after surgery until the body defenses are mobilized.

Home care and follow-up. Most patients treated with external fixation can be released to the owner within

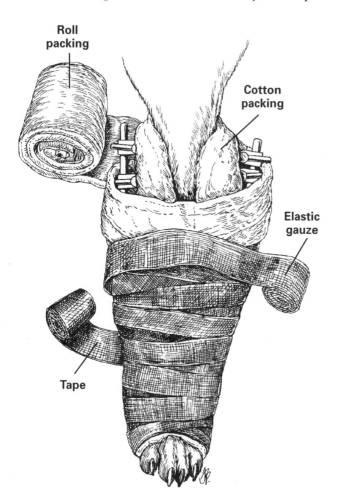

Fig. 5-42 Postoperatively, a bulky compressive bandage is used to control tissue swelling and stabilize the skin-pin interface.

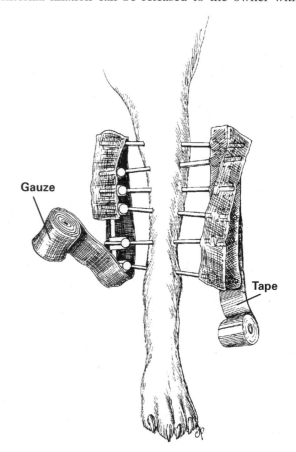

Fig. 5-43 Fixator cover constructed of gauze and tape to prevent entanglement and protect the environment. Space is left between the cover and skin to keep the skin dry.

2 to 4 days after surgery. The animal is released with instructions to limit exercise to leash walking and to take particular care to avoid fencing or other similar open structures that might catch the apparatus. Protection of the apparatus with a tape cover should be maintained until the device is removed. The owners are instructed to inspect the apparatus daily and advised to expect a small amount of dry crust to develop at the skin-pin interface. Although diverse opinion exists as to proper pin care,[4,45] we advise no or minimal cleaning of dry pin sites. Voluminous serous or serosanguineous discharge may indicate a serious problem (see Potential Complications). The patient should return for a recheck after 10 to 14 days for suture removal and to evaluate for loose clamps. Further rechecks are performed at 3- to 4-week intervals depending on the anticipated rate of healing, or sooner if problems develop.

Removal of the external fixator. When fracture healing is complete, the fixator can usually be removed with no or minimal sedation. The connecting clamps and bars are removed and the fixation pins pulled using a hand chuck or pin puller in a twisting motion. If threaded pins were used, they must be unscrewed with a Jacob's hand chuck. Full pins are removed by cutting off and cleaning one end and pulling through the other. Acrylic pin external fixator removal is achieved by cutting each fixation pin between the skin and acrylic column. Each pin is then removed using a hand chuck or pliers. After pin removal, a small amount of serosanguineous fluid often drains from the pin site, which can be cleaned up with hydrogen peroxide. The pin holes should not be sutured closed. Continued activity restriction for 6 to 8 weeks is usually indicated while the fracture remodels and the bone hypertrophies.

Potential Complications

Complications can develop during the course of fracture treatment when using an external fixator, just as with other forms of fracture treatment. Chapter 14 discusses general concepts of cause, avoidance, and treatment of such complications. Two complications unique to external fixation are discussed here.

The most common minor complication of fracture repair with external skeletal fixation is *drainage* around the fixation pins.[26] A loose fixation pin often results in pin tract drainage. The other major cause of drainage is related to excessive skin and soft tissue movement or tension against the pins. As with other complications, pin tract drainage is better avoided or minimized by careful attention to principles of fixator application. Treatment depends on the cause. A short course of broad-spectrum antibiotics and instructions for strict activity often alleviate minor drainage caused by excess soft tissue-pin motion and inflammation. Any skin ten-

sion against the pin should be relieved by sharp incision. However, if a fixation pin is loose, removal of the pin is the only permanent solution. Rarely, drainage persists after pin removal. This may result from a pin tract sequestra, which must be removed by curettage.[45] Soft tissue motion against pins and some drainage is unavoidable in certain locations, such as the distal femur, and additional activity restriction and cleansing the pin sites with 2% hydrogen peroxide may be necessary.

Loosening of the fixation pins in the bone occurs often with external fixation in veterinary orthopedics.[3,7,43] If too many pins loosen before adequate healing occurs, loss of fixation may result in failure of the bone to heal. Also, if bone resorption around a loose pin becomes too extensive, fracture of the bone through the hole can occur either while the fixator is in place or after its removal. Pin loosening is radiographically characterized by a lucent "halo" surrounding the pin and periosteal proliferation. Tightness of a pin can be assessed by loosening the connecting clamp and gently attempting to rotate the pin. Clinically, loose pins often lead to significant drainage and infection of soft tissues surrounding the pin.

Many factors can be responsible for fixation pin loosening. Most are related to application technique and can be minimized or avoided by careful attention to principles. Once a fixation pin is loose, little can be done to secure it again. Replacement with a larger pin in the same hole usually results in rapid loosening and a larger cortical defect. Loading the pin against one side of the hole by bending toward an adjacent pin again provides only transient stability before loosening recurs. If enough other pins remain secure, the loose pin may be removed. However, if overall fixation is in question or lost, additional pins should be inserted in new locations. This is accomplished by first removing the loose pin and the bolt and nut of the existing connecting clamp. The clamp's yoke is disinfected with chemical sterilant, and a new sterile bolt and nut are inserted. Finally, the skin is prepped and a new pin inserted using standard aseptic techniques.

BONE SCREWS

Bone screws are usually used as auxiliary fixation in combination with bone plates and occasionally intramedullary pins or external fixators in fracture repair. In some instances, bone screws may be used without plates as the primary means of repair, such as with fractures of the humeral condyle's lateral portion or fractures of the femoral neck.

Screw Types

Two types of bone screws are available to the veterinary orthopedic surgeon: cortex (cortical) and cancellous.

The differences between these two screws are primarily related to the width of the thread, the diameter of the screw's shaft, and the number of threads per unit of length of screw shaft. Cortex screws have a relatively smaller thread width, a relatively thicker shaft diameter, and more threads per unit of length than cancellous screws. The *pitch* of the thread (angle of the thread relative to a perpendicular orientation to the long axis of the screw shaft) determines the number of threads per length of screw shaft. Cancellous screws have a steeper pitch than cortex screws.

As the screw's diameter approaches 40% of the bone's diameter, the screw's holding power is significantly reduced. To accommodate the wide range of cortical bone diameters encountered in veterinary medicine, cortex screws from the AO/ASIF group have the following screw thread diameters: 1.5, 2.0, 2.7, 3.5, 4.5, and 5.5 mm (Fig. 5-44). All cortex screws are fully threaded throughout the shaft length. Cancellous screws have only 4.0 and 6.5 mm thread diameters (Fig. 5-45). Cancellous screws may be fully threaded or partially threaded. However, even when a cancellous screw is considered fully threaded, a small but significant nonthreaded area exists between the screw head and the start of the thread.

Screws may be either self-tapping or non-self-tapping. Self-tapping screws have a cutting edge at their tip that cuts a thread in the bone as the screw is inserted into the pilot hole. If a self-tapping screw is removed and reinserted, care must be taken to insert the screw at the original angle or it will cut a new thread in the bone, reducing the screw's holding power. The pilot hole for non-self-tapping screws must have threads cut in them with an instrument known as a "tap." Removal and reinsertion of this screw does not cut a new thread in the bone because the screw only engages the threads previously tapped. Currently, only the 4.5 mm cortex screw from the AO/ASIF group has a self-tapping version. However, it is expected other screws will eventually be developed with self-tapping tips.

Screw Functions

Cortex screws are intended for use in dense cortical bone, whereas cancellous screws are more appropriately used in either soft bones, such as the bone associated with a hypertrophic nonunion, or in the areas where cancellous bone is normally found. Cortex screws can also be used in areas where cancellous bone is found, but with a slightly increased risk that the screw will strip its threads during insertion.

Bone screws can have three different functions depending on how they are used in fracture repair: (1) plate screw, (2) lag screw, and (3) position screw. Fully threaded screws may have any one of the three functions, whereas partially threaded screws may function only as plate screws and lag screws. In some instances a screw may function as a plate screw and either a lag screw or a position screw at the same time.

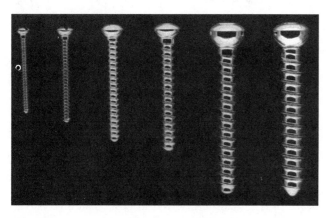

Fig. 5-44 A wide range of cortex screws are available. Named according to the diameter of their thread from left to right they are the 1.5 mm, 2.0 mm, 2.7 mm, 3.5 mm, 4.5 mm and 5.5 mm cortex screw.

Plate screw function. A screw has plate screw function when it passes through a plate hole and is used to secure the plate to the bone (Fig. 5-46). This is a screw's most common function. When the screw is tightened securely through the plate hole, the plate is compressed against the bone's surface, and friction is created between the plate and the bone and the plate and the screw. As long as the compressive load and the friction created by the inserted screw are greater than any other loads acting at this point, this part of the plate will remain securely fixed to the bone. If this holds true for all screws inserted through plate holes, the plate will remain fixed to the bone.

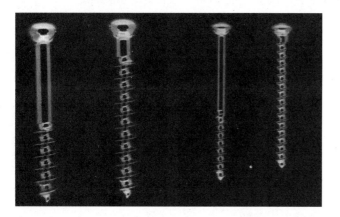

Fig. 5-45 Cancellous screws come in two sizes 4.0 mm (*right*) and 6.5 mm (*left*). They may be either partially threaded or fully threaded.

Lag screw function. A screw with lag function holds two bone fragments together and provides interfragmentary compression along the fracture line. Optimally,

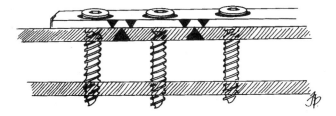

Fig. 5-46 A screw that functions as a plate screw secures the plate to the bone creating compression along contact points.

a lag screw should be placed 90 degrees to the fracture line to provide the best compression.

At one time there was concern that placing all lag screws 90 degrees to the fracture line in long oblique or spiral fractures would allow the fracture segments to shift along the lines of shear loads. Screws placed at 90 degrees to the bone's long axis would not allow the fragments to be shifted because these screws are the shortest screws that can be placed across the bone's cylindrical shape. With the bone fragments fixed by the shortest possible screws, the potential arc of motion for the fragments is the smallest arc possible. However, placing screws 90 degrees to the bone's long axis might cause the fragments to shift while the screws are being tightened if the compressive loads are applied unevenly along the fracture line. Thus it was proposed to have lag screws inserted at an angle halfway between 90 degrees to the bone's long axis and 90 degrees to the fracture line. For many years this compromised position was the guideline from the AO/ASIF group for placement of lag screws. It has become apparent, however, that this compromise is unnecessary. Almost all lag screws used in veterinary medicine are protected from shear forces by a primary means of fracture stabilization (e.g., bone plates and screws). Thus the sometimes confusing guideline that was used for so many years has been replaced by a simpler guideline that affords the best compression across the fracture line, that is, placing the lag screw 90 degrees to the fracture line.

For a screw to have lag function, the threads should only purchase (engage [engagement]) the cortex or cancellous bone in the bone fragment farthest from or opposite to the screw head (Fig. 5-47). One can easily see how this is accomplished with screws that have bare shaft immediately below the head. The bare shaft must cross the fracture line so that thread purchase is present only in the fragment opposite the screw head. In the diaphysis, this objective is achieved as soon as the screw threads clear the near fragment's cortical bone. In the metaphysis and epiphysis, the near fragment's cancellous bone must be cleared before compression is achieved.

If a fully threaded screw is to be used as a lag screw, it is necessary to drill a hole in the near fragment through all cortical and cancellous bone that is as wide as the

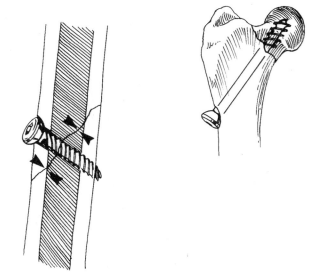

Fig. 5-47 For a screw to have lag function, the threads of the screw only purchase bone in the bone segment furthest from the head of the screw. When a cortex screw is used as a lag screw, a hole is created in the bone segment under the screws head that is the same diameter as the screw's thread. A partially threaded cancellous screw provides lag effect if all its threads cross the fracture line. Lag screws provide interfragmentary compression and increased fragment stability.

screw thread diameter (Fig. 5-48). This hole is referred to as the *glide hole*. The hole in the far cortex where the threads purchase the bone is known as the *thread hole*. The thread hole should be drilled with a bit that has the same diameter as the diameter of the screw shaft. The AO/ASIF bone screw systems require the use of a tap to cut threads in the bones that match the threads of the screw, except when a 4.5 mm self-tapping cortex screw is used. To be sure the thread hole is properly positioned relative to the glide hole, the drill sleeve is inserted in the glide hole until the far fragment of bone is contacted. This ensures that the thread hole is properly centered. The proper screw length is determined by a depth gauge. As the screw is tightened, only the bone in the thread hole is purchased, and the two fragments are drawn together. Complete tightening of the screw provides interfragmentary compression at the fracture line.

Position screw function. At times, placing a lag screw causes a fracture segment to collapse into the medullary cavity. This occurs when the two fracture surfaces can slide past each other and do not abut against each other when the segments are compressed. The occurrence is relatively rare. If the orthopedic surgeon suspects this will happen, the effects of compressing the fracture line should be tested before screw insertion. By carefully closing a pointed reduction forceps across the position where the screw is to insert, the fragments are observed to see whether compression or collapse of the fragments occurs. If collapse occurs, a screw with position function

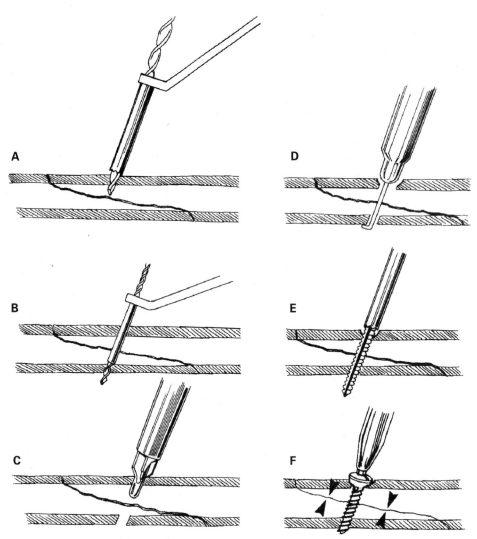

Fig. 5-48 The following steps are used to insert a cortex screw with lag function. **A,** A glide hole is drilled in the near bone segment with a drill bit the diameter of the outside diameter of the screw thread. The drill guide is used to protect soft tissues and align the drill bit. **B,** An insert sleeve is placed through the glide hole until the far bone segment is engaged. A thread hole is drilled with a drill bit the same diameter as the core of the screw. The drill sleeve keeps the thread hole centered relative to the glide hole. **C,** A countersink cuts a bevel in the cortical bone at the entrance point of the glide hole. This increases the contact area between the bone and the screw and decreases the exposed portion of the screw head. This step is not needed if the lag screw is placed through a plate hole. **D,** The length of the screw to be inserted is determined with the depth gauge. **E,** A tap cuts threads for the screw in the far bone segment. This step is not necessary if self-tapping screws are used. **F,** The screw is inserted creating interfragmentary compression as it is tightened.

is inserted (Fig. 5-49). In this instance, thread holes are drilled in the cortex of both the far and the near fragments. Both holes are tapped to the appropriate size, and when the screw is inserted, the position of the two fragments is maintained. An insignificant amount of distraction occurs along the fracture line when using a position screw.

BONE PLATES

Bone plates and screws are used to provide rigid fixation to fractures. If the basic principles of bone plate application are adhered to, this method of fixation most consistently allows the patient to have early limb function, which sometimes starts the day of surgery. Because the bone plate and screw system frequently allows a fracture

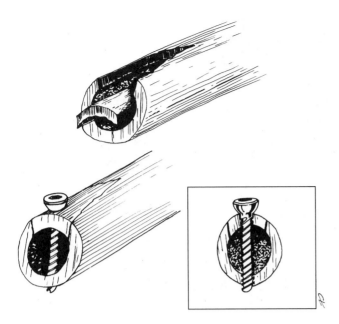

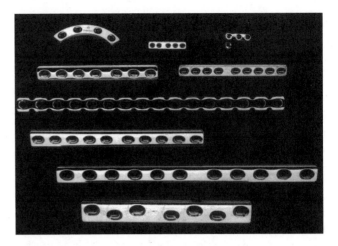

Fig. 5-49 Screws with position function purchase bone on both sides of the fracture line. This screw is used when compression of the fragments would cause one segment to collapse into the medullary cavity.

Fig. 5-50 Shown are only a few of the plates available to the veterinary orthopedic surgeon. Some plates are used for repair of very specific fractures such as the C-shaped acetabular plate (*top, left*), whereas others have more general use in long bone fracture repair. The type and location of the fracture and the intended function dictate the type of plate chosen for fracture stabilization.

to be anatomically reconstructed while providing compression along the fracture line, the fracture callus is usually minimal. Bone plating often provides the patient the greatest chance of achieving a healed fracture and normal function of the injuried limb.

Types of Plates

Many types and sizes of plates are available to the veterinary orthopedic surgeon (Fig. 5-50). Many plates are used for fractures in human medicine, but some have been specifically designed for veterinary use. The most frequently used bone plates are named according to the size of the cortex screw that is inserted in the plate hole, the configuration of the plate hole and/or plate, the number of plate holes present, and the width of the plate.

The plates used most often in small animal orthopedics accept the 2.7, 3.5, or 4.5 mm cortex screws. All the typically used plates from the AO/ASIF group have a plate hole known as a dynamic compression (DC) hole.* This hole is oblong and has a slope at one end. Screws inserted eccentrically in this hole create compression along the fracture line, as described below. Bone plates that have a width only slightly larger than the plate hole are referred to as *narrow plates*. Holes in these plates are arranged in a straight line along the plate's axis. Bone plates that are considerably wider than the plate hole are referred to as *broad plates*. Broad plates are also thicker than their narrow equivalent. The plate holes in these plates may be either in a straight line or staggered. The

DC narrow or broad plate has a centrally located wide metal section, which, whenever possible, is placed over the central portion of the fracture line. If the orthopedic surgeon selects a 10-hole, 4.5 mm broad DC plate, he or she knows that this plate accepts up to ten 4.5 mm cortex screws, that the plate is stronger than an equivalent narrow plate because there is more metal around the screw holes, and that the potential exists for providing interfragmentary compression along the fracture line with the proper use of the DC hole.

Specialty plates exist for specific areas of the body or for application to specific fracture situations. An example is the acetabular C plate, which comes in two different sizes, 2.7 and 2.0 mm. This plate is shaped like a "C" so that it can be more easily contoured to the dorsal rim of the dog's acetabulum. The reconstruction plate, rather than being a straight bar of metal with plate holes in it, like the DC plate, has indentations in the metal around each plate hole. This plate does not have a wide section of metal at its center. Because of its special configuration, the reconstruction plate can be bent in more planes more easily than the DC plate. The disadvantage of this particular plate is that the indentations in the metal make the plate weaker than a narrow DC plate of the same size. Because of this weakness, the reconstruction plate is used only for specific fracture situations. Very small plates in the shape of a T or L are available for fractures where one end of the bone is not long enough to accept at least two screws in a straight line. A very distal transverse fracture of the radius is a good example of where the T plate has application. Very small plates called miniplates are available and accept 1.5 and 2.0 mm cortex screws.

---

*Synthes (USA), Paoli, Pennsylvania.

Screws Used in Plate Fixation

As previously mentioned, plates are named for the size of cortex screw to be used in the plate hole. Cancellous screws can also be used with plates. The 6.5 mm cancellous screw can be placed in any hole in a 4.5 mm DC plate, and the 4.0 mm cancellous screw can be placed in any hole in a 3.5 mm DC plate. Because of the configuration of the DC hole, screws can be inserted at an angle in the plate hole. The maximum longitudinal angle is 25 degrees and the maximum sideways angle 7 degrees (Fig. 5-51).[7] The ability to place screws at an angle is necessary in some fracture repairs. It is also important to know that the next size of cortex screw can be inserted through the plate hole in any DC plate as long as the screw is placed perpendicular to the plate hole. Thus a 2.7 mm DC plate accepts a 3.5 mm cortex screw if the screw is placed perpendicular to the plate's long axis. This is helpful in saving a screw hole when the appropriately sized cortex screw has stripped the threads of the hole.

Plate Contouring

One of the important aspects of applying a plate to the bone is contouring the plate to the bone's shape. Contouring is accomplished with a bending press, twisting irons, or combination of the two. It is important to contour plates so anatomical relationships can be maintained as closely as possible. Taking a radiograph of the opposite limb in a view that is 90 degrees to the surface where the plate is to be applied provides a view of that surface. The plate can be contoured to the radiograph (Fig. 5-52). This can even be done preoperatively, after which the plate can be sterilized to help reduce the time taken to contour the plate during surgery. Slight adjustments usually have to be made to the precontoured plate once it is applied to the bone. Another technique that helps in contouring the plate is first to reduce the fracture and then mold an aluminum template to the bone's shape. The template can then be used as a guide for contouring the plate.

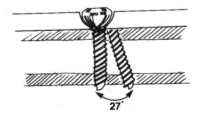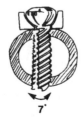

Fig. 5-51 Screws may be tilted in the Dynamic Compression Plate Holes. Tilting the screw is used to avoid fracture lines and to achieve a more favorable angle when placing a lag screw.

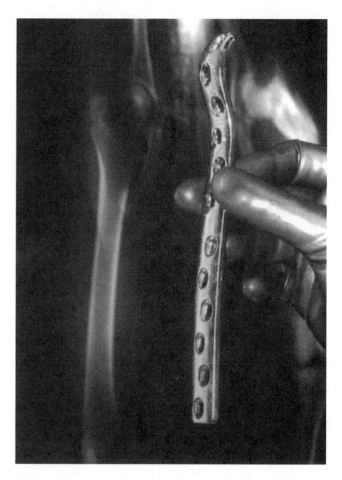

Fig. 5-52 Contouring the plate to the bone's normal anatomic configuration is critical in successful fracture stabilization. One method used to aid the surgeon in this process is taking a radiograph of the opposite normal bone. The radiograph should be oriented 90° to the surface the plate will be applied to.

When contouring the plate, bends must be made along a given length of the plate rather than concentrating the bend at one spot in the plate. The bends and curves in most bones are spread out over a portion of the bone, and thus the bends and curves in the plate should be spread out over the plate. It is sometimes necessary to put a twist in the plate to match a slope of the bone, particularly with the lateral humeral shaft. A plate that is not properly contoured can result in a malunion. If the malunion is great enough, significant alterations in anatomy result and may affect the function of other body parts. For example, a malunion of a femoral fracture may cause abnormal loading of either the stifle or the hock joint. A malunion of the mandible will cause uneven teeth wear because of malocclusion.

Number of Screws in a Plate

The number of screws in the plate on either side of the fracture line is very important to the rigid fixation of a fracture. A main fracture fragment under one end of the plate should never have just one screw in it. This fragment will have only one point of fixation, around which it can still rotate. To stop this fragment from rotating, it must have at least two points of fixation and thus at least two screws through two plate holes. Placing two screws beyond the fracture line in either end of the plate establishes axial alignment of two main bone fragments. If the mechanical loads acting at the fracture line are potentially high, as occurs with diaphyseal fractures, two screws per fragment are not adequate. In such a case a minimum of three screws should be present in a fragment (Fig. 5-53). However, if the distances between the ends of the bone and the fracture line are insufficient to allow three screws to be placed in the bone fragment, the minimum number of screws in a fragment becomes two, ensuring axial alignment of the fragment.

Once the two screws are placed at either end of the plate, establishing axial alignment, the next most important screw is the one placed closest to the fracture line. This screw negates the forces that act at the fracture line. A recent study using a 10-hole plate found no difference in the plate's ability to resist compressive forces when all 10 screw holes were filled versus filling the hole next to the fracture line and the two end holes in each segment, leaving two holes empty in each segment.[3] The plate's ability to resist compressive forces is significantly reduced if the third screw is placed in any hole other than the one directly next to the fracture gap.

Placement of Screws Through the Plate

In most instances the screw should be inserted through a pilot hole in both the near and the far cortices. This gives maximum screw purchase. The pilot hole is drilled through the appropriate drill guide, which is centered in the plate hole. (The various drill guides are discussed under Plate Function.) A depth gauge is used to measure the length of screw that will be inserted. A tap cuts the threads for the screw. The tap is inserted through the tap guide and turned continuously in one direction to cut the threads in the cortical bone. Periodically reversing the tap, which is sometimes done in human and equine bone, is not necessary in dog bone, which is relatively

thin and thus never allows debris to build up in the tap. Once the hole is tapped, the screw is inserted.

Occasionally it is necessary to place a screw through only one cortex. If the position of a lag screw outside the plate or the position of the fracture line indicates that the far end of the screw tip will either hit the lag screw or embed in the fracture line, and if good cortex exists underneath the plate, a short screw should be inserted that engages only the near cortex. In some instances there is a fracture gap underneath the plate hole but bone can be engaged in the far cortex. A screw that purchases the opposite cortex is placed through this plate hole. Plate holes are left empty if fracture lines in both the near and the far cortices lie where the screw would be placed, or if no solid bone exists in either the near or the far cortex under the plate hole.

Plate Function

Although many different types of bone plates are available, plate function cannot be determined until the plate is applied to a fracture situation. The types of possible plate function include (1) static compressive, (2) dynamic compressive, (3) neutralization, and (4) buttress. A bone plate can have one or more of these functions depending on its application.

Static and dynamic compressive functions. Short oblique or transverse fractures are repaired with plates that have static and/or dynamic compressive function. Static compression is applied at surgery. This is achieved by using the tension device, employing plate hole geometry, or prestressing the plate. All three of these techniques provide constant compression at the fracture site. Dynamic compressive function is achieved through the action of the animal's muscles and weight bearing. Plates with this function must be placed on the bone's tension side. Dynamic compression is cyclic in nature. A plate may have both static and dynamic compressive function at the same time.

The tension device is infrequently used because it requires an extended incision and extra equipment. Also, only the 4.5 mm plates accept the device. This device is attached to the end of the plate, and the plate is fixed to

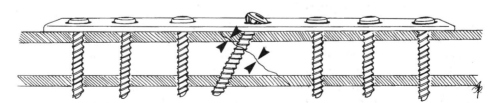

Fig. 5-53 The ideal minimum number of screws in each bone segment on either side of the fracture line for fractures of the shaft of long bones is three. In this example a lag screw through the plate was also used. Since it crossed the fracture line it did not count as one of the minimum three screws for either segment.

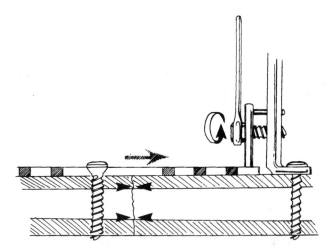

Fig. 5-54 Static compression can be applied to the fracture line with the use of the tension device. Use of this instrument requires a longer incision, enough bone beyond the plate to allow its application and application of a 4.5 mm bone plate. The most common use of the tension device is for compressing nonunions in large dogs.

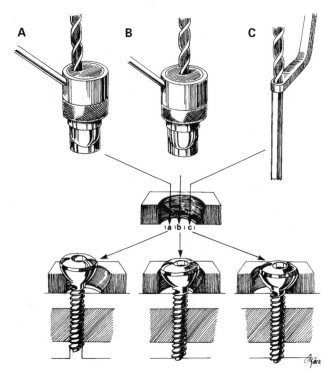

Fig. 5-55 The plate hole for Dynamic Compression Plate is depicted in the center of the illustration. There is a glide slope on the left side of the hole and a steep buttress wall on the right. **A,** When the load guide, which has a yellow central band, is used in the plate hole the screw starts in an eccentric position when it engages the plate. Tightening this screw provides static compression along the fracture line. **B,** The neutral guide, which has a green central band, places the screw in the center of the plate hole. Tightening this screw secures the plate to the bone but does not apply significant compression to the fracture line. **C,** The drill sleeve is used to place the screw in the buttress position. The head of the screw engages the steep buttress wall of the plate hole when it is inserted in this position.

the far bone fragment (Fig. 5-54). As the nut on the tension device is tightened, compression is created along the fracture line. The device is capable of providing a large amount of compression and can close a large gap. It is most effective in compressing a nonunion where the bone is very soft.

The most common way to provide static compression is with the mechanics of the plate hole in a Dynamic Compression Plate (DCP). (Dynamic Compression Plate is a trade name and does not reflect plate function. The DCP can have any of the four functions.) The hole is oblong with a glide slope at one end and a steep wall at the other (Fig. 5-55). The glide slope is located farthest from the central thick portion of the plate.

Two drill guides are designed to fit congruently in the plate hole of the DCP. One is banded with a green color and known as the *neutral guide*. When this guide is used, the pilot hole for the screw is located in the center of the plate hole (Fig. 5-55, *B*). A screw inserted in this hole in an anatomically contoured plate would secure the plate to the bone but would not significantly compress the fracture line.

Compression along the fracture line is achieved with the yellow-banded *load guide*. The plate is first fixed to the bone segment farthest from the hole to be loaded, using one or more bone screws. Any hole in the plate can be used to provide compression, but surgeons generally choose a hole close to the fracture line. The bone segment not secured to the plate by screws is fixed in proper alignment with bone clamps. The arrow on the load guide should point toward the fracture line. Centering the load guide in the plate hole when drilling

causes the screw pilot hole to be eccentrically located in the hole near the beginning of the glide slope (Fig. 5-55, *A*). When the screw is tightened, it engages the plate's edge at the glide slope. As the tightening of the screw continues, the plate on the side of the fracture where the screw is being inserted is pushed away from the fracture line. This pulls the plate and attached bone of the opposite segment toward the fracture line. The final tightening of the screw leaves the screw head in the center of the plate hole but not against the steep wall of the hole (Fig. 5-56). If the fracture is anatomically reduced, static compression is achieved at the fracture line. The screw head in the hole just loaded moves against the steep wall of the plate hole if a second screw is inserted in a loaded fashion. Thus, this procedure can be done two times on either side of the thick part of the DC plate. In 3.5 and

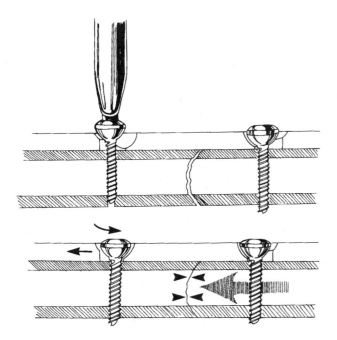

Fig. 5-56   If static compression of the fracture line is to be achieved using the load guide, one of the bone segments is first fixed to the plate with a screw or screws in the neutral position. The other bone segment is reduced and the load guide is used to eccentrically place a screw in the plate hole. The load screw engages the edge of the plate hole first. As the screw is tightened and slides along the glide slope, it moves the plate and the attached opposite bone segment closer to its position. If the gap between the segments is less than 1 mm, compression is achieved as the fracture surfaces are forced together.

4.5 mm plates, the plate is moved 1.0 mm each time the load guide is used, and 0.8 mm of movement occurs in the 2.7 mm plates.

Prestressing the plate indicates a slight overbend in the plate at the fracture line (Fig. 5-57). The overbend in an otherwise anatomically contoured plate creates a 1.0 to 2.0 mm gap between the plate and bone. The bone should be aligned as anatomically as possible with bone clamps before the plate is fixed to it. The plate is fixed to the bone through the end screw holes first, and the addition of subsequent screws to the fixation pulls the bone fragments toward the plate and into contact with each other. This causes the gap along the far cortex to close as the screws are tightened, which in turn creates static compression along the fracture line as the opposing cortices engage each other.

Dynamic compressive function is achieved during weight bearing and when muscles pull on the bone if the plate is applied to the bone's tension side (Fig. 5-58). This concept is most clearly understood when the eccentrically loaded femur is plated. Also, this principle is best applied to transverse or short oblique fractures because the cortical surfaces of the fragments can be anatomically reduced without any gap present. Any gap in the reduced fracture segments, especially in the cortex farthest from the plate, increases the load on the plate and can lead to cyclical failure of the plate. Since metal resists tension loads very well, a plate properly applied to the bone's tension side counters the tension loads created during weight bearing and muscle contraction. Compression is present along the congruent bone surfaces of the two fragments. The compression increases and decreases as the bone is loaded and

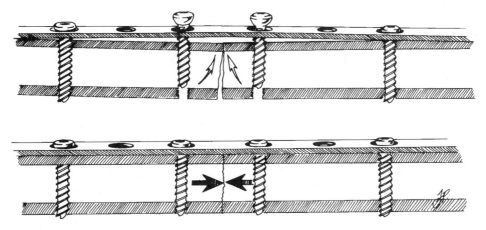

Fig. 5-57   The plate is prestressed if a slight overbend at the fracture site is applied to it in the contouring process. This creates a 1 to 2 mm gap between the plate and the bone when the first screws are put in the ends of the plate. Placing the screws next to the fracture line pulls the bone up to the plate and creates static compression along the fracture line. The fracture segments need to be reduced almost anatomically for compression to be achieved.

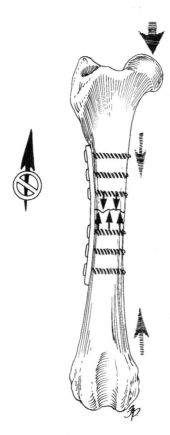

Fig. 5-58 By applying the plate to the tension side of the bone, dynamic compression at the anatomically reduced fracture line is achieved during weight bearing and when muscles are contracted on the side of the bone opposite the plate.

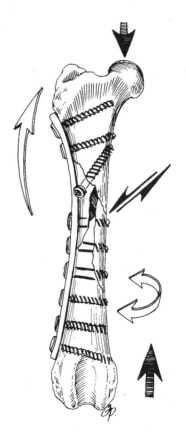

Fig. 5-59 The most common function for a plate to have is that of neutralization. The load transmission surfaces of the bone must be anatomically reconstructed and securely stabilized (usually with lag screws). The plate transmits most loads from one end to the other while protecting the reconstructed fracture.

unloaded, making it dynamic (cyclic) in nature. If a bone plate is applied to the tension side of a bone with a transverse fracture, and if static compression is created by one of the previously mentioned methods, the plate has both static and dynamic compressive functions.

Neutralization function. Neutralization function is the most common bone plate function. For a plate to have neutralization function, the fracture must be anatomically reconstructed so that load transmission points exist throughout the bone's length and the main fracture fragments are rigidly fixed, generally with the use of lag screws (Fig. 5-59). Cerclage wire reconstruction of a fracture that securely fixes the fragments and allows load transmission through the bone can also be protected by a plate with neutralization function. The plate protects the fracture fixation from loads generated during weight bearing and muscle contraction. However, the neutralization plate does not have to resist all the functional loads because the bone's load transmission surfaces have been reconstructed and stabilized with interfragmentary compression or cerclage wire. Small bone fragments that do not contribute to load transmission through the bone do not need to be reduced for a plate to have neutralization

function. Static compression can be achieved at the fracture line by application of the load guide in the DC plate hole. However, this is seldom done because applying static compression to a comminuted fracture may disrupt the fracture repair.

Buttress function. A plate has buttress function under two different circumstances: (1) when a gap exists through the complete circumference of the bone's load transmission surface and (2) when a fracture involves a joint or the congruity of a joint (Fig. 5-60). If the fracture cannot be reconstructed, or if fracture fragments that contribute to the bone's load transmission surface are missing, a plate with buttress function is used. This plate absorbs all the functional load applied to the bone until the process of bone healing creates contact points between all bone fragments. Because the plate is absorbing all the loads, it must be relatively strong. When a plate has buttress function across a gap or extensive comminution, some surgeons use the term *bridging plate*.

To reduce the possibility of fixation collapse, screws are placed in a buttress position in the plate holes (Fig. 5-55, *C*). The appropriate insert sleeve for the screw is positioned close to the steep wall of the plate hole in the

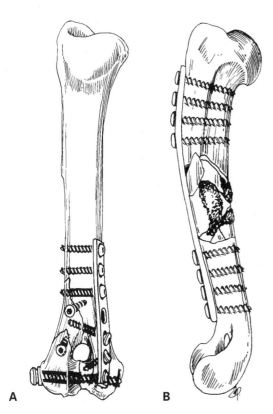

Fig. 5-60 A plate has a buttress function if it (**A**) maintains joint integrity or (**B**) spans a nonreconstructible fracture gap.

DC plate. The sleeve is the drill guide for the screw's pilot hole. The hole is drilled, measured, and tapped and the screw inserted. This places the screw head against the steep wall of the plate hole. Because the screw is as far forward in the plate hole as possible, the screw/plate complex is rigidly fixed. By doing this on both sides of the fracture line, the fracture gap is at less risk of collapse. When a gap exists in the bone, a cancellous bone graft at the fracture site is indicated.

Buttress function is present when a plate is used (1) to prevent the collapse of fragments in fractures involving joint surfaces or (2) to maintain joint integrity when the fracture involves the metaphysis or epiphysis. In some cases these fractures are totally reconstructed, whereas in others there are significant gaps in the bone. Just as buttresses are used in buildings to shore up walls or ceilings, these plates maintain joint alignment, integrity, and position.

REFERENCES

1. Anderson R: An automatic method of treatment for fractures of the tibia and fibula, *Surg Gynecol Obstet* 58:639-643, 1934.
2. Aro HT, and others: The effects of physiologic dynamic compression of bone healing under external fixation, *Clin Orthop* 256:260-273, 1990.
3. Aron DN, Toombs JP: Updated principles of external skeletal fixation, *Comp Cont Educ*, 1984, pp 845-858.
4. Aron DN, Toombs JP, Hollingsworth SC: Primary treatment of severe fractures by external skeletal fixation: threaded pins compared with smooth pins, *J Am Anim Hosp Assoc* 22:659-670, 1986.
5. Aron DN, and others: Experimental and clinical experience with an IM pin external skeletal fixator tie-in configuration, *Vet Comp Orthop Traum* 4:86-94, 1991.
6. Behrens F, Searls K: External fixation of the tibia: basic concepts and prospective evaluation, *J Bone Joint Surg* 68B:246-254, 1986.
7. Bennett RA, and others: Comparison of the strength and holding power of 4 pin designs for use with half-pin (type I) external skeletal fixation, *Vet Surg* 16:207-211, 1987.
8. Bjorling DE, Toombs JP: Transarticular application of the Kirschner-Ehmer splint, *Vet Surg* 11:34-38, 1982.
9. Briggs BT, Chao EYS: The mechanical performance of the standard Hoffman-Vidal external fixation apparatus, *J Bone Joint Surg* 64A:566-573, 1982.
10. Brinker WO, Flo GL: Principles and application of external skeletal fixation, *Vet Clin North Am* 2:197-208, 1975.
11. Brinker WO, Verstraete MC, Soutas-Little RW: Stiffness studies on various configurations and types of external fixators, *J Am Anim Hosp Assoc* 21:801-808, 1985.
12. Chao EYS: Biomechanics of external fixation. In Brooker AF, Cooney WP, Chao EYS, editors: *Principles of external fixation*, Baltimore, 1983, Williams & Wilkins.
13. Chao EYS, Pope MH: The mechanical basis of external fixation. In Seligson D, Pope MH, editors: *Concepts in external fixation*, New York, 1981, Grune & Stratton.
14. Coombs R: Introduction. In Coombs R, Green SA, Sarmiento A, editors: *External fixation and functional bracing*, London, 1989, Orthotext.
15. De Bastiani G, Aldegheri R, Brivio LR: The treatment of fractures with a dynamic axial fixator, *J Bone Joint Surg* 66B:538-546, 1984.
16. Egger EL: Static strength evaluation of six external skeletal fixation configurations, *Vet Surg* 12:130-136, 1986.
17. Egger EL, Runyon CL, Rigg DL: Use of the type I double connecting bar configuration of external skeletal fixation on long bone fractures in dogs: a review of 10 cases, *J Am Anim Hosp Assoc* 22:57-64, 1986.
18. Egger EL, and others: Type I biplanar configuration of external skeletal fixation: application technique in nine dogs and one cat, *J Am Vet Med Assoc* 187:262-267, 1985.
19. Egger EL, and others: Canine osteotomy healing when stabilized with decreasingly rigid fixation compared to constantly rigid fixation, *Trans Orthop Res Soc* 11:473, 1986.
20. Egger EL, and others: Effect of fixation pin insertion on the bone-pin interface, *Vet Surg* 15:246-252, 1986.
21. Egger EL, and others: Effects of destabilizing rigid external fixation on healing of unstable canine osteotomies, *Trans Orthop Res Soc* 13:302, 1988.
22. Ehmer EA: Bone pinning in fractures of small animals, *J Am Vet Med Assoc* 110:14-19, 1944.
23. Foland MA, Egger EL: Application of type III external fixation: a review of 23 clinical fractures in 20 dogs and 2 cats, *J Am Anim Hosp Assoc* 27:193-202, 1991.
24. Foland MA, Schwarz PD, Salman MD: The adjunctive use of half-pin (Type I) external skeletal fixators in combination with intramedullary pins for femoral fracture fixation, *Vet Comp Orthop Traum* 4:77-85, 1991.
25. Goodship AE, Kenwright J: The influence of induced micromovement upon the healing of experimental tibial fractures, *J Bone Joint Surg* 67B:650-655, 1985.
26. Green ST: *Complications of external skeletal fixation: causes, prevention, and treatment*, Springfield, Ill, 1981, Charles C Thomas.
27. Green ST: Combined internal and external fixation. In Coombs R, Green SA, Sarmiento A, editors: *External fixation and functional bracing*, London, 1989, Orthotext.

28. Green ST: History of external fixation. In Coombs R, Green SA, Sarmiento A, editors: *External fixation and functional bracing*, London, 1989, Orthotext.

29. Greenwood KM, Creagh GB: Biphase external skeletal splint fixation of mandibular fractures in dogs, *Vet Surg* 9:128-135, 1980.

30. Halloran WX: Motion. In Coombs R, Green SA, Sarmiento A, editors: *External fixation and functional bracing*, London, 1989, Orthotext.

31. Hierholzer G, and others: External fixation-classification and indications, *Arch Orthop Traum Surg* 92:175-182, 1978.

32. Hyldahl C, and others: Induction and prevention of pin loosening in external fixators in the sheep tibia, *Orthop Trans* 12:378, 1988.

33. Ilizarov G: Fractures and nonunions. In Coombs R, Green SA, Sarmiento A, editors: *External fixation and functional bracing*, London, 1989, Orthotext.

34. Ilizarov G: The tension-stress effect on the genesis and growth of tissues: the influence of the rate and frequency of distraction, *Clin Orthop* 239:263-285, 1989.

35. Johnson AL, Kneller SK, Weigel RM: Radial and tibial fracture repair with external skeletal fixation: effects of fracture type, reduction, and complications on healing, *Vet Surg* 18:367-372, 1989.

36. Latte Y: Treatment of radius curvus by Ilizarov apparatus, *Trans Vet Orthop Soc*, 1989.

37. Lesser A: Preliminary work with callus distraction, *Trans Vet Orthop Soc*, 1991.

38. Lewallen DG, and others: Comparison of the effects of compression plates and external fixators on early bone healing, *J Bone Joint Surg* 66A:1084-1091, 1984.

39. Matthews LS, Green CA, Goldstein SA: The thermal effects of skeletal fixation-pin insertion in bone, *J Bone Joint Surg* 66A:1077-1083, 1984.

40. Morshead D, Leeds EB: Kirschner-Ehmer apparatus immobilization following Achilles tendon repair in six dogs, *Vet Surg* 13:11-14, 1984.

40a. Müller ME, Allgöwer M, Schneider R, Willenegger H, editors: *Manual of internal fixation*, ed 3, Berlin, 1991, Springer-Verlag.

41. Ohashi T, Inoue S, Kajikawa K: External skeletal fixation using methylmethacrylate: current technique, clinical results, and indications, *Clin Orthop* 178:121-129, 1983.

42. Olds R, Green SA: Hoffmann's external fixation for arthrodesis and infected nonunions in the dog, *J Am Anim Hosp Assoc* 19:705-712, 1983.

43. Palmer RH, Aron DN: Ellis pin complications in seven dogs, *Vet Surg* 19:440, 1990.

44. Parkhill C: A new apparatus for the fixation of bones after resection and in fractures with a tendency to displacement, *Trans Am Surg Assoc* 15:251-256, 1897.

45. Prinz H, Blomer A, Echterhoff M: Pin-track infection. In Coombs R, Green SA, Sarmiento A, editors: *External fixation and functional bracing*, London, 1989, Orthotext.

46. Siris I: External pin transfixation of fractures: an analysis of eighty cases, *Ann Surg* 120:911-942, 1944.

47. Staumbaugh JE, Nunmaker DM: External skeletal fixation of comminuted maxillary fractures in dogs, *Vet Surg* 2:72-76, 1982.

48. Thommasini MD, Betts CW: Use of the "Ilizarov" external fixator in a dog, *Vet Comp Orthop Traum* 4:70-76, 1991.

49. Tomlinson JL, Constantinescu GM: Acrylic external skeletal fixation of fractures, *Comp Cont Educ* 13:235-240, 1991.

50. Toombs JP, Aron DN, Basinger RR: Angled connecting bars for transarticular application of Kirschner-Ehmer external fixation splints, *J Am Anim Hosp Assoc* 25:213-216, 1989.

51. Willer RL, Egger EL, Histand MB: A comparison of stainless steel versus acrylic for the connecting bar of external skeletal fixators, *J Am Hosp Assoc* (in press).

52. Williams EA, and others: The early healing of tibial osteotomies stabilized by one-plane or two-plane external fixation, *J Bone Joint Surg* 69A:355-364, 1987.

53. Wu JJ, and others: Comparison of osteotomy healing under external fixation devices with different stiffness characteristics, *J Bone Joint Surg* 66A:1258-1264, 1984.

SUGGESTED READINGS

1. Brinker WO, Hohn RB, Prieur WD, editors: *Manual of internal fixation in small animals,* Berlin, 1984, Springer-Verlag.

2. Brinker WO, Piermattei DL, Flo, GL: Fractures: classification, diagnosis and treatment. *Handbook of small animal orthopedics & fracture treatment*, ed 2, Philadelphia, 1990, WB Saunders.

3. Comte P, Straumann F: Influence of unoccupied holes on fatigue behaviour of bone fixation plates. In *Biomechanics: current interdisciplinary research*, Dordrecht, 1985, Martinus Nifhoff.

4. Dean PW: Stack-pinning. *Current techniques in small animal surgery*, ed 3, Philadelphia, 1990, Lea & Febiger.

5. DeYoung DJ, Probst CW, Pardo AD: Methods of internal fixation of fractures. *Textbook of small animal surgery*, ed 2, Philadelphia, 1993, WB Saunders.

6. Kraus KH: Tension band wiring. *Current techniques in small animal surgery*, ed 3, Philadelphia, 1990, Lea & Febiger.

7. Müller ME, Allgöwer M, Schneider R, Willenegger H, editors: *Manual of internal fixation*, ed 3, Berlin, 1991, Springer-Verlag.

8. Nunamaker DM: Methods of internal fixation. *Textbook of small animal orthopaedic.* New York, 1985, JB Lippincott.

9. Schatzker J: Concepts of fracture stabilization. In Sumner-Smith G, editor: *Bone in clinical orthopaedics*, Philadelphia, 1982, WB Saunders.

10. Straw RC, Withrow SJ: Cerclage wiring. *Current techniques in small animal surgery*, ed 3, Philadelphia, 1990, Lea & Febiger.

SECTION B Bone Grafting

Ann L. Johnson

Bone grafting, the technique of transplanting cancellous or cortical bone, has been used in veterinary medicine for many years. Autogenous cancellous bone grafts were first recommended as a treatment for management of nonunions and osteomyelitis.[18,19] Autogenous cancellous bone grafting is now considered a vital component of complete fracture management, helping the surgeon to achieve bone healing before implant failure. Cortical bone allografts have been used in veterinary surgery for the last 15 years as a treatment for long bone fractures with severe cortical bone loss and musculoskeletal tumors.[7] This section discusses the indications, techniques, and results of using the various types of bone grafts.

TYPES OF BONE GRAFTS

Bone grafts are named to indicate their structure and source. *Cancellous* bone graft comes from the trabecular bone found in the metaphyses of long bones and is a highly cellular, porous, three-dimensional network of bony plates and columns. *Cortical* bone graft is the relatively acellular, dense, compact bone that makes up the diaphyses of long bones. *Corticocancellous* grafts are composites, such as a rib or the wing of the ilium. *Osteochondral* grafts are composites of cortical bone, cancellous bone, and articular cartilage such as the proximal femur. *Vascularized* grafts are harvested with their blood supply intact and are implanted using microvascular anastomosis techniques that preserve the blood supply to the bone.

Bone transplanted from one site to another site in the same animal is an *autograft*. This type of graft is histocompatible with the host immune system and does not initiate rejection of the graft. Bone transplanted from one animal to another of the same species is an *allograft*. The cellular antigens of this type of graft may be recognized as foreign by the host immune system, setting up an immune response that may impair revascularization and remodeling of the graft. If transplanted bone is treated by freezing, freeze-drying, autoclaving, chemical preservation, or irradiation so that there is no cellular activity and decreased immunogenicity, it is an *alloimplant*. Bone transplanted from one animal to another of a different species is a *xenograft*. Bone substitutes of β-Tricalcium phosphate ceramics are available as extenders for cancellous bone graft.*

FUNCTIONS OF BONE GRAFTS

Bone grafts serve the functions of osteogenesis and osteoconduction.[5] In the *osteogenetic function*, they are a source of osteoprogenitor cells, either providing the cells directly or inducing the formation of osteoprogenitor cells from the surrounding soft tissues.[2,5,24] In the *osteoconductive function*, bone grafts provide varying degrees of mechanical support in the host bed, ranging from forming a space-occupying trellis for host bone invasion to supplying weight-bearing struts within the fracture site.[4,5]

The function varies with the type of bone transplanted. Cancellous autografts are highly cellular but mechanically weak. Therefore they provide superior osteoinductive capabilities but do not aid initially in the support of the fracture fixation. In contrast, cortical alloimplants provide excellent mechanical support to a fracture fixation but in most cases are acellular and stimulate little osteogenic response.[5] Partial decalcification of cortical allografts allows the release of bone morphogenetic protein to induce osteoprogenitor cells. However, partial decalcification weakens the cortical bone and decreases its capabilities of supporting a fracture

---

*Ossgraft, Miter, Inc., Columbus, Ohio.

fixation.[21] The type of bone graft used in a fracture repair is determined by the function needed for successful fracture treatment.

INDICATIONS FOR BONE GRAFTS

Bone grafting is very beneficial in the management of fractures. In addition, bone grafts can be used in other forms of orthopedic treatment. Most fractures treated with open reduction and internal fixation are candidates for cancellous bone autografts. Any gaps left in the reconstructed cortex should be filled with cancellous bone autograft to speed bone union and prevent premature implant failure caused by motion at the fracture site.[3] Fracture nonunions and delayed unions can be treated with adequate stabilization of the fracture and cancellous bone autograft.[1] Cancellous bone autograft is used after sequestrectomy and curettage to treat osteomyelitis.[18] Bone defects following curettage of cysts or resection of tumors are filled with cancellous bone autograft to promote bone healing.[16] Arthrodesis of joints is enhanced by the use of cancellous bone autografts.[15]

Cortical bone autografts, such as ribs and strips of bone from the ilial wing, are used to augment fracture repair of the mandible and long bones where mechanical support of the fracture is needed.[14] Cortical bone allografts are used when massive transplantation of cortical bone is needed to support large segmental defects in long bone diaphyseal fractures or for limb salvage techniques after tumor resection.[12,17,22] In addition, cortical allografts can be used to correct malunions that have resulted in limb shortening.[22]

AUTOGENOUS CANCELLOUS BONE GRAFT
Procedure for Cancellous Bone Harvest

Autogenous cancellous bone is the material most frequently used for grafting procedures. The wide range of indications, ease of harvest, advantages of use, and low associated complications make this procedure a routine part of orthopedic surgery. Cancellous bone can be harvested from the metaphyses of any long bone; however, the proximal humerus, proximal tibia, and wing of the ilium are most often used because of easy exposure and large amounts of available cancellous bone (Fig. 5-61).[9] The surgeon makes the decision to use cancellous bone graft before surgery and aseptically prepares the selected graft site. The graft site is selected because of accessibility when the animal is positioned for the fracture repair.

The approach to the proximal humerus is craniolateral, through the skin and subcutaneous tissue to the acromial head of the deltoid muscle. The muscle is retracted caudally, exposing the cranial lateral flat surface

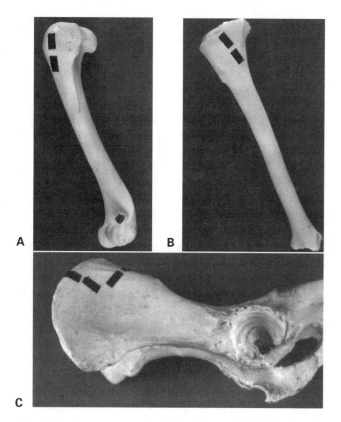

Fig. 5-61   Common sites for harvesting cancellous bone graft: **A**, proximal, craniolateral humerus; **B**, proximal, medial tibia; **C**, cranial dorsal wing of the ilium.

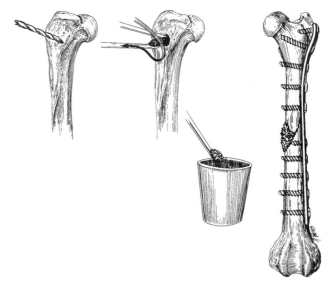

Fig. 5-62   Technique for harvesting a cancellous graft.

of the humeral metaphysis just distal to the greater tubercle. The approach to the proximal tibia is through a craniomedial skin incision. The subcutaneous tissue is incised and retracted, exposing the medial surface of the proximal tibial metaphysis. The approach to the ilial wing is made through a dorsal skin incision over the craniodorsal iliac spine. The subcutaneous tissue is incised and retracted, exposing the dorsal surface of the ilial wing. The gluteal musculature is elevated from the lateral surface of the ilial wing.

The equipment used for harvesting cancellous bone consists of an intramedullary pin or drill bit to penetrate the cortex, bone curettes to harvest the cancellous bone, and a stainless steel cup or sterile sponge to hold the cancellous bone. Size of instruments depends on the animal's size but should be large enough to permit easy recovery of trabecular bone. Alternately, an osteotome is used to excise a wedge of cortical bone from the ilial wing to expose the cancellous bone for harvesting (Fig. 5-61). The cortical wedge is macerated with a rongeur and used as corticocancellous bone chips.

Cancellous bone is usually harvested after fracture stabilization. The cancellous graft may be harvested before the primary orthopedic procedure if contamination of the donor site with infection or tumor cells from the pri-

mary surgical site is a concern. Alternately, a separate surgical team and instrumentation may be used to harvest the cancellous bone. The donor site is approached and the cortex penetrated with the intramedullary pin or drill bit. A round hole is made through the cortex to minimize the formation of a stress riser that could contribute to fracture development through the cortical defect. Care should be taken not to penetrate the opposite cortex or articular surface with the pin, drill bit, or curette. The cancellous bone is harvested with the bone curette and either placed directly into the recipient bed or stored in a blood-soaked sponge or stainless steel cup. Blood is added to the graft in the cup to keep it moist. The blood clots and forms a moldable composite with the graft, which aids in its handling. Cancellous bone graft should not be stored in saline or treated with antibiotics, both of which are toxic to the cells. The stored graft should be securely placed on the instrument table to avoid inadvertent disposal (Fig. 5-62).

The recipient fracture site should be flushed completely with saline, removing blood clots and necrotic debris. The cancellous bone graft is loosely packed in all defects and around fracture lines. The soft tissues are closed to hold the graft in position.

Fracture Healing with Cancellous Bone Autograft

Revascularization of the cancellous bone autograft begins as early as 2 days and is usually completed within 2 weeks. Transplanted osteogenic cells or differentiated primitive mesenchymal cells become active osteoblasts, lining the transplanted trabecular bone and depositing a seam of osteoid. The osteoid is mineralized, forming new host bone in the fracture site.[6] In addition, new bone is

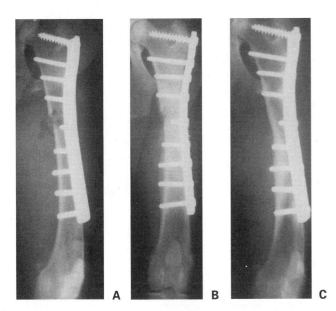

Fig. 5-63 Radiographs of **A,** fractured femur stabilized with a plate and screws with the gap in the medial cortex filled with autogenous cancellous bone graft; **B,** 1 month after surgery showing increased cancellous bone density in the graft area; and **C,** 6 months after surgery showing remodeled cortical bone.

formed that incorporates the graft into the host bone. Eventually the necrotic cores of trabecular bone are resorbed by osteoclasts, and the graft is totally replaced by host bone.[5,6] The trabecular new bone is remodeled into cortical bone in response to the mechanical environment. This healing response can be monitored radiographically by observing the filling of the defect with cancellous-type bone density followed by reconstruction of the cortex (Fig. 5-63).

The donor site heals by filling with a hematoma, which is replaced by fibrovascular granulation tissue. Osteoblasts migrate to the area and deposit osteoid. Cartilage and woven bone are formed within the defect, creating an endosteal callus. By 12 weeks, normal lamellar bone and hematopoietic marrow are present in the defect.[14]

Complications of Autogenous Cancellous Bone Graft

A low incidence of complications is associated with autogenous cancellous bone-grafting techniques. Pain at the donor site is not a common finding. Hematomas, seromas, or wound dehiscence may occur at the donor site. Iatrogenic infection or seeding of tumor at the donor site is very rare and can be prevented by proper sequencing of bone graft harvesting. Fractures through the donor site have been reported infrequently.[13] Complications at the recipient site, such as infection and instability, can result in failure of the graft to stimulate bone formation. The graft is resorbed rather than sequestered in these cases.

CORTICAL AUTOGRAFTS

Cortical autograft harvest is limited to areas of cortical bone that can be transplanted without adversely affecting the animal's function. Cortical bone can be harvested from the ribs, wing of the ilium, distal ulna, and fibula. Uses of cortical autografts include transplantation of a rib to form a segmental strut in a mandibular fracture, transplantation of the ilial wing for cervical vertebral fusion, or transplantation of ilial wing segments for arthrodesing joints or filling cortical defects.[20,23]

Cortical autograft harvest is done at the time of graft transfer. The donor site is aseptically prepared and the cortical bone isolated and resected. The cortical autograft is incorporated into the host site and held in place with implant fixation.

CORTICAL ALLOGRAFTS OR ALLOIMPLANTS

Cortical bone can be harvested and transplanted immediately as a fresh allograft.[1] It can also be harvested and banked to provide a ready source of cortical alloimplants.[10,12,22] Harvesting must be done under aseptic conditions unless the bone is sterilized after collection.[10,22] Donor animals should be mature and free of infectious disease. The procedure for aseptic harvest is euthanasia of the donor animal followed by aseptic preparation of sites for femoral, tibial, or humeral harvest. A surgical approach is made to the diaphyses of the selected long bones. The soft tissues are elevated and the diaphysis isolated. An oscillating bone saw is used to resect the diaphysis at the metaphyseal junctions. The marrow canal is cleaned and flushed with saline. The bone can be immediately transplanted into a fracture site. Alternately, the cortical bone is double-wrapped in presterilized containers and stored in a home freezer at –20°C for 6 to 12 months. Radiographs made of the harvested cortical bone serve as a record of bone size available in the bank. Microbiological cultures are made of one of the harvested bones to check the sterility of the harvesting technique. In another method of collection, cortical bone is cleanly harvested and double-wrapped in semipermeable packaging material for sterilization with ethylene oxide.[10,12] After sterilization, the bone is aerated to eliminate the toxic residues left after treatment with ethylene oxide. The cortical bone is stored at –20°C for 6 to 12 months.

Technique for Placing a Cortical Allograft in a Fracture

The ideal fracture for treatment with a cortical allograft is a middiaphyseal, severely comminuted, closed fracture because it fulfills the following criteria. Plate and screw fixation are needed to ensure stability of the host-graft interface for an adequate period to allow fracture healing and remodeling of the graft. Therefore, sufficient host bone must exist proximally and distally to the graft to secure at least three bone screws. A cortical allograft should be used only when insufficient host bone is available to reconstruct the fracture. Finally, the recipient site should be free of bacterial contamination, which eliminates animals with open fractures as candidates for cortical allograft techniques.

When a fracture meeting these criteria is identified, radiographs are made of the contralateral matching bone to determine the size and length of graft needed and to serve as a model for precontouring the plate. From the lateral radiographs, the length of the intact segments of the fractured bone is determined and subtracted from the length of the contralateral bone. The result is the length of graft needed to reconstruct the fracture. An appropriately sized (width and length) graft is obtained from the bank.

Adherence to aseptic technique is essential for successful use of cortical allografts. The fractured limb and a cancellous bone autograft site are prepared for aseptic surgery. The fracture is surgically approached, the fragments are removed, and the proximal and distal bone segments are resected perpendicularly to the bone's long axis with an oscillating bone saw, eliminating any fracture lines. The graft is also cut to the appropriate length perpendicular to the bone's long axis. This allows 360-degree contact between the graft and host bone. The graft is secured to the center of a precontoured plate using the appropriate number and length of cortical bone screws for the graft's length. The graft-plate composite is placed in the fracture gap and the bone segments reduced to the plate. The plate is secured to the host bone segments using cortical bone screws. The screws placed immediately proximal and distal to the graft in the host bone are inserted in a loaded manner to achieve compression of the host-graft interfaces. The rest of the screws are placed in a neutral position (Fig. 5-64). The fracture site is flushed with saline and a cancellous bone autograft harvested and placed at the host-graft interfaces. Samples for microbiological culture are taken, and the surgical wound is closed. Postoperative radiographs are made to document the position of allograft and metal implants. Postoperative care is the same as given to a fracture patient.

Fracture Healing With a Cortical Allograft

Fracture healing with a cortical allograft or alloimplant consists of filling of the host-graft interface with bone, vascularization of the graft followed by resorption of the graft, and replacement with host bone. The host-graft interfaces heal in 1 to 3 months.[11] Vascular invasion begins at the host-graft interfaces and progresses toward the graft's center. Osteoclastic activity results in resorp-

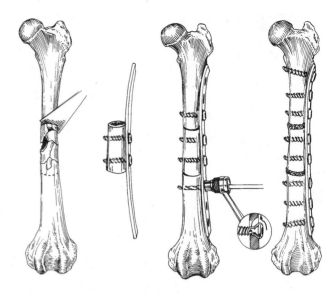

Fig. 5-64 Technique for placing a cortical bone allograft or alloimplant in a prepared segmented defect in a femur. One screw on either side of the graft is placed in a loaded position, resulting in compression of the host-graft interface when the screw is tightened.

tion cavities, which are then filled with host bone. The initial resorption phase results in a porous, mechanically weak graft. Allograft resorption is incomplete when spicules of dead graft are evident. These areas are mechanically strong but susceptible to fracture because of an inability to repair fatigue damage.[11,23,24] Remodeling of the graft takes months to years, depending on its length, and may never be complete. The process of remodeling can be monitored radiographically (Fig. 5-65). The host-graft interfaces fill with a cancellous-type bone. The graft changes from a cortical structure to a porous cancellous bone as resorption and remodeling proceed from the host-graft interface toward the graft's center. Eventually the host bone remodels into cortical bone. Because of the potential for weakening of the graft with the resorption phase of remodeling and the uncertainty of how much unremodeled graft remains, it is difficult to establish a correct time for plate removal. Premature plate removal may allow the graft to fracture. Plate removal should not be done until the entire graft shows radiographic signs of remodeling. Biopsy of the graft's center before implant removal may be useful to determine the amount of host bone invasion.[22] If no complications are observed with the metal implants, it may be prudent to leave them in place indefinitely.

Complications of Cortical Allograft

Complications associated with cortical allografts include infection, graft rejection, fracture repair failure, and graft

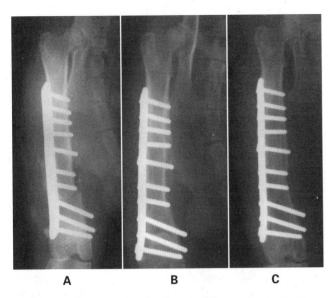

Fig. 5-65 Radiographs of **A,** fractured femur repaired with an ethylene oxide-sterilized cortical alloimplant, plate, and 10 screws (*arrows* are at the host-graft interface); **B,** 10 weeks after surgery showing filling and remodeling of the host-graft interfaces with new bone; and **C,** 34 weeks after surgery showing thinning of the graft's center coinciding with resorption and remodeling and thickening of the cortex at the ends of the graft.

fracture.[8,17,22] Graft infection usually results from contamination of the graft or fracture site coupled with instability. This results in a large sequestered piece of foreign material (the allograft) and must be treated by debridement and stabilization of the fracture site. This complication is seen most often in limb salvage techniques because of a compromised host bed, large surgical sites, and lengthy operating times.[17] Cancellous bone autograft may be used to fill the infected gap. Graft rejection is rarely noted as a clinical problem. Radiographic signs of rejection include failure of host-graft interface union and resorption of the graft without replacement. Loosened screws and broken implants resulting from instability in the fracture fixation have been reported.[17] Fracture of the graft can occur when the reduction and fixation of the host-graft interfaces are not adequate for support of the graft. Grafts can also fracture following premature plate removal.

REFERENCES AND SUGGESTED READINGS

1. Alexander JW: Use of combination of cortical bone allografts and cancellous bone autografts to replace massive bone loss in fresh fractures and selected nonunions, *J Am Anim Hosp Assoc* 19:671-687, 1983.
2. Bassett CAL: Clinical implications of cell function in bone grafting, *Clin Orthop* 87:49-59, 1972.
3. Brinker WO, Hohn RB, Prieur D: *Manual of internal fixation in small animals,* New York, 1984, Springer-Verlag.
4. Burwell RG: The fate of bone grafts. In Apley AG, editor: *Recent advances in orthopaedics,* Baltimore, 1969, Williams & Wilkins.
5. Goldberg VM, Stevenson S: Natural history of autografts and allografts, *Clin Orthop* 225:7-16, 1987.
6. Heiple KG, and others: Biology of cancellous bone grafts, *Orthop Clin North Am* 18:179-185, 1987.
7. Henry WB, Wadsworth PL: Diaphyseal allografts in the repair of long bone fractures, *J Am Anim Hosp Assoc* 17:525-534, 1981.
8. Henry WB, Wadsworth PL: Restrospective analysis of failures in the repair of severely comminuted long bone fractures using large diaphyseal allografts, *J Am Anim Hosp Assoc* 17:535-546, 1981.
9. Hulse DA: Pathophysiology of autogenous cancellous bone grafts, *Comp Cont Educ* 2:126-142, 1980.
10. Johnson AL: Principle and practical applications of cortical bone grafting techniques, *Comp Cont Educ* 10:906-913, 1988.
11. Johnson AL, Stein LE: Morphologic comparison of healing patterns in ethylene oxide–sterilized cortical allografts and untreated control autografts in the dog, *Am J Vet Res* 49:101-105, 1988.
12. Johnson AL, Roe SC, Harari J: Ethylene oxide sterilization of cortical bone for bone banking: technique and results in three dogs and one cat, *Vet Surg* 15:49-54, 1986.
13. Johnson KA: Cancellous bone graft collection from the tibia in dogs, *Vet Surg* 15:334-338, 1986.
14. Johnson KA: Histologic features of the healing of bone graft donor sites in dogs, *Am J Vet Res* 49:885-888, 1988.
15. Johnson KA, Bellenger CR: The effects of autologous bone grafting on bone healing after carpal arthrodesis in the dog, *Vet Rec* 107:126-132, 1980.
16. Knecht CP, Slusher R, Cawley AJ: Treatment of Brodie's abscess by means of bone autograft, *J Am Vet Med Assoc* 158:492-500, 1971.
17. LaRue SM, and others: Limb sparing treatment for osteosarcoma in dogs, *J Am Vet Med Assoc* 195:1734-1744, 1989.
18. Olds RB, and others: Autogenous cancellous bone grafting in problem orthopedic cases, *J Am Anim Hosp Assoc* 9:430-435, 1973.
19. Olds RB, and others: Autogenous cancellous bone grafting in small animals, *J Am Anim Hosp Assoc* 9:454-456, 1973.
20. Prata RG: Ventral decompression and fusion of the cervical spine in the dog. In Bojrab MJ, editor: *Current techniques in veterinary surgery,* ed 1, Philadelphia, 1975, Lea & Febiger.
21. Roe SC, Pijanowski GJ, Johnson AL: Biomechanical properties of cortical bone allografts: effects of preparation and storage, *Am J Vet Res* 49:873-877, 1988.
22. Sinibaldi KR: Evaluation of full cortical allografts in 25 dogs, *J Am Vet Med Assoc* 194:1570-1577, 1989.
23. Stevenson S: Bone grafting. In Bojrab MJ, editor: *Current techniques in veterinary surgery,* ed 3, Philadelphia, 1990, Lea & Febiger.
24. Urist MR: Bone transplants and implants. In Urist MR, editor: *Fundamental and clinical bone physiology,* Philadelphia, 1980, JB Lippincott.

SECTION C   Joint Fracture Repair

Larry J. Wallace

Intraarticular fractures are always a challenge to repair because anatomical reduction, rigid internal fixation, early weight bearing, and return to normal joint function are the intended goals. Therefore the articular fracture must be attended to as soon as the patient's overall physiological status allows. If other life-threatening emergencies such as ruptured urinary bladder, ruptured liver, diaphragmatic hernia, or spine fracture are present, they must be resolved first. In such cases the limb with the intraarticular fracture should be put in a splint or immobilization bandage until the articular fracture can be safely repaired. Failure to protect the affected limb may allow the articular fragments to rub on each other, causing further injury to the cartilage. This can lead to osteoarthritis, even if a perfect surgical repair is done. If the bony aspects of the articular fracture are allowed to move against each other, an abrasive loss of bone at the fracture surface also will occur. When reduced and fixed, these worn surfaces may result in gaps that prevent perfect anatomical reduction of the joint and loss of normal joint congruity. If this occurs, less-than-desired joint function can be expected, and osteoarthritis eventually develops.

If intraarticular fractures are not repaired early, excessive granulation tissue proliferates within the joint along with hematoma, which deprives the articular cartilage of its nutrition from synovial fluid. As with any fracture, intraarticular fractures are easier to repair within the first 24 to 48 hours after they occur. With increased time, muscle contracture and adhesion formation can further separate the fracture fragments, making anatomical reduction much more difficult, thus increasing anesthesia time.

SURGICAL APPROACH

Careful preplanning is essential to any orthopedic surgical procedure. Excellent-quality radiographs with at least lateral and craniocaudal radiographic views are a minimum requirement. Depending on the fracture and joint involved, oblique views may also be necessary. The surgeon must consider which surgical approach to the joint is best to repair a given intraarticular fracture. In some cases a limited approach to a joint is adequate (e.g., minimally displaced lateral condylar fracture of the humerus in a young dog), whereas in others (e.g., T or Y humeral condylar fracture) a more extensive surgical approach is necessary. Therefore, after carefully evaluating the fracture, the surgeon should select the surgical approach that allows the best visualization of the articular surface. This is critical in obtaining an anatomical reduction. In addition, the surgeon must be thoroughly familiar with the anatomy of the joint and periarticular structures.

All surgery must be done using strict aseptic technique. Hemostasis must be maintained by electrocautery or ligation. The surgical approaches and joint anatomy are well described in the literature.[1,3] Poor preplanning for intraarticular surgical procedure and inadequate visualization of the fracture can lead to technical failure and a frustrated, confused surgeon. To enhance exposure of the articular surface, osteotomy of a bony attachment of a tendon or ligament is often helpful. Osteotomy of the tibial tuberosity and upward reflection of the patellar

tendon provide a better exposure of the femoral condyles. Osteotomy of the olecranon process and reflection of the triceps tendon provide visualization of the entire width of the humeral condyle. Osteotomy of the greater trochanter of the femur is a common approach for exposing certain acetabular and femoral head fractures. These are only a few examples of what can be done to obtain added exposure to a joint for proper repair of intraarticular fractures.

INTRAOPERATIVE PRINCIPLES AND TECHNIQUES

All intraarticular fractures should be treated with open reduction and rigid internal fixation regardless of the fracture's location within the joint. Once the surgical approach is made and the fracture exposed, the soft tissue should be retracted using appropriate instrumentation. Moist gauze sponges should *not* be used in a wiping motion across the articular cartilage because this is abrasive; rather, a soft blotting method should be used. All exposed tissue must be lavaged periodically using lactated Ringer's solution to prevent drying. It is especially important to keep the articular cartilage moist. In studies on rabbits, the entire thickness of articular cartilage became necrotic after 60 minutes of drying; 30 minutes produced patchy necrosis that extended to the middle zone of the cartilage. In joints exposed to room air for 1 hour, necrosis of the chondrocytes was completely prevented by irrigating the joint every 5 minutes with lactated Ringer's solution.[2]

In another study, normal articular cartilage of the rabbit stifle was exposed to room air for 30 minutes. The articular cartilage was capable of recovery, as determined by special staining and ultrastructural evaluation 6 weeks after the arthrotomy.[4] It must be emphasized that in the latter study the articular cartilage had not been damaged by physical trauma, only by the trauma of room air exposure. These studies show that although normal untraumatized articular cartilage can recover from the effects of exposure to room air, it is best to keep the cartilage lavaged at least every 5 minutes with lactated Ringer's solution.

When fixing an intraarticular fracture, it is generally best to reconstruct the articular surface first. The osteochondral fragments can be manipulated much easier if they are not attached to larger fragments. Minor discrepancies in reduction of shaft fragments are less consequential than any discrepancies involving cartilaginous surfaces. Generally the osteochondral fragments in most fractures are fragile. The fragments can split easily if they are vigorously retracted or extensively levered in an attempt to achieve reduction. The muscle tension on fracture fragments usually can be decreased by flexing or extending the joint, which, along with proper exposure, allows easier and more exact anatomical reduction of the fracture fragments. The small osteochondral fragments generally can be properly fixed in place using multiple small Kirschner wires inserted at diverging angles. Lag screws are preferred for fixing and stabilizing larger fragments because they allow compression at the fracture surface. If necessary, the Kirschner wires or even very small lag screws can be introduced through the articular cartilage and countersunk below the articular surface into the subchondral bone. The small defect in the articular cartilage resulting from countersinking the Kirschner wires or small lag screws will fill in with fibrocartilage.

When repairing a comminuted articular fracture of the distal humerus or femur, the fracture is anatomically reduced and fixed first. The condyle(s) can then be reduced and properly fixed to the end of the specific long bone. Kirschner wire or small intramedullary pin fixation of avulsion fractures that are attached to a tendon or ligament should also be supported by a tension-band wire if the animal is mature or almost mature.

PRINCIPLES OF POSTOPERATIVE CARE

For the best results in dealing with the intraarticular fractures, early mobilization of the joint is desired. The precise postoperative management program varies among patients and is dictated by several specific factors. The amount of protection given to these fractures somewhat depends on the patient's size, age, and disposition; the degree of comminution of the fracture; fracture stability after fixation; degree of periarticular soft tissue and ligamentous injury; and especially the owner's ability and desire to follow the surgeon's instructions for postoperative home care.

A soft pressure bandage may be applied when applicable for up to 48 to 72 hours to decrease joint effusion and swelling of the lower limb. Joint movement should be encouraged as soon after surgery as possible to prevent formation of periarticular adhesions, which can drastically limit joint motion, especially in the elbow joint. Full weight bearing on the affected joint should be allowed to progress slowly. Intermittent passive joint motion, non-weight-bearing slings (Velpeau sling for the front leg, Ehmer sling for the rear leg) or a sling that allows only partial weight bearing, and a soft padded bandage with or without reinforced rods are methods of permitting some joint motion but guarding against excessive early loading of the articular surface. The more comminuted the fracture, the more care needs to be taken against premature loading of the articular fracture. Several studies have shown that articular cartilage viability and healing are enhanced by early passive joint motion after fracture repair. However, precautions must be taken in severe fractures to prevent excessive early

overloading of the joint and collapse of the repaired fracture.

In the postoperative period, restricted exercise (short leash walks) and no running or jumping must be minimum requirements until radiographic evidence shows a clinical union.

REFERENCES

1. Evans HE, Christensen GC: *Miller's anatomy of the dog*, Philadelphia, 1979, WB Saunders.
2. Mitchell N, Shepard N: The deleterious effects of drying on articular cartilage, *J Bone Joint Surg* 71A:89-95, 1989.
3. Piermattei DL, Greely RG: *An atlas of surgical approaches to the bones of the dog and cat*, ed 2, Philadelphia, 1979, WB Saunders.
4. Speer KP, Callaghan JJ, Seaber AV, and others: The effects of exposure of articular cartilage to air: a histochemical and ultrastructural investigation, *J Bone Joint Surg* (AM) Dec:72(10) 1442-1450, 1990.

SECTION D Osteotomies

Ann L. Johnson

Osteotomy describes a procedure in which bone is cut into two segments. Apophyseal osteotomies, such as trochanteric osteotomy or olecranon osteotomy, are done to enhance surgical exposure of a joint. Diaphyseal or metaphyseal osteotomies are performed to correct an abnormality in joint alignment or limb length. These procedures are termed *corrective* osteotomies, and this section discusses their indications, principles, and techniques.

INDICATIONS FOR CORRECTIVE OSTEOTOMY

The objective of a corrective osteotomy is to return a limb to normal function. Reasons to perform an osteotomy include (1) correcting excessive angulation of a bone, (2) creating an angulation in the bone to realign joint surfaces, (3) establishing adequate length of a bone, (4) correcting torsional deformity, and (5) improving articular configuration.

Trauma to the physes in an immature animal may result in complete or partial closure of the physis. Complete physeal closure in a single bone in an animal with growth potential results in a shortened limb. If the amount of limb shortening adversely affects the animal's function, a lengthening osteotomy may be done. Complete physeal closure in one of the pair of bones (e.g., radius and ulna) in an immature animal results in angular, rotational, and shortening deformities because of incongruent growth of the bones. Partial premature physeal closure results in angular and shortening deformities as the uninjured portion of the physis attempts to continue to function. Angular bone deformities cause a loss of the parallel alignment of the joints adjacent to the affected bone, which contributes to joint instability and development of secondary degenerative joint disease (DJD). Several osteotomy techniques, including oblique, wedge, and dome osteotomies, are designed to correct angular and rotational deformities that occur after premature physeal closure. Complete premature closure of the proximal or distal radial physis results in a shortened radius but may cause little or no angular deformity of the limb. In this case the elbow joint is unstable because the radial head fails to contact the humeral capitulum. A lengthening osteotomy of the radius is necessary to reestablish joint congruity. Table 5-1 lists deformities and corrective osteotomy techniques.

Developmental torsional abnormalities, such as femoral torsion or proximal tibial torsion, may result in unstable joints. Patellar luxation can be severe and may require osteotomy of the tibial tuberosity or, in certain cases, diaphyseal derotational corrective osteotomy to realign the quadriceps mechanism.

Joint surfaces must be properly aligned for optimum function. Again, loss of anatomical alignment leads to joint instability and development of DJD. In developmental diseases such as canine hip dysplasia, laxity or incongruity of the hip joint stimulates a degenerative response resulting in formation of osteophytes. Corrective osteotomy of the pelvis or femur results in improved joint alignment and prevents DJD.[8,10]

Animals with malunions of fractures resulting in angular, rotational, or shortening deformities are candidates for corrective osteotomy if the deformity is severe enough to interfere with limb function. The principles of corrective osteotomy can be applied to nonunions of long bone fractures.

Because the objectives of corrective osteotomy are to improve function and prevent DJD, the procedures should be done as early as possible, preferably before signs of osteoarthritis are present. Osteoarthritis does not contraindicate a corrective osteotomy, but the prognosis for normal function is diminished.

PRINCIPLES OF CORRECTIVE OSTEOTOMY

The goals of a corrective osteotomy are to realign joint surfaces, derotate the bone, and maintain or gain length. Preoperative planning is essential for achieving these goals. Craniocaudal and lateral radiographs are made of the affected bone, including the adjacent joints, and compared with radiographs of the contralateral bone. The radiographs are evaluated for (1) position and relationship of the joints at either end of the bone, (2) point of greatest curvature of the bone, (3) the degree of rotation, and (4) length of the bone compared with the normal bone. With this information, the surgeon chooses the corrective osteotomy technique that will best correct the deformities identified. Paper templates are made by tracing the radiographs. The surgeon uses the templates to plan placement of the osteotomy and the degree of correction desired.[7]

Interoperative planning is also important. Landmarks are identified or in some cases created with Kirschner ("K") wires and used to align the bone after osteotomy. When external fixation is used with oblique or transverse osteotomies, the most proximal and distal transfixation pins can be placed parallel to their respective joint and in the lateral-to-medial transverse plane. After osteotomy, these pins are aligned parallel to each other and in the same transverse plane, resulting in parallel alignment of the joint surfaces (Fig. 5-66). If internal fixation is used with a closing wedge osteotomy, the planned preoperative angle of osteotomy must be created exactly to ensure that the joint alignment will be correct (Fig. 5-67). For derotational osteotomies, prepositioned K wires at the metaphyses are used to indicate when the degree of desired derotation has been achieved (Fig. 5-68).

The appropriate surgical approach is made to the osteotomy site, preserving soft tissues, and the point of greatest curvature of the bone is identified. Osteotomies can be accurately and efficiently performed with an oscillating saw cooled with normal saline. An osteotomy can also be done by drilling holes through the cortex along the osteotomy line and using a Steinmann pin or K wire, then cutting the bone with an osteotome. The

Table 5-1 Deformities and Corrective Osteotomy Procedures

Deformity	Osteotomy technique
Shortening	Transverse lengthening
	Stairstep
	Continuous distraction of a transverse procedure
Angular	Oblique/open wedge
	Closing wedge
	Reverse wedge
Rotational	Transverse derotational
Combination of shortening, angular, and rotational	Oblique/open wedge
	Dome
Incongruent joint	Pelvic
	Intertrochanteric varus derotational
	Transverse lengthening
	Stairstep
	Release

Lateral view   **Cranial view**

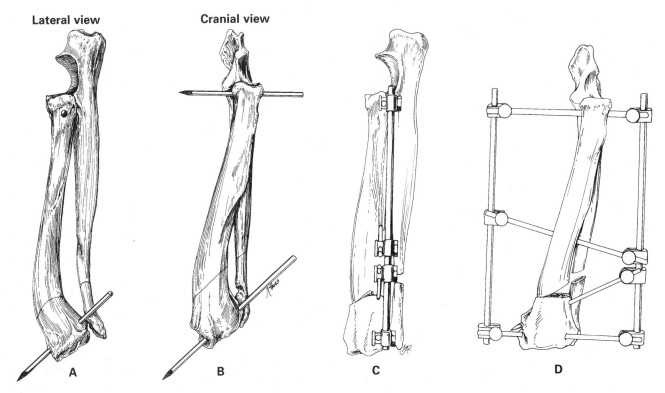

Fig. 5-66   Oblique osteotomy for correction of angular, rotational, and shortened deformity of a radius secondary to premature closure of the distal ulnar physis. **A** and **B,** Placement of the proximal and distal transfixation pins and location of the osteotomy. **C** and **D,** Corrected alignment following osteotomy and stabilization with an external fixator.

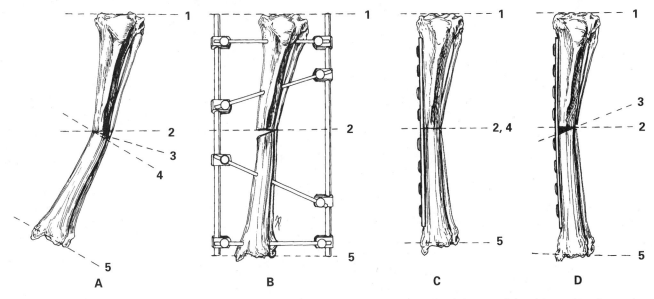

Fig. 5-67   Wedge osteotomy for correction of an angular deformity of the tibia. **A,** Angular deformity of the tibia. **B,** Opening wedge osteotomy stabilized with external fixation. **C,** Closing wedge osteotomy stabilized with internal fixation. **D,** Reverse wedge osteotomy stabilized with internal fixation.

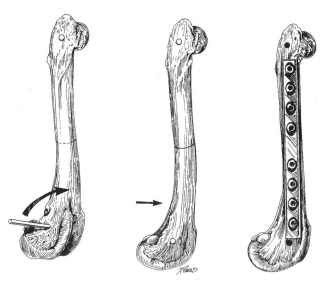

Fig. 5-68   Transverse derotational osteotomy of the femur. K wires are used as landmarks in the lateral transverse plane of the proximal and distal metaphyses. The osteotomy is made and the distal femur rotated until the K wires line up. The osteotomy is stabilized with internal fixation.

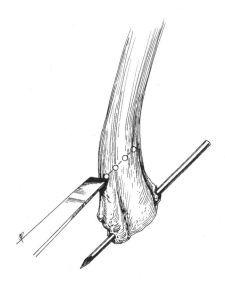

Fig. 5-69   Osteotomy performed using pin holes to outline the osteotomy line and an osteotome to create the osteotomy.

osteotome follows the path of least resistance created by drilling the pin holes (Fig. 5-69).

Although accurate alignment and cortical contact are important aids in stabilizing a fracture, the primary objective of most corrective osteotomies is to align the joints properly. In achieving this goal, especially with oblique osteotomies or open wedge osteotomies, a large gap will exist at the fracture site. This is also true of lengthening osteotomies. These gaps can be filled with autogenous cancellous bone to aid in fracture healing (Fig. 5-70). Fortunately, most corrective osteotomies are performed on young animals with good healing potential.

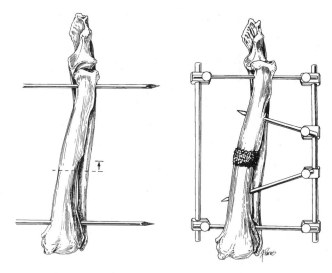

Fig. 5-70   Transverse lengthening osteotomy of the radius to reestablish humeroradial joint congruity. Cancellous bone autograft is packed in the osteotomy gap.

The principles of fixation are identical to those used for fixation of fractures. Rigid internal fixation with plates and screws or pins and wires must be achieved. External fixation splints are also used to achieve rigid fixation. Both axial and rotational stability must be obtained. Choice of implant depends on type of osteotomy created and surgeon's preference. Advantages of plate fixation are greater stability and quicker return to function, especially in corrective osteotomies of the femur. Advantages of external fixation devices are that they need a more limited approach and are more rapidly applied than plates. They also provide the flexibility to change the correction postoperatively, if needed, and allow easy removal of the appliance after bone healing.

Postoperative care is similar to that given to fracture patients. Postoperative radiographs are evaluated to determine if the deformity has been satisfactorily corrected. Because these animals are elective patients without systemic problems or acute injury, postoperative recovery is rapid. After surgery, the animal should be confined and physical therapy performed as needed. Daily care of the external fixation splint may be necessary. Monthly radiographic reevaluations are made to determine implant stability and degree of fracture healing.

OSTEOTOMY TECHNIQUES
Oblique Osteotomy

An oblique osteotomy consists of an oblique cut across the diaphysis at the area of greatest curvature and parallel to the distal joint surface in both the craniocaudal and the mediolateral planes.[4] Because this creates a transverse osteotomy line when viewed in relationship to the distal joint surface and an opening wedge line when the joint surfaces are aligned parallel to each other, this osteotomy can be considered an open wedge osteotomy. This is a versatile osteotomy, allowing simultaneous correction of deformities in three planes: craniocaudal axial angulation, mediolateral axial angulation, and rotational, while maintaining or gaining length. The procedure is frequently used for correction of radius curvus secondary to premature closure of the distal ulnar physis and can be used to correct angular and rotational deformity in any long bone. External fixation is used to stabilize the osteotomy. The most proximal and distal transfixation pins are placed parallel to their respective joint surfaces and in the correct medial-to-lateral transverse plane before performing the osteotomy. This provides a guide for the osteotomy and for aligning the joint surfaces.

The osteotomy is done at the location of greatest curvature of the diaphysis and parallel to the distal joint surface. The bone is aligned with the joint surfaces parallel and in rotational alignment by lining up the transfixation pins parallel to each other and in the same transverse plane. The tip of the proximal segment contacts the distal segment, preferably inserting into the marrow canal to aid in fracture stability. The rest of the fixation pins are placed to stabilize the fracture (see Fig. 5-66).

Dome Osteotomy

The dome osteotomy consists of a semicircular cut performed at the location of greatest curvature of the long bone's diaphysis. This osteotomy allows correction of deformities in three planes, without sacrificing length. In addition, the dome's shape allows it to function as a ball and socket. The cortical contact adds stability to the osteotomy site. This osteotomy is a technically demanding procedure used to treat angular and torsional deformities resulting from premature growth retardation or malunion of fractures. The advantages of increased cortical contact may be insufficient to offset the difficulties of performing this osteotomy when compared with the open wedge procedure.

Preoperative planning is essential. Tracings of the radiographic view that shows the greatest deformity are used to plan the dome. A line is drawn longitudinally down the center of the proximal and distal parts of the affected bone. At the point of intersection, a line is drawn across the diaphysis representing the diameter of a circle over the point of greatest curvature. The proximal portion of the circle is the outline of the osteotomy (Fig. 5-71). The osteotomy site is identified on the bone and the osteotomy outlined as a series of small drill holes made using a wire. The drill holes are connected using a high-speed air drill or oscillating saw. Using the dome as a pivot point, the deformity is corrected. The osteotomy site is stabilized with plate and screws or external skeletal fixation. If the osteotomy is in the metaphysis of the

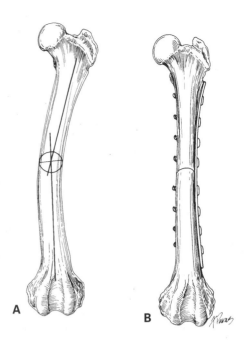

Fig. 5-71 Dome osteotomy for treatment of angular and rotational deformity of a femur. **A,** Preoperative planning lines. **B,** Osteotomy and correction of deformities stabilized with internal fixation.

long bone, cross-pinning may be used to stabilize the fracture.[9]

Transverse Derotational Osteotomy

The transverse osteotomy is a cut through the dorsal plane of the long bone's diaphysis. It is used for correcting torsional deformities. K wires are placed perpendicular to the bone's long axis in the proximal and distal segments and parallel to the lateral transverse plane of each joint. The osteotomy is made at the middiaphyseal area. The bone is aligned so that the K wires are in the same transverse plane, and the osteotomy is stabilized with a compression plate and screws (see Fig. 5-68).

Lengthening Osteotomy

A lengthening osteotomy consists of a transverse or stairstep cut through the bone's diaphysis followed by distraction of the segments. The gain in length can be achieved at surgery or by continual distraction done postoperatively. Indications for a lengthening osteotomy are shortened bones that adversely affect the animal's function. Most animals compensate well with a shortened long bone. Most dogs can lose 20% of the femur's length and still compensate by extending joint angles on the affected limb and decreasing joint angles on the contralateral limb.[2] A shortened radius caused by premature radial physeal closure results in a loss of articulation with the humerus and cannot be compensated for

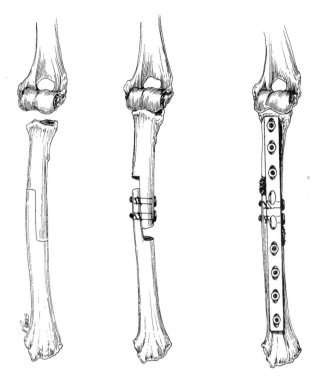

Fig. 5-72 Stairstep osteotomy for lengthening a radius to reestablish humeroradial joint congruity.

because the ulna's length is normal. A lengthening osteotomy of the radius and rearticulation of the radiohumeral joint is necessary to deter secondary DJD in the elbow.[4,11]

A *transverse lengthening osteotomy* is a transverse cut through the long bone's diaphysis followed by distraction of the bone segments to the desired length. The osteotomy is stabilized with plate and screws or an external fixator. The gap is filled with autogenous cancellous bone (see Fig. 5-70).

A *stairstep osteotomy* is a step-shaped cut through the long bone's diaphysis followed by distraction of the segments. Cortical contact and increased stability are achieved by securing the longitudinal portions of the step with a cortex lag screw. A plate and screws are used to stabilize the osteotomy. The gaps are filled with autogenous cancellous bone (Fig. 5-72).

Continuous lengthening can be done to treat shortened bones that require extensive elongation.[3,6,12] Following transverse osteotomy or corticotomy, external fixation is applied. Distraction at the rate of 1 mm per day is instituted 5 to 7 days later. Ideally, this should be continuous distraction, but practically, distraction of 0.5 mm every 12 hours can be used.[12] The use of stable fixation while allowing controlled axial lengthening results in a distraction osteogenesis, where bone is formed directly in the fracture gap. This eliminates the need for

cancellous bone grafting. The osteotomized bone is distracted to the proper length, then immobilized with the fixator until bone union is achieved. By distracting unevenly, angular deformities can be corrected while lengthening the bone.[3,12]

Wedge Osteotomy

The *closing wedge*, or *cuneiform, osteotomy* consists of cutting a predetermined wedge from the diaphysis of the long bone at the point of greatest curvature. This technique is used primarily to correct angular deformities, but some rotational correction can be achieved. The disadvantage of this technique is loss in length of the long bone. The closing wedge osteotomy is accomplished by resecting a predetermined-size wedge from the affected bone. Preoperative planning consists of obtaining tracings of the affected bone from craniocaudal and lateral radiographs. The size of the wedge is determined by drawing lines parallel to the joint surfaces. A perpendicular line is drawn from the joint surface lines to the location of greatest curvature of the diaphysis. Lines parallel to the joint surface lines are drawn, delineating the wedge that must be removed. The location of greatest diaphyseal curvature is surgically approached and the predetermined wedge resected with an oscillating saw. Care must be taken to recreate three-dimensionally the wedge described on two-dimensional drawings. When the wedge is removed, the fracture surfaces are apposed and the osteotomy is stabilized with plate and screws (see Fig. 5-67).

A *reverse wedge osteotomy* preserves bone length. The predetermined wedge is bisected, and half the wedge is removed, rotated 180 degrees, and reinserted, straightening and lengthening the bone simultaneously (see Fig. 5-67, *D*). The replaced wedge functions as a cortical bone autograft. The osteotomy is stabilized with plate and screws to ensure compression and rigid immobilization of the wedge.[7]

The *opening wedge osteotomy* maintains or increases length of the bone as the angular deformity is corrected. A transverse osteotomy is made parallel to the proximal joint surface. The bone is aligned so the joint surfaces are parallel, opening a wedge-shaped gap at the osteotomy site (see Fig. 5-67, *B*). The gap may be filled with cancellous bone, but this is not always necessary in young animals. Either internal or external skeletal fixation can be used to stabilize the osteotomy.[5,7]

Release Osteotomy or Ostectomy

An osteotomy may be done to remove the effect of a bone on an adjacent bone or on joint surface alignment. In premature closure of the distal ulnar physis in the

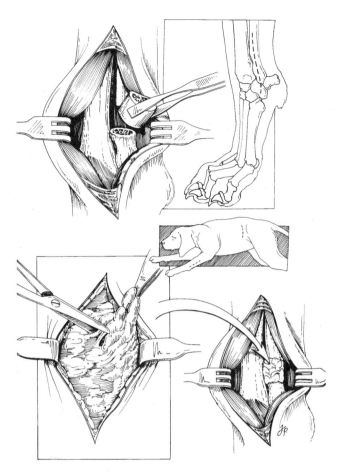

grow. A transverse ostectomy removing about 1 cm of bone of the distal ulna is done. The gap is filled with fat to prevent premature bone union (Fig. 5-73).[4] This procedure allows reestablishment of the incongruent humeroulnar joint and, if the animal has enough growth potential, may result in self-correction of the angular deformity of the radius. In mature dogs with humeroulnar subluxation, osteotomizing the ulna releases the tension on the ulna and may allow the humeroulnar articulation to realign more properly.

REFERENCES

1. Brinker WO, Piermattei DL, Flo GL: *Handbook of small animal orthopedics and fracture treatment*, Philadelphia, 1990, WB Saunders.
2. Franczuszki D, and others: Postoperative effects of experimental femoral shortening in the mature dog, *Vet Surg* 16:89, 1987.
3. Ilizarov GA: Clinical application of the tension-stress effect for limb lengthening, *Clin Orthop* 250:8-26, 1990.
4. Johnson AL: Correction of radial and ulnar growth deformities resulting from premature physeal closure. In Bojrab MJ, editor: *Current techniques in small animal surgery*, ed 3, Philadelphia, 1990, Lea & Febiger.
5. Johnson SG, and others: Corrective osteotomy for pes varus in the dachshund, *Vet Surg* 18:373-379, 1989.
6. Knecht CD, Bloomberg MS: Distraction with an external fixation clamp (Chamley apparatus) to maintain length in premature physeal closure, *J Am Anim Hosp Assoc* 16:873-880, 1980.
7. Newton DC, Nunamaker DM: Osteotomy. In Brinker WO, Hohn RB, Prieur D, editors: *Manual of internal fixation for small animals*, New York, 1984, Springer-Verlag.
8. Schrader SC: Triple osteotomy of the pelvis as a treatment for canine hip dysplasia, *J Am Vet Med Assoc* 178:39-44, 1981.
9. Sikes RI, and others: Dome osteotomy for the correction of long bone malunions: case reports and discussion of surgical technique, *J Am Anim Hosp Assoc* 22:221-226, 1986.
10. Slocum B, Devine T: Pelvic osteotomy in the dog as a treatment for hip dysplasia, *Semin Vet Med Surg (Small Anim)* 2:107-116, 1987.
11. VanDeWater AL, Olmstead ML: Premature closure of the distal radial physis in the dog: a review of eleven cases, *Vet Surg* 12:7-12, 1983.
12. Yanoff SR, and others: Distraction osteogenesis using modified external fixation devices in five dogs, *Vet Surg* 21:480-487, 1992.

Fig. 5-73   Release ostectomy of the distal ulna following premature physeal closure. The ostectomy gap is filled with autogenous fat to prevent premature bone union.

immature dog, the shortened ulna exerts an effect on the growing radius, causing cranial bowing, external rotation, and valgus angulation of the radius and incongruity of the elbow and carpal joints. Ostectomizing the ulnar in the growing dog allows the radius to continue to

6

Preoperative and Postoperative Care of the Orthopedic Patient

JONATHAN H. CHAMBERS

The amount of preoperative planning and postoperative care required for the orthopedic patient varies significantly depending on the disease problem, procedure, and the animal's age and overall health.

PREOPERATIVE EVALUATION
Evaluation of Patients with Nontraumatic Problems

The younger patient. A complete general physical examination should be performed on all patients.

Chapter 1 discusses the specifics of the complete orthopedic examination.

The younger patient (less than 4 years old) with a developmental orthopedic problem, such as patellar luxation, osteochondritis dissecans (OCD), or hip dysplasia, is rarely afflicted with other occult diseases that are life-threatening or preclude general anesthesia, but this should not lull the clinician into a false sense of security. Congenital problems are a good example of when a thorough physical examination occasionally uncovers a coexisting congenital disease that significantly alters the course of management.

Laboratory evaluation in the young, otherwise healthy orthopedic patient can usually be limited to a few well-chosen tests, such as packed cell volume (PCV), total plasma solids, and urinalysis. These three alone are quick, easy, and economical to perform and provide much information. For example, PCV picks up occult anemia and helps assess extracellular hydration. Likewise, measuring total solids helps in the baseline evaluation of extracellular hydration and plasma protein balance. Urine specific gravity is another important indicator of hydration status and is a relatively sensitive test of renal tubular function. The urine dipstick discloses common problems such as occult hematuria from urinary tract infection, or infrequent problems such as glucosuria from previously undiagnosed juvenile diabetes mellitus. I even diagnosed a case of unsuspected congenital portosystemic shunt in a juvenile with patellar luxation, simply by finding ammonium biurate crystals on routine urinalysis.

A few preoperative laboratory tests such as those already mentioned should be done on all patients, regardless of their apparent historical and physical health. These tests act as a screen to alert the surgeon to the potential of complicating conditions or at least the need for further laboratory tests. Other tests that might be considered routine include a heartworm check and fecal evaluation, depending on geographical area and the patient history.

The older patient. Older patients with degenerative orthopedic diseases, such as cruciate ligament rupture, degenerative joint disease, or disk ruptures, require as much or more attention to general history and physical examination as the younger patient. Just as the musculoskeletal system deteriorates with age, so do the other major organ systems, and any significant deficits must be recognized before they prove complicating to the anesthesia, surgery, or postoperative recovery. For example, pulmonary function decreases and the incidence of cardiac disease increases with advancing age,[8] and these two systems are not routinely evaluated with any laboratory tests.

Theoretically, older patients are more likely than younger patients to have occult diseases or marginal organ function and therefore require a more exhaustive preoperative laboratory evaluation. Many teaching hospitals require a complete blood cell count (CBC), blood chemistry profile, and urinalysis for all surgical patients older than 5 or 6 years, regardless of apparent general health. Although I am not aware of solid documentation in the veterinary literature supporting this practice, today's litigious American society has made this standard practice. A thorough history and physical examination are still the best screening tests for potentially complicating conditions, and the orthopedist should not become so dependent on clinical pathology as to view it as a replacement. Conversely, even seemingly minor positive findings such as recent inappetence or mild fever warrant complete laboratory investigation.

Preoperative Evaluation of the Orthopedic Patient with Traumatic Injury

Small animal orthopedic surgery involves treating many severely traumatized patients, many of which have been hit by automobiles. The veterinary orthopedist often becomes the primary care clinician, even when the orthopedic problem is of little or no life-threatening significance.

Multisystem injury often occurs concomitantly with traumatic forces of sufficient magnitude to fracture a major long or flat bone. The cardiovascular and pulmonary systems are most often affected. Many of these patients have been, are, or could easily lapse into hypovolemic shock from internal or external hemorrhage. Cardiac and lung injuries are also very common.[10] As many as 57% of dogs sustaining fractures have thoracic injury.[10] Unfortunately, the majority (79%) of these injuries go undiagnosed on routine physical examination, but radiography detects most (77%) of them.

Cardiac contusion can be present in as many as 17% of fracture patients and is not a radiographically detectable lesion. This is why many anesthesiologists recommend both a preoperative electrocardiogram (ECG) and thoracic radiographs for all orthopedic patients with high-energy trauma.

Intraabdominal injury is also frequently encountered with fracture resulting from high-energy trauma. Trauma to the stomach or intestine is rare, but hemorrhage from the liver or spleen or injury to the urinary tract is relatively common. In one study, 39 percent of dogs with pelvic fractures had radiographically detectable urinary tract trauma, and the injury was severe enough in 16% to warrant surgical intervention. One third of the urinary tract injuries were undetected on initial physical examination. Hematuria occurs often after high-energy impact and does not necessarily indicate a significant urinary tract injury, but persistent dysuria or anuria warrant timely investigation.[9]

Concomitant injury to the nervous system also occurs in fracture patients. The surgeon must be particularly watchful for radial nerve or brachial plexus injury in humeral fracture and sciatic nerve or lumbosacral plexus injury coincident with pelvic and sacroiliac fracture. Spinal fracture must always be ruled out in nonambulatory patients before focusing on a more obvious appendicular injury. Preoperative analgesics should be given if the patient is systemically stable and in pain, but only after a complete general and nervous system examination.

Serial reexamination of the trauma patient is important because potentially lethal injuries to some organs may only become apparent after several hours or even days. This is exemplified by small tears or vascular injuries to the gastrointestinal tract and ruptures of the biliary tree. Even small changes in the patient's status, such as malaise, inappetence, or fever, should be promptly investigated and never ignored.

Laboratory evaluation of the high-energy trauma patient should be exhaustive, including at least a CBC, serum chemistry profile, and urinalysis. Abnormal values should be assessed for significance in light of the physical findings and the need for additional tests determined. As with the physical examination, the first laboratory tests should be considered baseline and repeated whenever a change in the patient's status is suspected. Serial testing also helps to determine whether an abnormal finding is transient and resolving or progressive and possibly requires treatment.

Many patients with severe trauma have significant deficits in extracellular (intravascular) fluid volume and components. These preexisting lesions in water, acid-base balance, erythrocyte mass, and coagulation may have life-threatening consequences unless identified and managed in a timely, accurate manner.[8] Physical criteria such as heart rate, pulse character, capillary refill, skin turgor, mental alertness, and urine output should be carefully assessed for signs of shock or dehydration.

PCV and plasma protein (total solids) should be measured initially and frequently thereafter if significant deficits are detected or to monitor the response to therapy. Crystalloid fluids (lactated Ringer's, acetated Ringer's solution) should be used initially as volume replacement to resuscitate shock or correct dehydration. Hypertonic saline or colloid plasma expanders may also be indicated in patients with severe shock or who are otherwise unresponsive. Plasma can also be used as an albumin replacement to maintain intravascular colloidal osmotic pressure whenever the total plasma protein concentration is significantly less than 3.5 g/100ml.[16] Plasma is more predictable than colloid plasma expanders relative to the subsequent proportion of protein binding of anesthetic drugs. Specific component or whole blood replacement should follow as indicated after repeating the PCV and total solids. Packed red cell or whole blood replacement should be considered if the PCV is significantly less than 25%,[8] especially if the anemia is caused by acute hemorrhage. Platelet count and activated clotting time can be used as a minimum database for patients with suspected coagulation abnormalities,[4] such as disseminated intravascular coagulation brought on by massive tissue necrosis.

Regardless of the specific abnormality, it is best to delay relatively elective surgery such as open reduction and repair of closed fractures until the patient is systemically stable and the results of resuscitative measures can be assessed, usually 24 to 48 hours.[6]

Preoperative Coaptation

All acutely unstable injuries of long bones or joints in between should be coapted. The interrelated goals are to put the limb at rest, decrease pain, reduce displacement, improve circulation, decrease swelling, and prevent further damage to soft tissues, bone, and cartilage.

Fractures or luxations below the elbow or stifle should be splinted from the trunk to the toes. The Robert Jones–type dressing is best suited because it combines sufficient stiffness to prevent undue angulation and compliance to prevent or retard excessive swelling (Fig. 6-1, A). The Robert Jones dressing is contraindicated for femoral or humeral fractures because the top of the bandage acts as a fulcrum near the fracture site (Fig. 6-1, B); the same applies to any splint that terminates in the same location (e.g., Schroeder-Thomas splint). Fractures or luxations at the elbow or stifle can be temporarily stabilized with a Robert Jones bandage if the dressing can be extended high enough in the axilla or groin to control movement of the injured parts. If not, a spica splint should be used.

Fractures of the femoral or humeral diaphysis should be coapted with a spica splint. This is the only type of

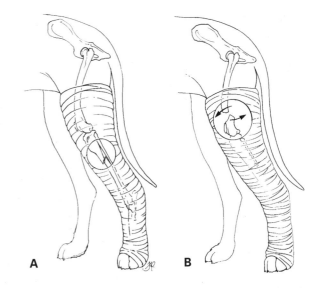

Fig. 6-1   A, Heavily padded Robert Jones bandage for the preoperative coaptation of unstable injuries below the stifle or elbow. **B,** Robert Jones bandage or any coaptation device that ends at the groin (or axilla) is *contraindicated* for femoral or humeral fractures. The top of the bandage becomes a fulcrum, encouraging angulation and motion at the site of injury.

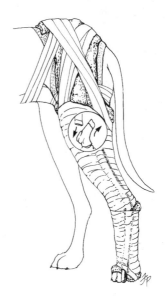

Fig. 6-2   Spica splint for preoperative coaptation of femoral or humeral fractures.

coaptation that extends a sufficient distance proximal to the fracture to neutralize bending forces and immobilize the hip or shoulder (Fig. 6-2). Fractures involving the shoulder or scapula can be stabilized with either a spica splint or Velpeau sling. Hip luxations or fractures can be temporarily managed in a similar manner, although sling immobilization may not be sufficient to prevent erosion of displaced articular surfaces if the patient is ambulatory.

IMMEDIATE POSTOPERATIVE CARE
Analgesia

Postoperative analgesic medication has been previously underutilized in small animal orthopedics. Although assessment of the intensity of an animal's pain is subjective and based on observations after various surgical procedures, invasions of the femur, humerus, and large muscle masses are obviously painful to animals.[11,12]

Opiates should be considered for at least the first 6 to 12 hours after a major orthopedic procedure. Administration before the animal shows signs of intense pain is often more effective than trying to relieve the agony later. Combining the initial dose of the analgesic drug with a tranquilizer or sedative usually diminishes the postanesthetic emergence delirium, smoothes the recovery, and may delay the need for a second dose of narcotic.[1,12] Patients with severe pelvic limb injury may benefit from regional (epidural) opiates, which have a longer duration than systemic administration and circumvent unwanted sedation. Opiates can usually be replaced with nonsteroidal antiinflammatory drugs by the second or third postoperative day if analgesia is still warranted.

Wound Care

Chapter 10 discusses the management of wounds associated with open injuries. The focus here is on care of surgical wounds after aseptic (clean) procedures.

Wounds with drains should be dressed to prevent contamination, but bandages for undrained wounds are optional depending on the surgeon's judgment and preference. Bandages should be considered whenever the position of the wound or other conditions are such that heavy contamination or trauma is likely in the early postoperative period. A fibrin clot effectively seals the normally healing wound within hours, and fear of external contamination beyond that point is unfounded, although immersion of the wound (e.g., hydrotherapy) is usually postponed for a few days. Dressings should be changed frequently to allow wound inspection, and the wound should be inspected immediately if a local or systemic change occurs in the patient's status.

Bandages can be used to prevent self-mutilation of the wound, but bad-tasting local topical medications or other restraint devices (Elizabethan collar, side brace) serve the same purpose but leave the wound exposed for observation. Circumferential pressure bandages help control postoperative swelling as a result of transudative edema,[15] but they also inhibit active and passive limb motion. Return to normal function is often the quickest and most physiological method of resolving edema, and dressings should be abandoned if the limb is stable and they serve no other purpose.

Postoperative Coaptation

A primary goal of surgical orthopedics is to ensure sufficient internal stability as to obviate coaptation, and all fixation plans should be aimed at achieving this goal. When coaptation is believed necessary, it is questionable whether an adequate procedure was performed or whether internal fixation was feasible from the outset. The disadvantage of postoperative coaptation is the combination of scarring and disuse atrophy with fixed joint angles (fracture disease). This may be elected as a permissible drawback in closed-fracture or luxation management, but to add surgical trauma and the resultant scarring is to invite unacceptable withering and ankylosis. If internal fixation is deemed insufficient, augmentative external skeletal fixation should be chosen over coaptation whenever possible, since the former still allows a degree of limb rehabilitation during healing (see Physiotherapy).

Exceptional situations exist in which coaptation is desired and cannot be replaced by external skeletal fixation after surgery, such as precarious repair of either hip or shoulder fractures, luxations, or fracture/luxations. The internal repair can be protected in these patients with a sling to prevent axial loading. Even then, the sling can be left loose enough to allow passive muscle stretching and possibly even graded weight bearing as the healing progresses. Another example is the very-short-term use of a soft, well-padded pressure dressing (Robert Jones type) to prevent swelling. Some surgeons believe swelling delays recovery from an injury, and therefore prevention and treatment are desired goals. However, the pumping action of muscular activity is also very beneficial to venous and lymphatic drainage, and thus exercise should be encouraged in the near term and not discouraged by the prolonged use of cumbersome dressings.

The one situation in which long-term postoperative coaptation is indicated is after arthrodesis, but even in this case, external skeletal fixation may prove as effective and easier to manage.

Detection and Diagnosis of Wound Complications

Dehiscence and seroma. Wound complications such as dehiscence and seroma often occur, and their cause and treatment are usually clear-cut. *Dehiscence* usually develops within the first few days of surgery and is not preceded by signs of excessive wound inflammation (as with infection). The cause can usually be traced to a technical problem (e.g., excessive tension) or patient self-mutilation. Preexisting factors that might impair normal wound healing, such as malnutrition or chronic corticosteroid therapy, must be considered.

Treatment for dehiscence is directed at correcting the primary problem, reclosure, and more arduous wound protection.

Seroma is a fluctuate collection of transudative fluid between the skin and underlying tissues. This can usually be traced to technical errors such as failure to obliterate dead space, excessive motion, or excessive intraoperative trauma. As with the otherwise uncomplicated wound dehiscence, seromas are nonpainful, and the wound should not appear particularly inflamed. If there is any question about the degree of associated inflammation, a sample of the fluid should be immediately analyzed to rule out infection.

Treatment of seroma is relatively elective depending on the size and location, but early elimination of large seromas often averts other problems such as dehiscence or prolonged hospitalization for aesthetic reasons.

Detection and diagnosis of wound infection. Wound infections are often insidious in onset, are difficult to differentiate from postoperative inflammation alone, and may go undetected except by the more astute, introspective surgeon. To diagnose a wound infection is to admit failure, either technically or in anticipating, identifying, and suppressing predisposing factors. However, to procrastinate in the face of even reasonable suspicion is to lose the opportunity to treat when the chances of prompt and complete resolution are the greatest.

Postoperative malaise is usually the first clinical sign of infection,[2] but this may be difficult to discern in the patient that has polysystemic trauma. A lack of return to normal demeanor should be interpreted as suspicious in these patients.

Fever is a relatively sensitive predictor of infectious complications,[13] and a temperature greater than 103° on or persisting beyond the first postoperative day should always alert the orthopedist and never be ignored. An abnormal leukogram showing leucocytosis and a left shift is highly suggestive of infection after clean elective surgery but must be interpreted in the light of the preoperative leukogram in the trauma patient. Most postoperative trauma patients have a mild to moderate neutrophilia from stress and tissue necrosis but usually no left shift;[8] thus a postoperative left shift is significant. A preoperative left shift sustained after surgery is more difficult to interpret, but the magnitude or additional changes in neutrophil morphology may signal a switch from traumatic inflammation to infectious. Even without a left shift, however, infectious complications cannot be ruled out on the basis of the leukogram alone.

The mainstay of wound infection detection is serial site inspection. The criteria are unexpected or excessive signs of inflammation, swelling, discoloration (redness), heat, pain (tenderness), and possibly poor return to function.

Antibiotic therapy or a change in a previous regimen is indicated when a wound infection is suspected, but not before an attempt is made to substantiate the diagnosis and characterize the organism. Suspicious wounds should always undergo needle aspiration(s) because cytology of the aspirate is usually conclusive. Nondegenerate neutrophils may be seen in varying numbers in nonseptic inflammation, but the presence of degenerate neutrophils is highly indicative of septic inflammation, even if organisms are not seen.[5] If the infection is of an exclusively cellulitis nature, it is doubtful that representative cells or organisms will be recovered. The negative aspiration confirms that the infection should respond promptly to appropriate antibiotic therapy alone, since the bacteria are in a rapid replication phase,[2] are not isolated in ischemic areas, and are thus most susceptible. This is rare in wounds after internal fixation, however, and a thick, superficial swelling often overlies an abscess that will be discovered by aspiration. Antibiotics alone in this instance may initially abate the clinical signs but rarely eradicate the infection, and thus potential exists for disastrous long-term consequences. These wounds require incision, inspection, debridement, and drainage. In addition to cytological evaluation, the aspirate provides a representative sample for culture, identification, and susceptibility testing of the causative organism so that antibiotic therapy can be directive rather than empirical.

LONG-TERM POSTOPERATIVE CARE
Physiotherapy

Broadly defined, physiotherapy is use of natural forces in the treatment of disease. In clinical orthopedics, it indicates the use of exercise, manipulation, cold, and heat in the rehabilitation of the injured musculoskeletal system. As all experienced orthopedic surgeons have learned, this phase of patient care is as important as the procedure in determining the eventual outcome. For example, a technically precise internal fixation still often ends in ultimate treatment failure if the patient does not, cannot, or will not use the limb after surgery. It is rarely a question of whether the bone will heal (it will), but rather how strong and serviceable the entire limb is after healing. Conversely, if the patient accepts a well-planned, vigorous physiotherapy program, this often does much to compensate for a less-than-optimum surgical procedure.

The goals of physiotherapy are to relieve pain, restore motion and strength, and ultimately return the limb to as near-normal function as possible and as quickly as possible. The prescription should be tailored to each patient and for each stage of healing. Good judgment must be exercised. For example, if internal fixation of a diaphyseal fracture is perfectly executed, the patient is usually relatively pain free within hours and should be expected to achieve limited axial loading immediately. In this instance the physiotherapy program can be fairly aggressive, such as long, slow leash walks within 48 hours of surgery. Less stable repairs of bone, ligament, or tendon may require a more conservative approach, with non-loaded exercise limited to passive motion or swimming. Some physiotherapeutic components are primarily valuable in the short term and others in the long term. The basic ingredients and indications are covered in the following discussion.

Cold. Cold therapy in the form of ice packs should be used in the *acute* phase of injury, which includes the first few days after surgery. Its beneficial effect is limiting inflammation by slowing the blood flow in the microcirculation and slowing metabolism. The specific clinical attributes are a decrease in pain, swelling (edema), and muscle spasm. Ice therapy is often helpful when used before or with passive stretching and massage of the acutely injured limb.

Crushed ice in a plastic bag is the easiest method of applying cold therapy because if conforms well and thus provides a broad, uniform contact surface. Commercially available refreezable ice packs also work well. The treatment regimen is empirical, but 20 minutes two or three times a day is often recommended.

Heat. Heat therapy in the form of hot compresses is primarily indicated in the more *chronic* phase of healing, which begins a few days after injury or surgery. Its general beneficial effect is a rise in blood flow by dilation of the microcirculation, which increases oxygen delivery and metabolism in injured tissues. The observed clinical effects are a decrease in pain and muscle spasm and an increase in muscle relaxation. Another common indication for heat is to help draw (drain) exudate from an infected wound.

A common misconception is that heat decreases acute swelling and is indicated in the immediate postoperative period. In this instance, heat may aggravate swelling and initiate delayed hemorrhage from wound edges. Therefore, heat should not be used until several days after surgery.

Heat is most easily applied with moist hot towels. The temperature should not exceed 105°F (40.5°C) but the towels should be changed frequently to maintain a warm temperature, and treatment should continue for at least 20 minutes. Moist heat can also be used in the form of whirlpool baths but should not be used in the immediate postoperative period for reasons previously stated.

Dry heat is also indicated to treat chronic inflammation and is applied as ultrasonic, incandescent, infrared, ultraviolet, or microwave radiation, but this requires special equipment and training.

Contrast cold and heat therapy. Using intermittent ice and hot compresses in 2-minute cycles is thought to help mobilize edematous swelling. A microvascular pump is created as the ice causes vasoconstriction, followed by heat-induced vasodilation. The cycles are continued for 20 to 30 minutes, always beginning and ending the process with ice. This type of therapy should not be used in the acute phase after injury (48 to 72 hours) because the heat aggravates swelling until the microvascular injury begins to heal.

Massage. Massage is purported to relieve pain and muscle tension, increase blood flow, and mobilize fluid and waste materials from injured limbs; the actual degree of beneficial effect is poorly understood and documented. Even so, massage appears to do no harm and is often combined with cold and heat therapy. Manual squeezing and kneading of the tissues is the most common means of massage, but whirlpool baths are also used.

Passive motion. Passive physiotherapy is probably best described as controlled *stretching* of muscle and other soft tissues. The primary purpose is to maintain or restore range of motion in the joints in the face of restriction or even ankylosis caused by swelling or fibrosis. It is done by gradually forcing the joints into maximum flexion and extension, with the goal of eventually attaining normal range of motion.

The usual technique involves gradually and slowly flexing the joint to the point of acceptable pain tolerance, holding it there for 10 seconds, then slowly releasing the pressure. The same is done for extension. The procedure is repeated through approximately 10 cycles. Stretching beyond minimum pain should be avoided, since this usually indicates tearing of fibrous tissue rather than stretching and leads to additional scar tissue formation. Mild analgesics and heat therapy are often combined with stretching. Heating of the tissue is thought to make it more plastic and easier to stretch.

A common misconception is that passive stretching is an acceptable replacement for active physiotherapy. No muscular work is performed, however, and therefore muscular strength and tone are unaffected. In addition, passive stretching is not as effective as active stretching in maintaining or restoring joint motion.

Active physiotherapy. Active physiotherapy, or "exercise," is when the patient performs the work of maintaining or restoring muscular strength and joint motion. In short, this is the most physiological and effective method of restoring function to an injured limb, and no substitute for it exists. Many active physiotherapy techniques are used on people that do not involve axial loading of the limb, but veterinary orthopedics is much more limited. Therefore, good judgment must be used when deciding when the patient's injury is stable enough to withstand ambulatory forces. However, the goal of operative orthopedics is always to repair the injury to as near-normal strength as possible so that the patient can resume function quickly. A better short-term and long-term clinical result is consistently achieved under these conditions, and the patient should not be deprived of the benefits of active physiotherapy.

Slow leash walks are the mainstay of early active physiotherapy. A towel or other sling device can be used initially to support part of the weight-bearing force if the limb is still mildly unstable or very painful. Analgesics should also be used if pain is hampering the physiotherapy, but the clinician should always be alert to an unexpectedly high degree of pain or an increasing pain pattern; this is often a warning of unacceptable instability or other major complication.

Patients must often be coaxed to use painful limbs, especially if lameness was a chronic preoperative problem. Increasing the length of the slow leash walks in both time and distance often brings about the desired effect. The objective is to create enough fatigue in the other limbs so as to divert attention away from the injured limb. Walking up and down hills or steps also produces the same fatigue factor and creates a gait obstruction that may stimulate use of the injured limb.

A useful tool to distract the patient's attention away from the injured limb involves taping an irritating but otherwise harmless object to the weight-bearing surface of the contralateral foot. The goal is a sensation similar to having a small pebble in a shoe. Any smooth, relatively round object of appropriate size can be used, but I prefer the plastic cap from a small syringe case. It is placed between the digital and metatarsal (metacarpal) pads before the walk. It may be occasionally necessary to use the same technique on both contralateral limbs or even all three of the uninjured limbs, especially if the injury is extremely chronic and the patient has become habitually dependent on them. Some clients initially object to this treatment, but they must be reoriented and reassured that it is for the pet's benefit. A similar technique of slinging the contralateral limb has been suggested, but I have not found this to be as beneficial and believe it might be dangerous if it causes the patient to be so uncoordinated as to cause a fall or otherwise apply too much force to the repaired limb.

Swimming is an excellent form of active physiotherapy and has the added advantage of building muscle strength and joint mobility without weight bearing.

Electrostimulation of muscles is another method that can be used in the early postoperative period when the patient will not or should not ambulate. It retards muscle atrophy, relaxes muscle spasm, maintains or increases joint motion, and increases local circulation. Newer designs of muscle stimulators are safe, easy to use, and offer a reciprocating mode for simultaneously working on muscle strength and joint mobility. I have found stimulators to be especially beneficial in early postoperative rehabilitation after articular and periarticular fractures of the elbow and stifle. Patient acceptance is usually good, but sedation or analgesia may be required.

Client Communication and Compliance

Effective client communication must include a thorough preoperative explanation of the disease, treatment options, prognosis, expectations, and potential complications. No assumptions should be made as to the client's wishes, financial capability, or expectations. For example, the orthopedist may be delighted when the patient with the spinal fracture finally walks again, but the client may not share the enthusiasm if the unrealistic expectation of return to performance athletics was never discussed.

Instructions to owners concerning nursing care and rehabilitation of the postoperative patient should be explicit and detailed and in both written form for the patient record and verbal form to ascertain understanding and give the client an opportunity to ask questions. Physiotherapy and other procedures such as wound and dressing care must be *demonstrated*, not just described. General statements such as "restrict the exercise" must be avoided and replaced with detailed instructions and explanations. Some clients have and use good judgment, whereas others may interpret restricted exercise as confinement to three acres of fenced-in yard because the animal was previously allowed to run free. If an orthopedic procedure is truly effective, usually a substantial lag occurs between return of pain-free normal function and true healing time, but many clients tend to forget or ignore this despite diligent counseling. The wise orthopedist overestimates the degree and duration of restricted activity in hopes of acquiring the minimum owner-patient compliance required for a successful result.

REFERENCES

1. Aron DA: Pain. In Lorenz MD, Cornelius LM, editors: *Small animal medical diagnosis*, Philadelphia, 1987, Lippincott.
2. Artz CP: Infections in surgery. In Artz CP, Harty JD, editors: *Management of surgical complications*, ed 3, Philadelphia, 1975, Saunders.
3. Bertoy RW, Johnson AL, Weigel RM: Organ system injury and postoperative complications in dogs and cats with two long bone fractures: a matched case design, *Vet Comp Orthop Traum* 4:140-143, 1989.
4. Blue JT, Short CE: Preanesthetic evaluation and clinical pathology. In Short CE, editor: *Principles and practice of veterinary anesthesia*, Baltimore, 1987, Williams & Wilkins.

5. Duncan JR, Prasse KW: *Veterinary laboratory medicine*, ed 2, Ames, Iowa, 1986, Iowa State University Press.

6. Houlton JEF, Taylor PM: *Trauma management in the dog and cat*, Bristol, 1987, Wright.

7. Meyer RE: Anesthesia for neonatal and geriatric patients. In Short CE, editor: *Principles and practice of veterinary anesthesia*, Baltimore, 1987, Williams & Wilkins.

8. Raffe MR: Fluid therapy, electrolyte and acid-base balance, and blood replacement. In Short CE, editor: *Principles and practice of veterinary anesthesia*, Baltimore, 1987, Williams & Wilkins.

9. Selcer BA: Urinary tract trauma associated with pelvic trauma, *J Am Anim Hosp Assoc* 19:785-793, 1982.

10. Selcer BA, and others: The incidence of thoracic trauma in dogs with skeletal injury, *J Small Anim Pract* 28:21-27, 1987.

11. Short CE: Pain, analgesics, and related medications. In Short CE, editor: *Principles and practice of veterinary anesthesia*, Baltimore, 1987, Williams & Wilkins.

12. Soma LR: Behavioral changes and the assessment of pain in animals, *Proceedings of the 2nd International Congress of Veterinary Anesthesia*, 1985, pp 38-41.

13. Stevenson S, Olmstead ML, Kowalski JK: Bacterial culturing for prediction of postoperative complications following open fracture repair in small animals, *Vet Surg* 15:99-102, 1986.

14. Swaim SF, Henderson RA: *Small animal wound management*, Philadelphia, 1990, Lea & Febiger.

15. Zaslow IM: *Veterinary trauma and critical care*, Philadelphia, 1984, Lea & Febiger.

II

STANDARD FRACTURE REPAIR

7

Fractures of the Skull, Mandible, Spine, and Ribs

THOMAS M. TURNER
PETER K. SHIRES

SECTION A   Fractures of the Skull and Mandible

Thomas M. Turner

Fractures of the skull and mandible, unlike long bone fractures, demand additional considerations in treatment because of their intimate association with other organ systems. Specifically, these considerations are the potential impairments to functions of the digestive, respiratory, and neurological systems The skull and mandible provide support for the dentition and associated soft tissue structures such as the tongue and adjacent musculature involved with the digestive process. The bony structure of the skull also forms the nasal cavities, which are the initial (facial) structures of the respiratory system. In addition, the skull bones also form the cranial cavity for encasement of the brain and associated neurological structures. The surgeon must consider these associated functions in performing definitive fracture treatment.

The purpose of this section is to focus specifically on the treatment of fractures of the skull and mandible. Dentistry, disease processes of the upper respiratory system, and neurology are only mentioned peripherally, and the reader is encouraged to consult other authorities for discussions relating to these systems.

ANATOMICAL CONSIDERATIONS

The bones of the skull, particularly the facial bones, generally are unicortical and relatively thin and thus structurally weak if isolated from the skull. However, the anatomical arrangement of these skull bones forms a structure that can resist considerable forces despite the relatively thin bone. In particular, the incisive, maxilla, nasal, frontal, and zygomatic bones form a critical buttress to support the dentition and palate. Forces created as a result of dental occlusion during mastication are transferred from the dentition through the nasal bones, principally the maxilla, to the mass of the skull (Fig. 7-1). These bones also define the nasal and frontal cavities of the skull.

The other principal component of the skull is the cranial cavity, which contains the brain and is formed by the frontal, parietal, sphenoid, temporal, and occipital bones.

The mandible is divided into symmetrical right and left halves, which are joined rostrally at the fibrous mandibular symphyseal joint. The horizontal portion (body) of the mandible contains the dentition, whereas the more vertical portion (ramus) provides for articulation with the skull and musculature attachments. When viewed from the cranial aspect, the mandibular body is inclined in the dorsolateral direction. The bicortical mandibular body can be further divided into cranial and caudal aspects. In the caudal aspect the body deviates into a prominent vertical ramus, which is composed of three prominent structures: coronoid, condyloid, and angular processes. The condyloid process articulates with the zygomatic portion of the temporal bone. The dorsal aspect of the ramus is very thin and unicortical, particularly over the broad masseteric fossa. The mandibular artery, vein, and nerve enter the body of the mandible at the mandibular foramen, which is located on the medial aspect of the ramus just cranial to the angular process. Neurovascular structures are contained within the mandibular canal through the mandible's length, providing blood supply and innervation to the dentition and mandible. The dentition lies along the dorsal aspect of the mandibular body; with the roots contained in the alveoli. The mandible's tension surface is along the line of the dentition.

FRACTURE TREATMENT METHODS
Fracture Repair Goals

The major goals of fracture treatment are to restore accurate anatomical alignment and concurrently achieve normal dental occlusion. The fracture should be rigidly fixed to maintain the anatomical alignment during the healing process and to achieve a normal and stable range of motion of the temporomandibular joint (TMJ). Failure to achieve normal dental occlusion can result in abnormal wear of the dentition, altered eating habits, degenerative joint disease of the TMJ, and poor cosmesis.

Fixation Techniques

In general, nondisplaced fractures of the skull, either of the nasal cavity or cranium, are treated conservatively. However, unstable or grossly displaced fractures can result in malocclusion of the dentition and should be stabilized with open reduction and fixation.

A variety of fixation techniques have been described for fixation of fractures involving the skull and mandible. These may be classified as (1) intraoral techniques, such as interdental wiring and intraoral splints; (2) internal fixation through interfragmentary wiring techniques, small-diameter fixation pins, or bone plates (intramedullary pinning is not as preferable as other methods of fixation); and (3) external fixation, which may be applied to the mandible or skull.

Interdental wiring. Interdental wiring techniques, such as Ivy and Stout loops or a modification of these, have been described for dogs. These techniques require that the teeth be healthy and stable within the alveolus at the fracture site. The technique consists of a continuous interconnected wire pattern that encompasses two

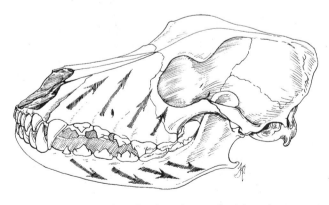

Fig. 7-1 Forces that develop during dental occlusion are transferred to the adjacent bony structures (arrows). The maxilla acts as a buttress to support the upper dental arcade. The fracture repair must be performed in a manner to counteract these forces that act on a given fracture.

or more adjacent teeth. Generally, 24-gauge wire is used, and loops of wire are passed from the lingual to buccal surfaces of the teeth at adjacent interdental spaces. The free caudal end of wire is passed behind the caudal tooth and passed beneath the projecting interdental wire loops on the buccal surface. The free end of wire on the lingual surface and the end of wire on the buccal teeth surfaces are twisted together and tightened against the next rostral tooth. The interdental wire loops are subsequently tightened to ensure that the entire wire splint is stable. This interdental technique does not counteract the rotational and bending forces acting on the fracture and other fixation techniques (Fig. 7-2). Fractures that occur in mandibles with diseased or absent dentition are not treatable by these techniques. These methods may also necessitate notching the teeth at the gingiva to prevent wire slippage, and attention must be directed to oral hygiene.

The three most frequently used fixation techniques are interfragmentary wiring, bone plates, and external fixtures. When using any of these methods, the surgeon must be careful to avoid damage to dental roots and projection of screws or pins into the oral cavity. If the mandibular artery and nerve are intact, further trauma of these structures also must be avoided.

Interfragmentary wiring. This technique can provide rigid fixation of the fracture fragments and is one of the most versatile methods available for treating skull and mandible fractures. In general, at least two wires should be applied across a fracture line. The wires are placed 90 degrees to the fracture line. Drill holes for

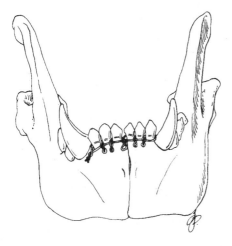

Fig. 7-2 Interdental wiring technique (modified Stout technique). A continuous wire is used to form loops that are passed through adjacent interdental spaces, and a free end of the wire is sequentially passed over the buccal surface of the teeth beneath the wire loops and tightened at the opposite free end. The series of interdental loops is subsequently tightened. This technique may be useful for stabilization of loose dentition or isolated alveolus fractures and to supplement other fixation techniques.

placement of the wire should be directed in a slight converging angle toward the medial aspect of the fracture, which aids in conforming the wire to the bone during tightening of the wire. The exact number and placement of the interfragmentary wires vary in fractures, but the surgeon must remember that the aim is to achieve compression of the entire fracture line. Wire of sufficient diameter should be used, preferably 0.8 mm wire in small and toy breeds and thin unicortical bone and 1.0 mm in larger breeds and bicortical bone. The use of inadequate-sized wire is a common error in treatment of skull and mandible fractures.

Wire should always be twisted under tension to achieve an even tightening and twisting of both strands. The twisted end of the wire is cut, leaving a length of at least four twists; the cut end is bent over to lie close to the bone and avoid projection into the soft tissues. When treating skull bone fractures, the surgeon should be careful not to overtighten the wire. This can result in tearing of the wire through the thin bones of the skull. In the skull, wires of no greater diameter than 0.8 mm and usually smaller-diameter wires are preferable. In the mandible, however, 0.8 mm and 1.0 mm wires are preferable.

Bone plates. The use of bone plates in the treatment of skull and mandible fractures can achieve rigid fixation of the fracture. However, this does demand precise contouring of the plate to the fractured bone. The aim is to achieve compression of the entire fracture line, and the surgeon must remember this occurs in three dimensions, therefore necessitating compression of the fracture in the axial, mediolateral, and ventrodorsal planes. Slight incongruities, which in a long bone fracture would be acceptable, can result in malocclusion of the dentition in mandible fractures. Plates are generally applied to the lateral aspect of the mandibular body and ramus.

The variety of available surgical implants, both in shape and size, helps the surgeon achieve the goal. Plates suitable for application to mandible and skull fractures are the standard Dynamic Compression Plate (DCP), finger plate and miniplate series, eccentric compression plate (ECP), and reconstruction plate. The reconstruction plate is now widely accepted in the treatment of fractures, particularly of the mandible. This plate offers the ability to contour in three dimensions. Conventional plates allow contouring by a longitudinal twist or bend. The reconstruction plate can be contoured in a longitudinal curve as well. This provides for an ideal contourability to the mandible's irregular architectural surface. When using plates in the skull, the surgeon should use only the 2.0 mm or 2.7 mm size, although mandible fractures may require 2.0 mm, 2.7 mm, or 3.5 mm size plates.

External fixation. The external fixtures are of particular benefit in highly comminuted fractures. They allow the surgeon to develop a fixation device that can easily be adapted to a variety of fracture types and severities. Individual pins or long screws are inserted into fracture fragments on either side of the fracture. Fragments are anatomically positioned and temporarily held in position using fixation forceps or by an assistant. The externally projecting ends of the pins or screws are then connected to a metallic bar or, more often, encompassed in an acrylic material such as methylmethacrylate. When using methylmethacrylate, the cement is applied in the dough stage, when it can be rolled into a long length of uniform diameter and pressed over the exposed ends of the projecting pins or screws. Alternately, the exposed ends of the pins or screws may be inserted into a length of vinyl tubing, which is easily deformable to the desired shape. The tube then is injected with the acrylic in a liquid state. The cement bar or vinyl tubing may range from ⅛ to ¾ inch in diameter, depending on the skull or mandible size (Fig. 7-3).

This method of external fixation can be very rewarding. It allows minimum implantation of metal, wide adaptability, and may function as a buttress, neutralization, or compression splint. However, the rigidity of the fixation may not be as great as that achieved with interfragmentary wiring or plating. Nevertheless, this technique deserves consideration, particularly in the treatment of severely comminuted fractures.

Wire mesh. Another technique in the treatment of fractures, particularly those of the skull, is the use of stainless steel wire mesh. This is used as an onlay to maintain the anatomical contour of a specific region that cannot be totally reconstructed because of severe comminution or bone loss. Using wire scissors, a section of wire is cut that is slightly larger than the fracture defect. This wire mesh is secured with small-diameter wires to the periphery of the defect (Fig. 7-6). Ultimately, the periphery of the wire mesh is incorporated in bone, and the portion over the defect is filled with fibrous tissue. Alternately, the retrieved comminuted fracture fragments may be overlaid on the wire mesh, or a cancellous graft can be applied.

Dentition Considerations

Since a primary goal of fracture repair is to achieve dental occlusion, both the health and the stability of the dentition at the fracture site must be evaluated. If the tooth and periodontal tissues are healthy and the tooth is secure in the adjacent alveolus, it should be allowed to remain in place because this can aid in reduction of the fracture and alignment. If the alveolus and periodontal tissues are healthy but the tooth is unstable, it may be wired in place using one of the interdental wiring techniques. Although a moderate percentage of these teeth do not reestablish stability in the alveolus, it is preferable to give the tooth the opportunity to reestablish integrity, removing it at a later date if it does not reattach in the alveolus. If the periodontal tissues and alveolus are unhealthy, whether the tooth is stable or unstable, it should be removed before fracture fixation and the adjacent tissues and alveolus debrided.

If extreme periodontal disease is present, the surgeon should use a minimally invasive fixation method (such as interfragmentary wiring or the external fixture) to provide support to the fracture. Extraction of any diseased teeth, debridement of periodontal and alveolar tissue, and dental prophylaxis are performed before application of the fixator.

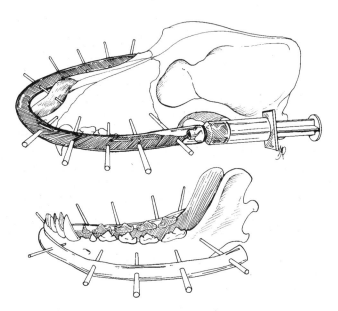

Fig. 7-3 External fixture may be developed by inserting small-diameter pins or screws into the fracture fragments after anatomical reduction of the fracture. The exposed external ends of the pins or screws then are encompassed in vinyl tubing, and acrylic cement is injected into the tube while the fracture fragments are maintained in anatomical position. Once the acrylic sets, a rigid fixation device adapted specifically to that particular fracture is achieved. Alternately, the acrylic may be allowed to develop into the dough stage, rolled into a uniform diameter and length, then molded over the exposed ends of the pins.

Surgical Preparation

A technique that can be extremely useful in reduction and fixation of jaw fractures is placement of an endotracheal tube through a pharyngotomy incision. The animal is first entubated in a standard manner. The site is identified for placement of a pharyngotomy incision caudal to the angle of the jaw and adjacent to the hyoid apparatus. Using blunt dissection, a large forceps is passed into the mouth, and the external end of the endotracheal tube without the adaptor is passed through the incision.

The adaptor is reconnected and attached to anesthesia. This allows closure of the mouth and normal interdigitation of the dentition. The dentition then acts as a splint, aligning the fracture fragments in an anatomical position. Any displacement of the dentition from the normal occlusion position during the repair alerts the surgeon to misalignment of the fracture fragments or improper contouring of the bone plate.

Fractures at the extreme rostral aspect, such as mandibular symphyseal fractures or fractures of the incisive bone, may be repaired with an oral or limited oral surgical approach. Fractures of the mandibular body and ramus should be approached from the ventral or ventrolateral aspect. Fractures of the nasal maxilla, frontal, parietal, temporal, or occipital bones are approached directly with incisions over the specific fracture line. If extensive fractures are present over the nasal bones, a midline dorsal approach is used.

FRACTURES OF THE SKULL
Incisive Bone

Longitudinal fractures of the incisive bone may be fixed using a cerclage wire passed transversely over the dorsal aspect of the incisive bone, twisting the wire behind the canine teeth. The twisted end is cut and bent to lie flat against the mucosa. Isolated fractures in which the fragment of the bone includes two or more teeth may be positioned and fixed using two or more Kirschner wires inserted in a converging manner, which may or may not be encompassed within a cerclage wire (Fig. 7-4).

Maxilla

Fractures of the bones involving the nasal cavity must be securely fixed to reestablish the buttress to the upper arcade of the dentition. Transverse and oblique fractures of the maxilla that involve the palatine portion may be fixed with intraorally placed interfragmentary wires. The protruding end of the wire twist must be bent to lie flat against the hard palate, or preferably the wire is placed in a more ventrolateral aspect, such that the wire twist does not lie over the palate but lies along the buccal aspect of the dentition.

Longitudinal fractures of the palate that are minimally displaced and stable may be treated conservatively. However, fractures displaced or associated with skull fractures must be stabilized. A small-diameter pin or Kirschner wire is inserted orally just above the premolar dentition and transversely through both maxillae. A heavy-gauge (0.8 or 1.0 mm) wire is placed over the exposed ends of the pin in a figure-eight pattern and tightened (Fig. 7-5).

Fractures of the maxilla proper frequently necessitate the use of multiple interfragmentary wires, particularly with extensive fragmentation of the maxilla. The recon-

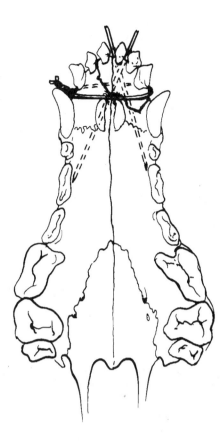

Fig. 7-4 Fractures of the incisive bone containing dentition may be stabilized using two or three crossed Kirschner wires. This may be further supported with a cerclage wire.

struction should begin by achieving normal occlusion of the dentition, then wiring the maxilla fragments sequentially with multiple wires. A useful technique is to preplace the interfragmentary wires, then tighten these, starting first with those closest to the dentition and moving to the more dorsal aspect of the maxilla. Fragments may also be stabilized by placing two small screws, one on either side of the fracture, and connecting these with figure-eight wire. Areas of the maxilla that have multiple fracture lines or that cannot be totally reconstructed may be bridged using a buttress plate (2.0 or 2.7 mm) (Fig. 7-6). The external fixator, using Kirschner pins and acrylic bars, can provide a satisfactory fixation method for treating maxilla and incisive bone fractures.

Zygomatic Bone

Fractures of the zygomatic bone may pose more of a cosmetic defect than functional impairment. However, extensive fragmentation or multiple fragments ventral to the orbit may allow ventral drift of the globe. An incision is made directly over the zygomatic bone, and the fragments are elevated from behind using a small periosteal elevator and fixed in place using a miniplate or small interfragmentary wires.

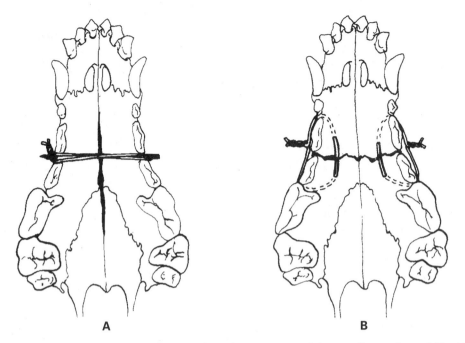

Fig. 7-5 **A,** Longitudinal fracture of the palatine portion of the maxilla may be stabilized by a transversely placed small-diameter pin inserted orally above the hard palate. An intraorally placed figure-eight wire is passed over the exposed ends of the pin. Tightening the wire causes compression of the longitudinal fracture. **B,** Transverse fracture through the palatine portion of the maxilla may be stabilized with interfragmentary wires using heavy-gauge wire (0.8 or 1.0 mm). The wires are placed such that the twist lies on the buccal surface of the gum.

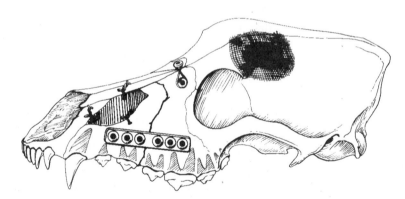

Fig. 7-6 Multifragment fractures involving the premaxilla, maxilla, and frontal bones may be stabilized with a series of preplaced interfragmentary wires. Likewise, small-diameter screws may be placed on opposing sides of a fracture line to serve as anchors for figure-eight wire. A 2.0 or 2.7 mm bone plate may be used to bridge areas of comminution or provide additional buttress support. Areas of severe comminution or bone loss may be covered using a stainless steel wire mesh, which is secured to the periphery of the defect with orthopedic wire sutures, thus restoring the anatomical contour.

Frontal Bone

Fractures of the frontal bone may result in an obvious cosmetic depression. If possible, the fracture fragments are elevated and the individual fragments stabilized in position using small-diameter interfragmentary wires. Care should be taken not to overtighten the wires because they can tear through the thin frontal bone. If only one or two large fragments are depressed, these may be elevated by drilling a small hole adjacent to the fracture line in the nonfractured frontal bone and elevating the fracture fragments from beneath into position and fixing with interfragmentary wires. Areas of small comminution may be bridged with a stainless steel mesh onlay after the small fragments have been removed (see Fig. 7-6). This provides cosmetic coverage of the defect. Graft may be placed over the mesh; however, this usually is not necessary because the mesh will be incorporated in bone and fibrous tissue.

Cranium

Fractures involving the bones of the cranial cavity are generally not fixed if they are stable and minimally displaced. In contrast, fractures that are depressed into the dura or brain tissue necessitate immediate surgical attention. The fracture fragments are gently removed, blood and damaged tissue are removed, and appropriate medical management is instituted using steroids, manmitol, and antibiotics. If large depressed fragments are present, these are elevated and, once the underlying neurological structures have been treated, loosely fixed in position so as not to impair swelling of the neurological structures. Defects that remain from highly comminuted fractures may ultimately be covered with a stainless steel mesh and soft tissue flap.

FRACTURES OF THE MANDIBLE
Symphysis

Fractures of the mandibular symphysis are frequently encountered. Symphyseal separations often occur with-

out other associated injuries. However, caudal mandible and ramus fractures also have a high incidence of concurrent symphyseal separation. Several different techniques have been advocated for the stabilization of this separation, ranging from intraoral wiring to the placement of a lag screw.

In the most efficient and effective fixation technique, a large-bore needle is inserted under the ventral aspect of the cranial mandible, with the point of the needle exiting just caudal to the canine tooth on the buccal surface of the cranial mandible. A length of either 0.8 or 1.0 mm wire is inserted into the needle, exiting at the point of the needle's entrance in the ventral midline. The same procedure is repeated on the opposite side of the mandible. Wire now passes over the dorsal aspect of the cranial mandible behind both canine teeth, with both strands exiting on the ventral aspect. The wire is pulled tight, the jaw closed so that the dentition is in normal occlusion, and the wire twisted tight (Fig. 7-7). The twisted end of the wire may be left exposed or bent to lie just under the skin.

Since this is a fibrous joint, the area usually heals within 6 weeks, and the wire may be removed within 8 weeks. The wire is cut on the intraoral exposed portion and pulled ventrally. In a fracture involving the incisors and a symphyseal separation, the use of two or more

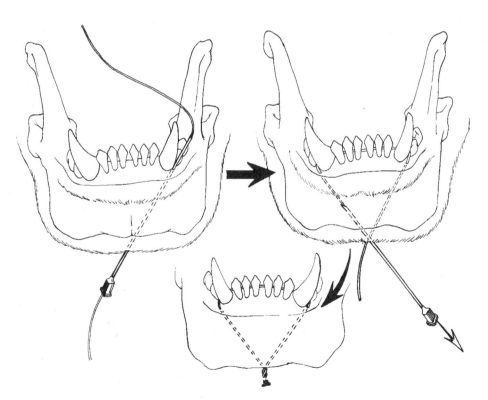

Fig. 7-7 Mandibular symphseal separation can be stabilized with a cerclage wire. The wire is inserted from the ventral aspect of the mandible, passing intraorally behind the canine teeth, with the twist remaining in the ventral mandibular area.

converging Kirschner wires combined with the cerclage wire can provide adequate fixation.

Cranial Mandible

Fractures of the cranial mandible generally are associated with a fracture into the lower canine alveolus. These fractures are preferably treated using an interfragmentary wiring technique. Two cerclage wires may be placed, extending from the buccal mandibular surface around the lingual surface; if necessary, a hole is drilled through the mandibular symphysis, with the wire passing from the buccal aspect of the canine tooth over the medial aspect. If the fracture line extends caudal to the alveolus, interfragmentary wires may be combined with the cerclage wires to achieve compression of the fracture line. Also, an intraoral figure-eight wire from the second premolar to encompass the canine tooth is advantageous, acting as a tension band and counteracting the distractive force on the canine tooth (Fig. 7-8).

Caudal Mandible

Fractures of the caudal mandible body may be treated using either an interfragmentary wiring technique or bone plates. Forces acting on the mandible tend to result in an opening of the fracture line along the dental arcade and displacement of the cranial mandible ventrally and caudal mandible dorsally. If interfragmentary wires are used, at least two wires must be used per fracture line, with at least one wire being close to the dental arcade.

All interfragmentary wires should be placed perpendicular to the fracture (Fig. 7-9).

Fractures of the caudal mandible are also well suited to the use of a reconstruction plate, which may be contoured to lie along the mandible's lateral surface, extending from the cranial aspect caudally and along the ramus vertically. Careful contouring of the plate is essential to anatomical fixation. Three screws of purchase should be obtained cranial and caudal to the fracture line. As the screws are tightened, the fracture should be evenly compressed (Fig. 7-10).

Fractures of the ramus may be treated with interfragmentary wiring. However, because of the thin texture of

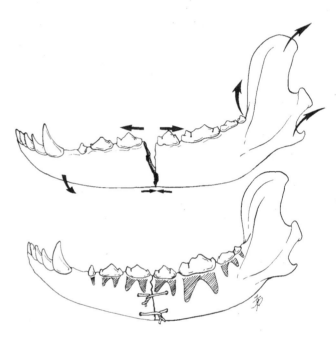

Fig. 7-9 Fractures of the mandibular body may be stabilized with interfragmentary wires using at least two wires per fracture. These should be placed perpendicular to the fracture line to counteract the distractive forces on the fracture.

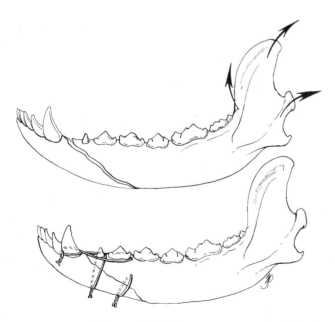

Fig. 7-8 Cranial mandibular fractures are most effectively fixed using a combination of cerclage and hemicerclage wires. If the fracture involves the canine tooth, supplementary fixation may be added using an intraoral figure-eight wire.

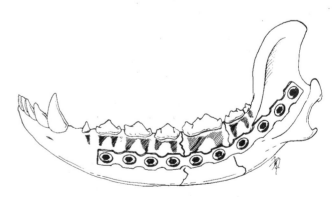

Fig. 7-10 Fractures of the mandibular body and caudal mandible or segmental fractures may be fixed using a reconstruction plate. This plate is useful because it may be contoured over a long segment of mandible in a longitudinal curve, twist, or bend.

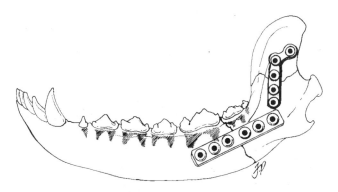

Fig. 7-11 Fractures of the caudal mandible and vertical ramus may be fixed using a combination of plates, such as a standard dynamic compression plate and a finger plate or miniplate.

the bone in this region, fractures also lend themselves to fixation using the finger plate series (2.0 or 2.7 mm). The surgeon must ensure that the fracture line is compressed across its entire length, especially along the cranial aspect of the ramus (Fig. 7-11). Segmental fractures involving the caudal mandible and ramus, as well as multifragment fractures involving this region, are preferably treated using a bone plate or combination of plates. The fracture fragments are sequentially aligned and fixed temporarily with fixation forceps or supplemented with interfragmentary wires or lag screws, followed by application of the contoured bone plate. Mandibular body fractures may also be fixed using an external fixture.

Temporomandibular Joint

The TMJ may be disrupted by a fracture of the condylar process or a luxation. If possible, the fractured condylar process is fixed to the mandible with interfragmentary wire or preferably a small finger plate. Fragmentation of the condyle necessitates condylectomy. Dislocation of the TMJ may result in rostral or caudal displacement of the condyle. These may be reduced by rostral traction on the jaw if a caudal displacement is present or by placing a pencil or small rod between the caudal molars and gently closing the jaw if there is rostral displacement. If the reduction is stable, the patient may be treated conservatively, feeding the animal only a soft diet.

If instability remains after reduction of the TMJ, supplementary fixation is indicated. A tape muzzle can be applied to allow only limited extension of the tongue but some occlusion of canine teeth. The muzzle must also be loose enough to allow the dog to pant; otherwise the animal may overheat. This technique requires owner compliance to keep the muzzle clean. Screws and elastic bands may also be used to maintain occlusion. The screws are placed in the maxilla and mandible caudal to the canine teeth and connected by elastic bands. The surgeon must

be careful to avoid the roots of the dentition, and the owner must be observant to replace the elastic bands, which frequently break. Alternately, the jaw can be maintained partially or completely closed with an interarcade wire. The animal may be fed a liquid diet through the limited opening or through a pharyngotomy feeding tube.

All techniques focus on maintaining the TMJ joint stable for 3 weeks. If recurrent instability is present, an excision arthroplasty (condylectomy) is indicated.

POSTOPERATIVE MANAGEMENT

The treatment of fractures of the skull and mandible, as with long bone fractures, is aimed at the rapid restoration of function while providing protection against the forces transmitted across the fracture. To achieve this goal with jaw fractures, although the animal is allowed to eat and drink, the food must be of a soft consistency. Since most mandible and maxilla fractures are open, prophylactic antibiotic therapy is indicated. An external fixture or intraoral wiring may need frequent cleaning. Severe head trauma may necessitate feeding by pharyngotomy tube until the animal can eat soft food.

Postoperative home care consists of instructions for a soft diet, the avoidance of any toys or chew items, strict attention to oral hygiene, administration of prophylactic antibiotics, and periodic reevaluation at 6-week intervals until the fractures have healed.

Removal of metal devices should be performed once the fractures are healed, particularly intraoral wires and external fixtures. Interfragmentary wires or bone plates used to repair fractures of the caudal mandible and ramus may be removed on an elective basis.

COMPLICATIONS

Failure to follow technical detail may result in malalignment of the fracture, resulting in malunion and malocclusion of the dentition. Fractures associated with extensive periodontal disease may result in osteomyelitis or infected nonunion, particularly in animals with substantial atrophy of the mandible.

Maxilla and mandibular fractures in which the dentition appears viable but the fracture line enters the alveolus may still result in ultimate instability or abscessed teeth adjacent to the fracture line. Thus, additional dental procedures and extraction of involved teeth may be required.

Failure to recognize instability in or to stabilize completely the TMJ can result in chronic luxation. Extensive trauma and multifragment fractures of the ramus and caudal mandible may result in fibrosis, leading to an inability to open the mouth. These conditions also result in malocclusion of dentition.

Highly contaminated open fractures may result in sequestra formation requiring debridement, bone grafting, and additional fixation procedures.

Fractures of the mandible that progress to osteo-myelitis, necrosis, or nonunion (septic or nonseptic) may require a partial mandibulectomy. However, animals can function adequately with a fibrous union of the fracture fragments provided a near-normal pain-free range of motion is present.

SUGGESTED READINGS

Brinker WO, Hohn RB, Prieur WD: *Manual of internal fixation in small animals*, New York, 1984, Springer-Verlag.

Dulisch ML: Skull and mandibular fractures. In Slatter DH, editor: *Small animal surgery*, vol II, Philadelphia, 1985, Saunders.

Hoerlein BF: *Canine neurology*, ed 3, Philadelphia, 1980, Saunders.

Manfra-Marretta S, Schrader SC, Matthiesen DT: Problems associated with management of jaw fractures. In *Problems in veterinary medicine*, vol 2, no 1, Philadelphia, 1990, Lippincott.

Newton CD: Fractures of the skull. In Newton CD, Nunamaker DM, editors: *Textbook of small animal orthopedics*, Philadelphia, 1985, Lippincott.

Piermattei DL, Greely RG: *An atlas of surgical approaches to the bones of the dog and cat*, ed 2, Philadelphia, 1980, Saunders.

Rudy RL: Fractures of the maxilla and mandible. In Bojrab MJ, editor: *Current techniques in small animal surgery I*, Philadelphia, 1975, Lea & Febiger.

Schrader SC: Dental orthopedics. In Bojrab MJ, Tholen M, editors: *Small animal oral medicine and surgery*, Philadelphia, Lea & Febiger, 1990, pp. 241-265.

SECTION B   Spinal Fractures

Peter K. Shires

The incidence of spinal fractures in small animal practice is about 1:1000 cases presented. Automobile trauma is the most frequent cause, followed by fall and "big dog–little dog" trauma. The type most often described is a vertebral body fracture. The most common treatment option is some form of spinous process fixation. The prognosis is only moderate for implant stability but good for clinical function in animals without serious neurological damage at presentation.

The increasing availability of both diagnostic modalities allowing precise preoperative determination of tissue disruption and implant options has caused a minor revolution in human spinal surgery. Recent investigations on nerve regeneration have suggested new, exciting possibilities regarding spinal injuries. It is hoped that this review will be out of date in a few years and will have to be adjusted for the advancements currently being made.

FUNCTIONAL ANATOMY

Since verterbral anatomy is functionally generated, a site-specific relationship exists between injury type and anatomy.

The cervical vertebrae, with their thin transverse processes, large vascular channels, and complex shapes, are at risk for multiple, lesser fractures. The low incidence of body fractures in cervical vertebrae probably reflects the reduced weight bearing of these vertebrae compared with other segments of the spine. In addition, the large-diameter vertebral canal also allows some freedom, resulting in a lower incidence of neurological involvement after fractures of the cervical spine. It is also likely that, because of the critical nature of the nerve tracts involved (respiration), a severe injury to the cord in the cervical spine usually results in rapid death and thus a reduced incidence of presentation and diagnosis in clinical practice. The comparatively high mobility of the cervical spine makes fixation a delicate balance between immobilization and reduced function. Implants have to be smaller because the bone is less bulky; complex movements are the norm, creating unusual stresses on the implants; and surgical exposure is potentially traumatic. The clinical result has been less frequent surgical repair of fractures.

A notable exception must be made with fractures involving the axis (second cervical vertebra, C-2). Because the dens is such a potentially devastating projection into the spinal canal, when the axis is unstable, fractures of C-2 are often repaired. This is a high-incidence area for injury, as is the junction between the head and spine. Dorsoventral movements are allowed by the atlantooccipital joint; at the end of the normal range of motion, the dorsoventral stress is transferred to the atlantoaxial joint, and the body of C-2 behind the dens is the weakest link (Fig. 7-12). In addition, the nuchal ligament acts as a "bowstring" contributing to axial body displacement. Fractures here cause angulation of the canal, and fixation is often necessary because of both instability and canal compromise by the angulation.

Stability of the thoracic spine is enhanced by the rib cage, the intercapital ligaments, and the long spinous processes with their muscular attachments. Some pro-

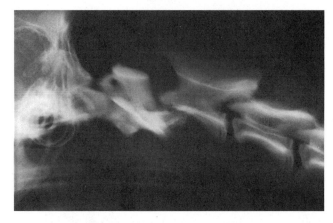

Fig. 7-12 Lateral radiograph of a cranial body C-2 fracture with dorsal displacement and compromise to the canal. Instability must be assumed in this case, even without severe neurological signs.

tection is afforded by the scapulae as well. The relative immobility of the thoracic spine reduces the incidence of displaced fractures and thus also indicates the magnitude of force involved when a displaced fracture is seen. The junctional area of static and mobile spine in the thoracolumbar area is described as a "stress concentrator" with an expected increase of incidence of fracture/luxation in this area (Fig. 7-13). However, a recent study found no incidence peak at this junctional area.

The mobile lumbar vertebrae are significantly larger in size compared with other vertebrae. The support required for propulsion from the hind legs is made possible by a strong but mobile spinal segment. The normal movement and force amplitude carried by this segment is intensified greatly by trauma, especially when escape is involved, resulting in a high incidence of fracture/luxation in the lumbar segment (Fig. 7-14).

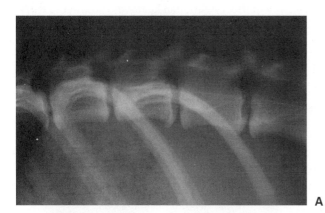

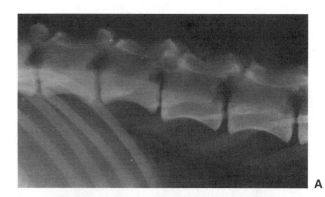

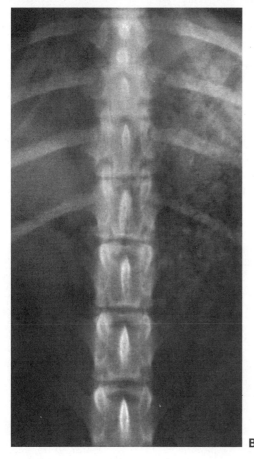

7-13   Lateral (**A**) and dorsoventral (**B**) radiographs of a T-13 vertebral body end-plate fracture with minimum displacement. Depending on neurological signs, this fracture could be stable enough to treat conservatively.

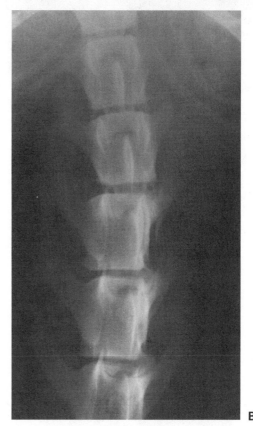

Fig. 7-14   Lateral (**A**) and dorsoventral (**B**) radiographs of an L-2 to L-3 fracture luxation of the annulus fibrosus, L-3 articular facet, and L-3 transverse process. The extent of the injuries, even with mild neurological signs, suggests this is an unstable or potentially unstable situation. Conservative management must be carefully monitored if elected as the treatment choice. A more aggressive approach, elective surgical stabilization, can be justified with this combination of injuries.

The junction between the mobile lumbar vertebrae and the immobile sacrum is another stress concentrator. Injury in this area tends to be less severe because of the reduced cord size and because nerve roots run through the canal, not "gray matter." Nevertheless, the incidence of fractures is high at this junction, and the clinical morbidity of urinary bladder dysfunction or fecal incontinence may be significant (Fig. 7-15).

Fractures farther caudal, in the coccygeal region, may occur because of the exposed nature of the tail; however, the significance of injury in this area is minimal and easily handled without compromise to the animal as a whole.

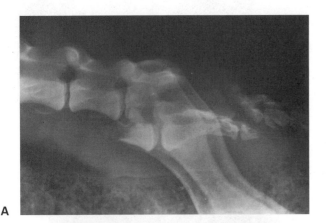

A

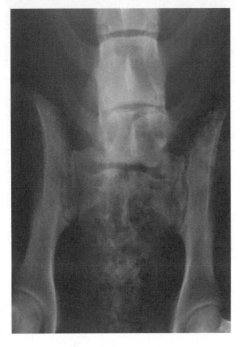

B

Fig. 7-15 Lateral (**A**) and dorsoventral (**B**) radiographs of an oblique L-7 and CX-1 fracture. Despite 100% displacement of the canal in the lateral view, neurological function was intact to the pelvic and pudendal distribution areas. The tail was anesthetic. Stabilization was essential for L-7 to prevent loss of function. The tail was amputated.

MECHANISM OF INJURY

The normal forces on any vertebra include compression, tension, torsion, and shear. The primary structures for coping with *compression* are the vertebral body, endplate, and intervertebral disc. *Torsion* and *shear* loads are dealt with by the articular facets and the vertebral endplate and disc. *Tension* is counteracted by ligaments and their attachments (spinous and transverse processes, etc.), the intervertebral disc, joint capsules of the articular facets, and the longitudinal ligaments within the canal.

When excessive force is applied, it is usually a combination of compression or tension and torsion or shear. The resulting fracture/luxation is often characterized by failure of the most vulnerable structure.

Compression forces most often cause vertebral body compaction and minimum displacement. When shear is involved as well, the body fracture is displaced, often seen as an end-plate or short oblique fracture "teardrop" (Fig. 7-16). Luxation of the articular facets can also occur with this type of injury, depending on the force and displacement involved. Torsional forces tend to luxate or fracture the articular facets and rupture the annulus or vertebral body (Fig. 7-17). Invariably, a compression or tension force is involved as well, and the vertebral body fracture is usually displaced at the time of injury.

Direct injuries to the spine cause local-process fractures (spinous and transverse processes, etc.), often without significant damage to the vertebral body or disk. Lamina fractures can also occur without major damage to the vertebral body. The significance of this differentiation lies in the therapeutic decision of whether to stabilize and decompress, stabilize only, decompress only, or perform no surgery. A rational decision-making process regarding the treatment of spinal fracture/luxation is emphasized in the remainder of this section.

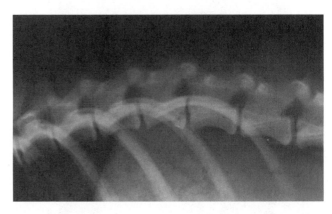

Fig. 7-16 Lateral radiograph of a "teardrop" fracture of the caudal end of the body of T-13. Conservative management was applied in this case with excellent long-term functional recovery.

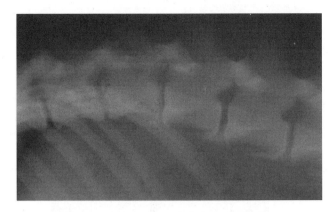

Fig. 7-17   Lateral radiograph of an end-plate body fracture of L-1 and displacement of the articular facets suggesting a rotational luxation. After a few days of cage rest, the neurological signs suddenly worsened and surgical stabilization was performed.

DIAGNOSIS

Two issues must be evaluated in every case of spinal fracture: (1) instability (orthopedic injury), to determine whether fixation is necessary or not, and (2) spinal cord compression (neurological injury), to decide whether decompression is appropriate or not.

Palpation

Assessment of instability is based on palpation, progress of neurological signs, and radiographs. Palpation is minimally effective and has considerable risk associated with overexuberance, especially in the sedated or anesthetized patient. An unstable, aligned fracture may become irretrievably malaligned and cause spinal cord damage with the wrong manipulation.

Neurological Examination

Neurological evaluation is valid, provided the changes in neurological signs between the injury and presentation are carefully assessed. This progression or static status offers the best, although tenuous, window for evaluating the stability of the spine, the prognosis, and the neuropathology involved in each case. The initial signs should always be reevaluated 4 to 6 hours after injury, since the incidence and extent of spinal shock in animals has not been clearly defined. *Spinal shock* is a clinical syndrome that can occur immediately after spinal injury. A temporary loss of function is not accompanied by visible pathological changes in the spinal cord. Recovery is usually evident in a few hours without treatment. If the neurological signs are still severe after 6 hours, further workup with radiographs and other studies is mandated, without further delay and repeated neurological exami-

nations. If clinical improvement in the neurological signs is documented in that time, spinal or hypovolemic shock may have influenced the initial evaluation.

A neurologically stable animal is less of an emergency than a deteriorating one. Neurological stability, however, may be short-lived in an unstable spinal fracture. This necessitates frequent reevaluation and an open mind to changing situations. A deteriorating clinical situation is the basis for a more aggressive therapeutic approach. A sudden change from a static to a deteriorating status is a strong indicator of instability and thus the need for surgical stabilization.

Loss of deep pain perception distal to the injury site that persists more than a few hours after injury is a serious prognostic indicator. Some of these animals may eventually recover some reflex or neurological function, but the chances of recovery are much less if pain perception is absent. A poor prognosis should be explained to the owner in light of prolonged bladder and bowel incontinence, urine scalding, dermatitis, self-mutilation, decubital ulceration of bony prominences, cystitis, and so on, all resulting from neurological dysfunction. Signs of improvement, if any occur, generally take months to develop.

Radiological Evaluation

Evaluating a dynamic situation, instability, with a static medium, radiography, can be highly inaccurate. The degree of displacement seen when taking the radiograph represents the injury status at that instant, which may be misleading. It does not allow evaluation of displacement at the time of injury or at any other time between injury and presentation. To minimize iatrogenic injury to an unstable spinal problem, it is necessary to take precautions while handling the patient during radiography. This is especially true when the patient is relaxed under sedation or anesthesia. Within the limitations that exist, significant displacement measurements may be used as a predictor of potential instability.

Any spinal canal decrease of 30% or more in either radiographic view can be considered potentially unstable. Displacement of 50% or more confirms that the potential for instability is high.

The vertebral body and intervertebral disc represent the most significant stabilizing structures in a vertebral motion unit. The bodies should be carefully examined for fracture lines, fragments, and displacement. Traumatic disc herniation is a distinct possibility, and a narrowed disc space should prompt further investigation with a myelogram if no other radiographic signs are evident and the animal's neurological condition dictates further investigation. Displacement of one vertebral body in relation to the next is evidence of luxation and rupture of the annulus that joins adjacent vertebrae. Loss of either the annulus or the vertebral body integrity significantly reduces the stability of the spine, perhaps in the range of 60% to 70%.

Biomechanically, the next most significant structures are the articular facets. These should be identified on the radiographs and inspected for damage or luxation. Luxation is often identified by a widened intraarticular space in the lateral view and malalignment of the spinous processes in the dorsoventral view. The facets contribute another 10% to 20% toward total spinal stability in research specimens.

The laminae surrounding the cord must be examined for displaced fragments of bone in an attempt to identify depressed fractures. A bone fragment identified within the spinal canal is an indication for decompressive surgery, depending on neurological signs. Fractures of the spinous and transverse processes, the accessory processes, ribs, and so on support evidence for a direct blow in the immediate area. This, in turn, should lead one to consider possible blunt spinal trauma and lamina fractures in the area.

Other Diagnostic Tools

Of the three diagnostic modes available for evaluating acute spinal cord trauma, serial neurological examinations provide the most current and dynamic assessment. Vascular compromise, local hemorrhage, edema, vasoactive neurochemicals, and direct pressure all influence the pathology present in the spinal cord and therefore the clinical signs seen. Other tools available for damage assessment include myelography, computed tomography (CT) scans, magnetic resonance imaging (MRI) scans, linear tomography, and microradioangiography. The information about spinal cord damage, canal invasion, and local ischemia can be greatly enhanced by these diagnostic tools.

Myelography is the tool most readily available to veterinarians and can be useful in localizing spinal cord compressive lesions. The limitations of a myelogram center around the almost universal presence of local swelling at the site of injury in acute spinal trauma. The myelogram does not always discriminate among compression injuries caused by disc herniation, cord edema, or other sources of local inflammation. When the site of injury is recognizable on plain x-ray films, a myelogram may be unnecessary because cord edema can be expected if neurological signs are present (Fig. 7-18).

The purpose of careful evaluation of the fracture site is to determine the degree of potential instability present and whether or not surgical reduction of a compressive lesion is necessary. On the basis of this determination and the results of serial neurological examinations, a medical or surgical plan can be developed.

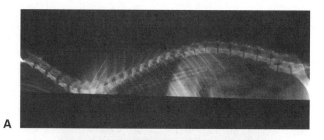

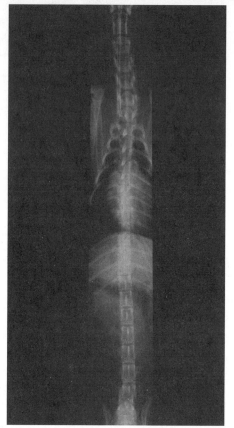

Fig. 7-18   Lateral (**A**) and dorsoventral (**B**) survey radiographs of an anesthetized patient allow evaluation of the entire spine in small animals. The L-6 body fracture can then be isolated with spot films for more complete evaluation.

THERAPY

The entire animal must be evaluated, and all critical injuries dealt with before spinal evaluation. Particular attention should be paid to the thorax, since concurrent injuries are common in this area.

The initial examination allows spinal fracture patients to be divided into two groups. Animals in the severely affected group are incapable of voluntary movement, in obvious and significant pain, or showing progressive deterioration of neurological signs. A therapeutic decision must be made immediately for these animals, and no observation period is recommended.

Most cases fall into the less critical second group. The neurological signs vary but are generally less than full motor paralysis. It is wise to stabilize a recently injured animal and repeat the neurological examination at regular intervals to exclude the possibility of spinal shock, which may obscure the true extent of the injury. In the less critical group, an observation period accomplishes several objectives. Neurological progress can be evaluated, medical and preanesthetic evaluations completed, the patient stabilized, and the client properly educated about the situation and potential prognosis. The acute observation period ends when a decision is reached or when the patient shows any neurological deterioration.

Conservative Management

This option is most often applied to patients with very minor injury or with an apparently hopeless prognosis. Mildly affected animals that are improving or are static are obvious choices for a conservative approach. Similarly, those that have no deep pain or perception, have no clinical signs of a painful condition, and do not have euthanasia as an option are relegated to medical management, since irreversible spinal cord injury must be assumed.

In the preacute stage after injury, several drugs have been used with some potential for reducing or limiting the effects of trauma to the spinal cord. The only one currently supported by research as having a positive effect is methylprednisolone. Given as an intravenous bolus, 30 mg/kg, as soon as possible after injury, methylprednisolone has been shown to improve the clinical and research results of spinal trauma. No consensus can be found as to whether extending the drug's 3½-hour half-life by continuous infusion at 5.4 mg/kg/hr is beneficial or not. It appears that the early effect of the single bolus is the most significant.

Dexamethasone has not been found to be effective in several comparative studies. Dimethyl sulfoxide (DMSO) has had mixed reviews; one investigator found no benefit, and another found benefit when it was combined with a myelotomy. Naloxone and thyrotrophin-releasing hormone showed some promise in a feline research model, but this has not been demonstrated in subsequent studies. Mannitol had a negative effect in a spinal trauma model. The current recommendation is for a single intravenous bolus of methylprednisolone as soon as possible after injury.

Drugs should never be used alone in the therapeutic stage. Any patient that has a spinal fracture and is receiving medication should be hospitalized or closely confined (caged) and repeatedly reexamined for signs of neurological change. Early recognition of a deteriorating clinical course is the key to success when one must

consider using a more aggressive therapeutic approach. The client must always be warned of the risks involved in a potential spinal instability situation.

External support is recommended as a supplement to hospitalization to reduce stress on the injured vertebrae. The most appropriate use of external bandages, splints, or casts appears to be for fractures or luxations of the cervical vertebrae. The neck's mobility can be significantly reduced without severe discomfort to the patient. The cervical spine is immobilized in extension (Fig. 7-19). The tolerance level is high, and a suitable splint that stretches from sternum to mandible can be constructed from a variety of light materials. Care must be taken not to compromise respiration and to hand-feed or give food and water in an elevated position while the splint is in place. Splints should remain in place for at least 2 and preferably 3 weeks to allow fibrous union and to reduce the risk of movement at the fracture site. After splint removal, activity should be restricted for 6 weeks more, and neck collars are no longer appropriate; a harness should be used instead.

Some propose external splints, body splints, body casts, and squeeze cages for patients with thoracolumbar spinal injuries as well. Anecdotal experiences suggest a less successful outcome with thoracolumbar fractures than with cervical fractures. Without consideration of the many factors that may contribute to this, one must recognize that body splints can be minimally effective,

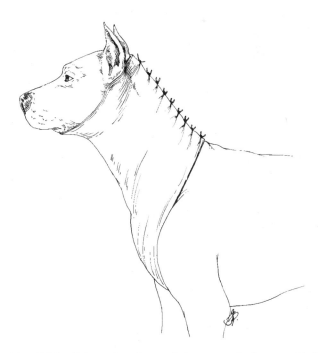

Fig. 7-19 Schematic of a neck brace made from padded Orthoplast or x-ray film; used for conservative management of some cervical fractures.

poorly tolerated, and difficult to maintain and may have a negative impact on the outcome. With this in mind, it is recommended to confine the patient to a hospital cage and to discourage activity by removing external stimuli (other dogs, owners, etc.) for at least 10 to 14 days, followed by confinement to a restricted, level area (playpen, dogpen) for another 6 weeks. Normal activity should only be resumed after fracture healing has been documented radiographically.

Careful handling while moving patients is a requirement in spinal injuries. Using a carrying tray (board, cage grid, etc.) while restraining the head is probably the best way to transport the injured animal. Tying or strapping them down usually leads to struggling and injury. Sedation is appropriate only when the animal is stable and constantly, physically restrained. Anesthesia is an unnecessary risk unless required for another purpose. When handling spinal fracture patients under anesthesia, all personnel should be mindful of the loss of muscle splinting around the fracture and resultant decrease in stability at the site of injury.

Conservative management can be effective for many patients if case selection is appropriate. A stable, mildly paretic animal that shows no progression of clinical signs in a 24-hour period is a candidate for cage rest, provided the radiological assessment suggests relative stability. Loss of an articular facet or a vertebral body fracture indicates instability and suggests that surgical stabilization may be appropriate, even when the clinical signs are not currently progressive.

The conservative management of a paralyzed animal must include frequent bladder emptying (preferably by manual expression) and prophylactic antibiotic therapy to prevent retention cystitis. Constant monitoring of the urine cytology can be used to delay the start of antibiotic therapy. Skin care should include regular bathing, topical treatment of skin problems, and soft bedding, frequent turning, or a water bed to prevent pressure sores. The animal must also be protected from the environment, including sharp objects, hot objects, insects, and other animals, because of regional anesthesia. Self-mutilation can also be a problem, frequently during long recovery periods, because reinnervation occurs haphazardly.

Surgical Management

The most frequent indication for surgery is spinal instability. Decompression is achieved by realignment of displaced vertebrae; therefore, laminectomy is not routinely performed unless a displaced fragment is within the canal or a herniated disc is causing compression. Realignment is accomplished by direct manipulation of the affected vertebrae. Bone clamps are placed on each side of the fracture/luxation on solid bone. It is frequently necessary to distract the fragments to realign

them. Sometimes a lever (Hohman Retractor) must be used to pry the fragments apart before realigning them. Great care must be taken to proceed slowly and gently to avoid further damage to the compromised spinal cord within the canal.

When the articular facets are displaced but intact, they provide a useful landmark for realignment. If both pairs of facets are lined up, usually the rest of the fracture/luxation has been reduced. The facet pairs can be clamped or skewer-pinned together with Kirschner wires to hold alignment while the primary fixation appliance is being implanted. Numerous implants are available for spinal stabilization. Based on in vitro biomechanical studies and clinical experience, the following are the most useful, practical, versatile, and effective implants. In general, combination techniques appear to be more secure than any single technique alone. The techniques are described next.

Surgical approaches. In general, to apply any of the following implants it is necessary to expose both sides of the dorsal lamina of the thoracolumbar spine down to the level of the transverse process. With cervical vertebrae, vertebral body fixation requires a ventral approach, whereas dorsal spine or articular facet fixation requires a dorsal approach. The dorsal approach again necessitates exposure of both sides of the dorsal lamina.

The surgical approaches used for spinal fixation are identical to those for dorsal and dorsolateral hemilaminectomies. The bilateral nature of the approach is the only significant difference. The length of the exposed area of the spine depends on the implants to be used; spinous process plating usually requires considerably longer exposure than vertebral body plating or application of pins and methylmethacrylate.

Fixation techniques

Vertebral body pins and methylmethacrylate. This is probably the most versatile of the techniques described, since it can be applied to any anatomical site in the spine. Dorsal placement is used for the thoracic and lumbar vertebrae, whereas ventral placement is required for the cervical vertebrae. Similar in function to a Kirschner external fixator apparatus, the pins are secured in solid bone on either side of the fracture/luxation. The free ends of the pins are notched or kinked and cut at an appropriate length. All the pin ends are embedded in a mass of sterile bone cement (methylmethacrylate). When the mass hardens, the vertebrae are held securely in a fixed position.

From a dorsal bilateral exposure of the thoracolumbar area, the pins are placed into the vertebral bodies starting at the lowest extremes of the spinal canal, at the level of the accessory or transverse processes. The pins are angled at about 30 to 45 degrees from the vertical and should just barely penetrate the transcortex of the vertebral body. An abrupt decrease in resistance to driving the pins indicates that the cortex has been penetrated. Power equipment makes it easier to drive the pins and evaluate their progress through the bone.

If a laminectomy is performed with this technique, the defect must be covered with a pad of fat when the methylmethacrylate is placed around the pins. The heat of polymerization damages the cord if it is not insulated. Many small-diameter pins are preferred to a few, larger pins. For most small and medium-size dogs, ⅟₁₆- to ⅟₁₈-inch-diameter pins are appropriate. Three or four pins can be placed in each vertebra, at least two pins on both left and right sides of the vertebral body, and at least three or four pins in the first complete vertebral body cranial and caudal to the fracture/luxation (Figs. 7-20 and 7-21). Threaded pins are less likely to loosen than smooth pins, provided the threads are onlay threads and not cut threads.

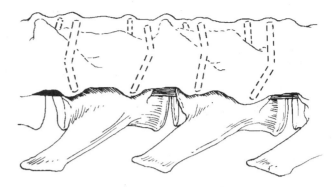

Fig. 7-22 Lateral view of a specimen with body pins placed bilaterally in two vertebrae. Bone cement has been molded around the exposed portions of the pins. The pin tips should be covered with cement. A "doughnut" formation of the cement is used if a dorsolaminectomy has been performed. A solid cement mass is appropriate if the lamina is intact.

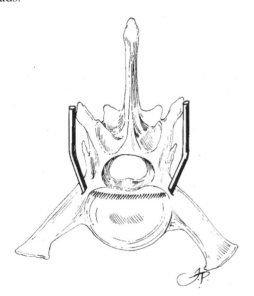

Fig. 7-20 End-on view of a lumbar vertebra with body pins placed at an appropriate angle outside the spinal canal.

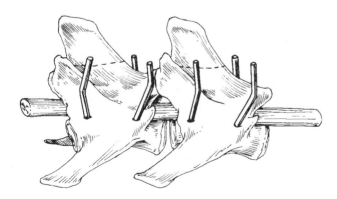

Fig. 7-21 Lateral view of two lumbar vertebrae with body pins placed in appropriate positions below the spinal canal.

The methylmethacrylate must be sterile, and 0.5 cefazolin is mixed with each 20 g cement to reduce the chance of infection being sequestered in the mass of acrylic. The acrylic powder is mixed with the solvent until it no longer sticks to a surgical glove. The cement mass can then be manually molded around the exposed pin ends. The pins should be completely encased in cement, being careful to mold the mass around the base of the pins close to the bone (Fig. 7-22). The cement mass should not project above the normal level of the spinous processes or laterally very far from the midline. Excessive cement makes closure very difficult and the result unsightly. The spinous processes are removed where the cement mass would enclose them—the blood supply to the bone would be compromised, and they add nothing to the strength of the fixation.

The primary complications associated with this technique are infection and pin loosening. If infection develops, the implant must be removed, a difficult process. Temporary suppression of the infection is possible with appropriate antibiotic therapy, but infection recurs until the implant is removed. Pin loosening in the bone is less significant because fracture mobility is usually still limited, which should allow fibrous union to develop despite the motion present. Ultimately the implant can be removed if it is causing discomfort, but this occurs infrequently.

Vertebral body plate. These plates are often used in conjunction with Lubra Plates to provide a more secure fixation than either can provide if used separately. The vertebral body plates are regular orthopedic plates, usually 3.5 or 2.7 mm Dynamic Compression Plates, used with cortical screws placed in the vertebral bodies. The plates are better suited to lumbar fractures caudal to T-11 and cranial to L-6, since the thoracic cavity, ribs, and ilial wings make placement more difficult at T-11 and L-6.

Ventrally placed cervical vertebral plates can be used, but screw placement is difficult because the spinal canal must be avoided.

Through a unilateral, dorsolateral exposure of the thoracolumbar area, the vertebral body is leveled just dorsal to the transverse processes for the length of the plate. The plate is placed on the vertebra at the lower extreme of the spinal canal (Fig. 7-23). Screw holes are drilled at a 30 to 45 degree angle through the body of the vertebra (Fig. 7-24). Two screws are placed in each intact vertebra cranial and caudal to the fracture/luxation. Plate length should be short because increased length makes the plate subject to "cycling" at each intervertebral space. The holes are measured and tapped, and appropriate-length screws are used to attach the plate to the vertebral bodies.

Care must be taken to avoid drilling through the spinal canal. If a screw strips out, it may be possible to replace it with a cancellous screw. Alternatively, injecting a small amount of liquid bone cement into the stripped hole, then reinserting the screw before the cement sets also holds a loose screw very well.

The primary failure mode of this technique is screw pullout. The vertebral bodies have thin cortices, and the screw-holding power is not very high.

Lubra plates. These polyvinyl chloride plates are used to trap the dorsal spinous processes and hold the vertebrae in alignment. This technique is effective where the dorsal spines are long enough and strong enough to accommodate the plates. Because the plates are flexible, lateral bending is possible but dorsoventral flexion is not. Some rotation can occur if the vertebral body is not stabilized as well. Adding a vertebral body plate to Lubra Plate fixation enhances the strength of the fixation.

Through a dorsal-bilateral approach to the fracture/luxation area, the unstable vertebrae are held in a reduced position while a Lubra Plate is placed on either side of the dorsal spinous processes in the area. At least three spinous processes on either side of the fracture must be trapped by the plates for the technique to be effective. The two plates are bolted together, passing the bolts in between the dorsal spines (Fig. 7-25). The roughened sides of the two plates are in contact with the dorsal spines and grip the bone securely when squeezed together by the bolts.

Two problems are associated with this fixation technique. Fracture of the dorsal spines is common after the implants have been in place for a time. Bone weakening under the plate makes this a weak link, and fractures occur frequently. Infection has also been associated with the roughened surfaces of the plates, which may have a tendency to trap bacteria and isolate them from the body's immune system.

Used by itself, the Lubra Plate system can provide a flexible stabilizing technique that often allows healing despite implant failure, dorsal spine fractures, and infections, which are all frequently encountered. Rigid fixation should not be expected using Lubra Plates alone.

Crossed pins. Crossed intramedullary pins, placed through a reduced vertebral body fracture/luxation,

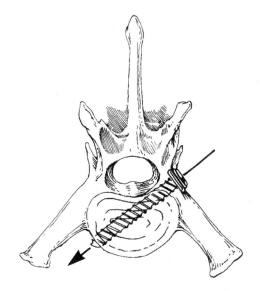

Fig. 7-23 Lateral view of lumbar vertebra with a body plate applied to the lateral aspect of the vertebral body. The screws are angled down to avoid the vertebral canal and spinal cord.

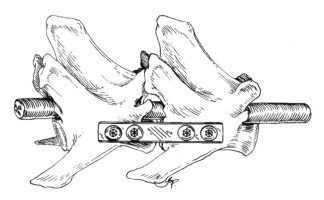

Fig. 7-24 Cross-sectional view of a lumbar vertebra with the body plate in place. The angle of screw placement is indicated.

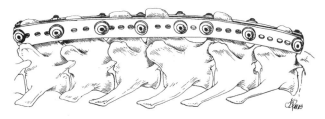

Fig. 7-25 Lateral view of the lumbar vertebrae held together with two Lubra Plates bolted to each other between the spinous processes. At least three spines on each side of the fracture/luxation should be trapped by the plates.

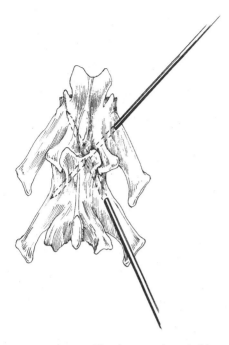

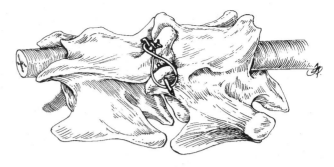

Fig. 7-27 Lateral view of cervical vertebrae held together with a K wire transfixing the articular facets, and a figure-eight wire compressing the facets together. The "skewer" fixation is weak and should be used as part of a more complex fixation construct.

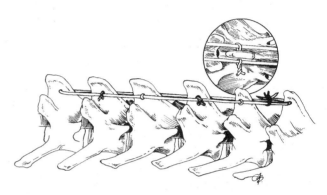

Fig. 7-26 Dorsal view of lumbar vertebrae held together with 1/8-inch Steinmann pins in a crossed (X) configuration. The pins are in the vertebral body, below the spinal canal. The free ends of the pins can be bent up and incorporated in the bone cement mass with body pins.

Fig. 7-28 Lateral view of lumbar vertebrae held together with a 5/64-inch Steinmann pins bent double at both ends and passed through holes drilled in the spinous processes. The intervening spinous processes are wired to the U pin for additional stability. Three spinous processes on each side of the fracture/luxation should be fastened to the pin. The strength of this device is such that it should only be used on small dogs and cats.

provide a weak and temporary stabilizing force. If incorporated into a methylmethacrylate mass in association with body pins, crossed pins may be beneficial but not essential to the construct. By themselves, crossed pins tend to migrate postoperatively with micromovement at the fracture site. Crossed pins should be used only as adjunct to fixation using another technique (Fig. 7-26).

Articular facet wiring and screw fixation. The facets are readily available for fixation with a figure-eight wire over a transfixation pin, hemicerclage wire alone, or screw fixation. Because the facets are relatively small, they cannot be expected to withstand all the forces exerted on an unstable spinal fracture segment. Facet fractures should be expected if these are the only fixation devices used. The best use of facet fixation is as a temporary fixator to hold the reduced fracture/luxation in place while the primary fixation technique is applied (Fig. 7-27). They can be used in conjunction with any of the previously described techniques. When incorporated into a methylmethacrylate cement mass, they will not fracture and therefore are a potential additive to the strength of the methylmethacrylate-pin unit.

U pins and longitudinal pins (spinal staple). These techniques require that intramedullary pins be attached to the dorsal spines, articular facets, or dorsal lamina of the vertebrae on either side of the unstable area using orthopedic wire (Fig. 7-28). In smaller animals the stability provided by this technique is probably suffi-

cient to minimize movement and allow healing. The primary difficulties with these techniques are the complex nature of their construction and the need to expose a considerable length of the spinal column to apply the implant. No biomechanical tests have been used to evaluate this group of fixators.

• • •

All the techniques described have been used with success in various circumstances. The diversity of applications suggests that no single technique can be defined as "the best." A common-sense approach to spinal fixation is required until an obviously superior technique is tried and tested. Most of these implants cause a limitation of movement during the development of a fibrous union at the site of instability. This prevents catastrophic spinal displacement, even if the implant fails at a later date; therefore, clinical success can be achieved in a variety of circumstances.

Decompression. Spinal cord decompression is essential when the cord has been compromised by significant vertebral displacement or by bone fragments in the spinal canal. Significant displacement has been described as greater than 30% narrowing of the spinal canal on either radiographic view. Because realignment and stabilization of a spinal fracture/luxation effectively eliminates the spinal cord compression caused by displacement, this alone may be sufficient to correct the problem. We have no conclusive method by which to evaluate the results of spinal cord decompression, other than by monitoring neurological progress after surgery. This may take days or weeks to show a change. The reported results in human and veterinary studies support the use of realignment alone as an effective means of decompression in most patients.

The inability to evaluate the degree of damage incurred at the time of injury or at any time before stabilization leaves the decompressive realignment approach open to error in some cases. Until a reliable quantitative and qualitative testing method for spinal function is proved, it is necessary to rely on neurological evaluation as a predictor and monitor of decompression.

It is currently recommended that only those patients that have depressed lamina fractures or bone fragments within the canal should be directly decompressed. Direct decompression can be achieved by dorsolaminectomy or hemilaminectomy. Biomechanical testing shows that when the vertebral body or disk has been disrupted, the additional removal of one and especially two articular facets significantly further destabilizes the fracture. This means that decompression of a fracture should always be accompanied by appropriate spinal fixation. Because none of the fixation techniques can be regarded as entirely secure, the decision to decompress must be made only after considering the consequences carefully.

COMMON FRACTURES
C-2 (Axis) Fractures

The dens and the cranial body of the axis are a pivot for movement of the head. Ligamentous support limits the range of motion, but excess force results in ligament and bony fractures. Whiplash is the most common etiology seen when a small animal is shaken by a larger animal. A common site of injury is the cranial body of C-2, with upward displacement of the caudal fragment (see Fig. 7-12).

A ventral approach to the body of C-2 allows gentle leverage of the caudal fragment back into alignment. Fixation can be achieved by placing several small pins (medium K wires) into the body of C-2, the body of C-1, and through the articulation between C-2 and C-1.

Positioning the pins is critical because the spinal cord, the vascular channels, and the occipital condyles must be avoided during pin placement.

At least two pins should be placed cranial and two caudal to the fracture. Methylmethacrylate is used to hold the pins, and thus the bone fragments, in place. Postoperative support with a neck brace is recommended for 3 to 4 weeks.

Cervical Fractures

A variety of cervical fractures can occur, but because of the anatomy of the vertebrae, process fractures occur most often. Direct trauma and bite injuries are the most common etiologies involved. It is usually possible to identify several spinous, transverse, or articular process fractures on the radiograph. The body can be fractured, but luxation is more common in this area.

If displacement is not significant, conservative therapy should be strongly considered. The large canal size and the ability to support the neck externally make this option viable in many cases. If the articular facets have been luxated, frequently in a rotational manner, surgical reduction and facet fixation can be applied in conjunction with a neck brace. When the vertebra body is fractured or a disk rupture has allowed body malalignment and instability, body fixation with pins and methylmethacrylate can be considered.

Surgical fixation is used much less frequently in cervical injuries than elsewhere in the spine, with satisfactory conservative management results in most cases. Neurological dysfunction is the main deciding factor as to whether fixation is required or not.

Thoracic Fractures

The long dorsal spinous processes and the ribs are prominent in the thoracic area making these vertebrae most vulnerable to direct trauma. Despite the protection provided by the paraspinal muscles, thoracic girdle, and ribs, the thoracic vertebrae are frequently subject to compression and rotation injuries. Body fractures and luxations can be dealt with conservatively only if the neurological deficit is mild and the disruption is inherently stable. Evaluating stability is difficult, so it is not unusual to change therapeutic direction when conservative management results in worsening of clinical signs.

To avoid entering the thoracic cavity, surgeons most often use spinous process plates or vertebral body pins and methylmethacrylate to fix thoracic fractures and luxations. Unless the local dorsal spines are all fractured, spinous process plating often provides enough stability to allow healing to occur without further neurological compromise. When the spines are all fractured, body pins and methylmethacrylate can be used. External support is not recommended because body braces usually cause discomfort, which in turn causes the animal to struggle and potentially disrupt the fixation. Cage confinement is a better option to reduce stress on the fracture device postoperatively.

Thoracolumbar Fractures/Luxations

This region of the spine is most vulnerable to injury because of its unprotected nature, its function in the propulsion mechanism, and the "bridge" support between the forelimbs and hind limbs. Despite the paraspinal musculature, a fracture/luxation in the thoracolumbar area is subject to significant displacement stresses, and instability often occurs.

In contrast to other spinal regions, the emphasis here is to fix the majority of vertebral body fractures and luxations. Cautious conservatism may be used with minimally displaced luxations, but when a fracture of the body is involved, surgical stabilization is probably more prudent than waiting for deterioration of clinical signs to develop. The canal diameter is unforgiving in this area of the spine, which makes a wrong decision permanent in many cases.

The entire range of spinal fixation techniques can be used in the thoracolumbar area because the body is accessible, the spinous processes sturdy, and the facets solid. Body pins and methylmethacrylate offer the most versatile technique for use in many different situations (Fig. 7-29).

Postoperative cage rest is again preferable to body splints or external bracing for postoperative immobilization.

L-6 and L-7 Fractures

Because the spinal canal in this region contains only nerve roots, it is possible for an animal to survive considerable displacement of a vertebral fracture without permanent dysfunction. The usual injury is an oblique body fracture of L-6 or L-7, with ventral displacement of the caudal fragment (see Fig 7-14, *B*).

Through a dorsal approach, the articular facets of the displaced adjoining vertebrae can be identified and realigned. Temporary fixation of the facets allows the permanent fixator to be applied. Longitudinal pins wired to the facets, lamina, and dorsal spines; transverse iliac pin fixation; or vertebral body pins in the vertebrae and the sacrum can all be used effectively to stabilize this fracture or luxation.

A relatively high success rate can be achieved with even the most severely displaced fractures, provided the neurological damage is not too severe. Postoperative cage rest is the most effective stress reducer after fixation.

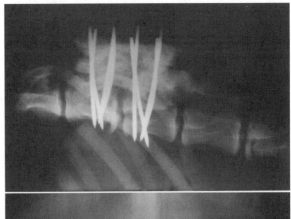

A

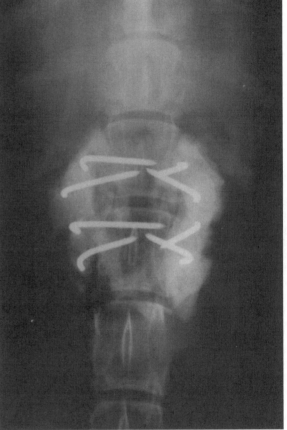

B

Fig. 7-29 Lateral (**A**) and dorsoventral (**B**) radiographs of a body pins and bone cement fixation used on a T-13–L-1 fracture/luxation. No implant failure or pin loosening has occurred over a 4-year postoperative period. Threaded pins are now recommended.

• • •

The complex nature of spinal fractures and the variety of techniques available to secure them have led veterinarians to be wary of injuries in this anatomical structure. No sinecure is currently available that can be universally applied to spinal instabilities. A logical approach to the selection of cases and fixation techniques must be used. Definitive decompression should be used only when essential, as indicated by radiographic signs of canal invasion by bone fragments. Increased use of alternate imaging techniques and spinal cord function tests may change our future approach to spinal fractures when we better understand the nature of the injuries involved.

SUGGESTED READINGS

Blass CE, Seim HB: Spinal fixation in dogs using Steinmann pins and methacrylate, *Vet Surg* 13:203-210, 1984.

Blass CE, Waldron DR, vanEr RT: Cervical stabilization in three dogs using Steinmann pins and methacrylate, *J Am Anim Hosp Assoc* 24:61-68, 1988.

Dulisch ML, Nichols JB: A surgical technique for management of lower lumbar fractures: case report, *Vet Surg* 10:90-93, 1981.

Gage ED: A new method of spinal fixation in the dog, *Vet Med Small Anim Clin* 64:295-303, 1969.

Gage ED: Surgical repair of spinal fractures in small-breed dogs, *Vet Med Small Anim Clin* 66:1095-1101, 1971.

Lumb WV, Brasmer TH: Improved spinal plates and hypothermia as adjuncts to spinal surgery, *J Am Vet Med Assoc* 157(3):338-342, 1970.

Matthiesen DT: Thoracolumbar spinal fractures/luxations: surgical management, *Compend Cont Educ* 5(10):867-878, 1983.

McAnulty JF, Lenehan TM, Maletz LM: Modified segmental spinal instrumentation in repair of spinal fractures and luxations in dogs, *Vet Surg* 15(2):143-149, 1986.

Renegar WR, Simpson ST, Stoll SG: The use of methylmethacrylate bone cement in cervical spinal stabilization: a case report and discussion, *J Am Anim Hosp Assoc* 16:219-223, 1980.

Rischen CG, Wilson JW, Swain CA: Effect of application of polyvinilidine plates on the dorsal spinous processes of dogs, *Vet Surg* 16(4):294-298, 1987.

Rouse GP, Miller JI: The use of methylmethacrylate for spinal stabilization, *J Am Anim Hosp Assoc* 11:418-425, 1975.

Selcer RR, Bubb WJ, Walker TL: Management of vertebral column fractures in dogs and cats: 211 cases, *J Am Vet Med Assoc* 198(11):1965-1968, 1991.

Shires PK, Waldron DR, Hedlung CS: A biomechanical study of rotational instability in unaltered and surgically altered canine thoracolumbar vertebral motion units, *Prog Vet Neurol* 2(1):6-14, 1991.

Shores A, and others: Combined Kirschner-Ehmer apparatus and dorsal spinal plate fixation of caudal lumbar fractures in dogs: biomechanical properties, *Am J Vet Res* 49(11):1979-1982, 1988.

Slocum B, Rudy RL: Fractures of the seventh lumbar vertebra in the dog, *J Am Anim Hosp Assoc* 11:167-174, 1975.

Smith GK, Walter MC: Spinal decompressive procedures and dorsal compartment injuries: comparative biomechanical study in canine cadavers, *Am J Vet Res* 49(2):266-273, 1988.

Swain SF: Vertebral body plating for spinal immobilization, *J Am Vet Med Assoc* 158(11):1683-1695, 1971.

Swain SF, Vamdevelde M: Clinical and histologic evaluation of bilateral hemilaminectomy and deep dorsal laminectomy for extensive spinal cord decompression in the dog, *J Am Vet Med Assoc* 170(4):407-413, 1977.

Turner WD: Fractures and fracture-luxations of the lumbar spine: a retrospective study in the dog, 23:459-464, 1987.

Waldron DR, and others: The rotational stabilizing effect of spinal fixation techniques in an unstable vertebral model, *Prog Vet Neurol* 2(2):98-105, 1991.

Walter MC, Smith GK, Newton CD: Canine lumbar spinal internal fixation techniques: a comparative biomechanical study, *Vet Surg* 15(2):191-198, 1986.

Yturraspe DJ, Lumb WV: The use of plastic spinal plates for internal fixation of the canine spine, *J Am Vet Med Assoc* 161(12):1651-1657, 1972.

SECTION C   Rib Fractures

Peter K. Shires

Single, multiple, and segmental fractures of the ribs are most often associated with thoracic automobile-induced trauma or direct blows or kicks to the chest.[3] The management of underlying lung, cardiac, and pleural injuries is essential.

Most rib fractures are treated conservatively. Limitation of activity, cage rest, or hospitalization for 10 to 14 days is generally sufficient to allow fibrous union to occur. Even when moderate malalignment is present, satisfactory healing and full return to function can be expected in most patients. External support is rarely indicated because constrictive, circumferential bandaging limits chest excursions and hinders pulmonary function. If used, bandages should be light and elastic.

Fracture fixation may be indicated when fracture ends are potential dangers to the lungs, vessels, and pleura. Because the ribs are non–weight bearing, emphasis should be placed on pain control and chest wall integrity, rather than rigid fixation. A fibrous or cartilaginous union generally allows normal thoracic function if anatomical continuity is established. This allows considerable latitude in choosing a fixation technique because most achieve stability. What must be avoided is the introduction of infection, vascular damage, or thoracic compromise through unnecessary, ill-advised, surgical manipulations.

Regional anesthesia, local block, or short-term general anesthesia is generally sufficient to allow most rib fracture fixation surgeries. Blind pinning techniques result in minimum intervention, and thus minimum contamination, and a satisfactory result in most cases. Because the ribs are curved, it is possible to start a medium to large K wire (0.045 to 0.062 inch or 1/16 inch) into the rib's medullary center at the fracture end of one of the displaced fragments. The pin is advanced up or down the rib until it penetrates the cortex and skin. The exposed end is then used to withdraw the pin until the other end is flush with the fracture end. The fracture is reduced using towel clamps to grasp the rib through the skin, and the pin is retrograded down or up the other fragment until it penetrates the cortex (Fig. 7-30).

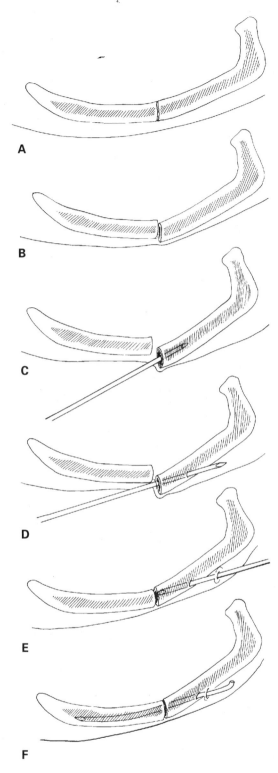

Fig. 7-30 **A,** Midshaft rib fracture. **B,** Displacement of the fracture to allow access to the medullary canal. **C,** Starting a small Steinmann pin up (or down) the medullary canal. **D,** Penetrating the lateral cortex of the curved rib to exit the skin. **E,** Withdrawing the pin until the end is flush with the fracture line. Reducing the fracture. **F,** Driving the pin distally down (or proximally up) the canal and seating in the corticocancellous bone; cutting the pin as short as possible and bending the tip over; and burying it under the skin.

Manually advancing the smaller, flexible pins slowly usually allows them to follow the medullary "canal" around the curvature of the rib. Using power equipment often results in penetration of the pin tip through the cortex. The free end of the pin can be bent over to prevent advancement migration and can be cut off short enough to reduce local irritation of the overlying tissues. Pin removal can be accomplished by direct cutdown under local anesthesia and withdrawal of the pin using a pair of pliers, once fibrous or bony union has been achieved.

Alternate techniques include cross pinning of the fracture with small pins, either blindly after closed reduction or through a limited open-reduction approach. The pins can be retrograded from the fracture site, the fracture reduced and aligned, and the pins driven into the other fragment. It is equally effective to drive the cross pins across the fracture site after reduction of the fracture has been accomplished. Wiring techniques require exposure of the fracture and drilling holes through the rib fracture ends. The wire is threaded through the holes, the fracture reduced, and the wires twisted tight. Many configurations can be used, including a single loop, a figure-eight loop, two loops, and a pin-wire tension-band technique.[2]

The wire should be orthopedic wire, at least 20 gauge, for dogs and cats. Heavy suture material has also been successfully used to maintain fracture alignment in rib fractures, but it cannot be recommended because of a propensity to fail before healing has been accomplished.

Postoperative management includes exercise restriction for at least 10 days.

Flail chest injuries can be repaired in a similar manner stabilizing both ends of the segmental fractures. An intramedullary K wire can often be used to traverse the entire segmental fragment and fix both fractures at the same time. When tissue loss is significant, chest wall defects may need filling with a Marlex Mesh[3] or other techniques.[2]

The least invasive technique that provides alignment of the fracture ends is generally the most successful.

REFERENCES

1. Bjorling DE, Kolata RJ, DeNovo RC: Flail chest: review, clinical experience and new method of stabilization, *J Am Anim Hosp Assoc* 18(3):269-276, 1982.
2. Krahwinkel DJ: Lower respiratory tract trauma. In Kirk RW, editor: *Current veterinary therapy VI*, Philadelphia, 1977, Saunders.
3. Schwartz A, Mehlhalf Schunk CJ: The thorax. In Harvey, Newton, Schwartz A, editors: *Small animal surgery*, Philadelphia, 1990, Lippincott.

8

Fractures of the Bones of the Front Limb

THOMAS M. TURNER

The forelimb, unlike the rear limb, does not rigidly articulate with the axial skeleton. Rather, the front limb is supported by the muscular sling formed by the trapezius, rhomboideus, serratus, and pectoralis musculature. This may partly explain the lower incidence of fractures to the front limb compared with the rear limb.

The front limb supports more of the body weight (60% to 66%) than the rear limb. This fact emphasizes the need for rigid fixation of front limb fractures, allowing a rapid return to weight bearing.

This chapter is organized according to specific bones. Shoulder fractures may involve the distal scapula or proximal humerus. Fractures of the elbow may encompass fractures of the distal humerus, proximal ulna, or radial head, since the elbow is a composite joint. Fractures of the carpus collectively may reflect fractures of the radial or ulna styloid, fractures of the radial or ulna carpal bones, the numbered carpal bones, or proximal metacarpals. For the specific details of a particular fixation device technique, such as bone plate, external fixator, or wiring techniques, the reader is referred to Chapter 5.

FRACTURES OF THE SCAPULA
Anatomical Considerations

Proximally, the scapula is a broad, thin expansive bone in the cranial-to-caudal direction that tapers to a narrow scapular neck distally. Projecting along the central aspect of the scapula on the lateral surface is a prominent scapular spine, which ends distally in the prominent acromion process. The area of greatest bone density is at the line of reflection of the scapular spine from the body and in the region of the scapular neck and glenoid. The scapular body supports the shallow glenoid. The glenoid articulates with the humeral head, forming the diarthrodial shoulder joint. The shoulder is supported by the medial and lateral glenohumeral ligaments and surrounding joint capsule. This support is supplemented by the biceps, supraspinatus and infraspinatus, subscapularis, and teres minor tendons, which cross the joint and provide stability, particularly during muscle contraction. These structures are tendons but function also as ligaments because they cross the joint and are thus referred to as "active ligaments."

The scapula overlies the cranial aspect of the thoracic cavity. Consequently, fractures of the scapula may be associated with concomitant trauma to the underlying soft tissue and bony structures. The extent of these injuries may range from nondisplaced rib fractures to damage of neurological structures, such as the brachial plexus or individual peripheral nerve components, and severe internal thoracic trauma, such as lung contusions, pneumothorax, or hemothorax. Therefore, as with any fracture, definitive fracture treatment must be preceded by a thorough preoperative examination with emphasis on the assessment of neurological and thoracic function.

Fractures of the scapular body and spine may be minimally displaced because of the support from the overlying musculature. These nondisplaced fractures may be treated conservatively by use of a non-weight-bearing or Velpeau sling (see Chapter 4).

Treatment

Fractures of the scapular spine. Fractures involving the scapular spine may occur as isolated injuries or associated with adjacent fractures of the body. Three techniques are used to stabilize the scapular spine to the body. First, the horizontal portion of a finger T plate, which has been contoured to 90 degrees, is attached to the spine and the vertical portion secured to the body. The plate may be applied either to the cranial or caudal surface of the spine. The surgeon should note that the scapular spine is somewhat concave on the caudal surface. This technique provides very rigid support of the scapular spine. Second, the scapular spine may be secured to the body using a hemicerclage wire passed through the body

and tightened over the scapular spine, thus compressing the spine to the body. Third, a lag screw may be inserted through the acromion portion of the spine and into the scapular body. One or more of these techniques can provide secure stabilization of the scapular spine to the body (Fig. 8-1).

Fractures of the acromion. Acromion fractures may result as isolated occurrences or, more frequently, may be associated with other scapular fractures. An osteotomy of the acromion process can also be reattached using the following techniques. Usually, the acromion is stabilized using a tension-band wire technique. One or two Kirschner wires are inserted through the acromion process into the scapular spine and body. The fragment is further supported with a tension-band figure-eight wire passed through the spine and over the exposed ends of the pins. Alternately, the acromion process may be stabilized using a simple interfragmentary wire technique of two or more wires passed through the process and the scapular spine (Fig. 8-2). In larger breeds an acromion process of sufficient size may be reattached to the body with a lag screw.

Fractures of the scapular body. These fractures tend to be displaced medially and dorsally, resulting in considerable overriding of the fracture fragments. Multifrag-

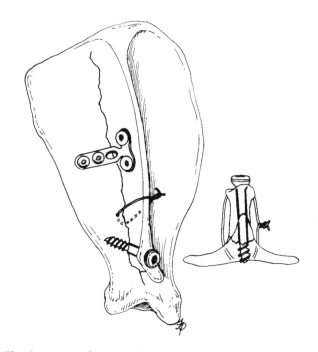

Fig. 8-1 Scapular spine fracture may be stabilized with any one of three techniques. A T plate (2.0 or 2.7 mm) is contoured to 90 degrees and applied to either the cranial or the caudal surface of the scapular spine. Additional fixation methods are the use of a hemicerclage wire or a lag screw inserted through the acromion process and into the scapular body.

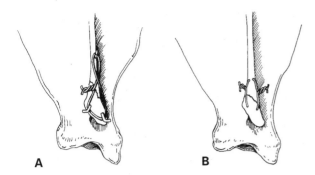

Fig. 8-2   **A,** Fractures of the acromion process or osteotomy of the acromion process may be stabilized using a tension-band wire technique with one or two Kirschner wires and a figure-eight wire. **B,** The acromion process may be fixed with two or more interfragmentary wires.

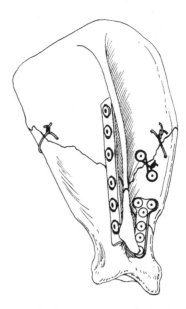

Fig. 8-3   Scapular body fractures may be fixed using standard finger plates or miniplates, bone plates, interfragmentary wires, or a position screw on either side of a fracture line connected with a figure-eight wire. When using a bone plate, the screws, if possible, should be inserted into the area of greatest bone density at the reflection of the spine from the body.

ment fractures of the scapular body can result in extensive overriding and collapse of the body, resulting in relative limb shortening if the fracture is not stabilized with internal fixation. In addition, the neurovascular structures medial to the scapular body may be traumatized as a result of the fracture and the unstable fragments. The scapular body can be problematic to obtain adequate screw purchase because of the thin bone, especially the extreme proximal aspect. Therefore, the relatively greater amount of bone stock present at the reflection of the scapular spine from the body should be used for screw purchase.

These fractures are stabilized easily by applying a bone plate to the scapular body just cranial or caudal to the scapular spine. Screws are inserted through the plate into the area of greatest bone density at the junction of the spine and body. This requires minimum plate contour, with the exception of the distal aspect of the scapula at the glenoid. If it is necessary to extend the plate distally, a slight lateral bend must be placed in the plate to follow the anatomical surface. Generally, 2.0 or 2.7 mm plates or cuttable plates are used for fixation of these fractures. A 3.5 mm plate may be used for a scapular body fracture in a large or giant breed.

Fixation of multifragment fractures involving the scapular body may be achieved by combining a variety of techniques. The fragments are sequentially aligned and stabilized in anatomical position using a combination of small plates, finger plates, or interfragmentary wires. Additionally, screws may be placed on each side of the fracture line and connected with a figure-eight wire (Fig. 8-3).

Highly comminuted fractures of the scapular body or gunshot injuries may be treated by using a larger-size plate to span the entire length of the scapular body from the glenoid to the proximal aspect. The plate functions as a buttress plate. The adjacent musculature acts to support the adjacent fragments, and if necessary, bone graft can be added.

Fractures of the scapular neck. The scapular neck is, in general, the weakest area of the scapula. These fractures typically are considerably displaced because of the contracture of the deltoid, pectoralis, and other adjacent shoulder musculature. This can result in considerable impingement on the adjacent neurovascular structures, particularly the suprascapular nerve. Likewise, the displacement of fragments also results in relative limb shortening and compromised shoulder range of motion.

The surgical approach must focus on identification and protection of the suprascapular nerve during internal fixation.

Typically, either standard Dynamic Compression Plates (DCPs) or finger plate series (2.0 or 2.7 mm) are used for stabilizing fractures in the neck area. The bone density in this area provides support for adequate screw purchase. Plates applied to this region must be contoured to allow for the metaphyseal widening over the glenoid surface. An improperly contoured plate can result in varus or valgus of the shoulder (Fig. 8-4).

Another method for stabilization of scapular neck fractures is the use of a crossed-pin technique. Kirschner wires are adequate for small breeds and small-diameter Steinmann pins for larger breeds. Pins are inserted in a converging pattern from the dorsolateral aspect of the distal scapular body into the caudal glenoid fragment and from the caudolateral aspect of the scapular body into the cranial glenoid fragment. Alternatively, two pins can be inserted in a diverging pattern from the cranial glenoid, in

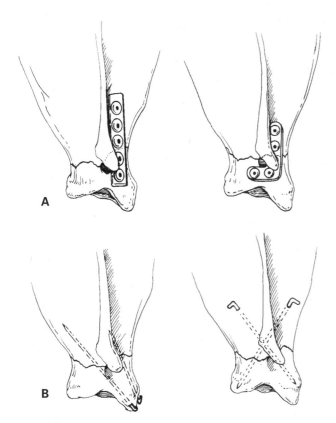

Fig. 8-4 **A,** Scapular neck fractures are preferably stabilized with a bone plate. Either a straight or finger plate design can be used, depending on the size of the distal fragment. **B,** Scapular neck fractures may also be fixed using crossed pins. Each pin must obtain purchase in the bone on either side of the fracture line. The suprascapular nerve must be protected during fracture repair.

a dorsocaudal direction, into the distal scapula to stabilize the neck. Pin placement can be problematic because of thin anatomy of the scapular body. The surgeon must ensure that the pins engage bone on either side of the fracture line.

Articular fractures

Fractures of the glenoid. Glenoid fractures are interarticular fractures and thus necessitate open reduction for direct visualization of the articular surface to ensure that anatomical reduction is achieved. The goals of fracture repair are to reestablish the articular surface and provide rigid fixation during the healing process. The suprascapular nerve is encountered in the surgical approach to the glenoid, as in scapular neck fractures, and must be identified and protected.

Occasionally, these fractures may be exposed by a standard craniolateral approach. However, an osteotomy of the acromion facilitates the fracture repair by providing a more adequate exposure. Once the fracture fragments have been anatomically aligned, initial stability is achieved by

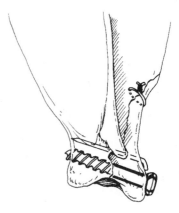

Fig. 8-5 Fractures through the glenoid involve the articular surface and require precise reduction of the fracture fragments. The fracture is fixed using a lag screw and supplementary Kirschner wire. Preferably, these are inserted parallel to the articular surface.

inserting a Kirschner wire in a craniocaudal direction parallel to the articular surface. A lag screw is inserted through the fragments parallel to the articular surface to achieve interfragmentary compression. The lag screw is inserted either from the cranial-to-caudal or caudal-to-cranial direction, depending on the fracture fragment size and position.

These fractures may extend into the scapular neck and body region. Depending on the extent of the fracture length, additional stability may be applied in the form of an additional pin or screw placement or hemicerclage wire (Fig. 8-5). Glenoid fragments are relatively thin in the medial-to-lateral dimension, and therefore smaller screw sizes should be used (2.7, 3.5, or 4.0 mm). The surgeon also must be careful that the screw does not penetrate the articular surface.

Avulsion of the scapular tuberosity. The scapular tuberosity (supraglenoid tubercle) lies at the extreme craniodistal aspect of the glenoid rim. This is the attachment site for the tendon of origin of the biceps muscle. Avulsion of this segment occurs almost exclusively in immature animals. Occasionally, it may be difficult to assess radiographically if the tuberosity is avulsed because it may be minimally displaced. A lateral radiograph of the suspect shoulder should be compared with lateral views of both the affected shoulder flexed and the opposite shoulder. The fragment is generally displaced into the intertubercular groove as a result of contraction of the biceps muscle. Since this is on the glenoid rim, it is also an articular fracture and necessitates accurate repositioning to restore the articular surface.

Osteotomy of the greater tubercle of the humerus provides the greatest exposure for surgical repair. Although these repairs may be approached without osteotomy of the greater tubercle, this can result in awkward manipulation of the tissues and further complicates the procedure.

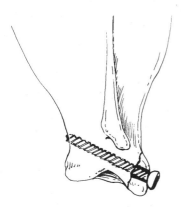

Fig. 8-6 Avulsion of the scapular tuberosity can be fixed using a lag screw (2.7 or 4.0 mm) or a tension-band wire technique with two Kirschner wires and figure-eight wire. Overtightening the lag screw must be avoided.

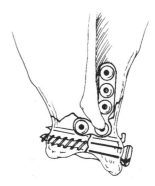

Fig. 8-7 A fracture of the scapular neck and glenoid (T-Y fracture) can be stabilized using a lag screw fixation supplemented with Kirschner wire for fixation of the glenoid fragment. The glenoid fragment is then stabilized to the scapular body with a bone plate, DCP, or finger plate, or crossed Kirschner wires.

Two techniques are available for fixation of the tuberosity. Preferably, the fragment is repositioned and fixed using a lag screw. Either a 2.7 mm or 4.0 mm lag screw should be used. A 3.5 mm screw requires overdrilling with a 3.5 mm drill for lag effect. Therefore, this screw should be used only in very large or giant breeds (Fig. 8-6). Careful attention should be directed not only to anatomical positioning of the fragment, but also to tightening of the screw. Overtightening can result in stripping the screw threads or iatrogenic comminution of the fragment. An alternate technique is the use of a tension-band wire. Two Kirschner wires are inserted through the fragment and directed into the scapular neck. In addition, a figure-eight tension-band wire is inserted through a hole drilled in the proximal fragment and over the exposed ends of the pin.

Comminution of the tuberosity or extreme trauma to the proximal end of the tendon may necessitate transposition of the biceps tendon of origin to the greater tubercle. A hole is drilled transversely through the proximal aspect of the greater tubercle, and the tendon of origin of the biceps is passed through the hole and sutured back on itself. Normal shoulder function can still be anticipated.

T-Y fractures of the distal scapula. A T-Y fracture is a combination of a scapular neck fracture and glenoid fracture. These fractures result from extensive trauma to the shoulder and in extreme cases can pose a formidable challenge for reconstruction. The glenoid fragments are generally displaced distally, and the humeral head is displaced proximally, overriding the scapular body. These fractures must be approached with an acromion osteotomy to achieve optimum exposure for fragment reconstruction. The primary aim of the reconstruction is to restore the glenoid's articular surface. Once the glenoid fragments are anatomically aligned, initial stability is achieved using one or more Kirschner wires for temporary fixation. A lag screw is then placed parallel to the

articular surface for interfragmentary compression. Once reconstructed, the glenoid fragment is reattached to the scapular body, preferably using a contoured bone plate. In most cases, 2.0, 2.7, or 3.5 mm standard DCPs or finger plate series can provide rigid stability. The osteotomized acromion is reattached as previously described. Before closure, the shoulder should be placed through a range of motion to ensure that this is not impinged and that metal does not project into the articulating surface (Fig. 8-7).

• • •

Despite the thin bone structures, fractures involving the scapula tend to heal in a short time, especially those of the scapular neck and glenoid. Implant failure is generally associated with failure to obtain adequate screw or wire purchase at the time of surgery. Iatrogenic complications, such as overtightening of the screw, particularly in the region of the glenoid, can result in the need for additional stabilization using multiple Kirschner wires. If adequate internal fixation is achieved, early weight bearing and function should be allowed to prevent soft tissue contractures. Malalignment of the fractured articular surface can result in compromised joint function. In addition, a malaligned scapular body fracture can result in varus or valgus positioning of the limb.

FRACTURES OF THE HUMERUS
Anatomical Considerations

The humerus is a long bone with considerable architectural irregularity. The humeral head articulates with the glenoid and makes up the opposing half of the shoulder joint. The humerus tapers from the wide proximal metaphysis to a narrow supracondylar region distally, which supports the cranially displaced humeral condyle. Most of the support to the humeral condyle is along the medial ramus. A large supratrochlear foramen is present in the supracondylar region. The lateral aspect of the humeral condyle is supported by a narrow lateral ramus. Therefore, the distal humerus is inherently weaker than the proximal aspect of the humerus, which accounts for the high incidence of fractures in this area.

The radial nerve lies over the lateral aspect of the distal humerus and is at risk for injury from fractures in this area and during surgical repair.

The humerus is unique in that it may be approached surgically from all four aspects. A *transolecranon approach* exposes the caudal condylar area and can be further developed to expose the caudal diaphysis to the proximal metaphysis. The ulnar nerve and, if the exposure is extended proximally, the radial nerve also must be identified and protected. A *cranial approach* can be used to expose the proximal humerus, diaphysis, and distal metaphyseal region. This approach necessitates protection of the radial nerve during exposure and fracture repair. The proximal metaphysis to the medial condyle can be identified through a *medial approach* to the humerus. The median and ulnar nerves are encountered and must be protected during fracture treatment. Laterally, the *craniolateral approach* to the condyle combined with a *lateral approach* to the shaft allows visualization from the humeral condyle to the greater tubercle and humeral head. The radial nerve must be carefully identified and protected during the approach and fracture repair.

Treatment

Fractures of the proximal humerus

Fractures of the humeral head. These fractures occur infrequently. In the young animal, these occur as a physeal fracture (Salter-Harris fracture) and are fixed using two or three smooth Kirschner wires or small-diameter Steinmann pins. In the mature animal, fractures of the humeral head can be fixed by inserting lag screws or pins through the cranial aspect of the proximal humerus into the humeral head. The screws or pins are directed in a proximal-to-caudal direction and perpendicular to the fracture line, taking care not to perforate the articular surface (Fig. 8-8).

Multifragment fractures of the humeral head or gunshot injuries should be treated by anatomically replacing the fragments and stabilizing them with multiple Kirschner wires or lag screws. The reconstructed humeral head is reattached to the metaphysis with lag screws or pins. Bone graft can be applied to bone-deficient areas. Fractures of the humeral head occurring with a proximal metaphyseal fracture may be stabilized by passing lag screws through a plate applied to the proximal cranial surface of the humerus (Fig. 8-9).

Tubercle fractures of the proximal humerus. Fractures of the greater and lesser tubercles also occur infrequently. In the immature animal the greater tubercle is anatomically

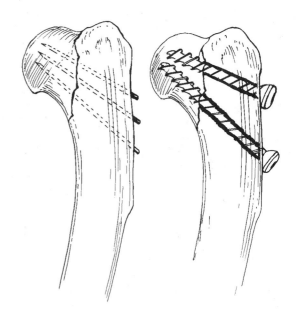

Fig. 8-8 Fractures of the humeral head can be stabilized using two or more smooth pins in the immature animal or lag screw fixation in the mature animal.

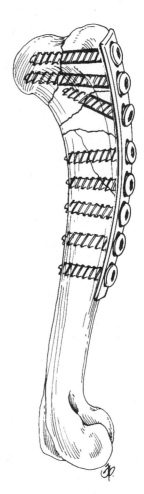

Fig. 8-9 Humeral head fractures concurrent with fractures in the metaphyseal region necessitate a cranially applied bone plate with lag screws inserted through the plate to stabilize the humeral head fracture.

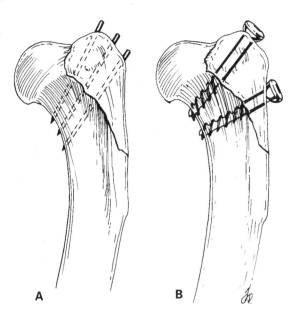

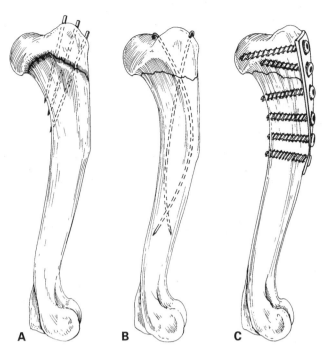

Fig. 8-10 **A,** Fractures of the greater tubercle may be stabilized with two or more smooth pins in the immature animal. **B,** In the mature animal, these fractures may be stabilized with lag screw fixation or pin fixation.

Fig. 8-11 **A,** Fractures of the humeral neck in immature animals (Salter-Harris types I and II fractures) are stabilized using two or three smooth pins inserted through the greater tubercle into the proximal metaphysis. **B,** Alternately, two pins may be inserted through the greater tubercle into the medullary cavity in a Rush pin technique. **C,** Humeral neck fractures in mature animals may be stabilized using a DCP applied to the cranial surface of the proximal humerus. This requires at least two screws purchasing the proximal humeral fragment.

positioned and fixed with two to three smooth pins. Lag screws or pins may be used to stabilize the fracture in the mature animal. The screws or pins are inserted in a caudodistal direction and engage the caudal cortex (Fig. 8-10).

Lesser tubercle fractures are generally an avulsion injury that can be associated with medial dislocation of the shoulder. Theses are identified through a craniomedial approach and fixed with a lag screw.

Fractures of the humeral neck. These fractures are most often seen in immature animals as a Salter-Harris type I or type II fracture of the proximal humeral physis. In the mature animal a fracture in this region occurs infrequently. Three techniques are available for fixation of humeral neck fractures.

In the immature animal, if the fracture can be reduced, closed fixation is achieved with closed pinning. The pins are directed through the greater tubercle into the caudal proximal cortex. However, precise anatomical reduction may be difficult to achieve because of hematoma and fracture debris within the disrupted physis. Therefore, open reduction and internal fixation are preferable to achieve accurate alignment of the fracture fragments. Once aligned, the fracture fragments may be stabilized by inserting two to three smooth pins from the cranial dorsal aspect of the greater tubercle into the caudal cortex of the proximal metaphysis (Fig. 8-11, *A*).

A second technique for stabilization of this type of fracture is the use of smooth pins inserted in a Rush pin technique. The pins are inserted in an alternating fashion through the lateral and medial aspects of the greater

tubercle, deflecting off the medullary aspect of the opposite cortex into the distal metaphysis (Fig. 8-11, *B*).

A third technique may be used in mature animals. A standard DCP or, in the case of a small proximal fragment, a T plate is applied to the cranial aspect of the proximal humerus. At least two screws must be inserted in the proximal fragment. The screws are inserted into the caudal aspect of the humeral head but do not perforate the articular surface. The remainder of the screws are inserted in a cranial-to-caudal direction. The use of the DCP allows compression of the fracture (see Chapter 5). As a result of the large cross-sectional area of the proximal humerus and the abundance of cancellous bone, fractures in this region heal rapidly (Fig. 8-11, *C*).

Fractures of the humeral diaphysis. The diaphysis, as with the distal humerus, may be approached from all four directions. The posterior approach may be combined with a posterior approach to the distal humerus; however, this is the most limited of the four directions. A cranial approach allows a plate to be extended from the greater tubercle to the supracondylar region. However, it is limited distally because of the supratrochlear foramen and the humeral condyle. Both the medial and the lateral approaches provide exposure from the level of the humeral head to the epicondylar region.

Paramount to internal fixation of humeral fractures are the identification and protection of the radial nerve. Likewise, the ulnar and median nerves must be identified and protected when using a medial approach.

A variety of fixation techniques may be applied to fractures of the humeral shaft, including closed-pinning techniques, open intramedullary pinning, bone plate application, and external fixators. Some fractures may be fixed adequately by a number of techniques, whereas others are best addressed by a particular technique.

Closed reduction and internal fixation may be applied to relatively nondisplaced transverse or slightly oblique fractures, particularly in immature animals. If a single pin is used, the diameter must approximate the diameter of the medullary canal at the shaft's distal aspect. The pin is inserted through the greater tubercle into the distal medial aspect of the metaphysis. This fixation may be supplemented with a half-splint external fixator (a half-pin inserted in the greater tubercle region and a half-pin inserted in the condyle, connected by a single bar laterally), which aids in maintaining rotational stability (Fig. 8-12, *A*).

Another method of fracture repair is stacked pinning, which consists of inserting two or more pins of smaller diameter normograde (preferably) or retrograde through the greater tubercle into the distal medial metaphysis or supracondylar region. The pins must not exit or project into the olecranon fossa or supratrochlear foramen (Fig. 8-12, *B*).

In mature large dogs the preferable treatment of this type of fracture is the use of a bone plate applied to the lateral, cranial, or medial surface to achieve interfragmentary compression and rigid stability (Fig. 8-12, *C*).

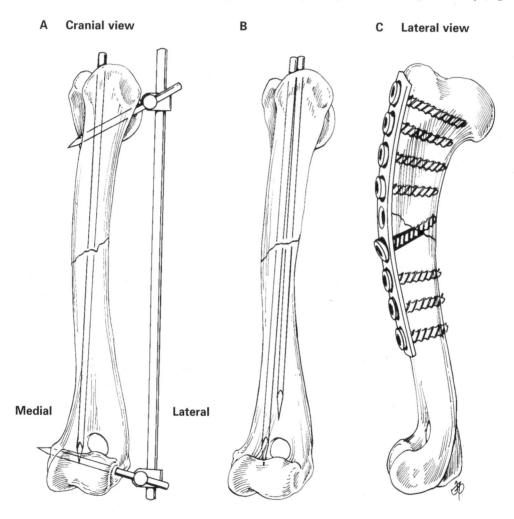

A Cranial view   **B**   **C** Lateral view

Medial   Lateral

Fig. 8-12 **A,** Fractures of the humeral diaphysis can be stabilized using a single intramedullary pin, with open or closed reduction supplemented with a half-splint external fixator. **B,** Alternately, two or more smaller-diameter pins inserted in a stacked pin configuration can be used to stabilize the diaphyseal fracture. The pins must not protrude into the olecranon fossa. **C,** A bone plate applied to the cranial (illustrated), medial, or lateral humeral surface may also be used to stabilize humeral diaphyseal fractures.

Long oblique fractures or fractures with small comminution involving the humeral shaft should be stabilized with internal fixation. Intramedullary pinning, either single or stacked pins, may be combined with lag screws or full-cerclage or hemicerclage wires. Application of cerclage wires in the humerus may necessitate shallow notching of the cortex to prevent the wires from slipping distally on to the narrow aspect of the humerus. Hemicerclage wires avoid this complication (Fig. 8-13, *A*). Application of a bone plate to either the lateral, cranial, or medial surface can provide excellent stability of this type of fracture. In addition, this can also allow for application of lag screws either through the plate or application outside the plate (Fig. 8-13, *B*).

Multifragment fractures are fractures involving a high degree of comminution or bone loss, such as gunshot injuries, and are preferably fixed with a bone plate or external fixator that spans the defect and functions as a buttress to support the proximal and distal fragments. The plate may be applied to the lateral, cranial, or medial aspect. Application to the lateral aspect may necessitate considerable contouring of the plate. The application of a bone plate necessitates a wide surgical exposure to approach the proximal and distal aspects of the humerus. Fractures with a resulting unreconstructable defect or bone loss require the addition of cancellous bone graft to fill the defect (Fig. 8-14, *A*).

Alternatively, multifragment fractures may be stabilized using a type I external fixator with or without an intramedullary pin. A type I fixator requires at least two half-pins and preferably three or four half-pins in the distal and proximal bone fragments, respectively. The extreme proximal pin is inserted in the greater tubercle area and the extreme distal pin through the epicondylar area. The connecting bar is attached to these pins with single fixation clamps. The connecting bar should have the additional number of single clamps loosely placed on the bar, but only the proximal and distal clamps should be tightened on the previously inserted pins. The remaining pins to be applied are inserted through the loose single clamps, then

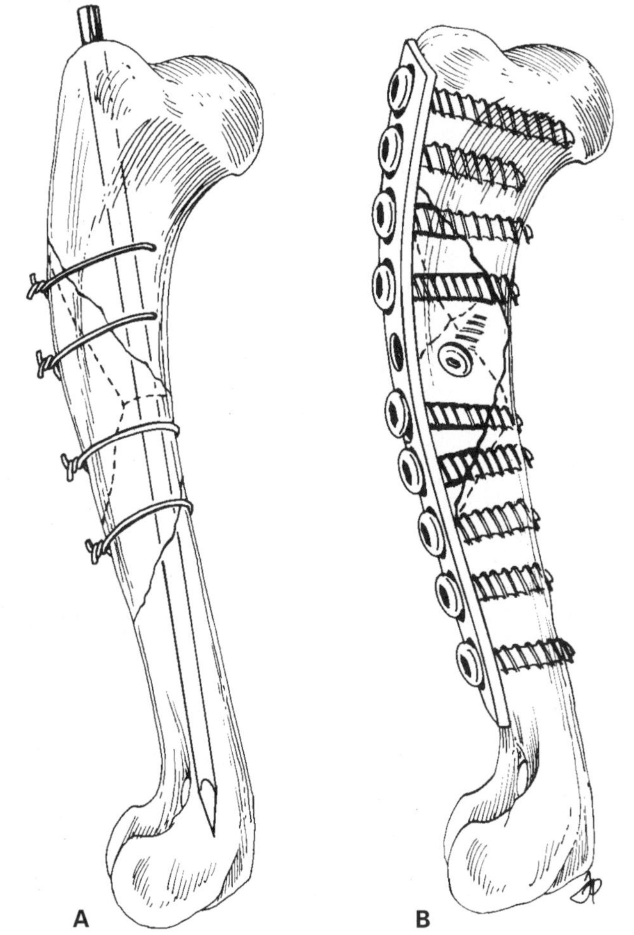

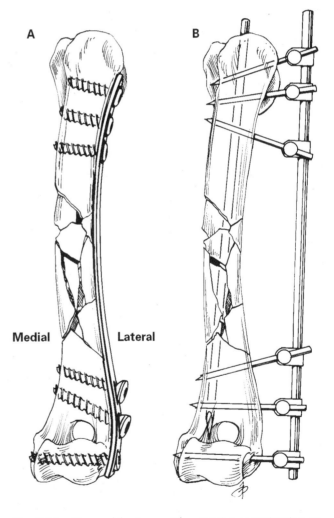

Fig. 8-14 Humeral fractures with extensive comminution or bone loss may be stabilized with **A,** a bone plate (buttress function), or **B,** an external fixator (type I) and intramedullary pin. At least two screws or two pins purchasing proximally and distally must be obtained.

Fig. 8-13 Comminuted fractures of the humeral shaft may be stabilized with **A,** intramedullary pins combined with cerclage or hemicerclage wires, or **B,** a DCP and lag screw fixation.

into the respective proximal or distal bone fragments. The single clamps are all tightened. This configuration results in all pins attached to the same connecting bar. The type I device so constructed results in a rigid fixation; (Fig. 8-14, *B*) if additional strength is needed, however, a second connecting bar may be applied adjacent to the existing bar.

Fractures of the distal humerus

Supracondylar fractures. The narrowing of the humeral shaft distally results in an inherently weak area at the distal humerus. Fractures through this region are some of the most frequently encountered fractures involving the humerus. In the immature animal, these occur as a Salter-Harris type I or type II fracture. Three techniques are typically used for fixation of these fractures. The supracondylar region may be exposed with a lateral approach, and a pin is inserted either retrograde through the distal humerus metaphysis or normograde from the greater tubercle to emerge at the distal medial metaphysis. The fracture fragment is anatomically aligned and the pin advanced into the caudal medial epicondylar area. A sec-

ond pin is then inserted obliquely into the caudal aspect of the lateral epicondyle to impinge in the medial distal cortex but avoiding the supratrochlear foramen (Fig. 8-15, *A*).

An alternative technique for fixation of supracondylar fractures is the use of smooth pins inserted in a Rush pin technique. Points of insertion are caudal to the lateral and medial epicondyle, respectively. This necessitates identification and protection of the ulnar nerve on the medial side. After the fragments are anatomically aligned, the pins are inserted in the distal fragment. Fragment reduction may be facilitated by placing the elbow in extension. The pins are advanced alternately using a back-and-forth twisting motion. The pins are inserted at a slight converging angle so that the medial pin deflects from the lateral cortex to impinge in the medial proximal cortex. Likewise, the lateral pin is inserted to be deflected from the medial cortex and impinge on the lateral proximal cortex (Fig. 8-15, *B*).

The application of a bone plate along the medial or caudomedial aspect of the distal humerus provides a third method of rigidly fixing a supracondylar fracture. Frequently, some degree of obliquity is associated with

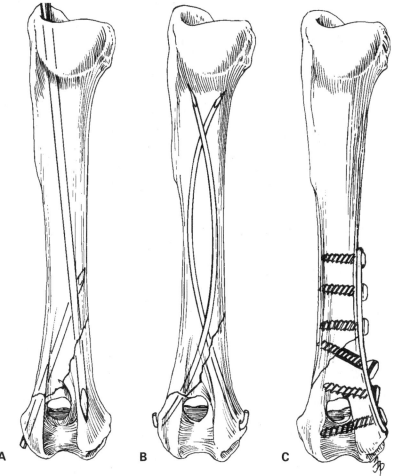

Fig. 8-15   Supracondylar fractures can be stabilized using **A,** a single intramedullary pin plus an obliquely inserted distal pin; **B,** two pins inserted in a Rush pin technique; or **C,** a bone plate applied to the lateral, caudal, or medial aspect of the humerus.

this type of fracture, which may extend into the medial metaphysis and shaft. Through either a lateral or caudomedial approach, the fracture is anatomically aligned and fixed with a lag screw. Performing this step initially greatly facilitates the application of the plate to the caudal or caudomedial aspect of the humerus. At least two screws are directed in either a medial-to-lateral or a caudal-to-cranial direction in the distal humeral fragment. With either method the surgeon must not allow the screws to penetrate the articular surface (Fig. 8-15, *C*).

Metal that protrudes into the foramen or fossa can impair elbow range of motion and abrade the cartilage, leading to degenerative joint disease. In the cat the median nerve passes through a medial supracondylar foramen. Added caution must be taken not to damage this nerve during fracture reduction and fixation. Occasionally, a supracondylar fracture in a cat extends into the foramen. This may necessitate gentle release and retraction of the nerve from the foramen by resection of the thin medial rim of the foramen.

Multifragment fractures involving the supracondylar and distal diaphysis are rigidly stabilized using bone plate fixation. The fracture fragments are anatomically positioned and sequentially fixed using lag screws, cerclage wires, or hemicerclage wires. The plate is contoured to lie along the lateral or medial aspect of the distal humerus and fixed with appropriate screws. If possible, lag screw fixation is preferable to wires for fragment stabilization. Fractures that result in an unreconstructable defect and the presence of bone loss, as in gunshot injures, necessitate cancellous graft applied to the fracture defects (Fig. 8-16).

Supracondylar fractures occurring in giant breeds occasionally may necessitate double bone plates. The plates are positioned on the caudal surface of the distal humerus along the lateral and medial metaphyseal ridges. This may be accomplished with or without an olecranon osteotomy (Fig. 8-17).

With all these techniques, the surgeon must ensure that metal does not extend into the supratrochlear foramen or the olecranon fossa or protrude from any of the articulating surfaces of the humeral condyle.

Condylar fractures

Lateral. The humeral condyle is well supported medially with a wide metaphysis. However, the radial head articulates with the capitellum on the lateral aspect of the condyle. As a result, this is the primary load-bearing surface of the condyle. This fact, combined with the supratrochlear foramen and the narrow lateral metaphysis, predisposes the lateral portion of the condyle to fracture.

One of the most common fractures of the humerus involves the lateral aspect of the humeral condyle. Typically, this occurs in the immature animal as a Salter-Harris type IV fracture. Although a simple fracture, this can result in disastrous results for elbow function if not accurately repaired. Since this is an interarticular fracture, it

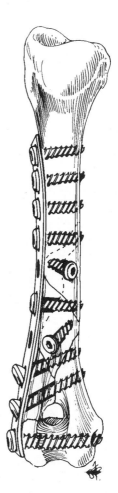

Fig. 8-16 Multifragment supracondylar fractures can be fixed using a DCP applied to the lateral, medial (illustrated), or caudal surface of the distal humerus.

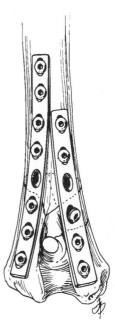

Fig. 8-17 Supracondylar fractures occurring in large and giant breeds may occasionally necessitate the use of double DCPs applied to the caudal aspect of the distal humerus.

necessitates open reduction and internal fixation. Although the use of a condylar clamp in a closed-fixation technique has been described, these fractures rarely can be managed accurately with this technique. Soft tissue interposition, hematoma formation, and musculature contraction can prohibit the accurate alignment of the articular surface that is so desirable for articular fracture repair. Also, the clamp can interfere with proper positioning of the lag screw across the condyle.

A craniolateral approach is advocated to visualize the articular surface and lateral ramus adequately during fixation. Once the fracture fragments are anatomically aligned, they may be stabilized temporarily with a transcondylar Kirschner wire inserted at or just proximal to the epicondyle. A transcondylar lag screw is then inserted. The point of insertion of the screw is just cranial and distal to the lateral epicondyle in the extensor fossa. Adequate tightening of the screw is determined by visualizing the compression at the fracture site as the screw is tightened. Overtightening the screw can result in iatrogenic comminution of the lateral condyle or loss of screw purchase. Conversely, in young animals, the soft bone may necessitate the use of a washer to distribute screw head forces and prevent the head from sinking into the bone. Additional fixation is achieved by inserting a Kirschner wire or small Steinmann pin from the lateral epicondyle obliquely through the lateral ramus into the medial cortex (Fig. 8-18). Alternately, if the obliquity of the fracture permits, a second lag screw is inserted in the metaphyseal region.

An alternative method for inserting the transcondylar screw is to drill the glide hole for the lag screw before fragment reduction. The fragment is externally rotated and drilled from the medial-to-lateral direction. The fracture fragment is then anatomically fixed with a Kirschner wire, and lag screw application is completed. Inadequate size of the screw or failure to obtain purchase with the screw results in failure of the fixation and nonunion of the fracture. The wide variation of screw sizes available (2.0 to 6.5 mm) gives the surgeon a good selection. A full range of motion and excellent functional results can be expected.

Medial. Fractures of the medial condylar region occur much less frequently than those of the lateral condylar region. Medial condylar fractures are usually associated with a long oblique fracture extending well up into the metaphysis and shaft. These fractures appear to occur more frequently in the chondrodystrophic breeds.

The fracture is approached craniomedially. Once anatomically aligned, the fracture is fixed using a transcondylar lag screw supplemented by either pin fixation or preferably one or two additional lag screws in the metaphyseal or diaphyseal region if a large fragment is present. A full range of motion and excellent functional results can be expected (Fig. 8-19).

Epicondylar fractures. Fractures of the medial or lateral epicondylar regions are generally avulsive injuries. These frequently are associated with subluxation or luxation of the elbow. It is important that these structures be securely fixed because these are the humeral attachments of the respective ulnar and radial collateral ligaments.

Three techniques for fixation may be used. Preferably, the fracture fragments are anatomically positioned and fixed using a lag screw or lag screw combined with a spiked washer, taking care not to allow the screw to protrude into the olecranon fossa. Second, the avulsed epicondyle may be positioned and fixed using two or more small Kirschner wires. Third, these Kirschner wires may be combined with a tension-band figure-eight wire (Fig. 8-20).

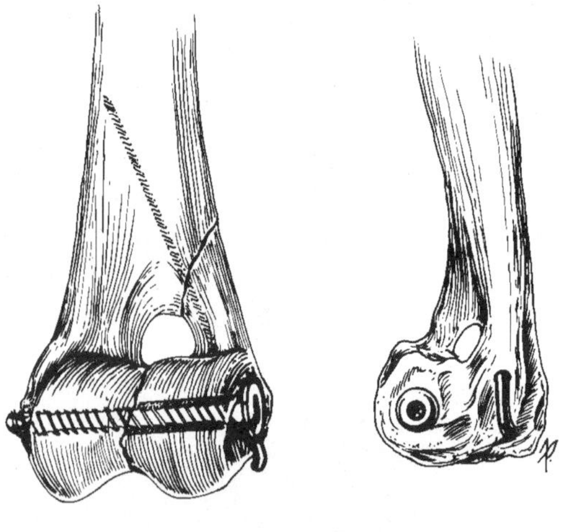

Fig. 8-18 Fractures of the lateral aspect of the humeral condyle involve the articular surface and require precise reduction of the articular surface. Fixation is achieved using a transcondylar lag screw inserted cranial and distal to the lateral epicondyle. This is supplemented with a smooth pin or additional lag screw inserted in the lateral ramus of the distal humerus.

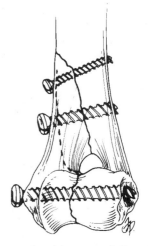

Fig. 8-19 Fractures involving a medial condylar area can be fixed with a transcondylar lag screw and one or two additional lag screws or small intramedullary pins.

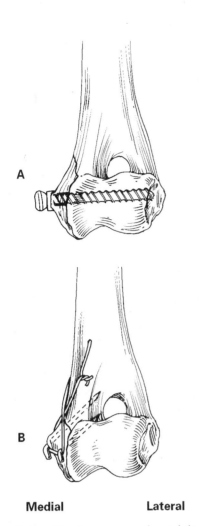

Medial   **Lateral**

Fig. 8-20 Epicondylar fractures may be stabilized using **A**, a lag screw with spiked washer, or **B**, small-diameter smooth pins and figure-eight wire.

Intercondylar (T-Y) fractures. A T-Y fracture of the distal humerus can be considered a combination of a condylar and supracondylar fracture. These fractures can be some of the most devastating for elbow function. Therefore, precise anatomical reconstruction and internal fixation are essential to the restoration of joint function. These fractures should not be attempted without some degree of orthopedic expertise.

Intercondylar fractures may be approached surgically through one of two techniques: a transolecranon approach to the caudal surface or a craniolateral approach. A transolecranon approach necessitates osteotomy of the olecranon, which should be performed as an oblique rather than a transverse osteotomy. This aids in stability of the reattached fragment by allowing compressive forces to act on the osteotomy. The ulnar nerve must be identified and protected when using this approach. This approach can be further developed exposing the posterior surface of the humeral shaft. The transolecranon approach prohibits the

surgeon from visualizing the cranial articular surface of the humeral condyle. However, this approach does provide a flat surface for application of a bone plate. On the other hand, the craniolateral approach allows exposure of the cranial aspect of the humeral condyle. It can be combined with a lateral approach to the shaft of the humerus to provide exposure from the humeral condyle to the greater tubercle. It is therefore beneficial not only for exposure of the humeral condyle, but also in highly comminuted fractures. The craniolateral approach necessitates the identification and protection of the radial nerve.

A simple intercondylar fracture (one fracture line in the condyle and one through the supracondylar region) may be reconstructed by one of two techniques. The condylar fragments may be anatomically aligned and fixed with a Kirschner wire and transcondylar lag screw. This reconstructed fragment is then reattached to the metaphysis using a lag screw and Kirschner wire, which is then supported with a laterally or caudally positioned bone plate. Using the transolecranon approach, the plate is applied to the caudal aspect of the distal humerus, and two screws are directed cranially or craniomedially into the humeral condyle, taking care not to allow the screws to perforate the articular surface (Fig. 8-21, *A*).

Alternately, through a craniolateral approach, the medial fragment may be anatomically aligned and fixed with a lag screw in the metaphysis. The lateral condylar fragment is then anatomically positioned and fixed with a Kirschner wire and transcondylar screw, as previously described for a lateral condylar fracture. The reconstructed fracture, although anatomical, is not sufficient to support weight and must be further supported with a bone plate applied along the lateral aspect of the metaphysis, with two screws (if possible) inserted into the condylar fragment. Using the standard DCP, the transcondylar screw cannot be inserted through the plate. However, the reconstruction plate allows contouring of the plate to follow the lateral aspect of the metaphysis proximally onto the humeral shaft (Fig. 8-21, *B*). In addition, it allows placement of the transcondylar screw through the distal hole in the plate, resulting in a very stable reconstruction. A disadvantage of the reconstruction plate is that its strength is less than that of a comparable-size DCP. However, the reconstruction plate is available in 2.7, 3.5, and 4.5 mm sizes. Therefore, if the surgeon is faced with a fracture that requires additional plate strength, he or she should select the next larger size reconstruction plate.

Another technique for stabilizing a T-Y fracture is a transcondylar lag screw combined with two crossed intramedullary pins. However, this fixation may not be as rigid as that obtained with plate techniques. The transcondylar lag screw is inserted through one of the previously described surgical approaches. The two small-diameter pins

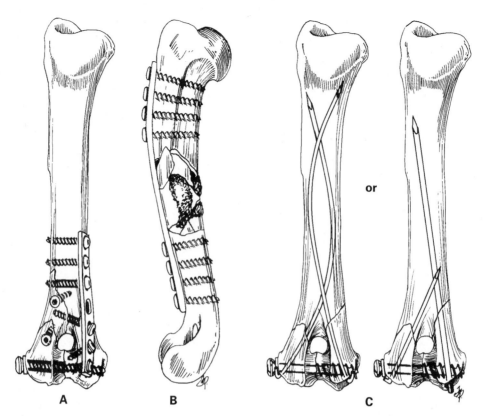

Fig. 8-21 **A,** Intercondylar fractures of the distal humerus (T fracture) may be fixed using a transcondylar lag screw supplemented with a DCP applied to the caudal or lateral aspect of the distal humerus. **B,** Alternately, use of a reconstruction plate, applied to the lateral surface, allows insertion of the transcondylar screw through the distal hole in the plate. **C,** Distal humeral intercondylar fracture may also be stabilized using a transcondylar lag screw in the condylar fragment, which is then stabilized to the humeral shaft with two smooth pins inserted in a Rush pin or cross pin technique.

are inserted retrograde or normograde as described in the section on supracondylar fractures. Once the fracture is anatomically reduced, the pins are advanced to stabilize the supracondylar portion of the fracture (Fig. 8-21, *C*).

After reconstruction and fixation of the fracture, the elbow should be placed through a normal range of motion to make sure metal does not project into the articulating surface or impinge on the olecranon fossa. If the transolecranon approach is used, the olecranon is fixed using a tension-band wire technique.

Any fractures involving the elbow should not be bandaged or supported postoperatively to allow rapid return to full range of motion and avoid the fibrosis that can frequently accompany these types of fractures.

FRACTURES OF THE ULNA
Anatomical Considerations

Although the major weight support of the forelimb is through the radius, substantial articulation with the humerus occurs through the ulna at the trochlear (semi-

lunar) notch. The ulna is one of the longer bones in the body and tapers to a narrow distal styloid process. Proximally, the olecranon is the site of attachment of a major muscle mass, the triceps. The trochlear notch is the major articulating surface with the humeral condyle.

Treatment

Olecranon fractures. Olecranon fractures occur as those involving the nonarticulating surface and those involving the articulating surface. Extraarticular fractures of the olecranon are preferably fixed using a tension-band wire technique. Two Kirschner wires or smooth Steinmann pins are inserted through the proximal caudal aspect of the olecranon into the cranial cortex of the ulna distal to the trochlear notch. A figure-eight wire is applied on the caudal aspect of the fragments, passing over the exposed pins and through a transverse hole in the distal fragment that is 1 to 1.5 cm from the fracture line. The figure-eight wire is tightened to achieve compression of the fracture and functions as a tension band. The wire used should be heavy-gauge wire, 0.8 to 1.2 mm and a twist on either side of the wire is preferable to obtain tightening on both arms of the figure eight (Fig. 8-22).

Articular fractures. Olecranon fractures involving the articular surface may also be fixed using the same technique as for extraarticular fractures. However, a more rigid technique is the use of a bone plate applied to the caudal aspect of the proximal ulna. The plate is contoured to obtain compression across the entire fracture line. At least two and preferably three screws of purchase must be obtained on either side of the fracture line.

Multifragment fractures involving the articular surface and proximal olecranon should be fixed using a bone plate. As with any articular surface, the articular fragments are anatomically aligned and fixed with lag screws or temporarily fixed with Kirschner wires. These wires may later be replaced with lag screws or permanently left in place. A plate is applied along the caudal aspect of the ulna to span the area of fragmentation. Areas of the frac-

ture that cannot be reconstructed or that have bone loss should be filled with cancellous bone, even if this involves an articulating surface. In these cases the graft should be packed well into the defect to restore the previous anatomical shape. Attention must be given to contouring the plate so that the trochlear notch is not closed or opened. A lateral radiograph of the intact opposite ulna can assist in contouring the plate. Closing of the trochlear notch results in impingement on the humeral condyle and subluxation, whereas opening of the trochlear notch results in elbow instability. Both conditions can result in impairment of elbow joint function and degenerative joint disease (Fig. 8-23).

Fractures of the ulnar diaphysis. Fractures of the ulnar shaft are frequently indirectly stabilized once the adjacent fractured radius is fixed.

The ulnar fracture can be stabilized using one of three techniques. A simple transverse or short oblique fracture can be stabilized with a single intermedullary pin inserted normograde or retrograde into the olecranon and driven distally to engage the distal ulna. The diameter of the

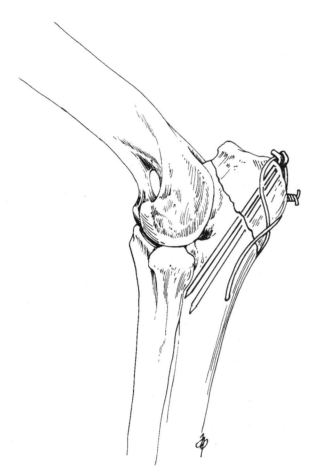

Fig. 8-22 Fracture or osteotomy of the olecranon should be fixed using a tension-band wire technique consisting of two Kirschner wires inserted through the olecranon into the cranial proximal ulna cortex, supplemented with a figure-eight wire placed on the caudal surface of the proximal ulna.

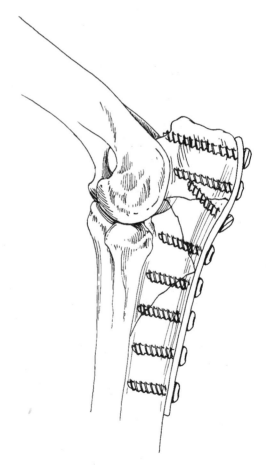

Fig. 8-23 Multifragment fractures of the proximal ulna may be fixed using a bone DCP applied to the caudal aspect of the proximal ulna, supplemented with lag screw fixation.

pin is dictated by the diameter of the distal ulna (Fig. 8-24, *A*). This fixation may be supplemented with a hemicerclage or figure-eight wire tightened on the caudal aspect of the ulna. In a stable ulnar fracture the figure-eight wire may be sufficient (Fig. 8-24, *B*). Long oblique ulnar fractures may be stabilized with two or more cerclage wires with or without an intermedullary pin or with two lag screws alone (Fig. 8-24, *C*).

Multifragment fractures involving the ulna or fractures involving the proximal aspect of the ulnar shaft are preferably stabilized using a bone plate applied to the caudal aspect or caudal lateral aspect of the ulna (Fig. 8-24, *D*).

Fracture/luxation of the ulna and radius. A fracture of the proximal ulna and concurrent luxation of the radial head, frequently referred to as a *Monteggia fracture*, is unique and always necessitates stabilization of the ulna. The radial head may be displaced in any one of four directions: lateral, cranial, medial, or caudal. The annular ligament is usually disrupted.

The treatment of this fracture necessitates reduction of the radial head followed by reduction and fixation of the ulnar fracture with one of the previously described methods. The radial head is then stabilized. If possible, the annular ligament is repaired with primary suture techniques. If a stable reduction can be achieved, no

further fixation is necessary. However, inability to reconstruct the annular ligament necessitates fixation of the radial head to the proximal ulna. This may be achieved preferably using a smooth pin inserted through the radial neck to project through the caudal cortex of the ulna. The pin is allowed to protrude slightly from the caudal ulnar cortex for removal at a later date. The pin is then cut flush with the cranioradial cortex (Fig. 8-25, *A*). Alternately, if a plate is applied to the ulna, the screw closest to the radial head may be inserted as a position screw to engage the radial head, as well as the ulna (both radial cortices must be engaged) (Fig. 8-25, *B*).

In either technique the pin or the screw should be removed at approximately 4 weeks postoperatively. In very immature animals, this should be removed at 2 weeks to avoid compromising ulnar and radial growth.

Distal ulnar fractures. These fractures normally occur with concurrent fractures of the distal radius. Occasionally, these may also occur with luxation of the radial head and even more infrequently occur as isolated fractures. If the fracture of the distal ulna occurs as an isolated injury, it may be treated with coaptation or tension-band wiring.

Fractures of the distal ulna occurring with radial fractures may also require stabilization if moderate instability

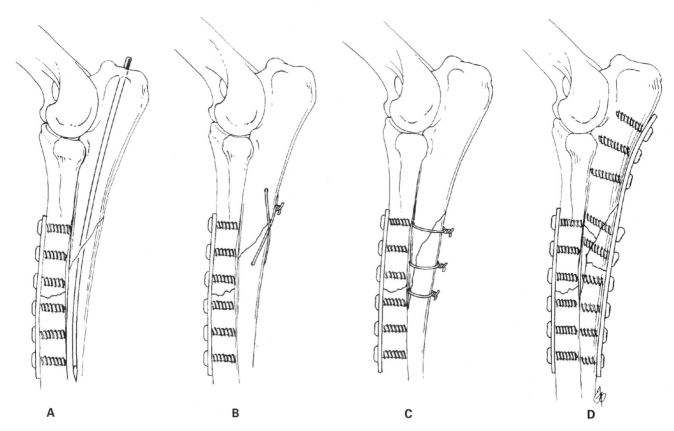

Fig. 8-24 Fractures of the ulnar diaphysis may be fixed with **A,** an intramedullary pin; **B,** figure-eight wire; **C,** cerclage wires; or **D,** a bone plate applied to the caudal aspect of the ulna.

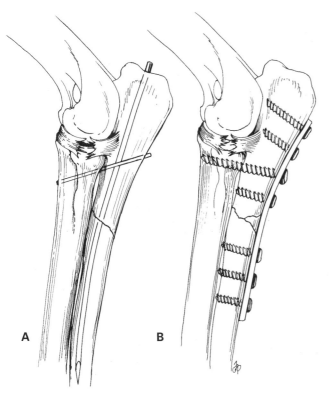

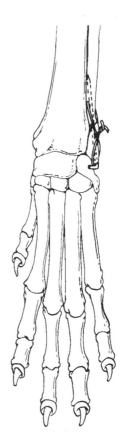

Fig. 8-25   A, Fracture of the proximal ulna and luxation of the radial head (Monteggia fracture) may be fixed with an intramedullary pin in the ulna and a smooth pin inserted through the radial neck and into the proximal ulna. **B,** Alternately, if a bone plate is used to stabilize the ulnar fracture, one lag screw may be inserted through the ulna and into the proximal radius.

Fig. 8-26   Fractures of the distal ulna and styloid process can be fixed using a smooth Kirschner wire and figure-eight tension-band wire.

is present after fixation of the radial fracture. Fixation may be achieved using either a figure-eight wire or an intramedullary Kirschner wire inserted through the ulnar styloid process.

The ulnar styloid is the site of attachment of the ulnar collateral ligament. Therefore, fixation of a fracture in this bony process is important to preserve carpal stability. Avulsion of the ulna styloid process should be fixed using a single Kirschner wire and figure-eight tension-band wire (Fig. 8-26).

FRACTURES OF THE RADIUS
Anatomical Considerations

The radius is the major weight-bearing bone of the forelimb and articulates with both the radial and the ulnar carpal bones distally and the lateral humeral condyle proximally. This, combined with the architecture of the radius, results in a structure into which it is difficult to insert an intramedullary pin properly. However, the cranial cortex provides a surface that is suitable to application of a bone plate. The radius can be approached from three directions: cranial, medial, and lateral. Thus, it lends itself well also to external fixator applications.

Any trauma that results in fracture of the radius and ulna in immature animals carries the risk of subsequent premature closure of one or more of the growth plates (see Chapter 13). The surgeon should inform the owners of this fact and the need to evaluate the animal periodically for any indication of premature physeal closure.

Treatment

Fractures of the radial head. Fractures involving the radial head occur rarely. Articular fractures of the radius should be approached as with any articular fracture, with the goal to restore the joint articular surface integrity. A craniolateral approach allows visualization of the articular surface. The fracture fragments are anatomically positioned and stabilized with Kirschner wires or lag screws. Even in comminuted fractures of the radial head, the surgeon should attempt to preserve the radial head because it is a major weight-bearing surface (Fig. 8-27).

Fractures of the radial neck are seen infrequently and generally in combination with a more comminuted fracture of the radius. Fixation is achieved using a bone plate and obtaining two screws of purchase in the proximal fragment. When the proximal segment is small, special T plates are used to allow placement of two screws in that

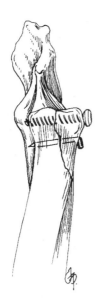

Fig. 8-27 Fractures of the radial head can be fixed with a lag screw and Kirschner wire after the articular surface has been anatomically aligned.

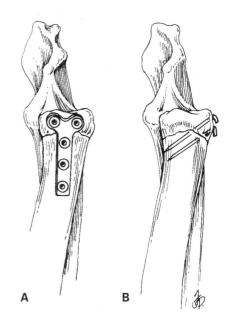

Fig. 8-28 Radial neck fractures may be stabilized using **A,** a small **T** plate (2.0, 2.7, or 3.5 mm), or **B,** two Kirschner wires.

segment (Fig. 8-28, *A*). If the fracture of the radial neck occurs as an isolated fracture, it may be fixed using two or more Kirschner wires inserted from the lateral or craniolateral periarticular area into the distal fragment (Fig. 8-28, *B*).

Radial diaphyseal fractures. Fractures of the shaft of the radius are frequently encountered. These fractures occurring in immature animals with minimum displacement may be treated with coaptation in a long leg cast. The surgeon must be careful not to position the distal limb in rotation, valgus or varus. A simple radial fracture can be stabilized with an external fixator (type I or II) applied either from the lateral, medial, or cranial surface.

Using a very limited approach to the fracture site, the fracture fragments are anatomically aligned and, if possible, fixed with a lag screw or cerclage wire or temporarily fixed with reduction forceps. To apply the external fixator, a half-pin is inserted at the extreme ends of the proximal and distal fragments and a connecting bar applied with two to four additional clamps on the bar. One or two additional half-pins are inserted per fragment. The half-pins are passed through the single clamps on the connecting bar, then into the respective bone fragments, and the clamps are tightened. This results in a series of half-pins that are all fixed to the same connecting bar, resulting in rigid fixation. The half-pins must be inserted carefully to avoid traumatizing the extensor tendons and fixing them to the bone. Application of the device on the medial surface of the radius avoids the soft tissue (Fig. 8-29).

A radial fracture may be fixed using a bone plate contoured to the cranial surface of the radius (Fig. 8-30). The surgeon must evaluate the limb periodically during fixa-

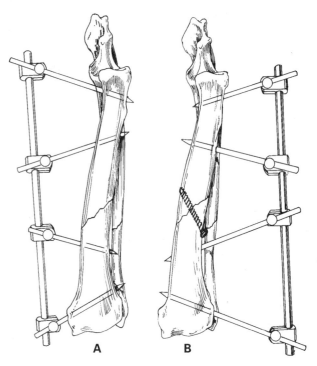

Fig. 8-29 **A,** Simple fractures of the radial shaft can be fixed using a type I external fixator applied to the cranial, medial, or lateral bone surface. At least two pins and preferably three or four pins per fragment should be used in the proximal and distal fragments. **B,** This may be supplemented using a smooth pin or lag screw inserted perpendicular to the fracture line.

tion and at closure to make sure that varus or valgus deviation has not occurred in the limb. This is important in small breeds, in which slight malpositioning of the fragments can result in marked varus or valgus of the lower limb.

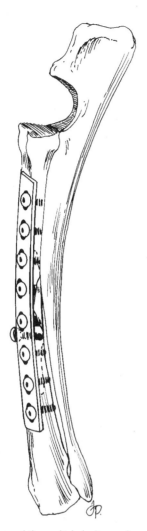

Fig. 8-30 Fractures of the radial shaft may be stabilized using a bone plate contoured to the cranial surface of the radius, supplemented with lag screws through or outside the plate.

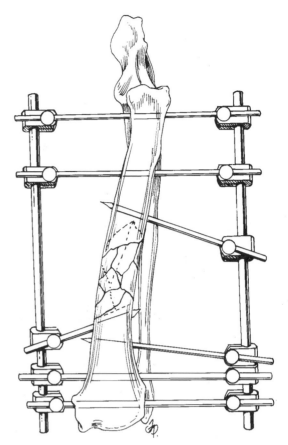

Fig. 8-31 Multifragment fractures of the radial shaft can be treated using a type II external fixator. At least two pins should be inserted in the proximal and distal bone fragments, preferably three or four. Some pins in the type II device should be inserted at either a converging or a diverging angle to avoid lateral or medial migration of the device during fracture healing. Unreconstructable areas of comminution should be filled with autogenous cancellous bone graft.

A transverse or short oblique fracture of the radial diaphysis can be supported by an intramedullary pin inserted in the distal cranial radius. The pin size is dictated by the craniocaudal dimension of the medullary canal. The point of insertion is lateral to the common digital extensor tendon. The surgeon must be cautious that the fracture is not forced into malalignment during pin insertion. The distal end of the pin is bent into a curve or cut short in order not to impinge on the radial carpal bone during extension.

Multifragment fractures involving the radius and the ulna may be fixed with either a bone plate or a type II external fixator. If a type II fixator is used, a full pin is inserted through the proximal and distal fragments closest to the articular surface. The radius and ulna are then placed in anatomical alignment, and an assistant applies medial and lateral connecting bars that contain two to four additional fixation clamps on each bar. The additional pins are inserted through the single clamps already on the connecting bars through the specific bone frag-

ment and into the single clamp on the opposite connecting bar. Some of the additional pins may be inserted as half-pins. A minimum of two and preferably three pins per fragment are necessary. At least one or two pins per fragment should be inserted in a converging or diverging pattern of 30 to 45 degrees to the long axis of the bone to counteract pin migration. With all clamps securely tightened, alignment is evaluated before closure (Fig. 8-31). In giant breeds a type III frame configuration may be necessary (see Chapter 5).

Fractures of the distal radius

Fractures of the metaphysis. Distal metaphyseal fractures of the radius and ulna are some of the most frequently encountered fractures of the front limb. In immature dogs, but not in cats, these fractures carry a high incidence of premature physeal closure, particularly of the distal ulnar physis. Although these radial fractures may be fixed with an external fixator, a preferred method of fixation is use of a bone plate. In most breeds, when using a narrow DCP, at least two screws can obtain purchase in the distal fragment. In small breeds, however, especially the toy breeds, it can be quite problematic to insert two screws into the small, short distal fragment. However, use of a T plate or mini T plate allows insertion of two screws distally in the horizontal plane. Careful attention must be given to the alignment of the fracture fragment, since a small amount of displacement of the distal fragment can result in noticeable varus or valgus deviation of the carpus (Fig. 8-32).

In small breeds, multifragment fractures that result in a small distal radial fragment may also be fixed with an external fixator using Kirschner wires and acrylic cement. Distally, two or more wires are inserted transversely in a lateral-to-medial direction parallel to the radial articular surface. Likewise, two or three wires are inserted proximally, with at least one wire adjacent to the radial head. The exposed portion of the pins may then be incorporated in acrylic bars on the medial and lateral aspects. This forms a type II fixator for the small radius (Fig. 8-33).

Articular fractures. Articular fractures of the distal radius occur infrequently, generally with extension of the fracture line into either the medial cortex or the cranial cortex. The fracture fragments are anatomically aligned with the distal radial articular surface visualized to ensure anatomical reconstruction. The fragments are fixed with Kirschner wires and at least one lag screw when possible. A slab fracture of the distal cranial radius may be fixed with two lag screws or supported with a buttress plate (T plate) (Fig. 8-34, *A* and *C*).

Avulsion of the radial styloid. The radial styloid is the site of attachment of the radial collateral ligament. Avulsion of this process results in medial instability of the carpus. Therefore, fixation is paramount to reestablishing carpal stability.

If the styloid process is of sufficient size, it may be fixed with a lag screw and spike washer. Alternately, it may be fixed with a Kirschner wire inserted through the fragment into the distal radius and supplemented with a figure-eight wire as a tension band (Fig. 8-34, *B*). If minimal osseous

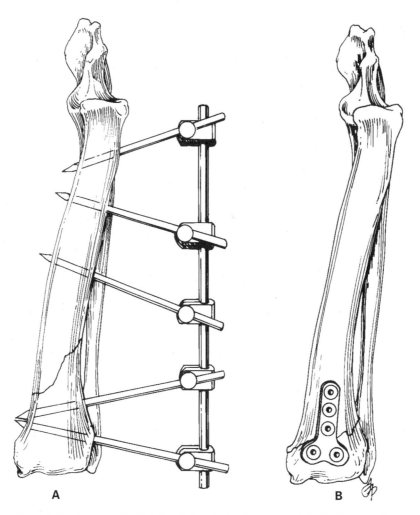

A **B**

Fig. 8-32 **A,** Fractures of the distal radial metaphysis may be stabilized using a bone plate or external fixator. **B,** If the distal fragment is very short, a **T** plate (2.0, 2.7, or 3.5 mm) allows the horizontal insertion of two screws in the distal fragment.

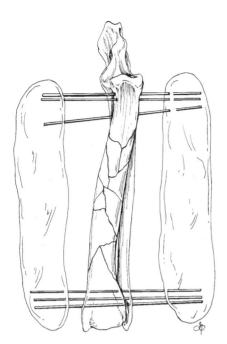

Fig. 8-33 Multifragment fractures of the distal radius, particularly in small breeds, can be stabilized using an external fixator developed by using smooth Kirschner wires incorporated in medial and lateral acrylic cement bars. The distal pins are inserted in close proximity, and even in extremely small breeds, two or three pins of purchase can be obtained in a small distal radial fragment.

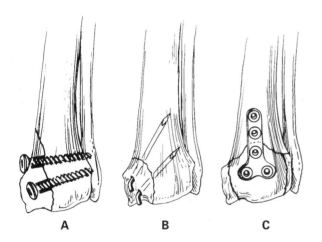

Fig. 8-34 **A,** Articular fractures of the distal radius are fixed using a lag screw supplemented with an additional lag screw or smooth pin. **B,** If the fragment is too small for a lag screw, one or two Kirschner wires should be used, supplemented with a figure-eight wire. **C,** Slab fracture through the cranial aspect of the distal radius may be fixed with lag screws or a T plate as a buttress plate.

tissue is present, the ligament may be reattached by using moderate-gauge stainless steel wire or monofilament suture in a Bunnell pattern in the ligament and passing the wire or suture through a drill hole placed in the remaining distal radial styloid.

FRACTURES OF THE CARPUS

Fractures involving the bones of the carpus occur infrequently in most pet animals. They are seen more often in working animals, such as sled dogs and particularly racing greyhounds. These fractures are generally created by compression and shear forces and do not heal unless they are rigidly stabilized to counteract those forces. Using a cast or splint on fractures of these bones does not usually lead to healing. Several factors combine to result in the poor healing that is seen without rigid fixation. The joint is a major load-bearing surface, and thus the bones of the carpus move frequently during weight bearing. The blood supply to these bones is relatively poor compared with that of the long bones. In addition, fracture surfaces are constantly bathed in synovial fluid. Many ligaments attach to the bones of the carpus and pull on a fracture fragment when the limb is loaded during weight bearing. None of these factors is conducive to bone healing. Unless they are rigidly stabilized, the bone and the cartilage fragments become free bodies that can cause significant degenerative joint disease.

Fractures of the carpal bones rarely occur as an isolated injury and typically involve more than one structure in the carpus. Most frequently, fractures involving these bones occur in either the radial carpal bone or the accessory carpal bone. Fractures of the numbered carpal bones and the ulnar carpal bone occur infrequently. If the fractures of these bones are small chips that cannot be stabilized, they should be removed. If the fragments are large enough, a lag screw or small Kirschner wires can be used to stabilize the fragments (Fig. 8-35). If possible, at least two points of fixation should be provided in each fragment. When Kirschner wires are used and their position could damage the adjacent articular surface, the wires should be countersunk below the articular surface. Because of the size of these fractures, the implants used are relatively small. Thus, this is one instance when the rule about not combining internal and external fixation is broken. After surgical stabilization, the carpus is placed in a short leg cast or a splint for 3 to 4 weeks. It may take 8 to 12 weeks for these fractures to heal completely. With severe fractures, the surgeon may consider primary arthrodesis of the joint.

Avulsion of the ulnar or radial collateral ligaments from the respective carpal bones may be reattached using stainless steel wire in a figure-eight pattern in the ligament and through a drill hole in the respective ulnar or radial bone. If the ligament is severely damaged, as in a shearing injury, it may be reconstructed using a figure-eight wire with position screws as anchors for the wire. For example, loss of the medial collateral ligament is treated by a screw in the medial distal radius and in the medial aspect of the radial carpal bone. A figure-eight wire (0.8 to 1.0 mm) is passed around the screws and tightened. Finding the center of the motion on the distal

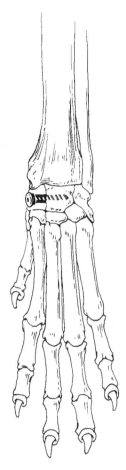

Fig. 8-35 Fracture of the radial carpal bone should be fixed with a small lag screw (2.0 or 2.7 mm), which can be recessed below the articular surface if necessary.

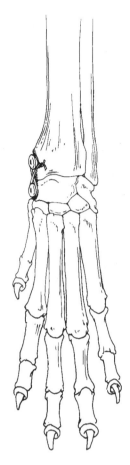

Fig. 8-36 Fractures resulting in severe ligament damage or total loss of the medial collateral ligament may be repaired using a screw in the distal radius and a screw in the radial carpal bone, which are connected by a figure-eight wire. Note that the point of insertion of the distal radial screw is critical to maintaining a maximum range of motion to the carpus. A wire may be placed around the screw in the radial carpal bone, and the optimum site for placement of the radial screw is determined by placing the carpus through a range of motion while holding the free end of the wire over the proposed point of screw insertion.

medial radius is important to maintain stability at flexion and extension (Fig. 8-36). Carpal injuries should be protected, with the carpus in a padded splint and slight flexion for 4 weeks.

FRACTURES OF THE METACARPALS AND PHALANGES

Fractures of the metacarpals occur frequently. If only one or two of the bones are fractured and relatively nondisplaced, a cast or splint can often be used successfully. The nonfractured metacarpals act as an internal splint. If coaptation is used, the splint or cast must extend from the level at the third and fourth digits to just below the elbow. Even if internal fixation is used, additional support in a splint for 3 to 4 weeks is advocated.

Fractures involving three or more metacarpals are preferably treated with internal fixation, particularly the more load-bearing third and fourth metacarpals. Intramedullary pins can be used to fix these fractures; the metacarpal-phalangeal joint is flexed and the pin inserted in the anterior distal metacarpal just above the articular surface. The pins are driven antegrade into the base of the metacarpal, avoiding perforation of the articular surface. The cut ends of the pins are bent over to avoid impairment of metacarpal-phalangeal joint function and to aid in removal after fracture healing. Oblique fractures may be stabilized by one or more lag screws. If the metacarpals are of sufficient size (medium and large breeds), small bone plates (2.0 to 2.7 mm) can be used to stabilize the fractures. Splint or coaptation support may be useful during the 3 to 4 weeks after surgery (Fig. 8-37, *A*).

Articular fractures occurring at the base or head of the metacarpals should be fixed using a single lag screw, a lag screw combined with a Kirschner pin, or two crossed Kirschner pins. If the fracture involves the attachment of

Fractures of P-1 are amenable to miniplate fixation only in large breeds. Generally, fractures of P-1 and P-2 involve the base or the head. These are interarticular fractures and may be fixed with lag screws or converging small Kirschner wires in medium-sized and large breeds. Fractures of P-3 are best treated with excision.

SUGGESTED READINGS

Bardet JF, Hohn RB, Olmstead ML: Fractures of the humerus in dogs and cats: a retrospective study of 130 cases, *Vet Surg* 12:73-77, 1983.

Berzon JL: Orthopedics of the forelimb—humeral fractures. In Slatter DH, editor: *Small animal surgery* vol II, Philadelphia, 1985, Saunders.

Bloomberg MS: Fractures of the radius and ulna. In Bojrab MJ, editor: *Current techniques in small animal surgery*, ed 2, Philadelphia, 1983, Lea & Febiger.

Brinker WO: Fractures. In Archibald J, editor: *Canine surgery*, ed 2, Santa Barbara, Calif, 1974, American Veterinary Publications.

Brinker WO, Hohn RB, Prieur WD: *Manual of internal fixation in small animals*, New York, 1984, Springer-Verlag.

Brinker WO, Piermattei DL, Flo GL: *Handbook of small animal orthopedics and fracture treatment*, ed 2, Philadelphia, 1990, Saunders.

Egger EL: Orthopedics of the forelimb radius and ulna. In Slatter DH, editor: *Small animal surgery*, vol II, Philadelphia, 1985, Saunders.

Jackson DH: Fractures of the humerus. In Bojrab MJ, editor: *Current techniques in small animal surgery*, ed 2, Philadelphia, 1983, Lea & Febiger.

Matthiesson DT: Fractures of the humerus, *Vet Clin North Am* 22(1):121-135, 1992.

Matthiesson DT, Walter M: Surgical management of distal humeral fractures, *Compend Cont Educ* 6:1027-1036, 1984.

Moore RW: Orthopedics of the forelimb—carpus and digits. In Slatter DH, editor: *Small animal surgery* vol II, Philadelphia, 1985, Saunders

Newton CD, Nunamaker DM: Fractures and dislocations. In Newton CD, Nunamaker DM, editors: *Textbook of small animal orthopedics*, Philadelphia, 1985, Lippincott.

Parker RB: Orthopedics of the forelimb-scapula. In Slatter DH, editor: *Small animal surgery*, vol II, Philadelphia, 1985, Saunders.

Piermattei DL, Greely RG: *An atlas of surgical approaches to the bones of the dog and cat*, ed 2, Philadelphia, 1980, Saunders.

Rudd RG, Whitehair JG: Fractures of the radius and ulna, *Vet Clin North Am* 22(1):135-149, 1992.

Ryan WW: Fractures of the scapula. In Bojrab MJ, editor: *Current techniques in small animal surgery*, ed 2, Philadelphia, 1983, Lea & Febiger.

Schwartz PD, Schrader SC: Ulnar fracture and dislocation of the proximal medial epiphysis (Monteggia lesion) in the dog and cat: a review of 28 cases, *J Am Vet Med Assoc* 185:190-194, 1984.

Turner TM, Hohn RB: Craniolateral approach to the canine elbow for repair of condylar fractures or joint exploration, *J Am Vet Med Assoc* 176:1264-1266, 1980.

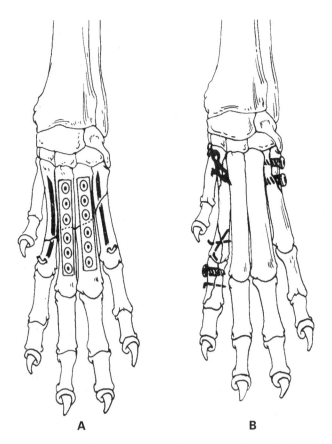

Fig. 8-37 A, Shaft fractures of the metacarpals or phalanges may be fixed using intramedullary pins, small DCPs or cuttable plates. **B,** Articular fractures involving the base or head of the metacarpals or phalanges may be stabilized using a lag screw and smooth Kirschner pin, two crossed Kirschner pins, or a tension-band wire using a smooth pin and figure-eight wire.

a ligament, as at the base of the second or fifth metacarpal, it is best to use the tension-band principle to secure the fragment and ligament. This can be accomplished with one or two pins and figure-eight wire or in large breeds a tension-band plate.

Severe trauma can result in compromised circulation to the paw. The surgeon should use a minimally invasive fixation technique to avoid further insult to the vascular supply. If marked swelling occurs, superficial fasciotomy incisions may aid in reducing pressure within the metacarpal area.

Fractures of phalanges, specifically P-1 and P-2, are generally treated with coaptation support for 6 weeks.

9

Fractures of the Bones of the Hind Limb

MARVIN L. OLMSTEAD

To treat fractures of the bones of the hind limbs successfully, the veterinary orthopedic surgeon must have a thorough understanding of principles of fracture repair (see Chapters 4 and 5) and be able to apply those principles to a given situation. Each fracture should be approached with a sound preoperative plan. However, the surgeon must have the versatility to change that plan if circumstances indicate the original plan will give the patient a less-than-optimal chance of having a normally healed bone and as normal limb function as possible. For each fracture, more than one method of fixation exists that gives a satisfactory result after an adequate convalescent period.

PELVIC FRACTURES

Pelvic fractures can present veterinary surgeons with some of their greatest challenges. Because 20% to 30% of all fractures in dogs and cats involve the pelvis, the surgeon must be able to select satisfactory treatment options for many different fractures. The choices range from nonsurgical patient management to total surgical reconstruction of the fractured bones. The final decision on a treatment plan depends on the severity of fragment displacement, the location of the fracture, and the degree of pelvic canal compromise.

Since almost all these fractures are caused by trauma associated with motor vehicle accidents, the loads creating a pelvic fracture can come from many different angles and have a wide range of magnitudes. Thus, pelvic fractures have varied configurations (Fig. 9-1). It is virtually impossible to have a single fracture in the pelvis because of its boxlike configuration. An animal hit directly from behind may have shear fractures in both iliac wings or bilateral sacroiliac luxations. A side blow may drive the head of the femur into the acetabulum, creating fractures in the acetabulum, ilium, and pelvic floor with medial displacement of the fragments.

Nonsurgical Versus Surgical Treatment

The decision to treat fractures nonsurgically or surgically is based on factors relating to the fracture, the effect of malpositioned fragments on the patient, and the patient's comfort. Nondisplaced, stable, fractures that are not painful and do not affect a vital structure or body function may be treated with cage rest. Any fracture appearing nondisplaced on initial radiographs should be reradiographed the next day. Often the fragments have moved, and the treatment plan should be reevaluated. A nonsur-

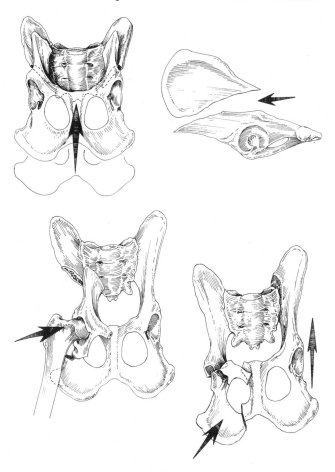

Fig. 9-1 Fractures of the pelvis vary depending on the direction of the force creating the fracture. Since most fractures are associated with motor vehicle–related trauma, impacts often occur from the rear or side and impart high energy to the bones.

gically treated patient often requires extensive nursing care, including physical therapy. A prolonged recovery period beyond that for the surgically treated patient is expected. The objectives of surgical treatment of pelvic fractures are to reestablish load transmission between the limb and the spine, recreate the pelvic canal, reestablish the acetabulum's articular surface, and shorten patient convalescent time.

Generally, fractures of the pubis and ischium do not need surgical repair. These bones support surrounding structures and do not directly transmit loads during weight bearing. They are surrounded by muscles that hold bone fragments in relative position. The pubis and ischium are seldom displaced in a manner that compromises any vital structures. However, marked ischial fragment rotation or displacement caused by muscle pull and wide separation of pubic fragments with an unstable pelvic floor may need surgical stabilization with wire and pins.

Ilial and acetabular fractures are best treated surgically. The ilium is often displaced medially in a manner compromising the pelvic canal and/or endangering the sciatic nerve or other structures in the pelvic canal. The ilium is also important in transmitting loads between the hind limb and the spine during weight bearing. Repair of these fractures also decreases pain and patient convalescent time. The patient will return to locomotor function much more quickly if these fractures are stabilized. Nonsurgical treatment should be considered only in patients with minimal fragment displacement that are already walking.

The acetabulum contains one of the articular surfaces of the coxofemoral joint. To maintain joint integrity, the acetabulum should be reconstructed if the joint's weight-bearing surface is involved. The cranial two thirds is accepted as the weight-bearing surface. Repair of fractures in the caudal one third of the joint is controversial. Although unrepaired fractures in this area result in coxofemoral osteoarthritis, it has not been definitively proven that repairing such fractures improves the patient's recovery. Fractures of the caudal one third of the acetabulum are often difficult to stabilize adequately, and the sciatic nerve is at risk of injury while the surgeon works in this area.

Sacroiliac luxations/fractures are treated surgically if they are very unstable, greatly displaced, or painful. A minimally displaced sacroiliac luxation adequately stabilizes with fibrous tissues after 2 or 3 weeks of cage rest.

Clinical Signs and Diagnosis

Dogs and cats with pelvic fractures generally have a history of an acute onset of lameness, usually non-weight bearing, in the affected limb(s). In some animals the lameness is mild even though the fracture appears to be moderate to severe on radiographs. After a general physical examination to establish the patient's current health status, a complete orthopedic examination should be performed. Whenever a pelvic fracture is suspected, careful digital rectal palpation of the pelvic canal is indicated. This should be performed as an isolated examination and with passive range of motion manipulations of the cox-ofemoral joint. The degree of canal narrowing and the location of fractures and bone fragments should be assessed throughout the canal's circumference.

Sacroiliac luxations and iliac fractures may be palpated externally as unstable bone segments or may disrupt normal hindquarter anatomic relationships. If an acetab-ular fracture is present, the normal spatial relationship between the ischium and the greater trochanter often is disrupted. The femoral head may have been driven into the acetabulum, displacing the trochanter medially, or if a concomitant iliac shaft fracture exists, the trochanter may be cranially displaced. A pain response is sometimes elicited by passive manipulation of a fractured coxofem-oral joint. However, lack of a pain response does not eliminate the possibility of an acetabular fracture.

Definitive diagnosis is established through radiographs of the pelvis. The two standard radiographic views of the pelvis for evaluating fractures are the ventrodorsal and lateral. Sometimes, an oblique view of the hemipelvis is necessary for better definition of fracture lines and fragment position. The oblique view is especially helpful when assessing acetabular fractures.

Surgical Techniques

Surgical treatment of ilial and acetabular fractures and sacroiliac luxations/fractures involves three steps: (1) exposure of the fracture site, (2) reduction of the fracture, and (3) fracture stabilization. The specific technique used for each step depends on the fracture's location and severity.

Exposure of the fracture site. To expose sacroiliac luxations, I prefer a dorsal midline approach. The animal is positioned on its sternum, and the hind limbs straddle sandbags or a positioning pad for this repair (Fig. 9-2). Such positioning usually makes manipulation and visual-ization of the bone fragments easier. The dorsal back mus-cles are reflected laterally off the spinous processes of the sixth and seventh lumbar vertebrae. The sacrum's lateral surface is exposed and the displaced ilium's dorsal aspect identified.

Ilial and acetabular fractures are more frequently treated surgically than sacroiliac luxations. The standard

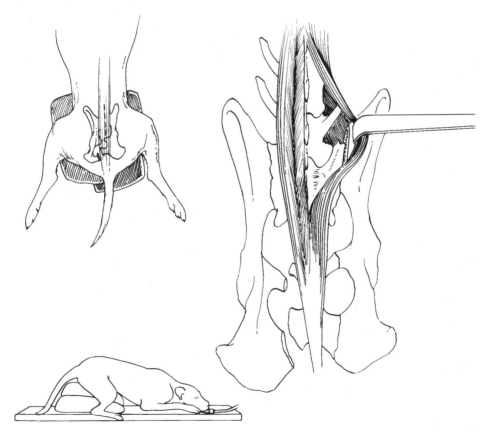

Fig. 9-2   Patients are positioned so that they straddle sandbags for surgical repair of sacroil-iac luxation/fracture. A dorsal midline approach is used to expose the area of trauma.

lateral approach works well for ilial fractures. The gluteal muscles' ventral margin is isolated, and the muscles are elevated from the ilial face to the extent that allows fracture repair. Acetabular fractures are approached either by a trochanteric osteotomy or by a caudal approach, which are described below. In most cases, I prefer the caudal approach to the classical trochanteric osteotomy. The caudal approach provides exposure of the acetabulum equal to that from the trochanteric osteotomy, does not require creation of a fracture site in the femur, and is more quickly closed than a trochanteric osteotomy.

Trochanteric osteotomy. Exposure of the acetabulum via a trochanteric osteotomy is achieved by isolating the superficial gluteal muscle, incising its insertion, and reflecting it dorsally. Next, an osteotomy of the greater trochanter is performed, starting at the level of the third trochanter and extending dorsally to the junction of the greater trochanter and the femoral neck (Fig. 9-3). The middle and deep gluteal muscles that remain attached to the greater trochanter are reflected dorsally. The deep gluteal and gemellus muscles over the acetabulum's dor-sal rim are elevated with a periosteal elevator, exposing the fracture site. The sciatic nerve must be protected.

After fracture repair, the greater trochanter is reattached to the proximal femur with a tension-band technique. The remaining layers are closed in a routine manner. I only use the trochanteric osteotomy when wide exposure of the cranial pelvis is needed for fracture repair, as when the ilial shaft and the acetabulum are both fractured on the same side.

Caudal approach. In the caudal approach the sciatic nerve should be identified and protected during the procedure. A tenotomy of the superficial gluteal muscle is performed at its insertion point on the third trochanter. The muscle is tagged with suture and retracted dorsally. The internal obturator and gemellus muscles are incised close to their insertion in the trochanteric fossa. These muscles are tagged and retracted caudodorsally, providing exposure to the caudal acetabulum and protection for the sciatic nerve.

The deep gluteal and gemellus muscles are elevated until the entire dorsal rim of the acetabulum is exposed.

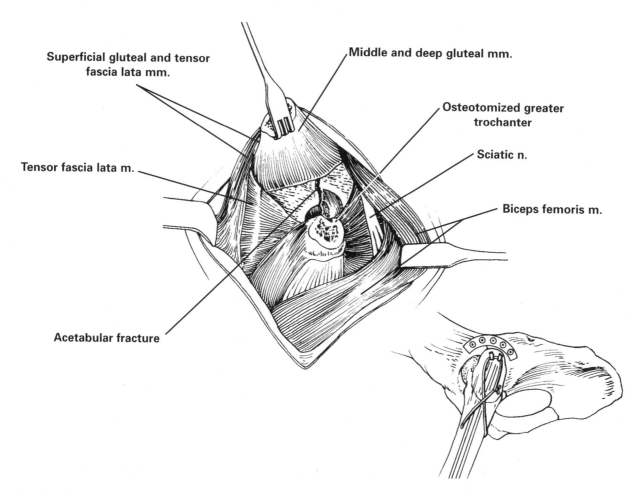

Superficial gluteal and tensor fascia lata mm.

Middle and deep gluteal mm.

Osteotomized greater trochanter

Sciatic n.

Tensor fascia lata m.

Biceps femoris m.

Acetabular fracture

Fig. 9-3   Trochanteric osteotomy is used to expose fractures of the acetabulum. The sciatic nerve should be identified and isolated before the osteotomy is preformed. After repair of the acetabulum, the trochanter is reattached with two pins and a tension-band wire.

The ilium's caudal aspect can be exposed by inserting the tip of a Hohmann retractor just ventral to the acetabulum's cranial border under the middle and the deep gluteal muscles. The retractor displaces these muscles distally. Maintaining the hip in an extended and internally rotated position provides maximum exposure to the acetabular rim (Fig. 9-4).

After the fracture is repaired, the internal obturator and gemellus muscles are sutured to fascial tissue near their original insertion point. The remaining tissues are closed normally.

Fracture reduction

Sacroiliac luxations/fractures. When using a lag screw for stabilization, fixation and reduction of the ilium to the sacrum can be accomplished simultaneously. Before the ilial segment is reduced, a thread hole is drilled in the sacral body. The sacrum's lateral surface is exposed by placing the tip of a Hohmann retractor under the sacrum's ventral point. The retractor is used to displace the ilial wing ventrally. The thread hole in the sacrum should be placed in the center of the exposed sacral surface to ensure that the screw is placed in the maximum available bone. A slight ventral angulation of the thread hole's position keeps the screw in the bone and out of the neural canal (Fig. 9-5). Positioning the thread hole away from the sacrum's center may place the screw in a thin part of the bone or in the sacrum's neural canal.

The middle gluteal muscle is reflected off its origin and the lateral iliac face at the caudodorsal iliac spine. The sacral

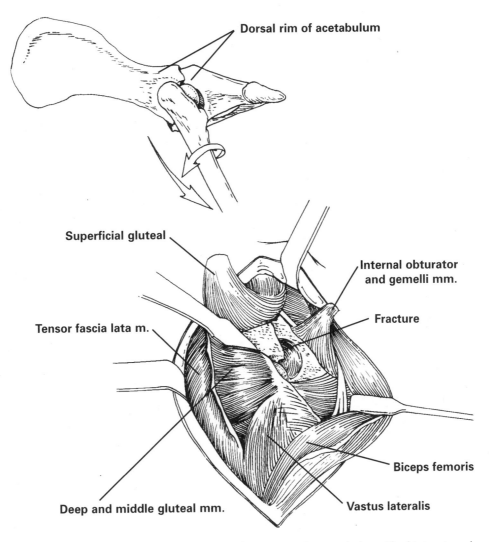

Dorsal rim of acetabulum

Superficial gluteal

Internal obturator and gemelli mm.

Tensor fascia lata m.

Fracture

Deep and middle gluteal mm.

Biceps femoris

Vastus lateralis

Fig. 9-4   Caudal approach to the hip is used to expose the acetabulum. The hip's external rotators are incised at their insertion in the trochanteric fossa. These muscles are retracted caudally to help protect the sciatic nerve. Extension and internal rotation of the femur enhance the exposure. A Hohmann retractor placed under the middle and deep gluteal muscles and hooked on the ilium's ventral edge is used to pull these muscles ventrally.

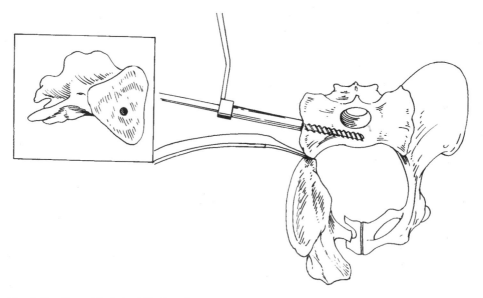

Fig. 9-5   Thread hole is drilled in the sacrum just ventral to the neural canal. The face of the sacrum is exposed by levering the ilium ventrally. The hole is started in the center of the sacrum and angled slightly ventrally.

articulation on the medial iliac surface is identified visually or with palpation. A glide hole is drilled from lateral to medial in the center of the ilium's sacral articulation. The ilium is reduced by grasping the dorsal iliac spine with a bone reduction forceps, such as a Kern bone clamp, and manipulating the ilium into near-anatomical position. The appropriate-sized screw is inserted through the glide hole. The screw is manipulated into position until its tip is in the thread hole. Tightening the screw reduces the luxation (Fig. 9-6). If the sacrum is large enough, a second lag screw or intramedullary pin is sometimes inserted into the sacrum.

Another technique used to reduce the ilium is to position a pointed reduction forceps with one point in the caudal sacrum and one point in the lateral ilial surface and then tighten the clamp. This technique is used when fixation techniques other than the one just described are used. The fully tightened clamp holds the ilium in place while the chosen fixation technique is performed.

Reduction of ilial and acetabular fractures. Fractures involving the ilium and the acetabulum are considered together because they often accompany each other and because the reduction techniques used on one often work for the other. Although reduction of the ilium does not need to be perfect, the acetabulum, because it is a joint surface, must be anatomically reduced if successful repair is to be achieved.

Fragment reduction can be the most difficult part of the surgery. Often the free segment of the pelvis is displaced cranially and/or medially. The fragment should be lateralized first and, if necessary, moved caudally. If the

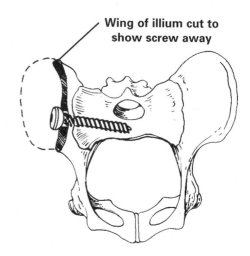

Wing of illium cut to show screw away

Fig. 9-6   Glide hole has been drilled through the ilium. Digital palpation of the articular surface on the medial ilial wall helps guide the position of glide hole. The screw is pushed partially through the glide hole before the luxation is reduced so that the screw's engagement with the thread hole in the sacrum can be visualized. Fully tightening the screw reduces the luxation.

fracture segments are collapsed medially, either a Lahey retractor or a Kern bone forceps is helpful in repositioning the fragments laterally. A Lahey retractor, which is blunt, strong, and bent 90 degrees, is passed along the medial wall of the free segment. The retractor's tip is kept on the bone as it is passed along the medial wall to avoid compromising the sciatic nerve. Pulling laterally with the retractor's handle moves the fracture segments laterally (Fig. 9-7).

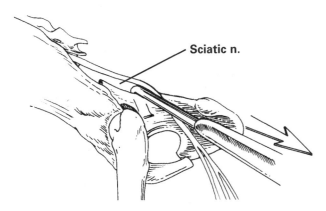

Fig. 9-7 Medially displaced fragments of a fractured pelvis can be moved laterally by placing the blunt blade of a Lahey retractor along the fragment's medial wall and pulling laterally.

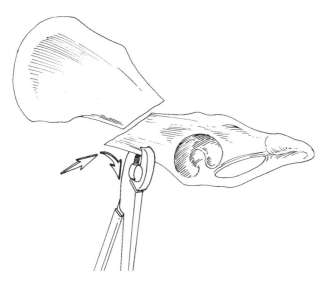

Fig. 9-8 Free ilial segments can be manipulated into position with a Kern bone clamp. The clamp's configuration provides four points of fixation in the fragment. This allows the segment to be pulled and rotated into proper alignment.

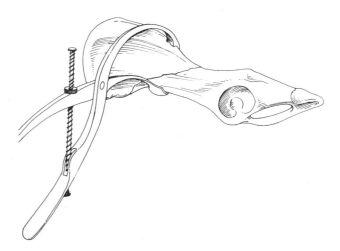

Fig. 9-9 Self-centering clamp can be used to reduce free ilial segments. One blade of the clamp is placed on the dorsal rim of the ilial segment that is still fixed to the sacrum. The other blade is placed on the ventral rim of the free ilial segment. Closing the clamp brings the free segment to the fixed segment. Adjustments in alignment can be done by using the self-centering clamp and the Kern clamp together. Reduction is maintained with the self-centering clamp, with a bone plate applied across the fracture line.

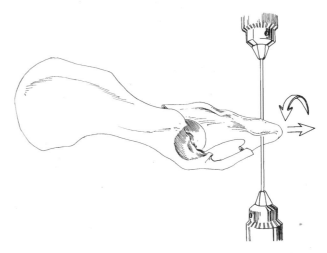

Fig. 9-10 Intramedullary pin driven through the ischium ventrally to dorsally can be used to apply caudal traction to a free pelvic segment. Flexing the hip while driving the pin moves the hamstring muscles out of the way.

If the fragment is large enough, the Kern forceps can be clamped along the ventral edge of the free ilial shaft, allowing the fragment to be manipulated (Fig. 9-8). If an ilial segment is cranially displaced, a self-centering reduction clamp can be placed with one part of the clamp on the secure cranial fragment and one part on the free caudal fragment. Closing this clamp will move the free fragment caudally (Fig. 9-9).

If the caudal fracture line is through the acetabulum and the bone segment is displaced cranially, it can be brought into a more caudal position by two different methods. These methods are also used to provide traction on an ilial fragment that is difficult to move when the acetabulum is not fractured.

In the first method, an intramedullary pin is driven with a pin chuck through the ischium just cranial to the ischial rim from a ventral-to-dorsal orientation. During this procedure the hip joint should be flexed. The pin should penetrate the skin on either side of the ischium. If a second pin chuck is attached to the portion of the pin exposed dorsally, the two pin chucks can be used as handles to pull the fracture segment caudally (Fig. 9-10). Some rotation of the segment can also be provided with this method.

The second method for providing caudal traction involves using a large Kern bone-holding forceps. An incision wide enough to allow insertion of the end of the Kern bone-holding forceps is made parallel with the ischial rim. Because the teeth of the Kern forceps provide four points of fixation, this instrument can be used for both caudal retraction and rotation of the segment (Fig. 9-11). Large Kern forceps are used in most midsized and all large dogs because small Kern forceps do not have a long enough lever arm to manipulate the fracture segment easily.

Reduction of the ilial fracture can almost always be maintained temporarily by positioning self-centering or Kern bone clamps dorsal to ventral across the fracture segments. Acetabular fracture reduction is maintained with pointed reduction bone forceps or by manually holding the fragments in place until the permanent stabilization procedure is completed. Reduction of an acetabular surface can be checked by placing ventral traction on the greater trochanter. This pulls the femoral head out of the acetabulum enough so that the acetabulum's articular rim can be observed through an incision in the joint capsule or an existing tear.

Fracture stabilization

Sacroiliac luxations/fractures. Primary fixation of sacroiliac luxations/fractures involves providing stability to the sacroiliac joint with the use of either a lag screw through the ilium into the sacrum, as already described (see Fracture reduction—Sacroiliac luxations/fractures) or a transilial pin(s). Positioning the animal and approaching the area as described earlier (see Exposure of the fracture site) allows good visualization of the surgical site and easy application of transilial pins.

The luxation pin is inserted. The pin selected for fixation should be easily bent and no larger than 1/8 inch in diameter. The transilial pin is inserted lateral to medial through the ilium on the side of the injury. The pin should pass dorsal to the seventh lumbar vertebra level with the base of the dorsal spinous process. It can pass either through the base of the dorsal spinous process or just caudal to the process. Once the pin is past the dorsal

spinous process, the hand chuck driving the pin is elevated, which lowers the pin's point. The pin is driven medial to lateral through the opposite ilium and the middle gluteal muscle until just enough of its point is exposed to be grasped. The pin should not penetrate the skin. The pin is bent dorsally as it is advanced. When the pin is advanced far enough, it is bent 90 degrees and is cut off, leaving a bend at the end. The pin is pulled back until the bend is buried in the gluteal muscle over the ilium opposite the injured side. The pin on the injured side is bent dorsally and cut off. The pin now has hooks on both ends and thus will not migrate (Fig. 9-12). If desired, a second transilial pin can be inserted in the same manner.

If the sacroiliac luxation/fracture is accompanied by an ilial fracture on the opposite side, the ilial fracture should be stabilized first, since this alone may result in reduction and adequate stability of the sacroiliac joint because of the box configuration of the pelvis.

Ilial shaft fractures. After the fractured ilium has been reduced as described above, the most effective method of maintaining stabilization during fracture healing is bone plating. Several types of plates developed by the the AO/ASIF group (see Chapter 5) can be used, depending on the animal's size and the degree of the fracture's comminution. For ilial fractures, minifragment T or L plates or standard Dynamic Compression Plates (DCPs), which accept 3.5, 2.7, or 2.0 mm screws, are available. The fragments' size governs the size of the implant used.

For ilial shaft fractures, the plates must be contoured to the concave shape of the ilium's lateral surface. If possible,

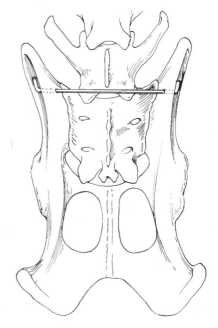

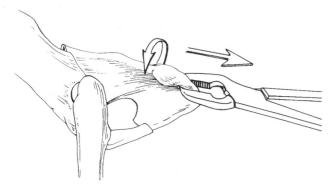

Fig. 9-11 Kern bone-holding forceps applied to ischium through an incision over the tuber ischia allows the free segment to be rotated and retracted caudally.

Fig. 9-12 Transilial pin is inserted through the wing of each ilium and dorsal to the seventh lumbar vertebra (L7). Both ends of the pin are bent to prevent its migration.

at least three screws should be placed in each fracture segment. If the screws are placed in the free fragment first, the plate will aid in reduction of the fracture when the screws are tightened in the cranial segment (Fig. 9-13). If the fracture is reduced and minimal collapse is present, the screws immediately on either side of the fracture line are placed first. The remaining screws are inserted alternately on either side of the fracture from closest to farthest from the fracture line.

An ilial fracture may be accompanied by an acetabular fracture. In such cases, I prefer to repair the ilial shaft before the acetabular fracture. Repair of the ilium is often done with a stronger system than is used on the acetabulum because generally, more screws and a longer and stronger plate can be applied. The reconstruction of the ilium does not have to be as anatomically exact as reconstruction of the acetabulum. When the acetabulum is repaired last, it is fixed to a solidly stabilized ilial segment. Also, its fixation is not subjected to additional loads that would be generated during manipulation of the ilial fragments if the ilium were fixed last.

Acetabular fractures. Although nonplating surgical techniques have been described for repair of acetabular fractures, none of them has proved to be as effective as or has provided the clinical results of plates. Two sizes of C-shaped acetabular plates from the AO/ASIF group (Synthes, LTD) are effective in the treatment of simple acetabular fractures. Minifragment plates and standard DCPs (Synthes, LTD) have been used to stabilize acetabular fractures. Some surgeons prefer to use the reconstruction plate for acetabular fractures because it can be bent in several different planes.

Plates must be perfectly contoured to the dorsal bone surface over the acetabulum. The bone fragments shift in position as the screws are tightened if the plate is not properly contoured because the plate is stiff. The C-shaped acetabular plates are easy to contour to the acetabulum's dorsal bone surface because of their special shape. Mini-plates are easy to bend because they are thin. However, this makes them relatively weak and limits the size of animal in which they can be used. The dorsal surface is used for plate placement because adequate bone is present and this is the bone's tension surface (Fig. 9-14).

It is sometimes helpful to bend the plate before surgery, using a model of an intact pelvis that is approximately the same size as the pelvis that needs repair. The prebent plate can be sterilized and minor contouring adjustments made during surgery. This technique reduces surgical time.

In all acetabular fractures, at least two screws should be located on either side of the fracture line and angled so that they do not penetrate the articular cartilage surface (Fig. 9-15).

One of the most difficult fractures to stabilize has a component of the acetabulum's medial wall fractured out. If a large section of this wall is involved, the femoral head will displace medially into the pelvic canal. If the fracture segment containing the medial wall extends far enough cranially, lag screw and/or intramedullary pin

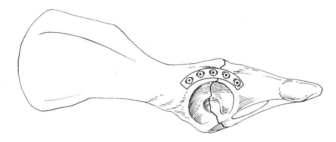

Fig. 9-14 Bone plates are placed over the dorsal rim of the acetabulum because it is the most accessible area of the acetabulum, has the largest visible bone surface, and is the tension surface.

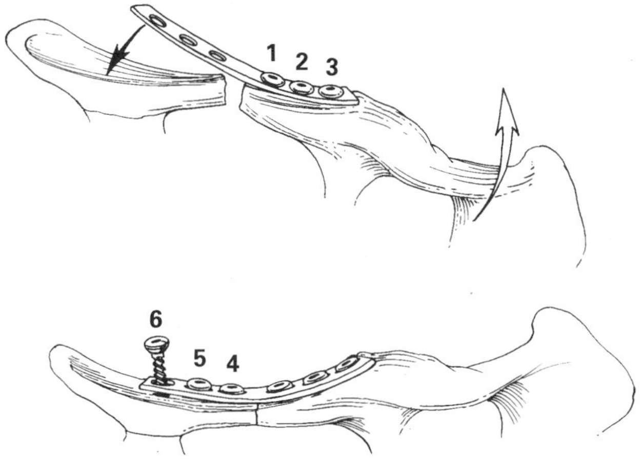

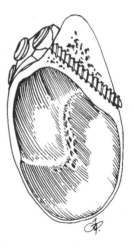

Fig. 9-13 By placing the screws in the order indicated, the bone plate can be used to move the free caudal ilial segment laterally.

Fig. 9-15 This cutaway view of the acetabulum shows proper angulation of the bone screw through the plate so that the articular surface is not violated.

fixation of the ilial segment should be done to bring the piece back into position. If the piece cannot be brought into position, a slight overbending of the plate, closing the diameter of the articular surface, makes it more difficult for the femoral head to displace medially. If the femoral head cannot be prevented from displacing medially, a salvage procedure, like an excision arthroplasty (see Chapter 17), should be considered.

For severe fractures when reconstruction is not possible, excision arthroplasty may be performed. This procedure is done only as a last resort because it sacrifices joint function but is intended to save limb function. If an acetabular malunion from an untreated acetabular fracture has resulted in degenerative joint disease in a dog weighing more than 14 kg, a total hip replacement may be considered (see Chapter 17).

FEMORAL HEAD FRACTURES

Fractures that involve the proximal femur are most frequently encountered in young animals and are classified either as intracapsular or extracapsular fractures. Intracapsular fractures involve either the head or the neck, whereas extracapsular fractures involve only the neck.

The attachment of the femoral head ligament to the femoral head is better able to resist traumatic loads than the physis of the proximal femur. Thus, when an animal incurs trauma, a physeal fracture is the most likely result. In some instances an avulsion fracture of the greater trochanter accompanies the femoral head fracture. The fracture segment of the greater trochanter is often obscure on radiographs because it is positioned behind the proximal femur.

When a fracture occurs in the proximal femoral physis, some surgeons are concerned that the animal will develop avascular necrosis of the femoral head. Although this concern has been expressed in the literature, this event occurs infrequently. Care must be taken when approaching a fractured femoral head or neck to preserve as much of the blood supply to the proximal femur as possible.

Preserving Blood Supply

Femoral head fractures are often exposed through a craniolateral approach. The gluteal muscles are elevated by the blade of an Army-Navy retractor, and an incision is made in the joint capsule to expose the fractured femoral head. The incision in the joint capsule should run parallel with the long axis of the femoral neck. The vessels in the joint capsule parallel this axis. Therefore, if the incision is made along this line, minimal damage is done to these vessels. The joint capsule often attaches to the ventral aspect of the femoral head. This should be preserved because it may be the only remaining primary blood supply to the femoral head once the fracture has occurred.

Some surgeons use a trochanteric osteotomy to expose this area. Although this gives greater exposure of the fractured femoral head and neck, it also disrupts more blood supply in the area. The craniolateral approach provides adequate exposure to see the alignment of the femoral head and neck and to stabilize the fracture in most patients.

Methods of Fixation

Two methods of fixation have been proposed for fractures of the proximal femoral physis. One is the use of three intramedullary pins in a triangulation pattern. A lag screw with an intramedullary pin has also been proposed as a method of fixation for this fracture. I prefer the three-pin technique.

With the lag screw, any growth potential that may still exist in the physis is eliminated by the screw's presence. Some argue that the trauma of fracturing has already damaged the physis such that growth will not continue. This may be true in some patients, but not in all. Thus, if an animal does have several months or more of growth left when the fracture occurs, placing a lag screw across the physis has the potential of damaging the femoral head by causing growth to stop in that physis. There is also minimal bone for the threads of the lag screw to purchase in the proximal fragment. The end of the screw should not penetrate the end of the femoral head because this would put the screw tip in the articular surface. An intramedullary pin to prevent fragment rotation should always be used with this lag screw, since the screw by itself cannot counter rotational loads.

When employing the three-pin technique, the pins should be driven approximately parallel with the long axis of the femoral neck. This means that the pins enter the femur distal to the third trochanter (Fig. 9-16). The vastus lateralis muscle will need to be removed from this

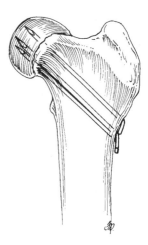

Fig. 9-16 To stabilize a Salter-Harris fracture of the femoral head, three intramedullary pins have been driven parallel with the femoral neck into the head.

area so the insertion point of the pins can be exposed. All three pins are placed before the fracture is reduced. The pins are driven out the exposed fracture surface so that their position can be assessed. Once their location has been determined, the pins are withdrawn until they are just below the fracture surface.

When reducing the fracture, it is helpful to abduct the limb while using the tip of a mosquito forceps on the ventral portion of the proximal fragment to help manipulate it into position. Care must be taken not to separate the proximal fragment from its ventral attachment to the joint capsule. It is sometimes difficult to tell when the proximal fragment is properly reduced because the fracture occurs at a cartilage-bone junction. This means that the fracture line will not be clearly demarcated as it would if the fracture were in dense lamellar bone. It may be necessary to lift the distal fragment off the surface of the proximal fragment using a bone clamp on the trochanter while manipulating the proximal fragment into position.

After the fracture is reduced, the limb should be held in an abducted position while the pins are driven. This helps lock the fragments in position while fracture fixation is established. The most central pin is driven into the femoral head first. The pin should not penetrate the articular cartilage. To determine if the pin has penetrated the articular cartilage, the femoral head should be put through full range of motion. The surgeon should feel for any scraping or limitation to free motion of the femoral head. If the pin has engaged the femoral head, it should move with the rest of the proximal femur. Visual inspection of part of the femoral head is also possible if traction is applied to the trochanter with a rake retractor. If it is determined the pin has penetrated the femoral head, the pin should be withdrawn until it is below the cartilage surface. The second and third pins are driven into the proximal fragment. A range of motion test is performed after each pin is inserted.

When all three pins have been satisfactorily seated, the pins should be bent so they lie flush with the lateral cortex of the femur. To bend the pins sharply, a hand chuck should be secured around the pin, leaving a distance of 6 to 8 cm between the bone surface and the chuck tip. The hand chuck can then be pushed in the direction of the desired bend. This will give a sharp bend on the pin as it exits the bone surface (Fig. 9-17). The pin-bone interface must be closely observed during this process because soft or thin bone may fail during the bending process. Once the pins are bent over, they can be cut off, leaving a short hook on the end of the pins. This hook ensures enough pin is present to be grasped if it later becomes necessary to remove these pins. By bending the pins over flush with the bone, there is less chance that the animal will be irritated by the pin tips if they lie on the side of the repaired femoral head. Placing the end of the hand chuck next to the bone when

bending the pins does not give a sharp bend to the pins and may cause the pins to be withdrawn a short distance. This could prove disastrous, since only a few millimeters of the pins are located in the proximal fragment.

Avulsion fractures of the femoral head occur with coxofemoral dislocations in mature dogs. If the fragment is too small to be adequately stabilized, it is excised at the time of open reduction of the hip. On the other hand, if the fragment is one-quarter the femoral head or larger, it can be reattached with the use of a lag screw and small intramedullary pin (Fig. 9-18). The lag screw is placed at

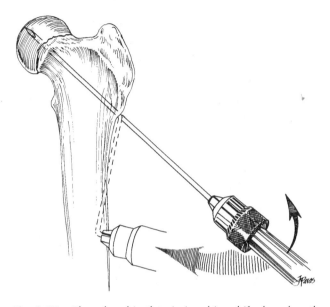

Fig. 9-17 Sharp bend in the pin is achieved if a long length of pin is left between the point where the pin enters the bone and where the hand chuck secures the pin. Pushing the hand chuck in the desired direction of bend produces a sharp bend in the pin.

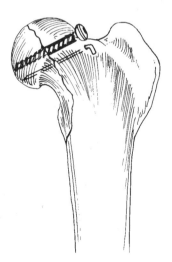

Fig. 9-18 Large avulsion fragments from the femoral head can be stabilized with a lag screw and an antirotation pin. The implants should be positioned so that their exposed portion does not interfere with normal hip joint articulation.

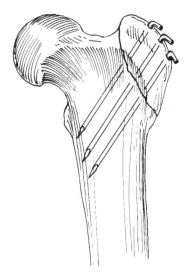

Fig. 9-19 In growing animals with an avulsion fracture of the trochanter, the fracture is stabilized with two or three intramedullary pins. A tension-band wire is not used because it would close the physeal plate.

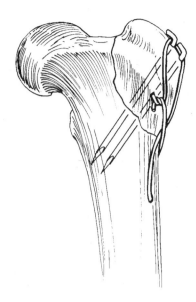

Fig. 9-20 In mature or nearly mature animals, a fracture of the trochanter is stabilized with two pins and a tension-band wire.

the margin of the head and neck and angled perpendicular to the fracture line. The pin is inserted beside the lag screw, providing a second point of fixation for the fragment and neutralizing rotational load.

GREATER TROCHANTERIC FRACTURES

A fracture of the greater trochanter is handled in two ways. If the animal is young and has significant growth potential left, the trochanter is secured with two or three intramedullary pins. These pins are driven through the trochanteric fragment and into the proximal femoral shaft. The pin should be placed perpendicular to the fracture line (Fig. 9-19). Absorbable sutures may be used in a cruciate pattern to secure the torn edges of the fascia and periosteum. Although a tension band would be the most ideal way to fix this fracture, growth potential prevents use of that technique. A tension band applied across a growth plate causes the growth plate to close. Fractures in growing animals stabilize and heal more rapidly; thus, the intramedullary pins are usually adequate to fixate the fracture until healing has taken place. The potential always exists that the trauma creating the fracture damaged the physis and growth will not continue. The status of the physis will not be known until after the fracture has healed.

Fractures of the trochanter in mature or nearly mature animals should be fixed with a tension-band technique (Fig. 9-20). The fracture is reduced and held securely in place with a pointed bone reduction forceps. Two intramedullary pins are driven through the trochanteric fragment into the proximal segment of the femur. A hole is drilled in the proximal femur distal to the fracture line,

perpendicular to the long axis of the femur and in the caudolateral aspect of the femur. A wire is passed through the hole and around the pins in a figure-eight fashion. The portion of the wire being twisted together should not lie underneath the continuous strand of the wire. Since the wire is twisted only on one side, it is important to pull the wire tightly around each pin. The tension band counters the pull of the gluteal muscles.

FEMORAL NECK FRACTURES

Fractures of the femoral neck occur most often in young animals but may occur in older animals as well. Whether intracapsular or extracapsular, these fractures are well suited for repair with a lag screw and a single intramedullary pin for rotational stability (Fig. 9-21). In most instances a cortex screw is used to provide the lag effect; however, the 6.5 mm partially threaded cancellous screw can be used in bones large enough to accept it. The glide hole should be drilled before the fracture is reduced. This ensures that the glide hole is centered in the fractured neck because the hole's exit point in the fracture surface can be visualized. The fracture is reduced and held in a fixed position while the thread hole is drilled in the proximal segment of the femoral neck. The proper insert sleeve is inserted in the glide hole, ensuring that the thread hole is centered properly.

The length of cortex screw to be used can be determined by using the depth gauge or by measuring the screw length from the radiographs. When using the radiographs, the magnification means that the measured distance should be reduced 2 to 6 mm, depending on the animal's size. The screw in the femoral neck should be

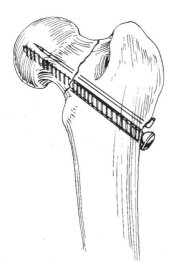

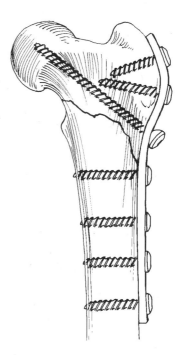

Fig. 9-21 Fractures of the femoral neck are stabilized with a lag screw and pin to prevent rotation of the fragment. The screw should be inserted parallel to the neck's axis. To achieve this alignment, the screw's insertion point is distal to the third trochanter. In animals with growth potential, the screw threads should not cross the physeal plate.

Fig. 9-22 When a subtrochanteric fracture of the femur is repaired with a bone plate, the plate should be contoured to fit over the trochanter. The screws in the proximal end of the plate are triangulated. If possible, one screw should be placed in the femoral neck.

placed parallel with the neck's long axis. When the bone is soft, as in a young animal, the screw head may sink into the femur as it is tightened. A metal washer can be used with the screw to prevent this.

It is sometimes helpful to insert an antirotation pin parallel with the lag screw before insertion of the lag screw. This keeps the proximal fragment from shifting in position during drilling and screw insertion. The proper-length screw is inserted but is not fully tightened until the antirotation pin has been completely withdrawn into the fragment with the glide hole. If the pin is not perfectly parallel with the lag screw, it will prevent full compression from being achieved if it crosses the fracture line while the screw is tightened. After the lag screw is then fully tightened, achieving maximum compression, the antirotation pin is reinserted into the proximal segment. The hip is placed through a full range of motion to ensure that neither the screw nor the antirotation pin has penetrated the articular cartilage of the femoral head. If the animal has growth potential left, the lag screw should not cross the area of the physis.

The three-pin technique also can be used on a fractured femoral neck, as previously described for fixation of the femoral head. This method does not provide compression along the fracture line but does give multiple points of fixation to the fracture fragments.

SUBTROCHANTERIC FRACTURES

If a subtrochanteric fracture of the femur exists and the animal is skeletally mature, intramedullary pins or bone

plates can be used to stabilize the fracture. In the immature animal, bone plates should not be used if screws would need to be placed across an open physis to secure the plate in position. Later comments on intramedullary pins (see Femoral Shaft Fractures) also apply to subtrochanteric fractures. Depending on the fracture configuration, it may be necessary to combine pin fixation with auxiliary implants such as orthopedic wire, figure-eight skewer pins, or external fixators. Plate fixation is most often combined with auxiliary screw fixation and/or orthopedic wire.

When the fracture is proximal in the femur, it is necessary to contour the bone plate over the trochanter. The plate is placed laterally after the main bone fragments have been made as stable as possible with lag or position screws and/or orthopedic wire. To ensure the presence of bone under the plate, the top and bottom screws in the plate should be inserted first. The most proximal screw is short because the trochanteric fossa limits the amount of bone available for screw purchase. By angling the screws in the proximal three or four plate holes, a triangulation effect is achieved. This provides solid fixation of the proximal fragment, especially if one of the screws is directed into the femoral neck (Fig. 9-22). The plate used for fracture stabilization should be long enough to allow at least three screws to be placed below the most distal fracture line.

If a fractured femoral neck exists with a subtrochanteric fracture, the fracture is repaired with a lag screw either through the plate or just caudal to the plate. This screw should be placed as described earlier when only a femoral neck fracture exists. All the other screws should be placed in the plate before this screw is inserted. An intramedullary pin placed outside the plate into the femoral neck should also be used to give the fractured neck another point of fixation and prevent fragment rotation.

FEMORAL SHAFT FRACTURES

Fractures of the femoral shaft are generally repaired with either plates and screws or pins or a combination of pins and wires and external fixators. Femoral shaft fractures should not be treated with a cast or splint because these methods of fixation are unable to control the proximal fragments and often place an unwanted fulcrum at the fracture site.

Bone Plates

Bone plates provide rigid internal fixation and allow the patient early controlled mobility. Bone plates are always applied to the lateral side of the femur because this is the tension side. With the eccentric loading of the femur during weight bearing, the tension forces that develop laterally and compression forces that develop medially are significant. Bone plates on the femur must negate the intense loads generated during even controlled weight bearing (Fig. 9-23). If significant loss of bone occurs or the load transmission surfaces of the femoral shaft cannot be reconstructed, a strong plate having buttress function and cancellous bone grafting should be used for fracture repair. If the load transmission surfaces of the femur can be reconstructed, the plate applied can be narrower than the plate needed in a buttress situation and will have neutralization function. Plates can be used with lag screws outside the plate or orthopedic wire when reconstructing the femoral shaft. Short oblique and transverse fractures can be stabilized with plates that have static and/or dynamic compressive function.

Intramedullary Pins

If intramedullary pins are chosen for the fixation method in the femur, they can be inserted normograde (orthograde), starting at the greater trochanter, or retrograde, in which they exit in the trochanteric fossa before being driven distally. The pins are seated distally in the cancellous bone at the level of the femoral condyles, but they should not penetrate the intercondylar groove. A single pin or stacked pins may be used (see Chapter 5).

The sciatic nerve must be protected when inserting intramedullary pins. The hip should be placed in extension

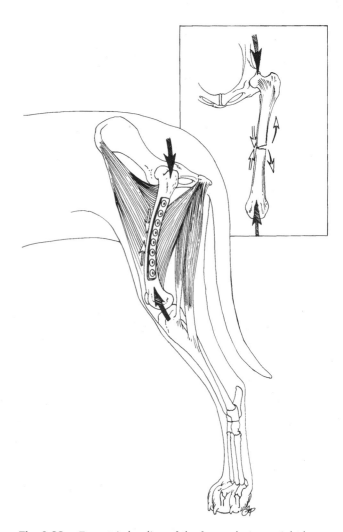

Fig. 9-23 Eccentric loading of the femur during weight bearing creates maximum tension loads on the femur's lateral side. Bone plates are excellent at resisting tension loads. Thus, bone plates are placed on the femur's lateral side.

and internal rotation. The limb should be adducted. These positions place the course of the pin during insertion as far away from the sciatic nerve as possible. Any animal with sciatic nerve dysfunction or extreme pain on hip extension after pinning should have the nerve explored.

If intramedullary pins are the sole method of fixation, the fracture must interdigitate and have transverse surfaces that will directly transmit compressive loads. A long oblique fracture can be stabilized with at least 2 cerclage wires and an intermedullary pin(s). If comminution is present, the bone fragments must be large enough to be reconstructed with orthopedic wires and/or figure-eight skewer pins for intramedullary pins to be used (Fig. 9-24). If the fracture cannot be stabilized by pins and internal auxiliary fixation, an external fixator should be added to the fixation (see External Fixators).

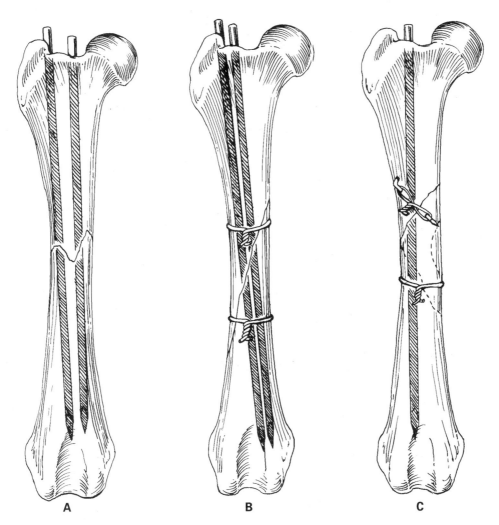

A   B   C

Fig. 9-24   A, If the fracture fragments interdigitate a in transverse fracture, intramedullary pinning may provide adequate stability to the fracture. **B,** To overcome shear loads in a long oblique fracture, at least two cerclage wires are combined with the intramedullary stabilization. Figure-eight skewer pins could be used in place of the cerclage wire. **C,** Comminuted fracture with large fragments can be stabilized with intramedullary pins and cerclage wires and/or figure-eight skewer pins.

Pins are left in place, as long as the fracture fixation is stable, until a healed fracture is confirmed with radiographs. Removal of intramedullary pins is performed by making a small incision over the pin as it exits in the trochanteric area. The pin is grasped with a pin puller and removed. The incision is closed with a subcuticular stitch.

External Fixators

External fixators are used as auxiliary fixation with intramedullary pins and as primary fixation without pins (Fig. 9-25). External fixators in the femur are applied to the lateral side of the bone with the outermost fixation pins anchored in the subtrochanteric area proximally and in the femoral condyles distally. External fixators are generally type I frames with one or two connecting bars.

When secure stability of a fractured femur cannot be achieved with a pin(s) and internal auxiliary fixation, an external fixator should be added. A good example is when an intramedullary pin is used on a transverse fracture. Collapse of the fracture is controlled because the surface of the bone segments abut against each other, but rotational loads are not controlled. Internal auxiliary fixation (e.g., cerclage wire) is not possible in this fracture. The addition of an external fixator with one fixation pin proximally and one distally makes this fracture stable (Fig. 9-26). If this fixation is used, the intramedullary pin must be small enough to allow for placement of the fixator's proximal fixation pin. The proximal femur is slightly wider than the shaft, and fixation pins can be inserted obliquely, making a combination of external fixators and intramedullary pins

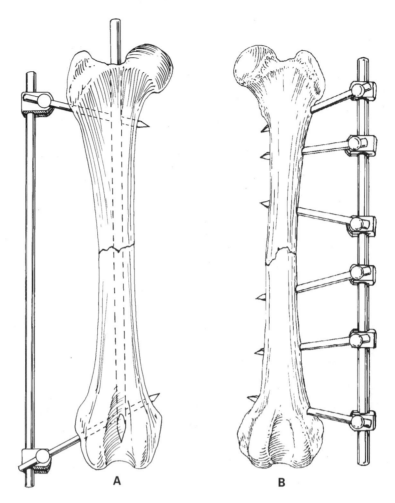

Fig. 9-25 **A,** External fixators are used with intramedullary pins to prevent fragment rotation or collapse. Two fixation pins and a connecting bar are often all that is needed when the external fixator is an auxiliary fixation device. **B,** External fixators can also be used for primary fracture stabilization. More fixation pins must be used when an external fixator is used as the primary fixation device.

possible. Distal fixation pin placement is not difficult because the condyles are wide and the intramedullary pin ends in the proximal portion of the condyle.

The external fixator can be removed after a fibrous callus has joined the two fragments together. This takes 2 to 6 weeks depending on the animal's age. The intramedullary pin is left in place until the fracture is determined to be fully healed based on radiographic evaluation.

When an external fixator is used as the primary stabilization of fractures, ideally at least three fixation pins should be inserted into the proximal and distal main fragments. If the dog is large and the fracture highly unstable, a second connecting bar should be used. Orthopedic wire and screws may be used as auxiliary fixation with external fixators. The external fixator used for primary stabilization should be left in place until radiographs show the fracture has healed. If the fracture is healing at a slower-than-anticipated rate, the fixator frame

can be partially destabilized by removing one or more pins or the second connecting bar, if present. This increases the load transmission through the bone and may increase the healing rate.

The external fixator causes lameness when used for fixation of femoral fractures because the fixation pins penetrate muscle as well as bone. This has caused some surgeons to use external fixators on femoral fractures infrequently or not at all.

DISTAL FEMORAL FRACTURES

The most common distal femoral fracture is a Salter-Harris I or II fracture of the femoral condyles. This occurs because the open physis is weaker than the ligaments of the stifle joint. Several methods using an intramedullary pin(s) have been described for stabilization of this fracture. Because this fracture is through an active physis

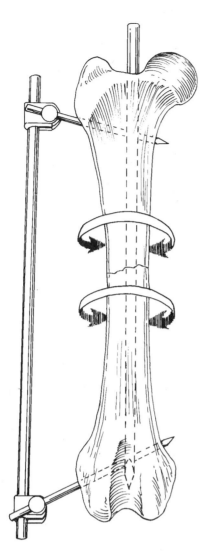

Fig. 9-26 Axial alignment of this transverse fracture is achieved with intramedullary pinning. The fracture will not collapse because the fracture surfaces are in complete contact around the shaft. With the pin alone, the fracture is not rotationally stable. The addition of two fixation pins and a connecting bar has eliminated rotational instability.

and the distal fragment is relatively small, the use of plates and screws is not recommended.

Fracture Approach and Reduction

A lateral approach with a lateral arthrotomy to the stifle joint is performed. The patella, femoral condyles, straight patellar ligament, and tibial tuberosity must all be identified before the arthrotomy is made. These structures are displaced caudally and possibly medially. If they are not identified before the incision is made, the straight patellar ligament is at risk of being inadvertently severed. The distal end of the proximal bone fragment (the distal femoral metaphysis) should also be exposed. This fragment sometimes penetrates the vastus muscle group and

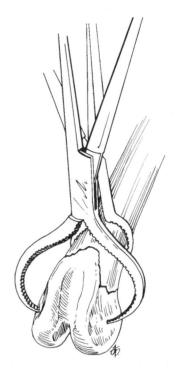

Fig. 9-27 Gentle manipulation of the distal segment of a Salter-Harris I or II fracture of the distal femur is required to reduce the fracture successfully. Excess force applied during reduction may make the fracture more complex. The fragments can be reduced by using a bone clamp to stabilize the proximal segment, while the distal segment is slowly levered into place with a Lewin clamp. The prongs of the Lewin clamp should be placed in the thick part of the condyle.

must be returned to its normal position caudal to muscles without further damage to the muscles.

The most difficult aspect of the condylar fracture can be reduction of the fracture segments, especially if more than 48 hours has passed since the original trauma. The effect of muscle contracture on bone fragment position is more prominent in young animals. The soft bone and cartilage of the young animal's femoral condyle are easily disrupted if manipulated even with typically used fragment reduction forces. The proximal segment is controlled by placing a bone clamp on the metaphysis just above the fracture line. The distal segment is gently manipulated into a partially reduced position. Some surgeons use a Lewin bone clamp, with its prongs purchasing the caudal portion of the femoral condyles to control this fragment (Fig. 9-27), whereas others use only their hands and fragment manipulation. The stifle is flexed and extended several times to help stretch any contracted muscles.

It is helpful when relaxing contracted muscles to hold the fully extended position for 30 seconds or more. The distal fragment often moves closer to a fully reduced position with each cycle. The joint can also be placed in a flexed position so that the tibia can be used to push on the condyle while the proximal segment is pushed caudally with the bone clamp on the metaphysis (Fig. 9-28).

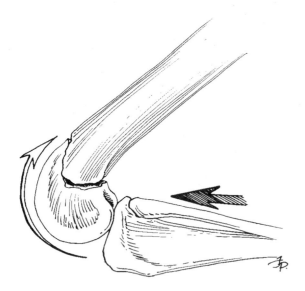

Fig. 9-28 If the fracture cannot be fully reduced as described in Fig. 9-27 or the bone is too soft for the use of a Lewin bone clamp, the stifle should be flexed and the tibia used to push the femoral condyle into place. The proximal femoral fragment needs to be stabilized to accomplish this.

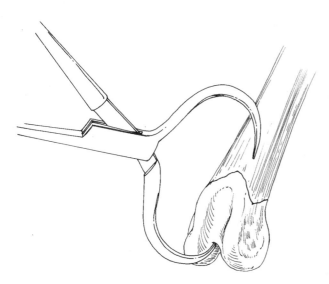

Fig. 9-29 Distal fragment may reduce to within a few millimeters of its anatomical location with the methods shown in Figs. 9-27 and 9-28 but cannot be completely reduced. In this instance, a pointed reduction forceps can be used to achieve the final reduction. One point of the forceps is placed at the origin of the caudal cruciate ligament and the other on the cranial surface of the proximal fragment. Closing the forceps should provide the force needed for the final reduction.

If the distal fragment does not completely reduce with these techniques, a pointed reduction forceps can be placed so that one point purchases the femoral condyle just cranial to the caudal cruciate ligament's origin and the other point is in the cranial metaphysis. Gently closing

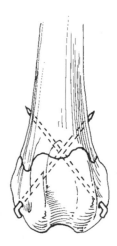

Fig. 9-30 Cross-pin technique used for stabilization of Salter-Harris I or II fracture of the femoral condyle.

these clamps almost always provides the final reduction of the fracture (Fig. 9-29). The clamp can be left in place while primary fixation is applied to the fracture. Levering the fragments into place with a pin or instrument should never be done because this will almost always create new fractures.

Fracture Stabilization

Once the fracture is reduced, an intramedullary pin(s) is (are) used for stabilization. In the cross-pinning technique, two pins are driven distal to proximal across the fracture line (Fig. 9-30). One of these pins is started laterally in the lateral femoral condyle caudal to the origin of the long digital extensor muscle. The pin is driven normograde across the fracture line into the medial metaphysis. The other pin is driven in the same manner, except it is started medially in the medial condyle and traverses to the lateral metaphysis. These pins may either exit the proximal fragment at the metaphysis or continue proximally along the endosteal surface. The angle of insertion and the flexibility of the pin determine the pin's course. The pins are cut off close to their insertion point inside the joint.

In another technique using two pins, the pins are driven normograde from cranial to caudal (Fig. 9-31). These pins are started in the cranial metaphysis and end in the condyles without exiting the distal fragment. The pins do not cross but traverse from the medial metaphysis to the medial condyle and from the lateral metaphysis to the lateral condyle. After the pins are seated, they are bent over and cut off at their insertion point.

A single pin can also be used to stabilize this fracture. Using the preoperative radiographs as a guide, a pin is chosen no larger than 50% of the femur's endosteal diameter. After the fracture is reduced, the pin is inserted

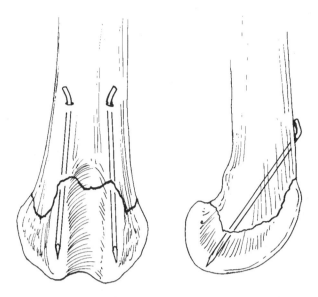

Fig. 9-31 Femoral condylar fracture is stabilized with two pins driven from the cranial metaphyseal surface of the proximal fragment into the condyles in the distal fragment.

normograde, starting at a point just cranial to the origin of the caudal cruciate ligament in the intercondylar groove. The limb is positioned as described earlier (Femoral Shaft Fractures—Intramedullary Pins) so that the sciatic nerve is protected. The pin is driven out the trochanteric fossa, ideally along its lateral margin. The pin is advanced through the skin over the hip until the chuck can be placed on the exposed portion. The distal end of the pin is cut off close to the cartilage surface. The pin is withdrawn slowly, using the chuck attached to the proximal end, until the distal cut-off end is 2 to 3 mm below the cartilage surface. A properly placed pin will engage caudal endosteal surface distally and cranial endosteal surface proximally (Fig. 9-32).

After the fracture is healed, the pin is easily removed via a small incision over the hip. One pin is almost always sufficient to stabilize this fracture because the fracture fragments interdigitate, negating rotational instability. If any instability exists, a pin driven from the distal fragment into the proximal metaphysis will eliminate it.

CONDYLAR FRACTURES

Rarely, an isolated fracture of either the lateral or the medial femoral condyle is encountered. After reduction, the fracture is stabilized with a lag screw(s) for interfragmentary compression and an intramedullary pin(s) for rotational stability (Fig. 9-33). The lag screws should be oriented 90 degrees to the fracture line. The screw should be placed where it will not interfere with joint motion. Screws are inserted either cranial to caudal or caudal to cranial and are always positioned obliquely in the bone.

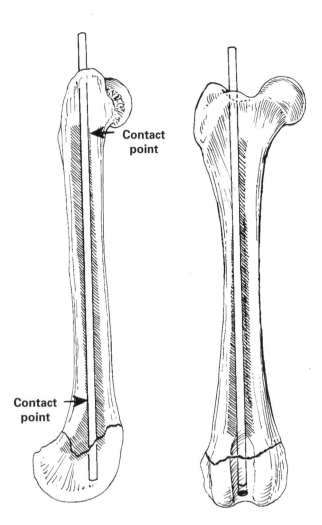

Fig. 9-32 Single intramedullary pin driven normograde from the femoral condyles and out the intertrochanteric fossa is used to stabilize a fracture of the distal femur.

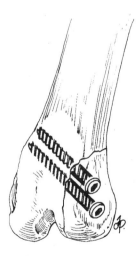

Fig. 9-33 Femoral condylar fracture is stabilized with at least one lag screw placed perpendicular to the fracture surface. A second point of fixation in the form of another lag screw or an intramedullary pin should be used to ensure this fixation is rotationally stable.

PATELLAR FRACTURES

Fractures of the patella are rarely encountered. The pull of the quadriceps muscles displaces the proximal fragment cranially, while the distal fragment is fixed in position by the straight patellar ligament. The fracture is approached by a lateral arthrotomy. The articular surface of the patella should be anatomically reduced, or degenerative joint disease will result.

In a two-piece fracture, a tension-band wire placed through the patella's fibrocartilage dorsally and the straight patellar ligament ventrally may provide adequate stabilization. Placing the stifle through a range of motion after the tension band is in place and observing the fracture line for motion will determine if the tension band alone is sufficient fixation.

A figure-eight skewer pin can also be used for stabilization (Fig. 9-34). The fragments must be held in anatomical reduction while the intramedullary pin is being driven. Power-driving the pin gives more accurate placement than hand-driving the pin in this small, dense bone. If the fracture is highly comminuted, small loose fragments can be removed and figure-eight skewer pin stabilization employed.

FIBULAR FRACTURES

Usually, fibular fractures occur with tibial fractures. Repair of the tibia adequately aligns the fibula. If an isolated fibular fracture occurs that does not involve the lateral malleolus, it can be treated with a support bandage and/or rest.

Fractures of the malleolar portion of the fibula are treated with tension-band fixation (Fig. 9-35). Unless the patient is a large dog, the surgeon can use only one intramedullary pin with the tension-band wire. In most cases the stabilizing intramedullary pin is driven through the malleolar portion of the fibula into the tibia. The wire is anchored through a transverse hole drilled in the tibia.

TIBIAL FRACTURES

Tibial fractures are treated with all forms of internal and external fixation. The use of casts and splints is limited to relatively nondisplaced fractures in young animals. The principles established in Chapter 4 for casts and splints apply here. Surgical fixation of tibial fractures is discussed next.

Intramedullary Pins

When pinning the tibia, a single pin approximately two-thirds the bone's radiographic endosteal diameter is chosen. Using a large pin tends to straighten the bone's normal S-like configuration, resulting in valgus deformity.

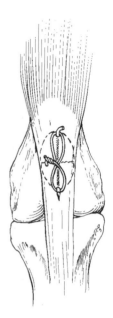

Fig. 9-34 Two-piece patellar fractures can be stabilized with an intramedullary pin and a figure-eight wire, which functions as a tension band.

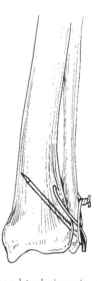

Fig. 9-35 Tension-band technique is used to stabilize fractures of the lateral malleolus. Usually only one pin can be inserted because the distal bone fragment of the fibula is small. The tension-band wire is anchored in through the tibia.

Too large a pin is also difficult to insert properly. Stacked pinning is not recommended for the tibia.

Intramedullary pins are inserted normograde from the medial side at a point halfway between the tibial tuberosity and the medial tibial condyle (Fig. 9-36). The insertion point is located just medial to the joint capsule, and the pin should be aligned parallel to the tibia's long axis. If the pin tends to slide along the bone's surface, the angle of insertion should be made more obtuse until the pin's cutting point is embedded into the bone. The angle can

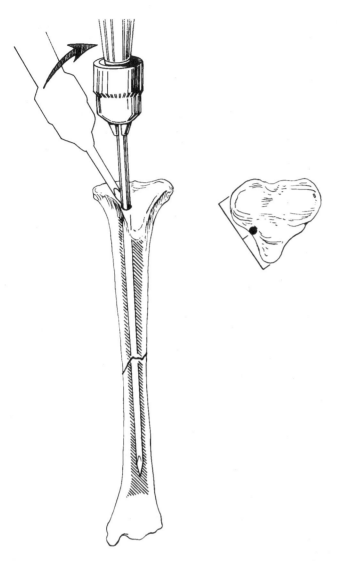

Fig. 9-36   An intramedullary pin placed in a tibia is always driven normograde. It should be started on the medial side of the bone halfway between the tibial tuberosity and the medial tibial condyle. The pin should be placed outside and immediately medial to the joint capsule. It may be necessary to start the pin at a large angle relative to the tibia's long axis and decrease the angle of insertion as soon as the pin purchases the bone.

be flattened as soon as adequate bone purchase has been obtained. Inserting the pin as described allows it to traverse in a straight line to the cancellous bone in the distal tibia.

Once the pin is seated, the hock should be put through range of motion and the pin measured against a second pin of equal length to be sure the distal tibia has not been penetrated. After it has been determined the pin is of proper length, it should be cut off as close to its insertion point as possible.

A pin should never be inserted retrograde in the tibia. Retrograde insertion of a pin causes it to exit the proximal tibia in the stifle joint, interfere with extension of the

joint, and damage the articular surface of the femur and/or patella.

It is almost always necessary to combine some form of auxiliary fixation with pinning of the tibia. Cerclage wires, figure-eight skewer pins, and external fixators are the most common types of fixations combined with pins.

Combining an external fixator with an intramedullary pin can present a challenge. The fixator's outer pins should be placed near the ends of the tibia. Ample bone exists in the proximal end to allow room for the intramedullary pin and the fixation pin. However, distal fixation pin placement can be compromised by the intramedullary pin if the fixation pin is placed in the distal diaphysis and not in the wider metaphyseal/epiphyseal area. The problem is avoided by identifying anatomical landmarks.

External fixators as auxiliary fixation help prevent rotation and collapse of the fragments. When a fibrous callus has joined the bone fragments, usually in 2 to 6 weeks, the fixator can be removed, leaving the intramedullary pin to continue as the primary means of stabilization.

External Fixators

External fixators are used as either primary or auxiliary fixation in the stabilization of tibial fractures. The previous section discusses their use as auxiliary fixation.

External fixators can be positioned on either the medial or the lateral side of the bone. At least three fixation pins should be inserted in each of the proximal and distal main bone fragments. Although type I fixators are adequate for fracture stabilization in some patients, a type II fixator is generally preferred for primary fixation (Fig. 9-37). The type II fixator is more rigid and cannot be pulled off if the animal should catch it on something. Fixation pins may be inserted from both sides of the bone with the type II fixator, making it easier to insert three pins in a fragment. Animals bear weight more readily with a type II fixator. Type III fixators are usually needed only for very large dogs with highly unstable fractures that cannot be reconstructed.

Bone Plates

Bone plates are applied to the medial side of the bone via a cranial approach. The cranial approach is used rather than the traditional medial approach so that the plate will not lie directly under the skin incision. After the incision is made, the skin is reflected caudally exposing the medial tibia, which is relatively flat, making plate contouring easier. The plate should be contoured to match the tibia's normal S-like shape (Fig. 9-38). A craniocaudal radiograph of the opposite normal tibia can be used as a guide for plate contouring.

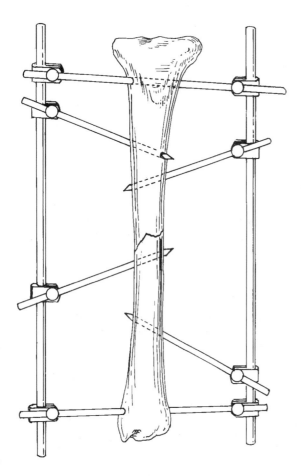

Fig. 9-37 Box configuration of the type II external fixator provides rigid fixation to tibial fractures. This configuration is often used when the external fixator is intended to be the primary fixation device.

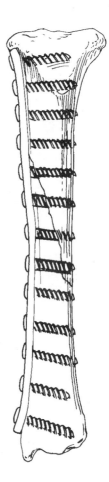

Fig. 9-38 Bone plates are applied to the medial side of the tibia because this area is easily approached and its relatively flat surface simplifies plate contouring.

If the plate extends to the tibia's distal end, the hock joint should be put through range of motion to determine the exact position of the distal end of the tibia and the proximal portion of the talus. The medial malleolus extends below the proximal talus; thus, the most distal screw in the plate should not be inserted in this area. The most proximal and most distal screws in the plate should be the first two screws inserted. Placing these screws first ensures there will be bone under the entire length of the plate.

Special Proximal and Distal Tibial Fractures

In the proximal tibia, avulsion fractures of the tibial tuberosity occur occasionally. These fractures are most often observed in young animals because the physeal plate is relatively weak and fails when excess tension is applied to it. Pressure applied over the tibial tuberosity during physical examination will elicit a pain response if the fracture is present. If the animal has no growth left or is almost grown, a tension-band wire with one or two

intramedullary pins (depending on the fragment size) is the most mechanically sound fixation for this fracture (Fig. 9-39). The pin(s) should be inserted 90 degrees to the fracture line from cranial to caudal through the avulsed fragment into the proximal tibia.

If the animal has significant growth left, the tension band should not be used because it will close the physis and cause a significant deformity to develop in the tibial plateau. In this patient, only two pins should be inserted to stabilize the fracture. If the pins are inserted 90 degrees to the fracture line and the germinal zone of the physis was not damaged by the trauma, the tibial plateau should continue to develop normally. The fracture line will heal in 2 to 5 weeks in a young animal. The client should provide cage rest until healing is complete.

A Salter-Harris fracture of the distal tibial physis can be challenging because the distal fragment is small. A small incision over the fracture site allows visualization of the fracture site so one can determine when reduction is achieved. Generally, digital manipulation and joint flexion and extension will reduce the fracture. Fracture fixation

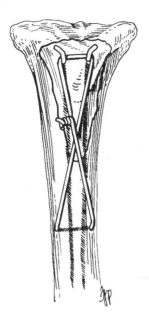

Fig. 9-39 Avulsion fractures of the tibial tuberosity in mature or nearly mature animals are stabilized with the tension-band technique. In animals with growth potential, two pins without the tension-band wire are used for fixation.

is achieved by inserting two small intramedullary pins in a crossing fashion. One pin is started at the medial malleolus and driven to the lateral tibial metaphysis, and the other is started at the lateral malleolus and driven through the fibula to the medial tibial metaphysis. This method of fixation and cage rest is generally enough to obtain a satisfactory result.

A fracture of the medial malleolus is repaired with a tension-band wire and one or two small intramedullary pins. Care must be taken when driving the pins because the distal fragment is usually small. The wire is anchored in a transverse hole through the medial tibia and passed around the pin in a figure-eight pattern.

TARSAL FRACTURES

Fractures involving the bones of the tarsus occur infrequently in most pet animals. They occur more often in working dogs, such as racing greyhounds and sled dogs. Most fractures in the tarsal bones, particularly in the central tarsal bone, are created by compression and shear forces. Tension is most frequently responsible for avulsion fractures of the calcaneal tuberosity.

Generally, these fractures do not heal well unless they are rigidly stabilized. Using a cast or splint does not usually lead to acceptable healing. Several factors combine to result in the poor healing observed when rigid fixation is not used. The joint has many major load-bearing surfaces, and thus the tarsal bones move frequently during weight bearing. The blood supply to these

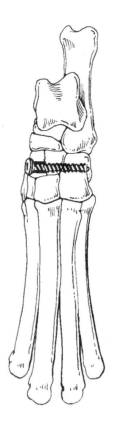

Fig. 9-40 Simple fractures of the calconeal tuberosity stabilized with 2 pins and a tension band wire. The tension band counters the pull of the extensor's of the hock.

bones is relatively poor compared with the long bones. The fracture surfaces are constantly bathed in synovial fluid. Many ligaments are attached to the tarsal bone and will pull on the fragments when the limb is loaded. Unless they are rigidly stabilized, the bone and cartilage fragments can become free bodies (joint mice), causing significant degenerative joint disease to develop. None of these factors is conducive to bone healing.

The most common tarsal fractures occur in either the central tarsal bone or the calcaneus. Fractures of the numbered tarsal bones and the talus occur infrequently. If the fractures of the central tarsal bone are small chips that cannot be stabilized, they can be removed surgically. If the fragments are large enough, a lag screw(s) can be used for stabilization (Fig. 9-40). If possible, at least two points of fixation should be provided in each chip. Because of the size of these fractures, the implants used are relatively small but are exposed to large loads during weight bearing. Thus, this is one case in which the rule about not combining internal and external fixation cannot always be followed. The lower limb may need to be placed in a short leg cast or a splint for 3 to 4 weeks. It requires 8 to 12 weeks for these fractures to heal completely. In patients with severe fractures, primary arthrodesis of the joint should be considered.

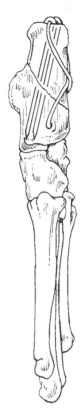

Fig. 9-41 Fractures of the central tarsal bone stabilized with 1 or 2 lag screws when the fragments are large enough.

Avulsion fractures of the calcaneal tuberosity are stabilized with a tension-band technique (Fig. 9-41). This counters the pull of the hock's extensor muscles. The tension-band wire, which is located on the calcaneal plantar surface, should not be placed over the superficial digital flexor tendon that caps the tuberosity. In large dogs with comminuted calcaneal fractures, a bone plate may be placed on the bone's lateral surface.

METATARSAL FRACTURES

Fractures of the metatarsal bones occur more frequently than fractures of the tarsal bones. If only one or two of the bones are fractured and relatively nondisplaced, a cast or splint can often be used successfully. The intact metatarsal bones act as an internal splint in these patients. Even if internal fixation is used to repair these fractures, it is often necessary to support them with a splint or short leg cast. If internal fixation is used, application of the cast or splint may be limited to 3 or 4 weeks. In all except young animals, it requires 8 to 10 weeks for these fractures to heal.

When three or four of the metatarsal bones are fractured, internal fixation is more of a consideration. Since the third and fourth metacarpal bones are the central weight-bearing bones of this region, they receive the primary attention with internal fixation. The surgeon must be careful not to disrupt too much vascular supply when fixing fractures involving these bones. These fractures are often created by a trauma that has compromised the circulation to the foot. Further insult to the circulation through the surgical approach and manipulation should be avoided. If marked swelling occurs after fixation of fractures in this area, it may be advisable to perform fasciotomy incisions to help reduce the pressure within the foot.

Intramedullary pins can be used to fix metatarsal fractures. The pins are inserted by flexing the metatarsal-phalangeal joints and starting the pin just above the articular surface in the distal metatarsus. The pins are driven normograde until they seat in the proximal metatarsus. Intramedullary pins are bent dorsally to keep them from damaging the phalangeal articular surface. This also aids in their removal after the fracture is healed. In large dogs, small bone plates may be used to stabilize metatarsal fractures.

PHALANGEAL FRACTURES

Phalangeal fractures are generally not treated surgically. A cast or splint for 3 to 4 weeks is usually adequate to allow enough healing so that the fracture is no longer painful. Continued limited activity after that period for an additional 3 to 4 weeks is advisable.

In rare instances a lag screw may be used in the fixation of phalangeal fractures. A small bone·plate may be applied to a fracture of the first phalanx in very large dogs. Internal fixation of phalangeal fractures is usually limited to working dogs.

POSTOPERATIVE CARE

If reconstruction of the bones of the hind limb is anatomical and the stabilization deemed adequate, immediate controlled weight bearing is usually allowed. The animal's activity level should be limited to walking and being outside only on a leash until radiographs indicate a healed fracture(s). This usually takes 3 to 12 weeks, depending on the animal's age and the fracture's severity. In those rare instances when fracture stability is uncertain, a non-weight-bearing sling may be employed for 2 to 3 weeks to allow early fracture healing without the stress of weight bearing (see Chapter 6). Passive flexion and extension of the hip while the animal is in the sling are recommended to help maintain articular cartilage integrity. With anatomical reconstruction of the fractures, adhering to sound surgical principles and early controlled limb motion, normal function with no or minimal secondary effects can be anticipated in most patients.

SUGGESTED READINGS

Betts CW: Pelvic Fractures. In Slatter D, editor: *Textbook of Small Animal Surgery,* ed 2, Philadelphia, 1993, Saunders.

Boudrieau RJ, Kleine LJ: Nonsurgically managed caudal acetabular fractures in dogs: 15 cases (1979-1984), *J Am Vet Med Assoc* 193:701-704, 1988.

Brinker WO, Piermattei DL, Flo GL: Fractures of the pelvis; Fractures of the femur and patella; Fractures of the tibia and fibula; Fractures of the tarsus, metatarsus, and phalanges. In Brinker WO, Piermattei DL, Flo GL:, editors: *Handbook of small animal orthopedics and fracture treatment,* ed 2, Philadelphia, 1990, Saunders.

Brinker WO, Braden TD: Pelvic fractures. In Brinker WO, Hohn RB, Prieur WD, editors: *Manual of internal fixation in small animals,* Berlin, 1984, Springer-Verlag.

Daily WR: Femoral head and neck fractures in the dog and cat: a review of 115 cases, *Vet surg* 7: 29-32, 1978.

DeCamp CE, Braden TD: The anatomy of the canine sacrum for lag screw fixation of the sacroiliac joint, *Vet Surg* 14:131-135, 1985.

DeCamp CE, Braden TD: Sacroiliac fracture-seperations in the dog: a study of 92 cases, *Vet Surg* 14:127-130: 1985.

Denny HR: Pelvic fractures in the dog: a review of 123 cases, *J Small Anim Pract* 19:151-155, 1978.

Gilmore DR: Internal fixation of femoral fractures. In Bojrab MJ, editor: *Current techniques in small animal surgery,* ed 3, Philadelphia, 1990, Lea & Febiger.

Hulse DA: Acetabular fractures. In Bojrab MJ, editor: *Current techniques in small animal surgery,* ed 2, Philadelphia, 1983, Lea & Febiger.

Johnson AL, Boone EG: Fractures of the tibia and fibula. In Slatter D, editor: *Textbook of small animal surgery,* ed 2, Philadelphia, 1993, Saunders.

Milton JL: Fractures of the femur. In Slatter D, editor: *Textbook of small animal surgery,* ed 2, Philadelphia, 1993, Saunders.

Piermattei DL: The hindlimb. In Piermattei DL, Greely RG, editors: *An atlas of surgical approaches of the bones of the dog and cat,* ed 3, Philadelphia, 1993, Saunders.

Olmstead ML: Surgical repair of acetabular fractures: In Bojrab MJ, editor: *Current techniques in small animal surgery,* ed 3, Philadelphia, 1990, Lea & Febiger.

Pope ER: Fixation of tibial fractures. In Bojrab MJ, editor: *Current techniques in small animal surgery,* ed 3, Philadelphia, 1990, Lea & Febiger.

Salter RB, Harris WR: Injuries involving the epiphysical plate, *J Bone Joint Surg* 45A: 587-591, 1963.

Slatter DH, editor: Methods of fracture fixation; Orthopedics of the hind limb; Pelvic fractures. In *Textbook of small animal surgery,* ed 2, Philadelphia, 1993, Saunders.

Slocum B, Hohn RB: A surgical approach to the caudal aspect of the acetabulum and body of the ischium in the dog, *J Am Vet Med Assoc* 65:167, 1975.

Tarvin GB, Lenehan TM: Management of sacroiliac dislocations and ilial fractures. In Bojrab MJ, editor: *Current techniques in small animal surgery,* ed 3, Philadelphia, 1990, Lea & Febiger.

Taylor RA, Dee JF: Tarsus and metatarsus. In Slatter D, editor: *Textbook of small animal surgery,* ed 2, Philadelphia, 1993, Saunders.

Vernon FF, Olmstead ML: Femoral head fractures resulting in epiphyseal fragmentation: results of repair in 5 dogs, *Vet Surg* 12:123-125, 1983.

III

COMPLEX FRACTURE CONDITIONS

10

Open Fractures

LAWRENCE W. ANSON

In human orthopedics, three rules of fracture treatment have been exalted by Brown: "(1) leave closed fractures closed; (2) leave contaminated or infected open fractures open; and (3) early return of the injured extremity to as near normal function as possible."[4] In veterinary orthopedics the last two rules should be followed, but strict adherence to the first is seldom possible. Early return to function often requires open reduction and internal fixation of fractures. Since veterinary patients cannot be expected strictly to control their activity and clients are sometimes uncooperative, open reduction and rigid fixation are the preferred treatments for many fractures. The result is that the veterinary surgeon is the primary cause of open fractures. However, since this is done in the operating room, the risk of complications should be minimal. Open fractures that have a greater risk of complications are the main focus of this chapter.

An open fracture is defined as a fractured bone that is in contact with the environment. Open fractures can be classified into three grades.[17] The use of this classification system has several advantages. First, communication about the severity of the open fracture is simplified. Second, the grade of the open fracture correlates with the degree of soft tissue damage associated with the fracture, and third, suppositions can be made about appropriate choices of implants for fracture fixation.

A *grade I* open fracture occurs when the bone penetrates the skin (Fig. 10-1). The tip of the bone may be projecting from the skin, or only a small puncture wound may be present. Careful inspection of the skin to observe the opening may be required. Long-haired animals may require clipping of the hair coat to identify the wound. Less damage to the soft tissues occurs including the vascular supply of the bone, than in higher grades of open fractures.

Skin perforation in a *grade II* open fracture occurs from the outside trauma (Fig. 10-2). A variably sized wound is contiguous with the fracture. Soft tissue injury is more extensive than that observed with a grade I open fracture, but extensive soft tissue damage, skin flaps, or avulsions are not present. This grade can include some low-muzzle-velocity gunshot injuries and some motor vehicle accidents.

The most severe open fractures are classified as *grade III* (Fig. 10-3). Extensive skin and soft tissue injury is present. Comminuted fractures, as a result of the dissipation of high kinetic energy, are common. High-muzzle-velocity gunshot injuries are an example. Shearing injuries of the distal extremities, sometimes caused by motor vehicle accidents, may result in loss of bone and extensive loss of skin and other soft tissues.

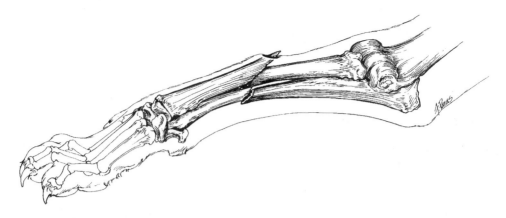

Fig. 10-1   Grade I open fracture. The open wound is the result of the tip of the bone penetrating the skin.

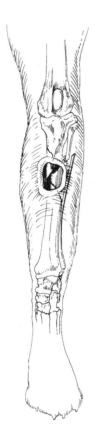

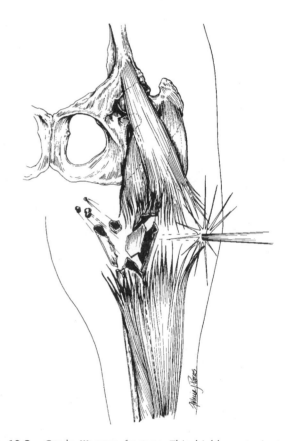

Fig. 10-2   Grade II open fracture. The open wound is the result of the trauma, not the bone penetrating the skin.

Fig. 10-3   Grade III open fracture. This highly comminuted fracture as a result of a gunshot has extensive soft tissue injury.

INITIAL EVALUATION

Since severe trauma may be associated with open fractures, "tunnel vision" must be avoided when treating these patients. The fracture is important, but the entire patient must be critically evaluated. Initial assessment of the patient should include evaluation of the airway, control of excessive hemorrhage, and appropriate cardiovascular support. Life-threatening injuries should be treated first. Care of the open fracture can be initiated once treatment of the more critical injuries has been instituted.

PATHOPHYSIOLOGY

The break in the integument that occurs with open fractures is an avenue for contamination. Soft tissue infection and osteomyelitis may occur. The risk of infection may also be increased by other factors. The vascular injury associated with open fractures may be significant. Depending on the fracture grade, extensive damage to the blood supply of the bone, muscle, fascia, and skin may be present. This local effect may be compounded by systemic injury, such as damage to other organ systems.

Hypovolemic shock as a sequela to blood loss may be present. Corticosteroids are often administered to these animals. This combination of local and systemic factors places these patients at a higher risk of infection at the fracture site.

Whether infection of the bone and soft tissue occurs depends on several factors. The fracture is in contact with the environment, and thus contamination may occur. Bacteria may reach the fracture by extension from an adjacent soft tissue infection or by direct contact of the bone with the environment.[13] However, contamination does not equal infection. The degree of trauma to the skin, soft tissues, and bone is important in the development of an infection. By definition, a grade I open fracture indicates less injury than a grade III. A grade III fracture results in a more conducive environment for bacterial colonization and growth. One must consider the importance of the local blood supply as a factor in the establishment of an infection. Minimum bacterial inhibitory concentrations of antibiotics may not be reached in the vicinity of the open fracture if a poor blood supply exists. The vascular damage associated with open fractures may also isolate the injured tissues from the body's defense mechanisms.

In addition to the local immune response, the systemic status of the patient's immune system is another critical factor. The animal treated with high doses of corticosteroids and stressed by trauma and shock may have a compromised immune response to bacterial contamination. The number of organisms per gram of tissue and the virulence of the organisms are important. Usually, an infection does not become established if less than 10^5 organisms are present per gram of tissue. Under normal circumstances, infection may not be caused by a highly virulent bacteria. However, the circumstances associated with an open fracture may create the ideal opening for a small number of these same bacteria to cause a clinical infection. Low virulence of bacteria combined with immunosuppression of the animal may also result in a clinical infection.

The final and perhaps most important factor in the establishment of infection is the clinical management of the case. Inappropriate treatment of an open fracture is likely to result in all types of complications, including infection. Appropriate clinical handling of the different grades of open fractures is discussed later.

Open fractures may be expected to have a protracted period of healing. This delay in clinical union may be expected for several reasons. The higher dissipation of kinetic energy that occurs with open fractures results in greater impairment of the circulation in surrounding tissues.[4] As a result of the local circulatory impairment, revascularization of the soft tissues and bone is delayed. Prolonged healing of the fracture results. An open fracture or open reduction of a closed fracture may lead to loss of the fracture hematoma. Delayed union may then occur, since organization of the hematoma is one of the early steps in healing.[4, 16] Soft tissue trauma and blood loss are increased with open reduction of a fracture. Further disruption of the vascular supply to the bone occurs with fracture fixation. Medullary circulation is disrupted by intramedullary pins and periosteal circulation is disturbed by bone plates.[23] Open reduction and internal fixation also introduce large metallic foreign bodies into the fracture site. The combination of open fracture, open reduction, and implantation of a foreign body may result in a clinical or subclinical infection. A delayed or aberrant healing process may then occur.[27] These factors all contribute to the longer average healing time of an open fracture compared with a closed fracture.

INITIAL MANAGEMENT

Owners often provide initial treatment of open fractures. If a sterile bandage is available, it should be placed over the wound. A clean cloth may be substituted if bandaging materials are not available. Hemorrhage can be controlled by direct compression. The pet should be transported to the hospital as expediently as possible. Care must be taken to prevent further injury to the animal. The owner should take precautions to avoid being bitten by the injured pet.

Physical Examination

On arrival at the clinic or hospital, a rapid but thorough examination should be completed. The neurological and vascular status of the limb must be carefully assessed. Abnormal neurological function or questionable vascularity to the limb may influence the client's decision on treatment of the injury. Historical information obtained from the owner should include the source of the trauma and the environment in which the injury took place. For example, a gunshot injury, when litigation may be a possibility, requires documentation and treatment. The risk of a clostridial infection in an open tibial fracture, as a result of being kicked by a horse, for example, influences decisions made about management of the case.

Stabilization of the patient should be followed by inspection of the open wound. Any previously applied bandage should be removed. The limb should not be manipulated more than necessary to avoid additional damage to the soft tissues. The wound must not be probed until the clinician is prepared to debride it. Violation of this principle may increase the risk of nosocomial infections.

Antibiotic Administration

Open fractures should be considered contaminated. Therefore, antibiotic administration can be considered an adjunct to appropriate case management. Selection of an appropriate antibiotic should be based on knowledge of bacteria typically isolated from osteomyelitis cases. Gram-negative isolates usually found are *Escherichia coli* and *Pasteurella*, *Proteus*, and *Pseudomonas* species.[5,26,28] Gram-positive isolates are *Streptococcus* species and the coagulase-positive *Staphylococcus* species.[5,26,28] Mixed infections of both gram-positive and gram-negative bacteria also may be found.[5,26,28] The conditions of devitalized muscle mass and damaged vascular supply, with an attendant decrease in tissue oxygen content, may create a local environment in which anaerobic bacteria flourish.[9] An intravenously administered broad-spectrum antibiotic that achieves therapeutic levels in both bone and soft tissue should be considered. Cephalosporins fulfill these requirements.[20]

Wound Debridement

A critical facet in the treatment of open fractures is adequate wound debridement. The conversion of a contaminated wound to a clean wound requires strict adherence to aseptic technique. One must ensure that no hair enters the wound while the limb is being clipped. While clipping, sterile lubrication jelly may be used to cover the wound. Alternately, towel clamps may be used to appose skin edges temporarily while clipping the hair. With grade I fractures, clipping the hair from the wound may be sufficient until definitive fracture care can be instituted. If the wound is more than a puncture, wound exploration and debridement are performed. Sterile instruments should be used and a cap, mask, and surgical gloves worn. Copious lavage of the wound is performed after surgical preparation of the limb to remove gross contamination. The remaining foreign material may be removed with debridement of the tissues. An 18-gauge needle and a 35 ml syringe can be used as a lavage system.[18] Sterile isotonic saline, either with or without chlorhexidine, is a satisfactory solution for lavage.[29]

Grossly devitalized soft tissue may be removed with sharp dissection during the initial debridement. If possible, extensive dissection under the wound edges should be avoided, but flaps of tissue should be looked under for hidden debris. After the initial debridement, surgical preparation should be repeated. The surgeon should then reglove and perform the final debridement, again using copious lavage. Good debridement requires adequate surgical exposure, but extensive soft tissue dissection should be avoided. Any bullets retrieved should be saved because of the potential for litigation.

Bacterial culture and sensitivity testing are recommended. In humans, infection is correlated with what is cultured from the wound at the *end* of debridement, not at the beginning.[15] Extrapolating this finding to animals is logical. If performed, culture and sensitivity should follow the final debridement rather than when the patient first arrives. During wound management, it may be necessary to debride a wound several times as questionable tissue dies or to control infection.

Bone debridement is usually accomplished during fracture stabilization. Gross contamination should have been removed during the initial debridement. All bone should be carefully cleaned. The primary clinical concern is the potential for formation of sequestrae. Clinical decisions concerning the debridement of bone must be made on a case-by-case basis. However, general guidelines for bone debridement follow. Small pieces with no soft tissue attachment may be removed. An attempt should be made to save any piece of bone with no soft tissue attachments that is integral to the reconstruction of the fracture. Pieces with soft tissue attachment that contribute to the stability of the fracture should be incorporated into the repair. Those fragments with soft tissue attachment that are not integral to the repair should be left in the fracture site. They will contribute to callus formation.

Fracture Stabilization

Open fractures below the stifle or elbow may benefit from temporary external support. The use of a padded support bandage lessens the chance for additional soft tissue trauma. Other benefits from temporarily stabilizing the fracture include increasing patient comfort and decreasing the formation of limb edema. This may make the surgical approach easier. A support bandage is contraindicated if the fracture is proximal to the elbow or stifle, unless the shoulder or hip joint is also immobilized. An inappropriately applied bandage may act as a pendulum, resulting in exacerbation of the injury. The use of a spica splint is recommended because this immobilizes the shoulder or coxofemoral joint. The use of a support bandage for temporary fracture stabilization depends on the patient's disposition and condition. Strict cage confinement, gentle handling of the limb, and tranquilization may constitute a better option than a bandage. Definitive fracture repair can be performed when the patient is stable.

Radiography

A minimum of two radiographic views of the fracture should be evaluated. These views are lateral to medial and cranial to caudal, including the joints above and below the fracture. Careful assessment of the radiographs for signs that may affect fracture management, such as fissures, is mandatory.

Anesthesia

Chemical restraint may not be required for radiographic evaluation and initial debridement of the wound. However, anesthesia is needed for definitive debridement of the wound and fracture stabilization. Options include local anesthesia, neuroleptanalgesia, regional anesthesia such as an epidural, or if the patient is stable, general anesthesia. The choice of anesthesia is dictated by the patient's condition.

FRACTURE FIXATION

Open fractures should be stabilized as soon as possible. Patient comfort is increased, making it easier to manage the open wounds and the patient. An important benefit of stabilization of the fracture is that it allows the soft tissues to begin to heal. Movement of the bone fragments is reduced or eliminated, with the result that the soft tissues begin to repair their traumatized blood supply and revascularization of the bone fragments begins. Therefore, the tissues heal more rapidly and subsequently are more resistant to infection.

External coaptation has limited use in managing open fractures. Splints and bandages may provide adequate temporary support until more definitive fracture treatment is performed. The best candidate for external coaptation is the patient with a stable fracture and an easily managed soft tissue wound. Splints and casts make wound care difficult. Excessive movement of the fracture may result if frequent changes of the support wrap are required. A restrictive cast or splint is contraindicated if the soft tissue injury includes skin with a tenuous blood supply.

Selected grade I and II open fractures may be stabilized with intramedullary pins (Fig. 10-4). Their principles of use are no different than when they are used in closed fractures. Theoretically, the potential exists to contaminate the medullary cavity when using an intramedullary pin. The risk of this complication in adequately debrided open fractures is low.

Rigid fixation of grade I and II open fractures may also be obtained with a bone plate and screws (Fig. 10-5). After stabilization the plate and bone should be covered with soft tissue. Plates are a less attractive option for grade III open fractures if extensive soft tissue dissection is required for their placement. The additional dissection translates into additional trauma to the tissues and their vascular supply.

External fixators are ideal in many grade III open fractures (Fig. 10-6). The transfixation pins may be placed away from the fracture site and the traumatized soft tissue, thus preserving blood supply and facilitating wound care. Autogenous cancellous bone graft should be considered when cortical defects exist. Bone plating may be considered if application can be accomplished without extensive vascular compromise.

A decision to amputate the limb may be made in some circumstances. Severe vascular compromise, permanent peripheral nerve injury, or economics may dictate amputation as the most expedient treatment.

After stabilizing the fracture, the surgeon must make decisions about closure of the open wound. Influencing

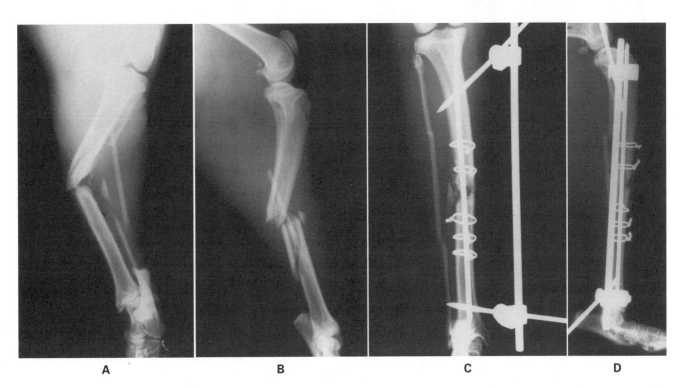

A   **B**   **C**   **D**

Fig. 10-4 **A** and **B,** Preoperative radiographs of a grade I open tibial fracture in a cat. **C** and **D,** Immediate postoperative radiographs of the open tibial fracture after repair with five full-cerclage wires, a single intramedullary pin, a type I external fixator, and an autogenous cancellous bone graft.

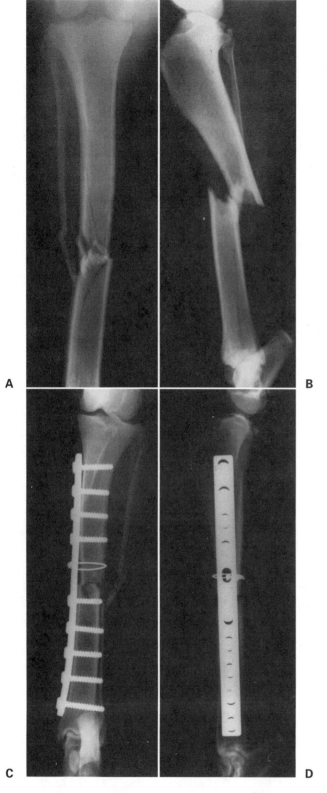

Fig. 10-5   A and **B,** Preoperative radiographs of a grade I open tibial fracture in a German shepherd. **C** and **D,** Immediate postoperative radiographs of the open tibial fracture after repair with a 10-hole bone plate, nine bone screws, and one full-cerclage wire.

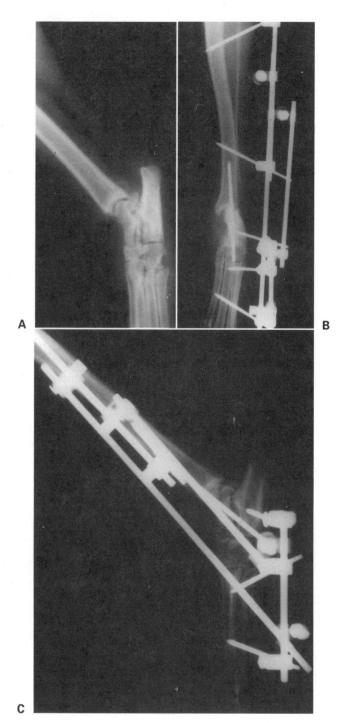

Fig. 10-6   A, Preoperative radiograph of a grade III open fracture of the hock and distal tibia in a dog. This was a degloving injury. **B** and **C,** Postoperative radiographs after application of an external fixator and a transarticular pin. Arthrodesis of this joint was the final outcome.

factors are the degree of soft tissue injury, the adequacy of the debridement, the environment in which the injury occurred, and the time elapsed since injury. Successful management of the soft tissue injury may depend on whether the wound is left open or closed. If doubt exists about closing the open wound, it should be left open. Grade I and II open fractures that are well debrided and clean are candidates for primary closure. There should be no devitalized tissue, good vascularity to the wound edges, no dead space, and no tension on the closure. If excessive dead space exists, closed-suction drains can be used with a primary closure.

Primary closure of grade III open fractures is rarely indicated and often impossible because of the extent of skin loss. The methods of choice are delayed closure or second-intention healing. The wound is covered with a sterile dressing after final debridement and culture. The tissues are kept moist with saline-soaked gauze sponges. Bandages are changed once or twice a day as required for appropriate wound management. Repeated debridement of the wound, if required, may be easily done if the patient is managed in this manner. In some patients an autogenous cancellous bone graft may be placed in areas of cortical defects to help speed union of the fracture, but not until after the wound is covered with granulation tissue.[3] Frequent reevaluation of the patient is required when treating a wound with delayed closure or second-intention healing. Treatment may be altered based on clinical assessment of the wound.

GUNSHOT FRACTURES

Open fractures sustained as a result of gunshots are a special problem. In many cases the clinician is unable to obtain specific information about the injury other than the animal having been shot. Careful evaluation of the wound, the bullet, and the radiograph of the fracture, coupled with a basic knowledge of ballistics, enables the veterinarian to reach some conclusions about the weapon and projectile used to inflict the injury. This information may then be applied to clinical management of the patient.

Ballistics

Ballistics is the science of motion of projectiles. It may be divided into interior ballistics, the motion of the projectile within the barrel of the weapon; exterior ballistics, the trajectory of the bullet through the air; and wound ballistics, the effect of the projectile moving through tissue.[30] The degree of damage to the tissues from the projectile is influenced by the weapon, the bullet, and the range from which the gun is fired. Additional factors influencing the wounding capability are the projectile's velocity, kinetic energy (KE), and stability in

flight.[19] Knowledge of these factors may be important in the clinical management of a patient.

Velocity is the speed of the projectile measured in feet per second (ft/s). Two velocities can be measured. The first is the *initial*, or *muzzle*, *velocity*. This is the speed of the projectile immediately after firing.[19] Weapons may be classified by their muzzle velocity. Bullets from low-velocity guns travel at less than 1000 ft/s. Medium-velocity projectiles travel 1000 to 2000 ft/s. Handguns fire bullets that are generally low-to-medium velocity. High-velocity projectiles travel faster than 2000 ft/s. Rifles fire bullets that are medium-to-high velocity[21] (Tables 10-1 and 10-2).

The second velocity that may be measured is *impact velocity*, the speed of the projectile when it meets the target.[19] The farther the tissue is from the gun's muzzle, the slower the impact velocity. Impact velocity is equal to the muzzle velocity for projectiles from low-velocity weapons that strike a target less than 50 yards away and those from high-velocity weapons less than 100 yards away.[19]

Velocity is the most important factor in wounding capability of a projectile. In humans, penetration of the skin requires a minimum impact velocity of 150 ft/s; 195 ft/s is required to break bone.[19] The velocity is an

Table 10-1 Comparison of Frequently Used Firearms and Bullets

Firearm	Bullet weight (grains)	Muzzle velocity (ft/s)	Muzzle energy (ft–lb)
HANDGUNS			
.32	71	863	91
.45	230	850	370
.45 Colt	250	860	410
.38 Special	158	1090	425
.357 Magnum	158	1415	695
.44 Magnum	240	1470	1150
RIFLES			
.22 Remington	40	1180	124
M–16	55	3200	1248
.22 Swift	45	4140	1825
.30–.30 Winchester	170	2200	1830
.303 British	215	2160	2230
Russian 7.62	150	2810	2635
M–14	180	2610	2720
M–1	172	2700	2785
8 mm Mauser	170	2530	2415
Mauser Modified 98	198	2650	3031
.357 H and H Magnum	270	2720	4440

From Ordog GJ: Wound ballistics. In Ordog GJ, editor: *Management of gunshot wounds*, New York, 1988, Elsevier.

Table 10-2 Caliber and Velocity of Commmon Air Guns

Brand name	Caliber	Muzzle velocity (ft/s)
PNEUMATIC RIFLES		
Beeman R1	.177, .22	940
ARH/Feinwerkbau F–12–cx	.177	820
Feinwerkbau 124 Sporter	.177	800
Beeman/Webly Vulcan	.177, .22	600-800
Crossman American Classic 766	.177 or BB	450-700
Beeman 400	.177	660
Feinwerkbau 300S	.177	650
Crossman Model One	.22	625
Beeman Falcon 1 and 2	.177	600
Crossman 2200 Magnum	.22	600
Weihrauch 55 target	.177	600
Powerline 850	.177 or BB	520
Sheridan CO_2	.20	514
Crossman 788 Scout	BB	462
PNEUMATIC PISTOLS		
Crossman 1322, 1377	.177, .22	530
Feinwerkbau F–80	.177	525
Beeman/Webly		
Hurricane	.177, .22	470
Tempest	.177, .22	470
Powerline CO_2 1,200 Custom	.177, BB	450
Beeman 700	.177	450
Daisy 780, 790	.177, .22	425
Crossman Mark 1	.22	405
Marksman Plainsman CO_2	.177, BB	400
Sheridan CO_2	.20	400
Crossman 1861 Shiloh CO_2	.177, BB	370
Daisy Match 777	.177	360
CONVENTIONAL RIFLES/PISTOLS		
Long rifle .22	.22	1,000
Short and long rifle .22	.22	800
ACP .32	.32	900
Long Colt .32	.32	755
S & W .38	.38	685
S & W .44 Special	.44	755
.45 Automatic	.45	850

From Ordog GJ: Wound ballistics. In Ordog GJ, editor: *Management of gunshot wounds*, New York, 1988, Elsevier.

important factor in the KE of the projectile. The greater the KE, the greater is the bullet's wounding capacity. The KE of a bullet may be calculated from the following formula:

$$KE = \frac{Mass\ (grains) \times Velocity^2\ ft/s}{2 \times g\ ft/s \times 7000\ grains/lb}$$

Where mass is the projectile weight in grains (7000 grains/lb), velocity is the impact velocity, and *g* is the gravitational force (32.16 ft/sec). KE is measured in foot-pounds (ft-lb). From this formula, one can see that the projectile's mass is also important, but not to the degree of velocity.

Pathophysiology

Wound severity also depends on the specific gravity (SG) of the tissue that the bullet strikes. Tissues with higher SGs absorb more KE, resulting in greater tissue destruction. Lung, which has an SG of about 0.4 to 0.5, would have less tissue damage than liver (1.01 to 1.02 SG), muscle (1.02 to 1.04 SG), and bone (1.11 SG).[19]

The bullet's angle of impact to the tissue is also important. At an acute angle of entrance, more surface area of the bullet strikes the tissue. The bullet decelerates more rapidly, with a greater dissipation of KE and more tissue destruction.[19]

The design of the projectile also influences the potential wounding capacity. Pointed bullets are less likely to lose velocity at greater distances. Therefore, at equal distances a pointed bullet has a greater KE on impact than one with a blunt tip. At short distances the shape of the tip is not much of a factor. Bullets that are unjacketed or partially jacketed are more likely to deform on impact, thus losing more KE in the tissues. Fully jacketed bullets are more likely to pass through tissue with less deformation. Therefore, there is less loss of KE and potentially less tissue damage. Hollow-point bullets, which have a concavity at the tip and are partially jacketed or unjacketed, are more likely to mushroom on impact, leading to rapid loss of KE and more extensive tissue injury.

As mentioned previously, the bullet's stability in flight influences the wounding capability. Bullets may be unstable during flight. Two important types of instability are yaw and tumbling (Fig. 10-7). *Yaw* is movement of

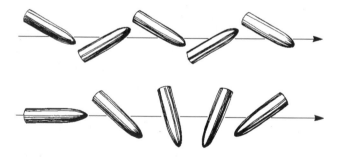

Fig. 10-7 Bullets may be unstable during flight. Two instabilities are yaw and tumble. The arrows indicate the direction the bullet is traveling. *Top*, Yawing is the deviation of a bullet in its longitudinal axis from the straight line of flight. *Bottom*, Tumbling is the action of forward rotation around the center of mass.

Redrawn with permission from Swan KG, Swan RG: *Gunshot wounds: pathophysiology and management*, ed 2, Chicago, 1989, Year Book.

the bullet from the longitudinal axis of its line of flight. *Tumbling* is forward rotation of the bullet around its center of mass. This same instability may occur in tissues. Instability in tissue depends on the angle of impact of the projectile and the tissue density.[19] The instability in the tissues decreases the projectile's velocity, resulting in greater dissipation of KE and greater tissue destruction.

Secondary missiles may also increase tissue destruction. Fragmentation of the bullet or fragments of bone may act as secondary missiles. These projectiles increase the damage done to the tissues.

The mechanism of tissue damage from gunshot wounds is related to the impact velocity. Low-velocity gunshot wounds cause laceration and crushing of soft tissues. The bullet moves the tissues directly in its path. The design of the bullet, its angle of impact, and its stability in flight also determine the amount of crushing and laceration in low-velocity gunshot wounds.[19] High-velocity bullets (faster than 2500 ft/s) produce additional damage by shock wave propagation in the tissue. The tissue ahead of the bullet is compressed in all directions by the high-energy shock waves produced.

At bullet velocities faster than 1000 ft/s, *cavitation* occurs. A cavity is formed by the tissues moving forward and laterally away from the bullet.[19] Subatmospheric pressure develops in the wound, and air, hair, and debris may be sucked into the wound. The force generated results in damage away from the path of the bullet, causing stretching, compression, and shearing of the tissues. Muscle fibers, connective tissue, and vascular elements are injured by cavitation.[7] After passage of the bullet, the cavity collapses, leaving a much smaller permanent cavity. These higher-velocity projectiles produce more tissue damage and a greater possibility of infection.

Different weapons produce different patterns of injury. Pellet guns and BB guns fire low-muzzle-velocity projectiles. The velocity is great enough to break the skin at close range and cause fractures. The degree of tissue damage from handguns and rifles depends on the velocity and the range. Shotguns fire multiple projectiles that disperse in a cone-like fashion. There is a rapid fall off in the velocity of the pellets. At close range there is a high muzzle velocity and thus high KE. A severe soft tissue wound is produced, and fractures may occur. The farther a target is from the shotgun, the greater the decrease in pellet velocity and effectiveness of the weapon. The dispersion of the pellets may result in only minor injury, and fractures become unlikely.[6]

The damage to the bone depends whether the projectile is low velocity or high velocity and whether the composition of the bone is primarily cancellous or cortical. Cortical bone that is hit by a low-velocity bullet typically sustains a butterfly fracture.[12] High-velocity projectiles that strike cortical bone cause comminution.[7] Cavitation occurs in addition to the fragmentation of the cortical bone. The fragments are carried to the edges of the large cavity. As the cavity collapses, most of the fragments return to the permanent cavity, but some act as secondary missiles.[1] Low-velocity gunshots of metaphyseal bone create a "drill hole" entrance with multiple fracture lines at the exit hole.[12] Metaphyseal bone that is struck by a high-velocity projectile becomes comminuted.[7]

Classification

In veterinary medicine, gunshot fractures have been classified by their radiographic appearance.[24] A *type I fracture* is caused by a low-velocity projectile. The fracture produced is transverse or oblique. No cortical defect is present, and minimal soft tissue injury occurs. A *type II fracture* is also caused by a low-velocity bullet. Radiographically, the fracture is comminuted, but no cortical defect exists. Soft tissue damage is minimal. A *type III fracture* occurs as a result of a high-velocity bullet. Severe comminution, cortical defect(s), and extensive soft tissue injury are present.

In humans, shotgun wounds have been classified by the degree of soft tissue damage.[25] Type I injuries result only in penetration of subcutaneous tissues or deep fascia. These are long-range injuries, with the pellets of low-velocity and the pattern dispersed. Fractures do not occur. Type II injuries penetrate structures beneath the deep fascia. Type III injuries occur at less than 3 yards, with massive tissue destruction. In extremity injuries, fracture is possible.

Case Management

As with any open fracture, complete patient assessment is mandatory. If the patient is unstable, resuscitation and supportive care are indicated. If the patient is stable, an orthopedic examination, including assessment of the neurological and vascular status of the limb, should be performed.

Low-velocity injuries. Management of the wound depends on the injury type. Low-velocity gunshot fractures (types I and II) have damage confined to the projectile pathway. Extensive debridement of the wound is not indicated. The entrance and exit wound (if present) should be covered. The hair is clipped and the skin cleansed. The tissue is debrided to convert a contaminated wound to a clean wound. Copious lavage and gentle handling of the tissues are required. After debridement, a sterile bandage is applied. The wound should not be closed.[11] These recommendations are only guidelines. The clinician should "read" the wound; more extensive debridement may be necessary. Good clinical judgment is needed. A culture should be obtained after the debridement is complete. Bullets are not sterilized by the act of firing. The bullet can carry organisms into the wound as a result of the subatmospheric pressure created by cavitation.[31] Administration of an appropriate antibiotic is indicated. Temporary support of the fracture by a splint or soft padded bandage is important. Immediate fracture fixation may be indicated depending on the circumstances and the animal's condition.

High-velocity injuries. Type III, or high-velocity, injuries have more extensive soft tissue damage, necessitating more aggressive debridement of the soft tissues. The initial care is similar to a type I or II gunshot fracture: debridement to create a clean wound. The clinician must be concerned about necrotic tissue, especially muscle. The tissue can be an excellent culture media for anaerobic bacteria such as *Clostridium* species. Decisions about muscle debridement may be based on the tissue's color, consistency, contractility, and capacity to bleed.[10,32] Muscle that has a healthy color, has normal consistency, contracts when stimulated, and bleeds when cut should not be debrided. Bacterial culture and sensitivity and appropriate antibiotics are indicated.

Fragments of bone with soft tissue attachments should not be removed. Large pieces of bone with no soft tissue attachment that are integral to the fracture repair should be saved. Small pieces of bone with no soft tissue attachment that are not integral to the fracture repair may be removed. At this time, fracture repair can be performed if dictated by circumstances. Cortical defects should be filled with an autogenous cancellous bone graft. This may be done at the time of primary fracture repair or delayed until the recipient bed is healthy. If possible, exposed bone and tendon should be covered with soft tissue.

The wound is initially left open. Further debridement may be necessary. A sterile bandage is applied to protect the wound. Delayed primary closure may be used after the tissues are healthy. In some cases, second-intention healing may be required.

Shotgun injuries. Injuries sustained from a shotgun may require different care. The range at which the injury was inflicted is important. At close range a large projectile mass with a small pattern produces severe injury.[6] In type III shotgun injuries of an extremity, massive muscle injury and vascular and nerve damage occur in addition to a fracture (Figs. 10-8 and 10-9).[14] A decision must be made on whether or not the limb may be salvaged. Vascular and neurological status of the limb *must be assessed.* If the vascular damage is severe and irreversible nerve damage is present (loss of deep pain sensation in the limb), amputation may be the most expedient solution. Radiographic assessment of the fracture and debridement of traumatized soft tissue must be performed. The wound should be left open and sterile bandages applied.

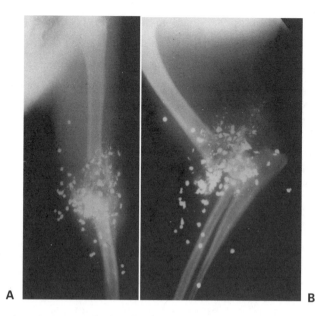

Fig. 10-8   **A** and **B,** Radiographs of a type III shotgun injury (grade III open fracture) of a distal humerus in a dog.

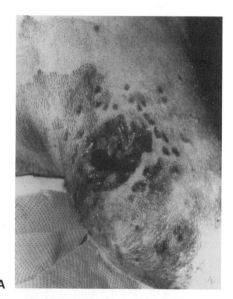

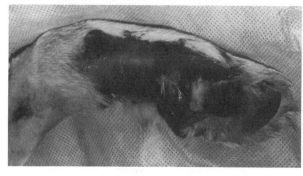

Fig. 10-9   **A,** Photograph of the entrance wound of the shotgun injury in Fig. 10-8. **B,** Photograph of the paw 3 days after injury. Gangrene is present. The limb was amputated.

Skin flaps or grafts may be required because of the degree of soft tissue injury.

Joint injuries. Joint injury from gunshots must be properly handled (Fig. 10-10). The joint should be explored. Lead is dissolved by synovial fluid, resulting in periarticular fibrosis, chondrolysis, and possible lead poisoning.[2, 22] Bullets outside the joint should be removed if easily found, but it is not necessary to explore for them extensively because they generally do no harm. The joint should be radiographed immediately before surgery, since the bullet may migrate. All foreign bodies and osteocartilaginous fragments should be removed. Reconstruction of the joint surface, if possible, should be attempted. Bacterial culture should be obtained. If adequate debridement is performed, primary closure of the wound is indicated. Otherwise, it should be treated as an open wound.

Accuracy of medical record. In every gunshot fracture, if litigation is a possibility, special attention must be paid to the medical record so that it accurately reflects the clinical findings. Photos of the wound may be helpful. Accurate descriptions of the injury, the surgical procedure(s), and clinical care should be recorded. Good-quality radiographs documenting the fracture, the repair, and the healing are important. Projectiles that are retrieved from the site should be identified and the chain of custody of the bullets documented.[8]

Fracture Fixation

The choice of an implant used to stabilize a gunshot fracture is at the surgeon's discretion. The selection depends on the severity of the fracture, the bone that is fractured, and the surgeon's experience. An external skeletal fixator is an excellent choice for many comminuted long bone fractures (Fig. 10-11). Placement must allow at least two transfixation pins above and below the fracture. Entrance and exit wounds may be more easily treated when an external fixator is used. A bone plate and screws may also be used. One drawback to bone plating is the further trauma to the soft tissues that occurs when applying the plate. In some type I gunshot fractures, intramedullary pin(s) and wire may be a good choice for fracture fixation.

The prognosis for gunshot fractures depends on the type.[24] The primary determinants of fracture healing are the degree of comminution and the stability of the fracture. A type I fracture has a good to excellent prognosis. Type II has a fair to good prognosis. Type III has a guarded prognosis.

As with all fractures, complications may occur with gunshot fractures. Type I and II fractures are unlikely to develop nonunions. Prolonged healing of types I and II is unusual. These fractures should heal in 8 weeks or less.[24] However, type III fractures have a greater potential to become a nonunion. A healing period of greater than 14 weeks is not unusual.[24] Reasons for this delayed healing include cortical defects, avascularity of the bone caused by soft tissue detachment, and inadequate fixation. Infection is also a greater risk in type III fractures because of the soft tissue injury and damage to the vascular supply of the bone. In some type III injuries, the loss of soft tissue may require reconstructive procedures to cover exposed bone. Finally, amputation may be necessary in some complicated cases.

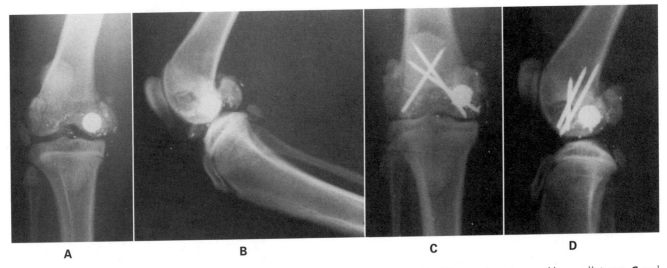

Fig. 10-10   **A** and **B,** Preoperative radiographs of an intraarticular fracture of the distal femur of a cat caused by a pellet gun. **C** and **D,** Immediate postoperative radiographs of the intraarticular fracture after repair with three small pins. The pellet was not removed because it was not intraarticular.

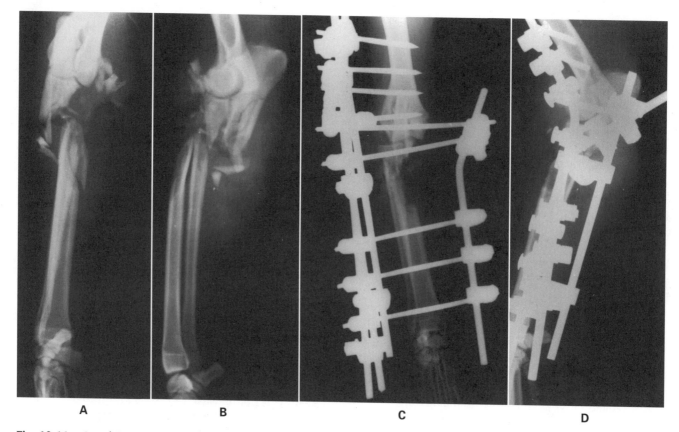

Fig. 10-11 **A** and **B,** Preoperative radiographs of a gunshot, grade III, open proximal radial and ulnar fracture in a dog. **C** and **D,** Immediate postoperative radiographs of the open radial and ulnar fracture after stabilization with a transarticular type II external fixator. The final outcome was limb amputation.

REFERENCES

1. Amato JJ, and others: High velocity missile injury: an experimental study of the retentive forces of tissue, *Am J Surg* 127:454-459, 1974.
2. Ashby ME: Low-velocity gunshot wounds involving the knee joint: surgical management, *J Bone Joint Surg (Am)* 56:1047-1053, 1974.
3. Bardet JF, Hohn RB, Basinger R: Open drainage and delayed autogenous cancellous bone grafting for treatment of chronic osteomyelitis in dogs and cats, *J Am Vet Med Assoc* 183:312-317, 1983.
4. Brown PW: The open fracture: cause, effect and management, *Clin Orthop* 96:254-265, 1973.
5. Caywood DD, Wallace LJ, Braden TD: Osteomyelitis in the dog: a review of 67 cases, *J Am Vet Med Assoc* 172:943-946, 1978.
6. DeMuth WE Jr: The mechanism of shotgun wounds, *J Trauma* 11:219-229, 1971.
7. DeMuth WE Jr, Smith JM: High-velocity bullet wounds of muscle and bone: the basis of rational early treatment, *J Trauma* 6:744-755, 1966.
8. Dixon DS: Gunshot wounds: forensic implications in a surgical practice. In Ordog GJ, editor: *Management of gunshot wounds,* New York, 1988, Elsevier.
9. Evarts CM, Mayer PJ: Complications. In Rockwood CA Jr, Green DP, editors: *Fractures in adults,* ed 2, Philadelphia, 1984, Lippincott.
10. Gustilo RB, Anderson JT: Prevention of infection in the treatment of one thousand and twenty-five open fractures of long bones, *J Bone Joint Surg (Am)* 58:453-458, 1976.
11. Hennessy MJ, and others: Extremity gunshot wound and gunshot fracture in civilian practice, *Clin Orthop Rel Res* 114:296-303, 1976.
12. Huelke DF, Darling JH: Bone fractures produced by bullets, *J Forensic Sci* 9:461-469, 1964.
13. Kahn DS, Pritzker KPH: The pathophysiology of bone infection, *Clin Orthop* 96:12-19, 1973.
14. Ledgerwood AM: The management of shotgun wounds, *Surg Clin North Am* 57(1):111-120, 1977.
15. Merritt K: Factors increasing the risk of infection in patients with open fractures, *Trauma* 28:823-827, 1988.
16. Mizuno K, and others: The osteogenic potential of fracture haematoma, *J Bone Joint Surg (Br)* 72:822-829, 1990.
17. Muller ME, Allgower M, Willenegger H: Compound fractures in the adult. In Muller ME, Allgower M, Willenegger H, editors: *Manual of internal fixation: technique recommended by the AO-group,* New York, 1970, Springer-Verlag.
18. Ndikuwera J, Winstanley EW: High pressure pulsatile lavage and high pressure syringe lavage in the treatment of contaminated wounds in dogs, *J Small Anim Pract* 26:3-15, 1985.
19. Ordog GJ: Wound ballistics. In Ordog GJ, editor: *Management of gunshot wounds,* New York, 1988, Elsevier.
20. Patzakis MJ, Wilkins J, Moore TM: Use of antibiotics in open tibial fractures, *Clin Orthop* 178:31-35, 1983.
21. Pavletic MM: Gunshot wounds in veterinary medicine: projectile ballistics. Part I, *Compend Cont Educ Pract Vet* 8:47-60, 1986.
22. Renegar WR, Stoll SG: Gunshot wounds involving the canine carpus: surgical management, *J Am Anim Hosp Assoc* 16:233-239, 1980.
23. Rhinelander FW: Blood supply of healing long-bones. In Newton CD, Nunamaker DM, editors: *Textbook of small animal orthopaedics,* Philadelphia, 1985, Lippincott.
24. Schwach RP and others: Gunshot fractures of extremities: classification, management, and complications, *Vet Surg* 8:57-62, 1979.

25. Sherman RT, Parrish RA: Management of shotgun injuries: a review of 152 cases, *J Trauma* 3:76-86, 1963.

26. Smith CW and others: Osteomyelitis in the dog: a retrospective study, *J Am Anim Hosp Assoc* 14:589-592, 1978.

27. Smith MM, Vasseur PB, Saunders HM: Bacterial growth associated with metallic implants in dogs, *J Am Vet Med Assoc* 195:765-767, 1989.

28. Stead AC: Osteomyelitis in the dog and cat, *J Small Anim Pract* 25:1-13, 1984.

29. Swaim SF, Lee AH: Topical wound medications: a review, *J Am Vet Med Assoc* 190:1588-1593, 1987.

30. Swan KG, Swan RC: *Gunshot wounds: pathophysiology and management,* ed 2, Chicago, 1989, Year Book.

31. Thoresy FP, Darlow HM: The mechanisms of primary infection of bullet wounds, *Br J Surg* 54:359-361, 1967.

32. Ziperman HH: The management of soft tissue missile wounds in war and peace, *J Trauma* 1:361-367, 1961.

11

Osteomyelitis

KENNETH A. JOHNSON

Osteomyelitis is defined most narrowly as inflammation of bone and the soft tissue elements of marrow, endosteum, periosteum, and vascular channels. In most cases, however, bacterial infection is also present. Postoperative osteomyelitis is a severe complication of orthopedic surgery that concerns all surgeons. Traditionally, animals and humans with osteomyelitis have had a poor prognosis for cure because of the difficulty of completely eliminating bacteria. With recent advances in our understanding of the pathogenesis of osteomyelitis and improved treatment methods, successful control of the disease can be achieved more often. However, such treatment is not without cost, since it may be prolonged, expensive, and frustrated by recurrences.

Osteomyelitis can be classified in several ways, including by its duration and etiology. It is designated as being either acute or chronic, based on duration of clinical signs, and the physical and radiographic findings. Whereas acute hematogenous bacterial osteomyelitis is a common serious disease affecting children, it is rarely diagnosed in small animals.[41] Acute osteomyelitis in small animals occasionally follows open fractures, bite wounds, and internal fixation of fractures. However, in the vast majority of cases, osteomyelitis is not diagnosed in small animals until the disease is chronic.

ETIOLOGY

Most cases of osteomyelitis are bacterial, but occasionally, fungi, viruses, loose or degraded surgical implants, and corroded metal implants contribute to initiation of the disease. It is important to appreciate that these agents require a favorable tissue environment that potentiates development of wound infections and osteomyelitis.[44] Infection is acquired by direct inoculation, by extension of existing infection, or hematogenously (Box 11-1). Bacterial contamination during open reduction of fractures is the leading cause of osteomyelitis and was responsible for more than half the cases in several surveys.[10,22,60] Traumatic open fractures may be the source of contamination in some of these cases, but most frequently, wound contamination occurs during surgery.

BOX 11-1
ROUTES OF INFECTION IN OSTEOMYELITIS

Open reduction and internal fixation of closed
fractures
Open fractures and traumatic injuries: infection from
the scene of accident, patient, and hospital
acquired
Elective orthopedic surgery
Extension to bone of soft tissue infection: periodon-
tal disease, rhinitis, otitis media, paronychia
Animal bite and claw wounds
Penetrating foreign bodies: sticks, grass awns
Gunshot wounds
Hematogenous infections

Although these complications are serious, they are not
sufficient reason to abandon internal fixation in favor of
closed fracture treatment. An infection rate in fracture
surgery of less than 1% is a reasonable expectation for
surgeons working in proper facilities, using meticulous
aseptic techniques and atraumatic soft tissue handling.

Bacteria

Infections with β-lactamase-producing *Staphylococcus*
species predominate in bacterial osteomyelitis. *Staphylococcus* species have been isolated from 40% to 50% of
cases of osteomyelitis, often as monomicrobial infections.
More than 40% of bone infections are polymicrobial,[10,34]
but involvement of *Staphylococcus* species in these
mixed infections is unusual. Most polymicrobial bone
infections have mixtures of *Streptococcus* species, gram-
negative bacteria (*Escherichia coli, Pseudomonas,
Proteus, Klebsiella*), and sometimes anaerobic bacteria.
Many of the gram-negative organisms isolated are resistant to a wide range of antibiotics. *Nocardia, Brucella
canis,* and tuberculosis are sporadically associated with
osteomyelitis, sometimes as a hematogenous infection.[4,9,47,49]

Because of the difficulty in isolating anaerobic bacteria, some earlier studies underestimated their contribution to osteomyelitis.[10,22,49] Recent studies indicate that
anaerobic bacteria are present in at least 15% to 18% of
bone infections overall[34,55] and in 64% to 74% of cases
when appropriate methods are employed in an attempt
to isolate them.[34,60] Anaerobic bacterial infection may be
caused by a single type of organism, but more often
there is a mixture of anaerobic, facultative anaerobic, or
aerobic bacteria. Some common anaerobic isolates from
osteomyelitis in small animals are *Actinomyces, Pepto-*

streptococcus, Bacteroides, and *Fusobacterium* species.[27,34]
Other anaerobes isolated have included *Clostridium*
species and *Wolinella recta*.[27,49] Although anaerobes have
been isolated from a variety of osteomyelitis cases, they
are especially common in bone infections caused by bite
and fight wounds. This probably reflects anaerobic bacteria being normal resident flora of the canine and feline
oral cavity. Anaerobes are potent stimulants of pyogene-
sis and produce toxins that cause tissue damage.
Anaerobic infections should be considered in animals
with osteomyelitis, especially if there is foul-smelling discharge, gas in the soft tissues, extensive tissue necrosis,
and no response to aminoglycoside and quinolone antibiotic therapy.[12] Failure to culture bacteria aerobically,
especially when multiple morphological forms of gram-
stained organisms are seen in tissue smears, suggests an
anaerobic infection.[12]

Implant Corrosion

Use of a combination of internal fixation implants manufactured from different metals can produce an elec-
trolytic reaction in vivo. This can occur between
implants made from stainless steels that deviate from the
316L specification, between stainless steel and chrome-
plated steel, or between stainless steel plates and
Vitallium alloy screws.[1,46] Electrolysis accelerates corrosion, dispersing metal ions into the surrounding tissues
and producing a gray-black discoloration. Increased production of wear particles caused by fretting corrosion
between implants of different hardness contributes to
this process. Sequelae to this include marked osteolysis
of bone surrounding the implant, neoplasia, and chronic
osteomyelitis.[1,46] Although bacteria are usually isolated
from this type of chronic osteomyelitis, infection is considered to be a secondary event.

Loose Implants and Foreign Material

Loose screws, plates, pins, and wire, as well as retained
foreign material such as surgical sponges and bone wax,
cause tissue irritation and incite chronic inflammation
and localized bone resorption.[35] This facilitates development of bone infection by bacteria that contaminate the
original wound and persist intracellularly, arrive hematogenously, or colonize draining sinus tracts.[51]

Fungi

Fungal infections are often multicentric and disseminated hematogenously after pulmonary inoculation.
Systemic mycoses that often cause osseous lesions
include *Coccidioides immitis, Blastomyces dermatitidis,
Histoplasma capsulatum,* and *Cryptococcus neofor-
mans.*[59] Disseminated aspergillosis caused by infection

with *Aspergillus terreus* and *A. deflectus* causes widespread skeletal lesions[11,26] in German shepherd dogs. Single and multifocal bone lesions caused by several other ubiquitous saprophytic fungi, including *Aspergillus fumigatus, Penicillium verruculosum,* and *Phialemonium obovatum,* have been sporadically reported in German shepherd dogs.[31,37,57] Treatment of mycotic osteomyelitis is primarily based on chemotherapy.[59]

Viruses

Limited evidence indicates that some bone diseases may be viral. Canine distemper viral transcripts were detected in osteoclasts and osteoblasts from metaphyseal bone of three dogs with hypertrophic osteodystrophy.[33] Although affected dogs also have other signs of viral disease, including systemic illness and pyrexia, further conclusive research is needed.

PATHOPHYSIOLOGY
Bacterial Contamination

Bacterial contamination of bone occurs by one of several pathways (see Box 11-1). Fortunately, normal bone is quite resistant to bacterial contamination. Experimentally, osteomyelitis cannot be created readily by just injecting bacteria into bone, without also injecting sodium morrhuate (a sclerosing agent), traumatizing the marrow cavity, creating a sequestrum, injecting acrylic bone cement, or creating an unstable fracture.[3,14,32,62] Therefore, in addition to bacterial contamination, decisive factors in the initiation of osteomyelitis are soft tissue injury, bone necrosis, fracture instability, foreign material, and altered host tissue defenses.

Bacterial contamination of fracture sites, detected by culture during surgery for open reduction and internal fixation, was demonstrated in 40% of closed canine fractures and 75% of open fractures. Despite this high rate of contamination, osteomyelitis developed in only 5% of patients overall.[50] Even in fractures that heal without complications, bacteria introduced at surgery colonize the surface of metallic implants and persist despite an effective host defense system and antimicrobial chemotherapy. The same species of bacteria can be detected by culture several years later, at the time of implant removal, but osteomyelitis develops infrequently.[48]

Soft Tissue Injury and Bone Necrosis

Soft tissue coverage of bone is very important for its contribution of blood supply to normal bone, as well as for its contribution to the healing of fractures and resolution of infection.[58] External trauma, energy dissipated by fracturing bone, and surgical intervention may damage the muscles and periosteum surrounding bone, thereby diminishing bone blood flow and causing ischemia and bone necrosis. In open reduction and internal fixation of fractures, atraumatic technique is paramount in minimizing soft tissue injury. Common sources of surgical tissue injury are excessive and circumferential elevation of periosteum, forceful muscle retraction, rough application of bone reduction forceps, heat of drilling, and tissue desiccation. Loss of soft tissue coverage, especially the periosteum, through trauma or surgery, and exposure of cortical bone usually result in death of the outer part of the cortex. Although revascularization of the outer region of the cortex can occur, large pieces that separate are at risk of sequestration.[5,7] Although a sequestrum is strictly defined as an avascular cortical bone fragment, by common use sequestrum implies concomitant bacterial infection and osteomyelitis. Bone and soft tissue necrosis, sequestra, hematoma, and edema favor the localization and proliferation of bacteria.

Fractures of the radius, ulna, and tibia are at increased risk for development of postoperative osteomyelitis.[50] The minimal soft tissue coverage of distal limb bones is probably a contributory factor to the development and persistence of osteomyelitis. In humans, rotation or transfer of vascularized muscle flaps to cover exposed bone in chronic osteomyelitis, nonunions, and defects is performed to increase vascularity of bone and stimulate bone healing.[44] Muscle flap coverage of avascular cortical bone segments accelerates both revascularization and formation of new intracortical bone.[42]

Sequestration and Draining Tracts

Normally in the course of fracture healing, fragments of cortical bone devoid of soft tissue attachment and blood supply are revascularized and then either resorbed or incorporated into the callus and remodeled. In osteomyelitis, however, sequestra are colonized by bacteria, surrounded by exudate, and remain avascular. Without soft tissue attachment, sequestra are free of callus, are not subject to osteoclastic resorption, and remain unchanged in appearance radiographically for long periods. Bacteria bind to the exposed collagen matrix proteins and hydroxyapatite crystals of damaged bone.[24] Bone sialoprotein acts as a ligand and binds specifically with bacterial receptors, which ensures their adhesion in osteomyelitis.[45]

Accumulating inflammatory exudate in osteomyelitis is forced along Volkmann and Haversian canals, into the medullary cavity, and under the periosteum. This causes further necrosis of the fracture fragments and perhaps formation of additional sequestra. In young animals the periosteum is thick and easily detached from bone, which allows extensive spread of exudate along the diaphysis, with consequent sequestration of the entire diaphyseal cortex (Fig. 11-1, *A*).

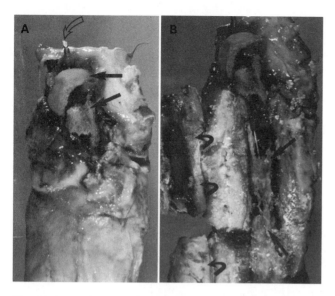

Fig. 11-1   A, Osteomyelitis of the femur in an immature dog, after open reduction and internal fixation of a fracture with an intramedullary pin (curved arrow). The femoral head and neck have sequestrated (*straight arrows*), and a thick layer of periosteal bone forms an involucrum around the diaphysis. **B,** Removal of the involucrum (*curved arrows*) reveals the intramedullary pin and sequestration of diaphyseal cortex (*straight arrows*).

Involucrum is new bone, formed predominant by the periosteum and response to infection. It encapsulates the infection and sequestrum. The quantity of involucrum is greatest in growing animals, whereas it may be negligible in adults. Regardless of the extent of involucrum, it is invariably incomplete and fenestrated, and these openings are called *cloacae*.[61] In young animals, along with involucrum formation, there may be progressive resorption of the sequestrated cortex, so the cylindrically shaped involucrum becomes the new diaphyseal cortex (Fig. 11-1, *B*).

Draining exudate from the bone follows sinus tracts that progress along fascial planes and open through the skin in a more dependent location. Flow of exudate from sinuses is usually intermittent, and in interim periods, sinuses heal. Draining sinuses are colonized by skin organisms that frequently do not represent the true pathogens involved in the osteomyelitis.[39]

Fracture Instability

Fractures and instability are each important factors in potentiating osteomyelitis whenever bacterial contamination of bone occurs. The trauma associated with fracture compromises bone blood supply, causes inflammation, and creates dead space for the accumulation of inflammatory exudate and hematoma. Instability of a fracture may be intrinsic to the method of fracture fixation or may result from implant failure or loosening. Unstable frac-

POST-TRAUMATIC OSTEOMYELITIS
THE PERPETUATING TRIAD

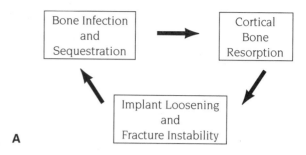

A

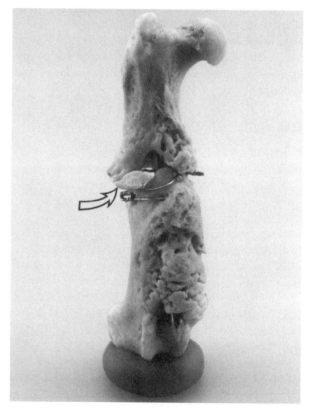

B

Fig. 11-2   A, Cyclical events that perpetuate osteomyelitis in an unstable fracture. **B,** Femoral fracture with chronic osteomyelitis 12 weeks after open reduction and internal fixation with an intramedullary pin and cerclage wires. The implants are loose, and the pin protrudes into the trochlear groove. The fracture is unstable and contains a sequestrum (*arrow*), and the cortex at the fracture has been resorbed and rounded off. Irregular, spiculated periosteal new bone, typical of chronic osteomyelitis, extends along the diaphysis.

ture fixation techniques, such as external coaptation and inadequate intramedullary pinning, allow continued interfragmentary motion (Fig. 11-2, *A*). Resorption of cortical bone at the fracture follows interfragmentary motion, and this causes widening of the fracture gap and additional instability. Implant failure and loosening are caused by technical errors in implant application, continued interfragmentary motion and bone resorption around the implant. These events in disturbed fracture healing are recognized complications of fracture instability.[56] However, when osteomyelitis is compounded upon fracture instability, bone necrosis and resorption at the fracture and around implants are greatly exacerbated[43] (Fig. 11-2, *B*).

Under some circumstances, fracture healing can occur in the presence of infection. Critical determinants are the stability of the fracture repair, preservation of soft tissue and bone blood supply, the timing of bacterial contamination with respect to fracture occurrence and internal fixation, and the chronicity of the osteomyelitis. Anatomically reduced fractures stabilized by a bone plate with interfragmentary compression that subsequently develop osteomyelitis may still proceed to fracture healing by primary union.[19,43] This knowledge is based on experimental studies of fractures that were created and repaired before bacterial contamination was introduced.[43] This is not always the situation in clinical practice. Often, bacterial contamination of the bone occurs at the time of fracture before surgical fixation. In grade III open fractures and in active osteomyelitis, the environment for fracture healing is much more hostile. Rigid fracture stabilization is needed. However, internal fixation techniques that further compromise soft tissues and bone blood supply in the region of fracture (e.g., bone plate, reamed interlocking nail) potentiate infection and delay fracture union and are contraindicated. External fixator stabilization of this type of fracture is preferred because it provides the necessary fracture stability, without surgically traumatizing the region of the fracture and osteomyelitis further.

Surgical Implants, Adherence, and Persistence of Bacteria

Surgical materials such as sponges and bone wax, as well as traumatically introduced material from the environment such as wood, soil, and asphalt, incite a foreign body response in the tissues and interfere with local host defenses.[17,35] In the presence of bacteria, these foreign materials promote development of soft tissue infection, as well as osteomyelitis when bone is nearby. Even though surgical implants composed of stainless steel, titanium, and methylmethacrylate are relatively biocompatible, they also potentiate infection in the presence of bacteria.[15,21] Bacteria successfully colonize inanimate material because of their unique mechanisms for chemical bonding of bacterial extracapsular structures to implant surfaces. The attachment of bacteria to biomaterial and development of infection involve similar mechanisms found in osteomyelitis. Both biomaterial infection and osteomyelitis occur concurrently in infected fractures with internal fixation and failed joint prostheses.

Immediately after implantation, the surfaces of biomaterials such as joint prostheses, nonabsorbable suture,

plates, and screws that are not integrated with tissue cells become coated with matrix and serum proteins, ions, cellular debris, and carbohydrates (Fig. 11-3). One of these proteins, fibronectin seems especially important in bacterial binding to biomaterial. *Fibronectin* is a ubiquitous serum and matrix protein that normally contributes to cell-to-cell attachments, cellular adhesion to implants, and clot stabilization. Staphylococci, as well as some other species of gram-positive bacteria, possess numerous cell membrane receptors for binding fibronectin molecules.[24] Staphylococci also bind fibrinogen, laminin, collagen, and fibrin.[52] Gram-negative bacteria are less effective at binding biomaterial, and binding is via a different mechanism, with pili and fimbriae specifically binding cellular proteins, matrix proteins, and glycolipids.[24]

Once adherent, bacteria have several mechanisms that ensure their persistence. Two important ones are slime production and phenotypical transformation to more virulent strains.[23,24,40] Adherent staphylococci and several other bacterial species form microcolonies and produce a slime composed of extracellular polysaccharide, ions, and nutrients. Slime, together with host-derived material, enshrouds bacterial colonies, and this material is called *biofilm* or *glycocalyx* (Fig. 11-3). Biofilm is a virulence factor because it increases adherence of bacteria to biomaterial, protects them from the action of host defenses, especially phagocytes and antibodies, and modifies antibiotic susceptibility.[24] Not all biofilms are the same, and the composition of slime is influenced by the species of bacteria producing it and the type of biomaterial. Although most antibiotics readily diffuse through biofilm, some biofilm contains increased concentrations of β-lactamase, which increases bacterial resistance. Biofilm does more than provide physical protection for the bacteria. Biofilm causes adherent bacteria to be altered phenotypically and become more virulent. Also, adherent bacteria are routinely more resistant to antibiotics than the same bacteria when assayed in culture media in vitro.

Therefore, although fractures can heal in the presence of infection provided the implants are stable,[43] removal of all implants after fracture union is usually necessary for complete resolution of osteomyelitis, since their presence provides a favorable environment for bacterial proliferation.

Antimicrobial Therapy

The traditional dogma was that osteomyelitis is difficult to cure because a blood-bone barrier prevented the passage of antibiotics from the vascular capillaries into the interstitial fluid filling the extracellular fluid compartment of bone canaliculi and Haversian and Volkmann canals. Recently, this explanation has been disproved, and the factors discussed in the previous sections are of

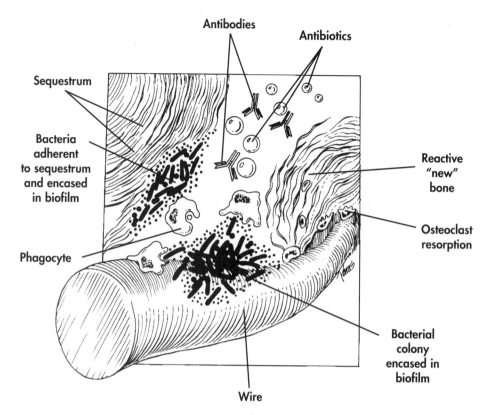

Fig. 11-3 Some gram-positive bacteria have specific receptors that bind with host-derived matrix and serum molecules on the surface of implanted biomaterials. Adherent bacteria produce a slime that, together with the host-derived material, forms a protective coating called biofilm. Colonies of adherent bacteria phenotypically transform to become more virulent and less susceptible to antibiotics and host defenses. These factors ensure persistence of infection in chronic osteomyelitis.

greater importance in explaining the refractoriness of osteomyelitis. Beta-lactam agents (penicillin, moxalactam, cephalothin, cefazolin, cefamandole), tetracycline, and aminoglycosides (gentamicin, tobramycin, netilmicin) readily traverse the capillary membrane in both normal and infected bone and are widely distributed in the interstitial fluid.[15] Peak tissue concentrations of these antibiotics are reached 25 to 45 minutes after intravenous administration in both normal and infected bone, and bone levels closely reflect the serum concentration of the antibiotic.[15] Therefore, factors other than antibiotic penetration of bone should dictate selection of an antibiotic, including toxicity, activity against the bacteria isolated, in vitro sensitivity tests, and cost.

CLINICAL SIGNS

The types of abnormalities detectable by physical examination are influenced by the duration of the bone infection. Animals with acute osteomyelitis display signs of systemic illness, including pyrexia, inappetence, dullness, and weight loss, together with neutrophilia and left shift. Heat, pain, redness, and swelling in the soft tissues, especially muscle and periosteum surrounding the infected bone, may be evident. Cortical bone, however, is incapable of displaying these classical signs of acute inflammation. Pain is a consistent feature throughout all stages of osteomyelitis, and lameness and disuse atrophy result. Fracture of the bone may contribute to pain and lameness.

After orthopedic surgery, pyrexia exceeding 48 hours, excessive pain, inflammation, and exudation may be the first signs of impending acute osteomyelitis. Deep postoperative wound infections are often indistinguishable from acute osteomyelitis because no radiographic changes are seen. The point of transition from acute to chronic osteomyelitis is somewhat arbitrary but occurs after about 8 to 15 days, beyond which time radiographic signs of bone change are evident.

The predominant sign in chronic osteomyelitis is abscess with single or multiple sinus tracts, which intermittently burst open and drain mucopurulent exudate.[10] Scar tissue may cover inactive tracts. Scarring can also result from previous surgery, open fracture, trauma, foreign body penetration, or fracture fixation by intramedullary pins or external fixator. Lymphadenopathy may be evident. Muscle atrophy, fibrosis, and contracture are also features of chronic disease. Systemic signs of inappetence, lethargy, and pyrexia, or hematological changes are frequently not present. Pathological fracturing of a vertebra or the spread of infection can cause spinal cord injury and neurological deficits. Peripheral nerve deficits can result from soft tissue swelling, but more often they are produced by the original trauma or surgery that led to osteomyelitis. Limb deformity and crepitus are present when fracture or nonunion coexists with osteomyelitis.

DIAGNOSIS

The clinical signs of acute and chronic osteomyelitis can mimic those of other diseases, such as panosteitis, hypertrophic osteodystrophy, and neoplasia, so additional diagnostic aids may be required. Usually the diagnosis can be made from the history, physical examination, radiology, bacteriology, or some combination of these.

Radiology

Radiographs are essential in the diagnosis of osteomyelitis and for evaluation of sequestra, involucra, and concomitant fractures.[17,54] The findings depend on the stage of disease (acute or chronic), age of animal, type of bone involved, cause of osteomyelitis, and types of organisms involved. In acute osteomyelitis, only soft tissue swelling is seen initially. A change occurs in the external contour of the limb soft tissues, as well as loss of definition between fascial and muscle planes.

Discospondylitis is usually a hematogenous osteomyelitis, although the acute phase is rarely recognized in animals. Discospondylitis can occur at any level of the spine and involve multiple sites. Most cases are caused by *Staphylococcus* species, and 75% of dogs have positive blood cultures.[28] In some geographical regions, *Brucella canis* is involved. Radiographic changes are localized to the intervertebral disk, end-plates, and adjacent vertebral bodies.

Chronic osteomyelitis is said to be present when radiographic evidence of bone changes is seen. In immature animals, these changes are seen as early as 5 to 10 days because of the responsiveness of the periosteum, but in adults they appear later. Periosteal new bone formation is an early sign. Unlike the smooth callus formed after trauma and fracture surgery, it tends to be more extensive, spiculated, and radially orientated on the bone's surface. This new bone, or involucrum, can partially encapsulate the cortex and focus of bone infection and may cause the bone to appear sclerotic. Bone resorption is another early finding, and cortices subsequently become osteoporotic, thinner, and rounded off at fracture lines. Resorption of medullary bone appears as a patchy radiolucency, with scalloping of the endosteal cortex. In young animals the entire diaphyseal cortex may be quickly resorbed and replaced by a shell of involucrum (see Fig. 11-1). The finding of sequestrated cortical bone, free of any surrounding callus, is common and virtually diagnostic for chronic osteomyelitis (Fig. 11-4). Sequestra may be small and obscured by surrounding involucrum, making them difficult to appreciate. However, sequestration should always be suspected in cases of persistent bone infection. Several radiographic examinations at long intervals may be needed to identify a sequestrum. Increased medullary density indicates endosteal new bone formation, and although a sign of bone response to infection, it is not an accurate predictor of infection resolution. Radiographic changes lag several months behind events at the cellular level and thus should be interpreted in conjunction with other findings before concluding that osteomyelitis has resolved.

In internally fixed fractures that are complicated by osteomyelitis, the key signs are evidence of fracture instability and implant loosening. Infection delays fracture healing, although union can occur provided the fracture remains stable. Signs of instability are widening of the fracture gap, loss of fracture reduction, rounded ends of bone, increased opacity of bone ends, a halo of radiolucency in the bone around implants, and change in position of implants relative to the bone or one another. Fracture nonunion from instability can be difficult to distinguish radiographically from nonunion caused by infection, and bacteriology becomes essential in these cases.

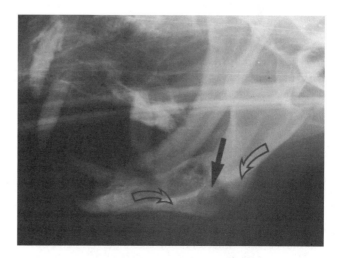

Fig. 11-4 Chronic osteomyelitis caused by anaerobic bacteria involving the mandible in a cat. A localized area of lysis containing a sequestrum (*arrow*) is surrounded by a buttress of periosteal new bone (*curved arrows*). The overlying soft tissues are swollen.

Reproduced with permission from Johnson KA and others: Osteomyelitis in dogs and cats caused by anaerobic bacteria, *Aust Vet J* 61:57-61, 1984.

Contrast radiography is sometimes useful for delineation of the course and extent of sinuses, as well as the location of radiolucent foreign bodies. The aim is to trace the sinus back to the bone and precisely identify the region of actively infected bone or sequestrum. This information is helpful in planning surgical drainage and debridement when extensive lysis and new bone production have occurred throughout the bone and it is not clear which region is currently active. A sinogram is performed by slowly injecting 10 to 20 ml of a water-soluble contrast media such as Angiovist 292 through a Foley catheter. A Foley catheter is inserted into each sinus opening, and the balloon of each catheter is inflated to prevent leakage of contrast onto the skin. Contrast leakage produces confusing radiographic images. Incomplete filling of sinuses with contrast is the major source of false-negative studies.

Radionuclide imaging of the bone after Indium-111 labeling of leukocytes is the most sensitive and specific noninvasive means of detecting osteomyelitis. Indium-111 imaging is especially useful in the diagnosis of acute osteomyelitis before radiographic changes are seen, as well as in chronic osteomyelitis when radiographic signs are equivocal. Although expensive and not widely available for use in animals, this technique may become useful in the future.[29]

Cytology

Cytology is valuable in the early detection of acute osteomyelitis and postoperative wound infection before radiographic changes are obvious in bone. Smears of serum, hematoma, or inflammatory exudate obtained by sterile aspiration centesis are stained with Difco Quick to look for toxic neutrophils and phagocytosed bacteria.

Bacteriology

Isolation of bacteria from suspected bone infections should be attempted. Bacterial identification is helpful in confirming the diagnosis. More importantly, in vitro sensitivity testing is a valuable guide to selection of antibiotic chemotherapy. In chronic osteomyelitis, antibiotic therapy should be withheld for at least 3 days before attempting bacterial culture and sensitivity testing.

Cultures of pus from externally draining tracts are an inaccurate indication of the true pathogens involved in osteomyelitis because draining tracts become colonized by skin organisms and gram-negative bacteria. In suspected surgical wound infections, cultures can be made of fluid collected by sterile aspiration from deep within the tissues. In chronic infections, fluid, necrotic tissue, and sequestra collected from deep within the wound at the time of surgical debridement provide the most accurate source of information on the pathogens involved.

Both aerobic and anaerobic cultures should be done routinely. Samples for aerobic culture that can be taken to the laboratory and plated out on agar within 10 to 15 minutes are collected into a sterile container. Fluid for anaerobic culture is aspirated into a syringe, all air is expelled, and the needle is capped with a rubber stopper to exclude oxygen. Specimens for anaerobic culture require special handling because even minutes in an aerobic environment can kill some sensitive anaerobes and prevent subsequent isolation.

If the delay in plating out samples is more than 15 minutes, tissue samples and swabs are placed into a reduced Cary-Blair, solidified anaerobic holding media (BBL Port-A-Cul tubes) so that oxygen is excluded. Fluid samples are injected through the rubber stopper into anaerobic transport vials containing reduced Cary-Blair media (BBL Port-A-Cul vials). Specimens transported in these anaerobic media can be used for isolation of aerobes and anaerobes because, except for some *Pseudomonas* species, aerobic bacteria are facultative anaerobes. Regular bacterial transport media are not suitable for isolation of anaerobes.

Histopathology

Histopathological examination of tissue and bone biopsies is performed to differentiate neoplasia and other

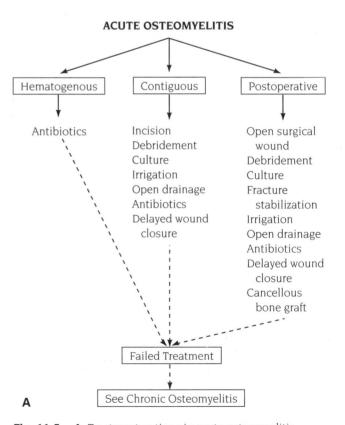

Fig. 11-5 **A,** Treatment options in acute osteomyelitis.

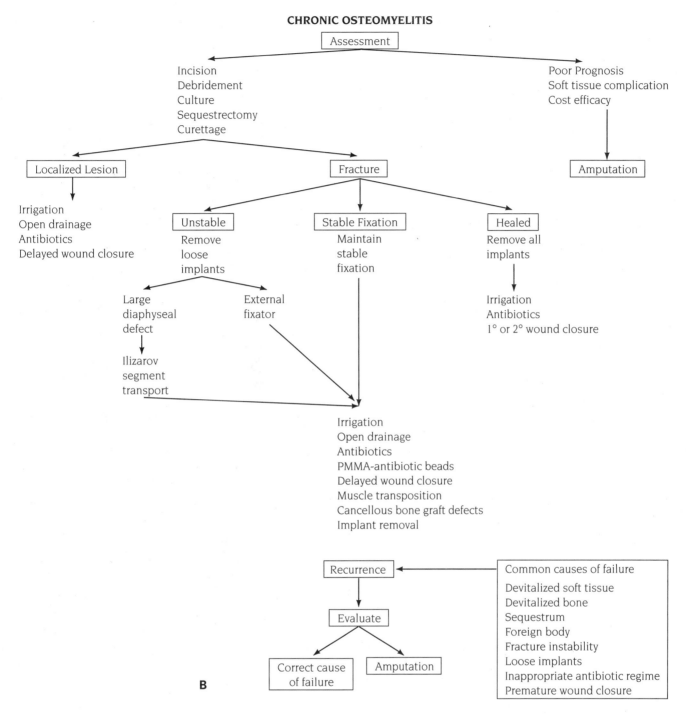

CHRONIC OSTEOMYELITIS

Fig. 11-5, cont'd. **B,** Treatment options in chronic osteomyelitis.

diseases from bone infection. Methenamine silver and periodic acid-Schiff-stained tissue sections are used to demonstrate fungal hyphae.

Hematology

Alterations in the hemogram may be consistent with systemic infection in acute osteomyelitis, but the hemogram is invariably unremarkable in chronic osteomyelitis.

TREATMENT

Having established the diagnosis, successful resolution can be a challenge. A treatment regimen is planned, taking into account the etiology, chronicity, location, and severity of the bone infection. Basic treatment options are summarized in Fig. 11-5. With more difficult cases, such as chronic bacterial osteomyelitis with concurrent fracture, clients must be well informed from the outset about the implications of embarking on such a course.

Physical examination and assessment of soft tissues, especially in regard to vascularity, peripheral nerve injury, muscle contracture, joint stiffness, and pain, may determine immediately if a cure is feasible or amputation is indicated. In phalangeal osteomyelitis, immediate digit amputation is an accepted treatment. Also, chronic osteomyelitis localized to the sternum, thoracic wall, mandible, or maxilla can be treated by en bloc resection of the infection with a margin of healthy tissue and primary wound closure.[18]

Acute osteomyelitis and chronic discospondylitis can be cured with antibiotics alone provided there is limited bone necrosis and no fracture. Discospondylitis is treated by antibiotic therapy for at least 4 to 6 weeks. Except for animals with neurological deficits, it is debatable whether surgical intervention or curettage of the disk is necessary.[28]

Except in the cases just mentioned, the temptation to treat osteomyelitis with antibiotics alone should be resisted. A cure is more likely when the following principles are considered and applied appropriately.

Debridement and Drainage

Soft tissue infections developing after surgery or associated with open fractures, trauma, and bites are immediately managed as if acute osteomyelitis exists, since delays in appropriate treatment invariably lead to chronic osteomyelitis. Infected surgical wounds are extensively opened by removal of the sutures using aseptic technique. Necrotic muscle, fascia, hematoma, foreign material, and nonfunctional sutures are debrided. Similarly, bites and traumatic wounds are opened and drained using a surgical incision that preserves vital structures and allows dependent drainage. Atraumatic technique and preservation of soft tissue and periosteal viability are paramount. Viable periosteum should not be removed from the bone, and any exposed bone is covered with viable muscle, if possible.

Chronically infected bone is exposed by a conventional surgical approach to remove sequestra and debride necrotic soft tissue. Necrotic muscle can be debrided vigorously, but a conservative approach is taken to removal of periosteum, ligament, and tendon. In fractures, loose unattached fragments of cortical bone usually must be removed. However, in the main fracture fragments, the demarcation between viable and dead cortex is not easily distinguished because cortical bone normally has a relatively low blood flow. Some devitalized cortical bone can be later remodeled if fracture stability and healing are achieved. Therefore, repeated surgical debridement with sequential resection of bone may be necessary until it becomes clear exactly how much cortex must be excised. A careful search for sequestra is crucial for suc-

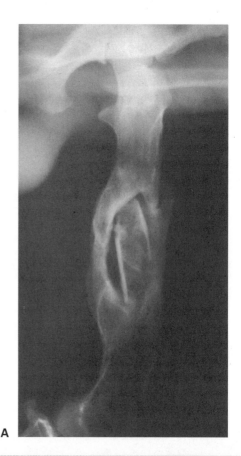

A

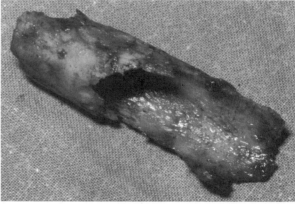

B

Fig. 11-6   A, Healed middiaphyseal femoral fracture that had been originally stabilized with an intramedullary pin. After 4 months, a chronic discharging sinus developed at the caudolateral aspect of the stifle joint. A large sequestrum, lying in a lytic cavity surrounded by an involucrum, is diagnostic of chronic osteomyelitis. **B,** Sequestrum removed at surgery.

cess. Sequestra are usually completely free of soft tissue or bone attachments, surrounded by pus or granulation tissue, and yellow colored (Fig. 11-6). The involucrum is elevated with an osteotome only if necessary to reach sequestra and establish drainage. Otherwise, this healthy reactive bone is preserved. It contributes to fracture union and is remodeled once the infection is resolved.

Sequestra and samples of pus and necrotic tissue are collected for bacteriology. Sequestra may migrate and become trapped within a draining sinus some distance from the original infection. Since draining sinuses are lined by modified fibrous tissue and not a secretory lining, it is unnecessary to excise all of them. The main reason to follow the tracts with a probe is to find migrating sequestra. Intravenous injection of vital dyes such as methylene blue or disulphan blue before surgery to aid identification of sequestra has been described. However, acute renal failure is a potential complication of intravenously injected methylene blue, so the technique is best avoided.[36]

Irrigation

Wounds are irrigated intraoperatively with 1 to 2 L of sterile physiological saline, under pressure with a 60 ml syringe. At the end of debridement, wounds are left open for drainage and irrigation. Closure with sutures is contraindicated. Metallic implants can be left exposed but should be covered with a sterile dressing. The value of this method of open wound treatment cannot be overstated. Closed-suction drainage systems and Penrose drains are contraindicated because they provide inconsistent drainage and potentiate ascending infections and abscessation.

Daily irrigation with sterile saline or 0.05% chlorhexidine in sterile water (1:40 dilution) is repeated using sterile technique until infection is controlled (Fig. 11-7). Sedation with acetylpromazine (0.05 to 0.1 mg/kg intramuscularly) and oxymorphone (0.01 to 0.02 mg/kg intramuscularly) may be adequate to accomplish daily irrigations, but general anesthesia is needed for more extensive debridement. Between wound treatments, the open wound is protected with wet-to-dry dressings of saline-moistened sterile gauze sponges and a dry, thick, padded outer layer of absorbent dressing. Coverage of denuded bone, neurovascular bundles, ligament, tendon, and articular cartilage with saline-moistened gauze prevents desiccation. Incisions on the trunk or upper limbs are protected with a tie-over bandage. Elizabethan collars provide further wound protection. After 5 or more days, wound closure with granulation tissue begins to occur. In fact, this may occur too rapidly and prevent proper drainage and irrigation, necessitating reopening of the wound.

Fracture Stability

Bone can heal in the presence of infection provided there is stable fixation, although union is delayed. If the fracture fixation is stable, osteomyelitis is treated without

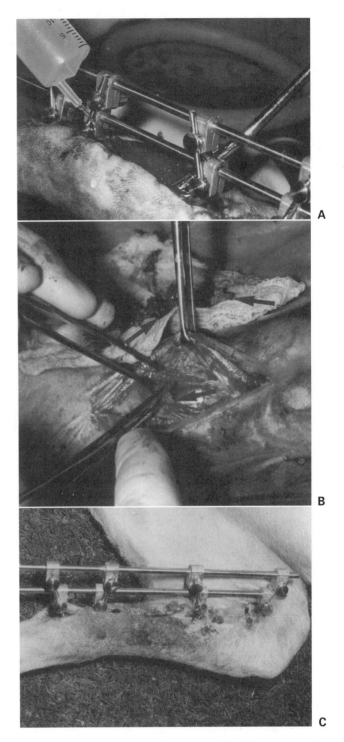

Fig. 11-7 **A,** Osteomyelitis in an open tibial fracture 2 weeks after debridement and stabilization with a type I double-bar external fixator. The open wound, which is now filled with healthy granulation tissue, is being lavaged with sterile saline. **B,** Autologous cancellous bone grafting (*arrows*) of the fracture via a separate approach through normal tissues on the lateral side of the tibia. **C,** Healed tibial fracture and wound after 10 weeks of treatment.

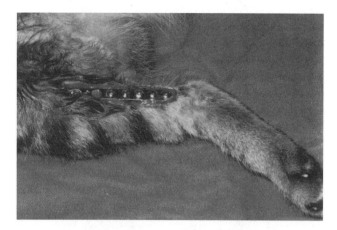

Fig. 11-8 Healed comminuted tibial fracture 6 months postoperatively, just prior to plate removal. Acute osteomyelitis had complicated the initial fracture fixation. Although the plate became exposed, it maintained fracture stability and was therefore maintained until the fracture was completely healed.

removal of the implants, until fracture healing or implant loosening occurs. Even plates that have become exposed should be left in place, if stable, until the fracture is healed (Fig. 11-8).

Loose implants lead to the triad of fracture instability, persistence of infection, and bone resorption. Loose implants are removed immediately, and the fracture is stabilized with some other device. Also, implants composed of dissimilar metals responsible for corrosion and osteomyelitis must be removed. External skeletal fixation is the preferred method of providing both temporary and definitive fracture stability in the tibia, mandible, and radius/ulna when active osteomyelitis exists (see Fig. 11-7). Advantages of external skeletal fixation are that fracture stability is maintained while easy access to the soft tissues is permitted for wound management. The large muscle groups surrounding the femur and humerus allow the application of a type I or biplanar external fixator. These configurations may not provide sufficient stability for complete healing of a fracture because of excessive pin-bone stress, soft tissue necrosis around pins, pin tract osteomyelitis, and premature pin loosening. However, plate fixation can be used secondarily once infection becomes quiescent, and the external fixator is no longer effective.

Bone Defects

Cortical deficits caused by debridement, osteomyelitis, or fracture are grafted with autologous cancellous bone after 7 to 10 days once a bed of granulation tissue has been established. Cancellous bone harvested from the humerus or tibia (see Chapter 5) is inserted into the bone deficit, either under the granulation tissue of the wound or via a separate surgical approach (see Fig. 11-7). This

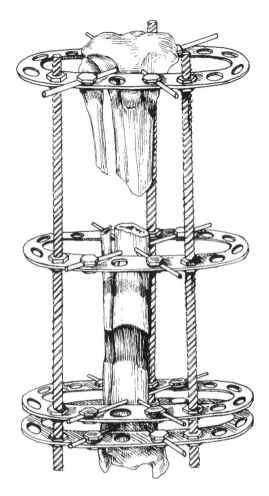

Fig. 11-9 Ilizarov technique of bone segment transport to fill a deficit after osteomyelitis. The transfixation wires are tensioned and attached to the rings with clamps to provide fracture stability and alignment. The bone segment is advanced by the progressive movement of the central ring along the threaded rods and the resultant tension in the two wires. The bone deficit created distally is filled with callus by a process of distraction osteogenesis.

approach is a modification of the Papineau technique.[2] The granulation tissue permits rapid vascularization and incorporation of the graft. Because of their porous structure, cancellous bone grafts are not at risk of sequestration and are a potent stimulus to osteogenesis.

For large diaphyseal bone deficits, the Ilizarov bone transport technique provides fracture stability and brings cortical bone into the deficit.[13,30] Ilizarov devices designed for small animals are available (Jorgensen Laboratories, Loveland, Colorado). An osteotomy is made through healthy bone in the distal metaphysis, and after a lag period of 5 to 8 days, the segment of bone is advanced proximally at a rate of 0.5 mm every 12 hours or 0.25 mm every 6 hours to fill the deficit and ultimately heal the fracture[13] (Fig. 11-9). Application of this device in small animal orthopedics has not yet gained widespread acceptance. In humans, fracture healing can be achieved by this method without any other bone grafts.[53]

Antibiotics

It is useless to proceed with the treatment of chronic osteomyelitis with antibiotics alone. Surgical drainage, sequestrectomy, microbiological culturing, and fracture stabilization must be performed meticulously if antibiotic therapy is to succeed. In the first few days after cultures are taken, when results are pending, antibiotics should be given, but the choice is empirical. The ultimate selection of an antibiotic should be one that is the least toxic, most active, and cost-effective bactericidal antibiotic of those identified by the culture and sensitivity results.[6] Cloxacillin, cefazolin, clindamycin, or amoxicillin-clavulanate may be appropriate for infections of β-lactamase-producing *Staphylococcus*. However, of this group of antibiotics, amoxicillin-clavulanate and clindamycin are the only ones that are also consistently effective against anaerobic bacteria. Approximately 20% of *Bacteroides fragilis* are resistant to the β-lactam and penicillin antibiotics. Metronidazole is highly effective in the treatment of anaerobic osteomyelitis, is bactericidal to all strains of *Bacteroides,* and is given orally.

A quinolone or aminoglycoside antibiotic is given for gram-negative infections. Although these antibiotics have some broad-spectrum activity against gram-positive bacteria, they are ineffective against anaerobes. Nephrotoxicity and ototoxicity are potential complications of the aminoglycosides, especially with long-term therapy. Another disadvantage is that they are not given orally. Ciprofloxacin, a new quinolone, may be the antibiotic of choice for serious gram-negative osteomyelitis because it can be given orally and it does not cause toxicity as do the aminoglycosides.[20,25] The principal contraindication to its use is in young animals, since ciprofloxacin may cause articular cartilage erosion.

Most of the frequently used antibiotics achieve therapeutic levels in infected bone.[15] Antibiotics are given at therapeutic dosages by intravenous or intramuscular injection for 1 week, then orally for 4 to 6 weeks[6] (Table 11-1). It may be necessary to treat with two antibiotics simultaneously. For a mixed infection of anaerobic and gram-negative bacteria, metronidazole and ciprofloxacin may be a suitable combination.

Chains of methylmethacrylate beads containing antibiotic such as gentamicin or tobramycin are effective in the local treatment of chronic osteomyelitis.[8] Once sequestrectomy and surgical debridement are complete, the beads on a stainless steel suture wire are packed into the dead space cavity. Antibiotic is eluted into the tissues for approximately 20 days. After the chain of beads is removed from the wound, the healthy granulation tissue that has formed is an ideal bed for cancellous bone graft-

Table 11-1 Antimicrobial Agents Used For Osteomyelitis

Agent	Dose (mg/kg)	Route	Interval (hours)
β-LACTAMS			
Amoxicillin	22-30	IV, IM, SC, PO	6-8
Amoxicillin-clavulanate	22	PO	6-8
Cloxacillin	30	IV, IM, PO	6-8
Oxacillin	22	IV, IM, SC, PO	6-8
CEPHALOSPORINS			
Cefadroxil	30	PO	12
Cephalexin	30	PO	12
Cefazolin	20	IV, IM, SC	6
MACROLIDES			
Clindamycin*,†	11	IV, IM, PO	8-12
QUINOLONES			
Ciprofloxacin	5-11	PO	12
Enrofloxacin	5-11	PO	12
AMINOGLYCOSIDES			
Amikacin‡,§	15	IV, IM, SC	24
Gentamicin‡,§	6	IV, IM, SC	24
Metronidazole	15	PO, IV	12

IV, Intravenous; IM, intramuscular; SC, subcutaneous; PO, oral.
*Parenteral dose every 8 hours; PO dose every 12 hours.
†Painful on intramuscular injection; can cause phlebitis if given IV.
‡Nephrotoxic and ototoxic. Renal function must be monitored throughout use.
§Limit use to 1 week.

From Budsberg, SC, Kemp, DT: Antimicrobial distribution and therapeutics in bone, *Comp Cont Educ Pract Vet* 12:1758–1762, 1990.

ing. Beads can be custom made from methylmethacrylate bone cement and an antibiotic, using a simple mold.[16]

Implantable pumps that infuse antibiotics locally into sites of chronic bone infection, along with debridement, are effective in the treatment of osteomyelitis.[38] Although expense currently limits their use, these devices may have future application.

Skin Grafts and Compound Myocutaneous Flaps

After debridement and irrigation, most wounds close with granulation tissue and contraction (see Fig. 11-7). No special wound management techniques are needed in these cases. Although second-intention healing can take weeks to months to close the wound, the final scar is often only slightly larger than that produced by a primary closure. In extensive open wounds on the distal limbs that fail to close by second-intention healing, skin grafts or myocutaneous flaps are indicated.

Implant Removal

Radiographs are taken at 2 to 4 week intervals to evaluate the fracture fixation, healing of fractures, and progress of osteomyelitis. Biofilm on the implants harbors bacteria, and thus all implants usually need to be removed once the fracture is healed to resolve the infection completely.

Recurrence

The first evidence of recurrence of chronic osteomyelitis is lameness and discharging sinuses. This can occur weeks, months, or years after the last treatment. The recurrence of osteomyelitis indicates the need to look again for sequestra, repeat debridement, or reestablish drainage, reevaluate fracture stability, perform a bone graft, repeat bacteriology, or change the type of antibiotic. Animals with osteomyelitis have a worse prognosis in cases of persisting sequestra, very extensive soft tissue and bone necrosis, concurrent fracture, large bone deficits, malnutrition, or older age.

REFERENCES

1. Bagnall BG: Reaction of dissimilar metals used in orthopaedic surgery, *J Small Anim Pract* 13:201-206, 1972.
2. Bardet JF, and others: Open drainage and delayed autogenous cancellous bone grafting for treatment of chronic osteomyelitis in dogs and cats, *J Am Vet Med Assoc* 183:312-317, 1983.
3. Braden TD, and others: Posologic evaluation of clindamycin, using a canine model of posttraumatic osteomyelitis, *Am J Vet Res* 48:1101-1105, 1987.
4. Bradney IW: Vertebral osteomyelitis due to *Nocardia* in a dog, *Aust Vet J* 62:315-316, 1985.
5. Brown PW: The fate of exposed bone, *Am J Surg* 137:464-469, 1979.
6. Budsberg SC, Kemp DT: Antimicrobial distribution and therapeutics in bone, *Comp Cont Educ Pract Vet* 12:1758-1762, 1990.
7. Burri C: *Post-traumatic osteomyelitis*, Bern, 1975, Hans Huber.
8. Calhoun JH, Mader JT: Antibiotic beads in the management of surgical infections, *Am J Surg* 157:443-449, 1989.
9. Carpenter JL, and others: Tuberculosis in five basset hounds, *J Am Vet Med Assoc* 192:1563-1568, 1988.
10. Caywood DD, and others: Osteomyelitis in the dog: a review of 67 cases, *J Am Vet Med Assoc* 172:943-946, 1978.
11. Day MJ and others: Disseminated aspergillosis in dogs, *Aust Vet J* 63:55-59, 1986.
12. Dow SW, Jones RL: Anaerobic infections. Part II. Diagnosis and treatment, *Comp Cont Educ Pract Vet* 9:827-839, 1987.
13. Ferretti A: The application of the Ilizarov technique to veterinary medicine. In Bianchi Maiocchi A, Aronson J, editors: *Operative principles of Ilizarov*, Baltimore, 1991, Williams & Wilkins.
14. Fitzgerald RH: Experimental osteomyelitis: description of a canine model and the role of depot administration of antibiotics in the prevention and treatment of sepsis, *J Bone Joint Surg (Am)* 65:371-380, 1983.
15. Fitzgerald RH, and others: Pathophysiology of osteomyelitis and pharmacokinetics of antimicrobial agents in normal and osteomyelitic bone. In Esterhai JL, Gristina AG, Poss R, editors: *Musculoskeletal infection*, Park Ridge, Ill, 1992, American Academy of Orthopaedic Surgeons.
16. Flick AB, and others: Noncommercial fabrication of antibiotic-impregnated polymethylmethacrylate beads, *Clin Orthop* 223:282-286, 1987.
17. Fossum TW, Hulse DA: Osteomyelitis, *Semin Vet Med Surg Small Anim* 7:85-97, 1992.
18. Fossum TW, and others: Partial sternectomy for sternal osteomyelitis in the dog, *J Am Anim Hosp Assoc* 25:435-441, 1989.
19. Friedrich B, Klaue P: Mechanical stability and post-traumatic osteitis: an experimental evaluation of the relation between infection of bone and internal fixation, *Injury* 9:23-29, 1978.
20. Greene CE, Budsberg SC: Veterinary use of quinolones. In Hooper DC, Wolfson JS, editors: *Quinolone antimicrobial agents*, ed 2, Washington, DC, 1993, American Society for Microbiology.
21. Grewe SR, and others: Influence of internal fixation on wound infections, *J Trauma* 27:1051-1054, 1987.
22. Griffiths GL, Bellenger CR: A retrospective study of osteomyelitis in dogs and cats, *Aust Vet J* 55:587-591, 1979.
23. Gristina AG, Costerton JW: Bacterial adherence to biomaterials and tissue: the significance of its role in clinical sepsis, *J Bone Joint Surg (Am)* 67:264-273, 1985.
24. Gristina AG, and others: Molecular mechanisms of musculoskeletal sepsis. In Esterhai JL, Gristina AG, Poss R, editors: *Musculoskeletal infection*, Park Ridge, Ill, 1992, American Academy of Orthopaedic Surgeons.
25. Hessen MT, Levison ME: Ciprofloxacin for the treatment of osteomyelitis: a review, *J Foot Surg* 28:100-105, 1989.
26. Jang SS, and others: *Aspergillus deflectus* infection in four dogs, *J Med Vet Mycol* 24:95-104, 1986.
27. Johnson KA, and others: Osteomyelitis in dogs and cats caused by anaerobic bacteria, *Aust Vet J* 61:57-61, 1984.
28. Kornegay JL, Barber DL: Diskospondylitis in dogs, *J Am Vet Med Assoc* 177:337-341, 1980.
29. Lamb CR: Bone scintigraphy in small animals, *J Am Vet Med Assoc* 191:1616-1622, 1987.
30. Lesser AS: Segmental bone transport for the treatment of bone deficits, *J Am Anim Hosp Assoc* 30:322-330, 1994.
31. Lomax LG, and others: Osteolytic phaeohyphomycosis in a German shepherd dog caused by *Phialemonium obovatum*, *J Clin Microbiol* 23:987-991, 1986.
32. Mader JT: Animal models of osteomyelitis, *Am J Med* 78 (suppl 6B):213-217, 1985.
33. Mee AP, and others: Canine distemper virus transcripts detected in the bone cells of dogs with metaphyseal osteopathy, *Bone* 14:59-67, 1993.
34. Muir P, Johnson KA: Anaerobic bacteria isolated from osteomyelitis in dogs and cats, *J Vet Surg* 21:463-466, 1992.
35. Nelson DR, and others: The promotional effect of bone wax on experimental *Staphylococcus aureus* osteomyelitis, *J Thorac Cardiovasc Surg* 99:977-980, 1990.
36. Osuna DJ, and others: Acute renal failure after methylene blue infusion in a dog, *J Am Anim Hosp Assoc* 26:410-412, 1990.
37. Oxenford CJ, Middleton DJ: Osteomyelitis and arthritis associated with *Aspergillus fumigatus* in a dog, *Aust Vet J* 63:59-60, 1986.
38. Perry CR, and others: Local delivery of antibiotics via an implantable pump in the treatment of osteomyelitis, *Clin Orthop* 226:222-230, 1988.
39. Perry CR, and others: Accuracy of cultures of material from swabbing of the superficial aspect of the wound and needle biopsy in the preoperative assessment of osteomyelitis, *J Bone Joint Surg (Am)* 73:745-749, 1991.
40. Proctor RA: The staphylococcal fibronectin receptor: evidence for its importance in invasive infections, *Rev Infect Dis* 9 (suppl 4):S335-S340, 1987.
41. Read RA, and others: Generalized osteomyelitis in a dog: a case report, *J Small Anim Pract* 24:687-694, 1983.

42. Richards RR, and others: The influence of muscle flap coverage on the repair of devascularized tibial cortex: an experimental investigation in the dog, *Plast Reconst Surg* 79:946-956, 1987.

43. Rittman WW, Perren SM: *Cortical bone healing after internal fixation and infection: biomechanics and biology*, Berlin, 1974, Springer-Verlag.

44. Roesgen M, and others: Post-traumatic osteomyelitis, *Arch Orthop Trauma Surg* 108:1-9, 1989.

45. Ryden C, and others: Selective binding of bone matrix sialoprotein to *Staphylococcus aureus* in osteomyelitis, *Lancet* 2:515, 1987.

46. Sinibaldi KR, and others: Osteomyelitis and neoplasia associated with use of the Jonas intramedullary splint in small animals, *J Am Vet Med Assoc* 181:885-890, 1982.

47. Smeak DD, and others: *Brucella canis* osteomyelitis in two dogs with total hip replacements, *J Am Vet Med Assoc* 191:986-990, 1987.

48. Smith MM, and others: Bacterial growth associated with metallic implants in dogs, *J Am Vet Med Assoc* 195:765-767, 1989.

49. Stead AC: Osteomyelitis in the dog and cat, *J Small Anim Pract* 25:1-13, 1984.

50. Stevenson S, and others: Bacterial culturing for prediction of postoperative complications following open fracture repair in small animals, *J Vet Surg* 15:99-102, 1986.

51. Teague HD, and others: Two cases of foreign-body osteomyelitis secondary to retained surgical sponges, *Vet Med Small Anim Clin* 73: 1279-1286, 1978.

52. Vercelotti GM, and others: Extracellular matrix proteins (fibronectin, laminin, and type IV collagen) bind and aggregate bacteria, *Am J Pathol* 120:13-21, 1985.

53. Villa A: Nonunion: principles of treatment. In Bianchi Maiocchi A, Aronson J, editors: *Operative principles of Ilizarov*, Baltimore, 1991, Williams & Wilkins.

54. Walker MA, and others: Radiographic signs of bone infection in small animals, *J Am Vet Med Assoc* 166:908-910, 1975.

55. Walker RD, and others: Anaerobic bacteria associated with osteomyelitis in domestic animals, *J Am Vet Med Assoc* 182:814-816, 1983.

56. Weller S: Instability of osteosynthesis and disturbed fracture healing, *Vet Comp Orthop Trauma* 2:92-97, 1989.

57. Wigney DI, and others: Osteomyelitis associated with *Penicillium verruculosum* in a German shepherd dog, *J Small Anim Pract* 31:449-452, 1990.

58. Wilson JW: Vascular supply to normal bone and healing fractures, *Semin Vet Med Surg Small Anim* 6:26-38, 1991.

59. Wolf AM, Troy GC: Deep mycotic diseases. In Ettinger SJ, Feldman EC, editors: *Textbook of veterinary internal medicine*, ed 4, Philadelphia, 1995, WB Saunders.

60. Wong WT, Mason TA: Survey of 44 cases of canine osteomyelitis, *Aust Vet Practitioner* 14:149-151, 1984.

61. Woodard JC, Riser WH: Morphology of fracture nonunion and osteomyelitis, *Vet Clin North Am Small Anim Pract* 21:813-844, 1991.

62. Worlock P: An experimental model of post-traumatic osteomyelitis in rabbits, *Br J Exp Pathol* 69:235-244, 1988.

12

Malunion, Delayed Union, and Nonunion

C. WILLIAM BETTS

MALUNION

A malunion results when a bone heals in an abnormal position.[34] Malunions can be classified as functional or nonfunctional, depending on whether the bone heals in a physiological or nonphysiological position (Fig. 12-1).[24,30] Some breeds of dogs tolerate rotational and angular deformities, limb shortening, or a combination better than other breeds because of their inherent conformation. A bassett hound with more than 10 degrees of external rotation and lateral angulation in one forelimb beyond what is normal for the breed may function well. A narrow-chested, straight-legged breed such as an Afghan hound might develop carpal joint and ligament problems from the same degree of abnormal limb position.

Many malunions do not interfere with limb function but are not acceptable to owners critical of breed conformation. In general, external rotational deformities less than 10 degrees cause little problem, but internal rotation is more difficult for the animal to adjust to and may cause a clinical problem. Many physeal injuries result from fractures that heal normally, but the premature physeal closure causes an angular limb deformity. The surgical correction may not totally reestablish normal bone conformation, but the healed fracture is not considered a malunion.

Cause

Asynchronous growth. Types I to IV Salter fractures may result in a malunion with angular or rotational components from asynchronous growth within the injured

277

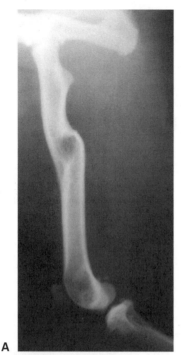

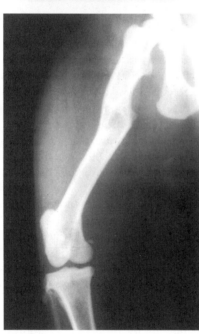

Fig. 12-1 Malunion of the femur. **A,** Lateral view of a healed femoral malunion. **B,** Craniocaudal view of a healed femoral malunion. Note the lateral angulation of the distal femur with external rotation of the femoral condyles.

physis during fracture healing. Type V fractures cause limb shortening in a one bone system such as a distal femoral physeal injury but also may cause rotational and angular deformity in a two-bone system (see Chapter 13). The latter is not considered a malunion, since the deformity develops after the fracture healing. Closed

management of physeal injuries is acceptable if the fracture is well reduced, but early reduction and stabilization are essential to reduce the chance of developing a malunion or worse, a nonunion.[17]

Insufficient/inappropriate fixation. In the distal limb, coaptation may cause a malunion if special attention is not paid to reestablishing normal limb alignment. Most often, a valgus position of the limb results if the animal is in lateral recumbency with the coapted limb uppermost. If the person applying the splint is right-handed, the left forelimb is externally rotated and the right forelimb internally rotated. Animals supinate more than they pronate. An assistant can easily counter these rotational forces, and the lateral deviation can be corrected by molding the coaptation device. If these tendencies are not recognized and prevented, the limb may be coapted in external rotation and be laterally deviated. This problem can be avoided by placing the dog with the injured limb down and wrapping in the direction of pronation. The olecranon, the accessory carpal pad, and the toes should all be in a neutral alignment with the limb. It is acceptable for the foot to be in slight varus, especially in immature animals.

Open reduction and fixation do not ensure that a malunion will not develop. The forces acting on a given fracture must be countered. Because of the pull of the iliopsoas muscle and the external rotators of the hip, the proximal fragment of a fractured femur externally rotates. This is most difficult to appreciate in comminuted fractures with denuded fragments when anatomical reconstruction is not possible. The external rotation of the proximal fragment should be anticipated and the distal fragment(s) positioned accordingly when it is not possible to use fracture reconstruction as an alignment guide. If the pull of the external rotators of the hip is not countered, the hip comes back to a normal position, causing internal rotation of the stifle when the fracture heals. The limb appears to be knock-kneed, and abnormal stress is placed on the stifle and tarsal joints. Transverse to slightly oblique femoral shaft fractures move to this position after anatomical reduction with an inadequate implant, such as an intramedullary pin used alone, because rotational forces are not countered. Angular deformities can also result when implants are too small or malpositioned.

Treatment

Nonsurgical management. If the function of the affected limb is acceptable, the owner should be encouraged to accept the malunion. The animal's weight should be kept down and its activity supervised if there is concern that abnormal stress is placed on adjacent structures, especially joints.

It is preferable to avoid a malunion when possible rather than correct one. Fractures managed by closed reduction and coaptation or by open reduction and internal fixation should be evaluated by making immediate post-reduction radiographs and then following the progress of fracture healing at accepted intervals. If a problem is seen, axis (angular) or rotational malalignment can often be corrected early with minimal disruption of ongoing healing.[34]

Surgical correction. It is possible to surgically correct established malunions that are causing limb dysfunction if attendant soft tissue changes do not preclude satisfactory return to function.[30,50] When surgery is performed on a healthy animal with healthy intact bone, good results are anticipated. Corrective osteotomies are required, and careful planning should be done before surgery. These procedures can be technically demanding and often require sophisticated equipment. This creates an open fracture, and all the sequelae of infection, delayed union, and nonunion can result.[34] The decision to recommend a corrective osteotomy should be considered carefully and the client advised accordingly.

Postoperative management. Osteotomy for correction of a malunion requires the same postoperative management provided for any fracture repair. Because of soft tissue changes that may have developed as a result of the malunion, physical therapy may be a more important component of the postoperative management than with primary fracture repair. As with all fracture repair, early return to function is desired. This mandates stable fixation.

DELAYED UNION

Delayed union is an intermediate stage in fracture healing that can proceed to union or nonunion, depending on the surgeon's skill and knowledge.[7] A fracture is considered a delayed union when it fails to heal within the normal time for the particular bone, type of fracture, location within the bone, age of the animal, and the type of fixation used.[9,22] Delayed union therefore can be defined as the condition that exists in a fracture that has not healed (or is not healing) in the time normally required for that particular bone and that type of fracture.[2]

The anticipated times for fracture healing of different bones are influenced by several factors. Fractures heal more rapidly in young animals, in metaphyseal and epiphyseal areas because of abundant blood supply, and when periosteal callus supports cortical callus.[9] Increased healing time should be expected when there is extensive comminution with devascularized fragments, cortical defects after repair, rigid internal fixation with anatomical reduction that results in primary bone

healing, and when cortical allografts are used. This does not establish that the particular fracture should be considered a delayed union unless it is not healing in the expected time that similar fractures under similar circumstances have healed.

The diagnosis of a delayed union is established by considering the previous factors relative to the time involved, physical examination parameters, and the evaluation of the radiographic appearance of the fracture.[2,18] On clinical examination, the animal may be reluctant to bear weight on the limb or may be lame. Muscle atrophy is evident on palpation, and crepitus and pain may be elicited at the fracture site. Instability may be present but is usually obscured by the fixation device. Radiographic assessment demonstrates a persistent fracture line, absence of bone healing evidenced by lack of a bony or bridging callus or some nonbridging callus, an open marrow cavity, and most importantly, no significant sclerosis of the bone ends (Fig. 12-2).[2,18]

Cause

Histology. Fractures that have reached the stage of delayed healing termed *delayed union* have the capacity to heal. Delayed unions that exhibit some attempt at bridging callus have an established fibrocartilaginous area between fragment ends. An avascular zone corresponds to the radiolucent zone evident on a radiograph made at this time. Histologically, an active vascular invasion of the fibrocartilage and replacement by new bone are seen in the external callus.[34]

The eminent orthopedic surgeon Sir Reginald Watson-Jones attributed delayed union of bone to interrupted immobilization, traction and distraction, infection, persistent angulation, too-early weight bearing, and loss of blood supply to the fragments.[49] He emphasized that overtraction amounting to only ¼ inch in reduction of femoral fractures caused serious delay in bone healing. It was acknowledged that overriding fractures of the tibia united more rapidly than fractures reduced perfectly by traction.

Traction is not a practical modality available to the veterinary orthopedic surgeon, but distraction of fragments should be avoided. If distraction is necessary to maintain limb length but creates a fracture gap (buttress plating of severely comminuted shaft fractures), a prolonged healing time can be anticipated. The use of skeletal traction in repair of tibial fractures in humans triples the time to union if the distraction amounts to ¼ inch, even if it is corrected within a few days.[49]

Fracture forces. In biomechanics, forces can be divided into two categories. Forces that come from outside a structure are called *loads*, whereas those generated within a structure's substance by loads are called *stresses*.[19]

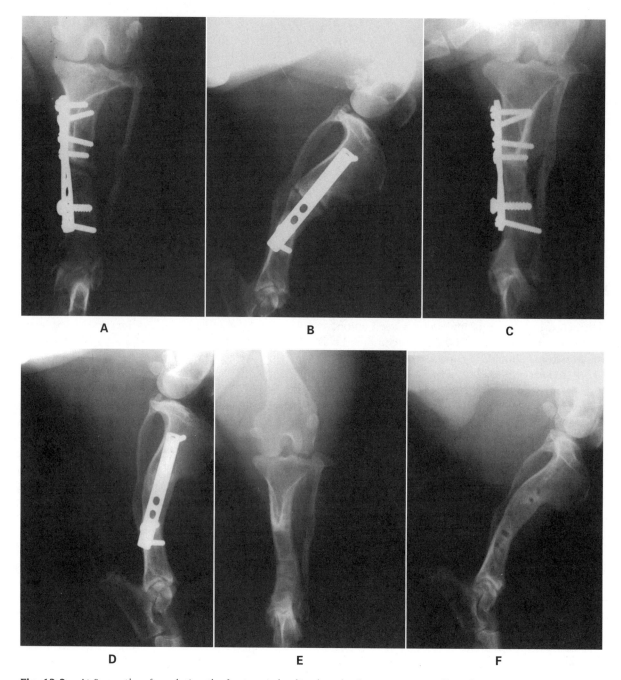

Fig. 12-2   At 2 months after plating the fracture is healing but the fracture gap is still evident. Progression was slow over the next few months, and the fracture was considered a delayed union. Increased levels of controlled activity were encouraged to stress the bone. **A,** Craniocaudal view at 2 months after plating. The plate is functioning as a buttress plate, and the fracture gap is smaller. **B,** Lateral view at 2 months after plating. The callus is progressing, but the fracture gap is still evident. At 7 months after plating, the fracture has healed. **C** and **D,** craniocaudal and lateral views of the healed fracture. **E** and **F,** Craniocaudal and lateral views of the healed fracture after plate removal. Note the improved alignment and filling of the fracture gap.

Fractures are subjected to a variety of fracture forces or loads, depending on the type of fracture and the means of fixation employed. More than one load can act on a fracture, but one load usually predominates after fixation. The ability of the fixation device to resist the fracture load is an extremely important factor in determining whether the fracture heals, becomes a delayed union, or worse, a nonunion. Most surgeons consider instability to be the main cause of delayed union. Additional factors include (1) a fracture gap from bone loss, distraction, malposition, or soft tissue interposition; (2) vascular damage from original trauma or surgery; (3) infection; and (4) systemic or local tissue disease.[9]

Blood supply. Fracture forces and instability from inadequate fixation have a profound effect on maintenance of blood supply to fracture fragments and the establishment of bone healing. Other factors that negatively influence the availability of blood supply to the fracture fragments include the interposition of soft tissue through the fracture area, disruption of contiguous soft tissue, and severe soft tissue trauma. In areas of minimal soft tissue coverage, the vascular supply may not be reestablished.[34]

Disruption of the interfragmentary repair tissue is affected by the degree of motion and the size of the fracture gap as well as the maturity of the tissue. Granulation tissue can elongate approximately 100% before rupturing, which enables it to tolerate relative immobilization of the fracture fragments. The developing fibrocartilage that fills in the fracture gap as bone healing ensues can tolerate approximately 10% elongation before rupturing. The increased stability from the callus maturing is necessary to prevent exceeding the elongation curve of the cartilage bed. As healing progresses, bone fills in the fracture gap to establish bone union. This bony tissue tolerates only 2% elongation before rupturing. Therefore, a large gap of many millimeters can change its dimension by 100% before disrupting early granulation tissue.

Rigid reduction with a plate should afford better reduction and a smaller fracture gap. Small amounts of motion acting on this gap have a greater deleterious effect than the same amount of motion on large gaps.[34] Because of the interrelated dynamics of motion, tissue tolerance, and bone healing, early diagnosis and intervention are important when a delayed or nonunion is diagnosed.

Infection. A delayed union can develop from infection's effect on wound and bone healing. The infection may develop from a primary open fracture or secondarily as the result of surgery. The presence of dead bone with infection seriously hinders bone healing and may result in sequestrum formation.[2]

Additional factors. The animal's general health should always be evaluated. Old age alone is not the reason fractures in older animals heal more slowly. Osteopenia associated with old age and inactivity may affect healing. Poor nutrition in any age animal coupled with a negative nitrogen balance has a direct adverse effect on bone healing. Other causes include metabolic defects, chronic corticosteroid use, anticoagulants, and radiation therapy.[2]

Treatment

Neutralization of fracture forces; enhancement or correction of fixation. With delayed union, a slight modification of the coaptation device and the animal's activity may provide better immobilization of the fracture site.[34] This often provides a sufficient decrease in tissue disruption for a return to normal healing. The morbidity of continuing the same treatment for a longer period, even if the fracture heals, may be justification for surgical intervention. The addition of an external fixator to a transverse fracture that exhibits delayed union because of rotational forces acting on an intramedullary pin often changes a delayed union to a healed fracture in a few weeks.[13,26,41] The external fixator also decreases soft tissue and joint morbidity by enabling the animal to bear weight and to use the joints above and below the fracture.

If the existing fixation is so poor that auxiliary fixation is not sufficient, it may be necessary to provide rigid internal fixation through plating. Plating provides the most reliable means of countering all fracture forces.

Promotion of blood supply. Delayed unions are viable fractures and have the essential ingredients for bone healing. In most cases, eliminating the instability responsible for disruption of blood supply is sufficient. In fractures with a large fracture gap or in bones with minimal soft tissue covering, addition of an autogenous cancellous bone graft promotes vascularization of the site. One of the most desired elements of the cancellous bone graft is the transfer of capillary buds to the fracture site.

Antibiotic therapy. Most delayed unions occur in healthy animals with a healthy tissue bed where the use of antibiotics is not justified. Perioperative antibiotic treatment may be indicated if major surgical intervention is necessary. If a low-grade infection exists, providing stability for the fracture is sufficient for bone healing to occur. The infection resolves when the fracture is healed and the implants are removed. If an active, aggressive infection exists, the problem is osteomyelitis and should be treated as such (see Chapter 11).

Postoperative management. Patient management is dictated by the means employed to convert the fracture to union. If an external fixator is added to the initial repair, advice is given on managing the fixator and avoiding its attendant problems. Additional activity might be allowed, however, as long as there is adequate supervision. If plating is done, it is hoped an early return to function is possible. It is extremely important to continue monitoring the animal's progress both physically and radiographically. The initial intervention may be insufficient, and more aggressive methods may be needed to prevent a nonunion.

NONUNION

A succinct definition of a nonunion that provides room for the various forms of nonunion encountered follows: "a nonunion is a fracture in which the apposed ends have failed to unite, and all signs of repair have ceased."[7,45] Different sources give similar definitions for a nonunion, which vary from an arrest of the bony fracture repair process with the formation of a fibrous, cartilaginous, or synovial false joint[9]; the condition that exists in a fracture when signs of repair have ceased[2]; to the consideration of a fracture as a nonunion when no progression toward healing is seen on two to three successive radiographs taken at monthly intervals.[7,21,48]

A general diagnosis or suspicion of a nonunion is obtained by correlating the history with the physical findings. If the mechanism of trauma, the signalment of the animal, and the means of fixation are known, the time for fracture healing can be reasonably estimated (Table 12-1). When this time is exceeded, one must decide if the fracture has become a delayed union or a nonunion. If appropriate steps are not taken at the time of delayed union, conditions worsen at the fracture site and a nonunion results.

Clinical signs vary with the type of nonunion present, the chronicity of the injury or time since surgery, and the type of fixation, if any, used. Physical examination findings may include disuse muscle atrophy, limb deformity (angular, rotational, or limb shortening), pain, and reluctance or inability to use the limb.[2,4,7] An animal may be able to bear weight and demonstrate little pain with marginal use of a long-standing nonunion despite gross instability. Fracture location is an influencing factor, even if all other factors could be kept constant. In one study, the distal radius and ulna of small dogs was the most common site for delayed unions and nonunions to develop. This location was followed by the tibia and the femoral shaft (25% and 15%, respectively).[3] In areas where large breeds predominate, nonunions of the femur are seen most often. Nonunions do occur in the cat, but infrequently and usually from mismanagement.

Nonunions are classified by their radiographic and histological appearance. The final diagnosis is made by radiographic evaluation combined with a consistent history. Some fractures might have the radiographic appearance of a nonunion, but because of the time involved, the fracture could be at the delayed union stage. Radiographically, two types of nonunions are seen that have varying degrees of change in each category. The radiographic appearance determines whether the fracture is considered a biologically active (viable, vascular, or hypertrophic) or a biologically inactive (nonviable, avascular, or atrophic) nonunion. Radiographic features common to both types of nonunion include sclerotic fracture ends, a gap between fragments, a sealed marrow cavity, and fracture surfaces that are usually smooth and well defined (Fig. 12-3).[2]

The classification devised by Weber and Cech is useful for the clinician because it helps determine the treat-

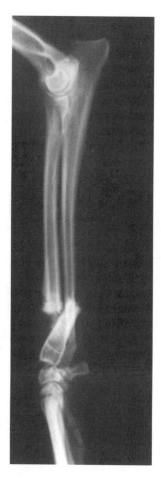

Fig. 12-3 Many radiographic features common to nonunions are seen in this nonunion of the distal radius that resulted from coaptation. Note the sclerotic fracture ends, the fracture gap, the density in the marrow cavity, and the smooth appearance of the fragment ends.

Table 12-1 Rate of Union in Terms of Clinical Union

Age of animal	External skeletal, and intramedullary pin fixations	Fixation with bone plates
< 3 months	2-3 weeks	4 weeks
3-6 months	4-6 weeks	2-3 months
6-12 months	5-8 weeks	3-5 months
> 1 year	7-12 weeks	5 months-1 year

ment needed.[45] The two major groups undergoing a disturbance in union are either (1) capable of biological reaction, or "viable," or (2) incapable of biological reaction, or "nonviable." Viable nonunions are subdivided into three categories based on the amount of nonbridging callus produced:

1. A hypertrophic nonunion has produced an abundance of callus rich in blood supply and is known as an "elephant foot" nonunion because of the expanded fragment ends (Fig. 12-4, *A*).
2. A slightly less hypertrophic nonunion is termed a "horse hoof" nonunion and depicts a less well vascularized callus (Fig. 12-4, *B*).
3. An oligotrophic nonunion does not display fracture callus, but the ends of the fragments are viable when checked by scintigraphy (Fig. 12-4, *C*). Instead of appearing sclerotic, the fracture ends round off after 2 to 3 months, resorb, and later decalcify.

Nonviable nonunions are divided into four categories[45]:

1. *Dystrophic nonunion* has an intermediate fragment that has healed only to one major fragment because of a disruption in blood supply. This can occur when the blood supply of the distal fragment is avulsed at the time of fracture. The distal end of the intermediate fragment has an inadequate blood supply and cannot provide sufficient osteogenesis to bridge the gap to the large avascular major fragment (Fig. 12-4, *D*).
2. Severe fractures with multiple fragmentation may develop a *necrotic nonunion* because of devascularized fragments. When stabilized, these fragments do not form a callus even though a gap may not be visible radiographically. With time, the pieces appear more radiopaque than the adjacent bone and may cause sequestration (Fig. 12-4, *E*).
3. When a small or large section of bone is lost because of the original trauma, sequestrectomy, or cancer excision, a *defect nonunion* is created. The remaining viable bone ends cannot bridge this gap without supplementary surgery (Fig. 12-4, *F*).
4. The worst condition arises when an *atrophic nonunion* results from one of the first three nonviable nonunions. Osteoporosis develops from inactivity, and loss of osteogenic activity occurs secondary to the loss of vascular supply (Fig. 12-4, *G*).[45]

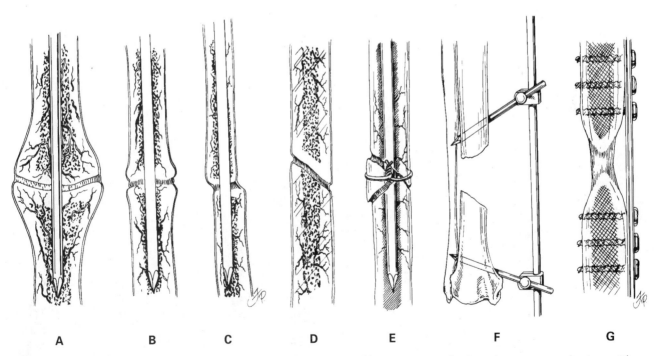

| A | B | C | D | E | F | G |

Fig. 12-4 The following examples typify the different degrees of viable nonunions. Fixation of a transverse fracture with an intramedullary pin subjects the fracture to a rotational load. The larger the pin is relative to the medullary diameter, the less effect transverse shear and bending loads have on the fracture healing. **A,** Elephant foot. **B,** Horse hoof. **C,** Oligotrophic nonunion. The following examples typify the different nonviable nonunions. **D,** Dystrophic. Despite adequate reduction and coaptation, this fracture is not healing. **E,** Necrotic. The devascularized segment is not stable and is preventing healing of the fracture. **F,** Defect. This segmental defect is too large for gap healing without grafting. **G,** Atrophic. The denuded fragment ends held rigidly apart by the plate have not revascularized.

Cause

It is essential to identify causative factors and eliminate them when treating a nonunion. The following major factors predispose the fracture to becoming a nonunion: (1) initial displacement of the fracture, (2) extent of soft tissue injury, (3) comminution (including loss of bone substance), (4) distraction, and (5) infection.[48] Other important predisposing factors include devascularization, an open and comminuted fracture, poor reduction, and poor fixation. Excessive concern over and attention to soft tissue without concurrent treatment of the involved fracture can also delay or impede fracture healing. Occasionally, a delay in weight bearing, or excessive weight bearing too early, can contribute to nonunion formation. In one study, primary closure of open tibial fractures was associated with a 73% incidence of infection, thus predisposing these fractures to nonunion.[48]

As these factors are evaluated, one can see that the causes of nonunion fall into the categories of biomechanical, biological, or a combination of the two[4,9,22]:

1. In veterinary orthopedics, inadequate stabilization that allows motion at the fracture site is the most common cause of nonunions (Fig. 12-5).
2. A fracture gap caused by bone loss from trauma, intraoperative removal of bone fragments, or distraction by external fixation devices or implants may exceed the fragment's ability to form bridging callus. The gap fills with fibrous and/or cartilaginous ingrowth, which does not convert to bone without help.
3. Primary loss of blood supply to the fragments and adjacent soft tissue from the initial trauma and the dissipation of impact force, alone or combined with surgical trauma to the remaining blood supply, has a significant effect on the time necessary for fracture healing. Surgical factors deleterious to available blood supply and revascularization include excessive periosteal stripping, excessive retraction of the soft tissue, allowing the exposed tissue to dry out, and overuse of cautery. The two events are additive and underline the necessity for gentle tissue handling and preservation of existing blood supply.
4. If infection develops, the lowered local pH tends to put calcium into solution. This impairs revascularization of devitalized fragments, which become sclerotic and may cause sequestration. The fractures heal in the presence of infection when stable fixation and adequate blood supply are present, but the implants are more likely to loosen in an infected tissue bed. This again emphasizes that instability, and thus motion, is responsible for maintaining both infection and nonunion.
5. Other factors that contribute to the development of a nonunion act locally or systemically. These include loss of initial fracture hematoma by surgical

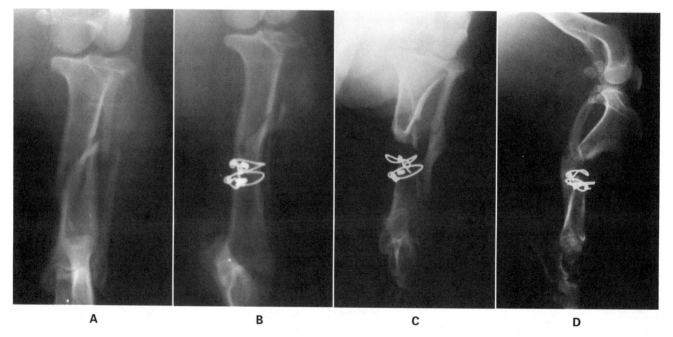

Fig. 12-5   An oligotrophic nonunion of an oblique midshaft fracture of the tibia in a 5-year-old female dachshund. The subsequent correction and development of a delayed union with final union is seen in Figs. 12-2 and 12-7. **A,** Preoperative craniocaudal view. **B,** Immediate postoperative craniocaudal view. Note the cerclage wire and transfixation K-wire fixation. **C,** Craniocaudal view at 14 weeks. The fracture gap is evident, and the implants are in the fracture line. **D,** Lateral view at 14 weeks. The caudal angulation of the proximal fragment is evident.

manipulation, reaction to metallic implants, improper use of cerclage wires, an excessive amount of implanted material in the wound bed, osteoporosis, neoplasia, starvation, radiation, steroids, antimetabolic drugs, metabolic or nutritional disturbances, senile changes, anticoagulant drugs, hyperemia, ischemia, and compression of the fracture hematoma by an unpadded cast. The latter situation is of importance in small-breed dogs with small, fragile bones and minimal soft tissue coverage to accommodate swelling.[7]

Histology. Little difference exists histologically between a delayed union and spontaneous healing. The major difference is the time required to establish bone union between fragments. When the mechanical forces acting on the fracture site exceed the fragments' biological capacity to produce adequate immobilization through callus and interfragmentary fibrocartilage formation, a nonunion develops. The extent of this effort to combat the instability determines the type of nonunion formed. The development of "elephant foot" or "horse hoof" nonunions is a reflection of persisting interfragmentary instability in an area of tremendous bone activity. Despite the sclerotic appearance of the fragment ends, scintigraphy confirms a high rate of metabolic activity.[33,42,45]

The initial bone that forms subperiosteally and in the medullary cavity is produced by endochondral ossification, with later formation of fibrocartilage between the fragment ends.[33] This fibrocartilage is unmineralized and may develop fissures, which eventually form the equivalent of a joint space that defines the late stage of a nonunion known as a *pseudoarthrosis*. At this stage the fragment ends are very active biologically, but the vascular resorptive canals are not able to penetrate into the fibrocartilage. Therefore, the fibrocartilage stays unmineralized and impedes further chondral ossification.[42,45] Nonunions with absent or minimal external callus have poor osteogenic activity at the fragment ends but sufficient activity to seal the medullary canal. Interestingly, when atrophic nonunions are evaluated scintigraphically, they have a reasonable level of metabolic activity.[33]

Access to scintigraphy is limited in veterinary practice. An acceptable alternative well within the capabilities of most veterinarians is *osteomedullography*. Biopsy to determine activity at the cellular level is not acceptable, but the technique of osteomedullography is similar to performing a small-bone biopsy and is thus a familiar technique. In a normally healing fracture, the injected contrast medium demonstrates interosseous flow between the fragment ends 3 to 10 weeks after the fracture. An Esmarch bandage or an inflatable tourniquet (pressure of 200 mm Hg) can be used to prevent the escape of contrast medium into soft tissue veins. A bone marrow biopsy needle or sternal puncture needle with an internal diameter

of 1.5 mm can be used. The puncture is made in the distal metaphysis approximately 1 cm proximal to the physis in immature animals. Sterile technique is mandatory to avoid creating osteomyelitis. Any routine iodinated contrast medium can be used. Three to five milliliters of a full-strength medium (400 mg I_2/ml) is sufficient for injection. An immediate radiograph is made and one at 5 to 10 seconds. If the contrast medium does not cross the fracture gap from the distal fragment into the proximal fragment, the osteomedullography is interpreted as negative. A positive osteomedullogram is seen when intraosseous veins are seen crossing the fracture gap, as demonstrated by flow of contrast medium into the proximal fragment.[44] If no contrast medium crosses the fracture gap by 12 weeks, grafting should be considered. The osteomedullogram does not present a normal picture for 9 to 18 weeks because of the medullary cavity being plugged by endosteal new bone growth. A fracture that is healing normally has abundant venous flow across the site even when the fragments are displaced.[45]

Fracture forces and fixation methods. All fractures result from a bone being subjected to biomechanical forces that exceed the bone's ability to absorb energy without fracturing. When analyzed, these forces produce somewhat predictable fracture patterns and consequently are subject to specific fracture loads that must be countered to maintain stability after repair. It is surprising how consideration of these basic forces can decrease the chance of a nonunion resulting. Most of the nonunions referred to referral practices and institutions could have been prevented with some forethought, evaluation of the forces acting on that fracture, and the decision on the best means available to counter those forces successfully.

The simplest example is the nonunion that results from unsuccessfully countering the rotational load acting on transverse fractures. Intramedullary pins cannot counter rotational loads but are often incorrectly used alone for repair of transverse fractures. Stack pinning has been shown to be minimally more resistant to countering rotational loads and is not a statistically significantly superior method to routine pinning with one pin.[12] It should be recognized that an intramedullary pin of correct size is capable of resisting bending, transverse shear, and axial compression forces on a given fracture but has no effect on rotational forces. If the fracture interdigitates or is impacted, some resistance to rotational forces occurs, but postoperative exercise must be strictly managed if an intramedullary pin is the sole means of fixation.

For transverse fractures of the distal extremity (radial/ulnar and tibial fractures), augmentation of the intramedullary pin with a suitable coaptation device may counter the rotational forces, but patient management may be more difficult and attendant soft tissue problems more manifest. Fracture disease may be a complication to this approach. The fracture heals, but limb function is severely compromised. By adding an external fixator to the initial repair, these problems can be avoided. The external fixator provides the distinct advantage of countering rotation and enabling the animal to use the joints above and below the fracture. Now the fracture heals, and soft tissue problems can be avoided.

The external fixator is a great addition to the orthopedic inventory but still has limitations and brings its own unique problems, which influence aftercare and client education. For some fractures, bone plating is the best choice to ensure stable fixation, to counter all fracture forces, and to decrease the amount of aftercare.

It is important to evaluate each individual fracture during surgery for the fracture forces to be countered. Oblique fractures are subject to shearing forces, which are poorly countered by an intramedullary pin. Proper use of cerclage wire to provide anatomical fragment apposition for oblique fractures that interdigitate may be sufficient augmentation of intramedullary pin fixation. If the fracture fragments do not interdigitate and have a tendency to slip in an axial direction, the cerclage wire usually proves insufficient, and shearing forces cause motion. A better choice is to provide neutralization plating with lag screws either through or outside the plate. If the veterinarian is not competent with these techniques or does not have the necessary equipment, the patient should be referred. If an inadequate method is used, the veterinarian is responsible for the resulting instability and creation of a nonunion.

Blood supply, fracture location, and animal's age.
It is common knowledge that an infected fracture heals if it is stable.[4] The fracture must have adequate blood supply, however, regardless of the stability or lack of healing. An unstable fracture that has adequate blood supply often heals but must produce a large callus to gradually gain the stability necessary for maintaining continuity of the vascular channels across the fracture.

The location of the fracture has a definite influence on the prognosis for healing and the length of time involved, primarily because of available blood supply to the fragments at different locations within a given bone. Metaphyseal fractures, especially of the humerus and femur, seldom become nonunions because of the abundant soft tissue structures and attachments in the area. Proximal fractures of the radius/ulna and tibia are less apt to become nonunions than are distal metaphyseal fractures. Toy and miniature breeds of dogs are notorious for developing nonunions of the distal radius and ulna. This problem is attributed to their small bones and sparse soft tissue covering,[9] which makes it very difficult to avoid stress protection of the fractures with most implants (Fig. 12-6). At the same time, revascularization

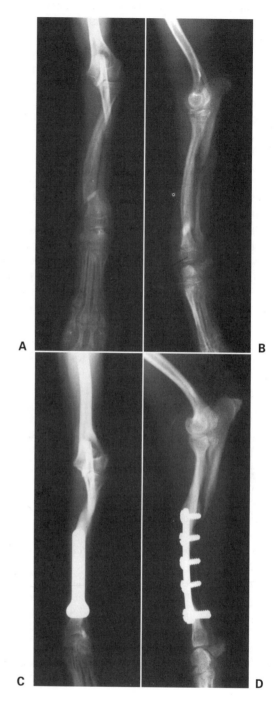

Fig. 12-6 An ulnar osteotomy was done to alleviate the effect of premature distal ulnar closure in an immature toy poodle. The dog subsequently fractured the distal radius. **A,** The slightly oblique distal fracture of the radius is seen on the craniocaudal view. **B,** The atrophic distal fragment of the ulna is noted on the lateral view. There is minimal craniocaudal displacement of the fracture. **C,** The small ASIF T plate obscures the radius as seen on the craniocaudal view. **D,** Lateral view 2 months after surgery. The distal ulna has practically resorbed, and the radius under the central third of the plate is extremely osteopenic. This reflects the stress protection afforded by too large a plate.

of the fracture site proceeds slowly, even though the repair provides stability.

The animal's age influences the relative time for fracture healing (see Table 12-1). An understanding of the bone-healing response with different repair methods coupled with the anticipated time for a fracture to heal in that age group of animal facilitates diagnosing delayed and nonunions.

Infection. Rigid fixation is essential for healing of infected nonunions. When possible, the infection's activity should be decreased before stabilization.[32] When an infection is present, the problem is usually chronic and one of the major factors responsible for the nonunion. Because of chronicity, the offending organisms are often resistant to most antibiotics. This is further complicated by evidence suggesting that although antibiotics can penetrate osteomyelitic bone, they cannot penetrate avascular bone surrounded by fibrous tissue.[15] With previous surgery, the associated scarring makes it more difficult to treat the infection effectively. Many fractures of this nature would have resulted in the limb being amputated in people before the advent of microvasculature transplantation.[20] The absolute importance of sufficient blood supply for bone healing under any circumstances, especially adverse ones, is a recurring theme for addressing delayed and nonunions.

Treatment

Neutralization of forces. Ossification of the fracture site occurs when tension and compression forces act together on the scaffolding of the bridging callus in the absence of opposing forces.[45] Fractures seemingly can withstand a considerable degree of bending, compression, and some tension at the fracture site without impeding healing. Torsional forces, however, delay and impair healing, and severe torsional forces disrupt the uniting fibroblastic network. This explains the success or failure of some radial/ulnar fractures to heal when placed in a cast. Rotational (torsional) forces are resisted by casting the forelimb from above the elbow to the foot with the elbow held in standing flexion and the carpus placed in slight varus. If the limb is cast in an extended position, torsional forces are poorly countered initially and not at all after disuse atrophy ensues. The human fibula is a substantial bone compared with the fibula in dogs and cats. An intact fibula can contribute to formation of a tibial nonunion by acting as a spring, thus creating alternating compression/expansion ("squeezing") forces. The invading microcapillaries are alternately squeezed and sheared, causing occlusion and severance of the neovascularization. In time a layer of fibrocartilage occludes the medullary cavities of the major fragments, and sometimes fibrous bone forms.[45]

Obtaining bone union when treating most nonunions is relatively easy. If one can identify the missing ingredient necessary for promoting union and supply it, the fracture heals. Unfortunately, in many patients the remaining fracture disease prevents the limb regaining full function. Once again, it is always better to intercede before the stage of nonunion when possible. Most nonunions are iatrogenic and reflect an error in judgment: selection of the incorrect implant(s) to combat the fracture forces present, inadequate client education and patient exercise restriction, or a combination of both. Surgical correction of these nonunions may involve adding an external fixator to the initial repair.[11,13,26,41] Some nonunions may need the rigid fixation and compression afforded by dynamic compression plating.* For articular fractures, the addition of lag screw fixation may be sufficient to resist existing fracture forces and promote union.[16,39]

Enhancement or correction of fixation. In fractures subject to rotational forces, the addition of an external skeletal fixator satisfactorily counters the rotation. This, in turn, enables vascular channels to establish continuity across the fracture site followed by mineralization of the fibrocartilaginous callus. In oblique fractures, subject to shearing forces, the addition of cerclage wire or preferably lag screws improves fragment apposition but is not necessarily sufficient to resist all the shearing loads. Adding an external fixator or a suitable coaptation device augments the initial repair and resists the shear forces that prevent revascularization and the formation of bridging callus. On occasion, replacing a small implant with a more appropriately sized implant suffices to stabilize the fracture site. This technique is most successful if the fracture is impacted.

Many clients are concerned about subjecting their pet to more surgery and may insist on the most effective method being done regardless of additional expense. If the nonunion is not infected and is a nondisplaced diaphyseal fracture, greater stability can be achieved through compression plating. Minimal soft tissue disruption is done, and all previously placed implants are removed. A sufficient amount of callus is removed for accurate plate placement, and a dynamic compression plate is used in a tension-band or compression mode. If the fracture gap is too wide for the compression capacity of the plate used, the tension device should be used to achieve maximum compression of the pseudoarthrotic tissue and stability at the fracture site.[9] The use of fully threaded cancellous screws may be necessary to gain secure purchase in osteoporotic bone. If these screws strip, the screw holes or medullary cavity can be filled with methylmethacrylate to provide secure screw purchase.[9,47] No infection can be

---

*References 1, 18, 21, 23, 25-27, 38.

present in the area of the bone cement. If the fracture is oblique, neutralization plating with the use of lag screws provides interfragmentary compression, but axial compression may be difficult to achieve without interdigitation of the major fragments. Step-cutting of the bone ends to convert shear to axial compression[9] is advisable, unless considerable bone shortening would result.

If the diaphyseal nonunion is displaced, greater exposure is necessary to gain access for correction of the axial alignment and plate placement. The previously mentioned steps can be done to achieve stability. To achieve reduction, the pseudoarthrotic tissue must be removed, along with opening the sclerotic ends of the major fragments by reaming to facilitate revascularization.[9]

Noninfected metaphyseal and epiphyseal nonunions are often more difficult to treat than diaphyseal nonunions because of concurrent joint stiffness and loss of cancellous bone.[9] Arthrolysis, joint manipulation, and intensive postsurgical physical therapy are necessary to regain joint function in humans, and the same principles apply to animals.[27] These fractures have excellent intrinsic healing capability because they occur in anatomical regions with normally abundant circulation. Stable fixation provides the best results when coupled with cancellous bone grafting for defect nonunions.[27] The surgical approach may have to be aggressive to enable freeing of the joint stiffness by capsulotomy/capsulectomy and debridement of restrictive hypertrophic bone. Anatomical reconstruction of the joint surface should be attempted by the use of a compression plate and/or lag screws.

Promotion of blood supply. Viable, noninfected, aligned nonunions have a good blood supply. Resection of the intervening fibrous tissue and the addition of a cancellous bone graft are unnecessary if compression and stable, rigid fixation can be accomplished. Mineralization of the interfragmentary fibrocartilage can proceed once the blood supply is maintained by eliminating motion at the fracture site.[7] Compression is not essential but does provide the most ideal circumstances for primary bone healing, which can occur secondary to repair of a nonunion. If the fracture is not well aligned, it is necessary to remove just enough callus to align the fracture. In both instances, the surgeon should achieve stable, rigid fixation even if compression is not possible.

Nonviable (biologically inactive) fractures need the same alignment and stability, but additional steps are necessary to encourage revascularization. If the medullary canal is sealed by fracture callus, it should be reamed to permit the invasion of new blood vessels across the fracture site in both viable and nonviable nonunions. In dense sclerotic bone, decortication (shingling) is done to expose viable bone and stimulate osteogenesis.[7,9,45] Small holes can be drilled in the cortical wall to facilitate penetration of the cortex by extraosseous blood supply from the surrounding soft tissue.

The key factor in promoting vascularization of nonviable nonunions once stability is achieved is the addition of a cancellous bone graft. Many delayed and nonunions can be prevented by harvesting and placing a cancellous bone graft in and around the fracture site at the time of initial repair. The usual excuse of "it takes too much time" is not valid unless the animal is doing poorly under anesthesia and it is critical to end the procedure immediately. The graft can be harvested by one surgeon while the other surgeon is finishing implant placement. If one is operating alone, a cancellous bone graft can be harvested easily in 5 to 10 minutes. The additional time pays back dividends for weeks. When treating a nonviable nonunion, it is imperative that proper planning is done and that the grafting is done as a major component of the treatment plan. It is best to collect the graft just before wound closure and transfer it immediately to the recipient bed. All the advantages of a cancellous bone graft come into play, but the capillary buds within the matrix of the graft may be the most important (Fig. 12-7).

Electric stimulation. Some interest exists in using electric stimulation of bone healing for nonunions in animals. It is accepted that osteogenesis is supported by or associated with the maintenance of electronegativity. New bone growth occurs in the vicinity of the negative electrode (cathode) and osteolysis at the positive electrode (anode). The anode can be implanted in soft tissues or on the skin distant from the bone to avoid bony destruction but still allow osteogenesis at the cathode.

Electric stimulation is used primarily for fracture healing of symptomatic, unstable, radiographically confirmed nonunions. To be successful, the nonunion must demon-

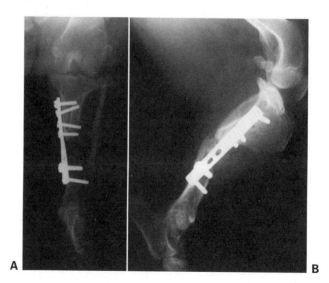

Fig. 12-7 This dog was referred to the NCSU-CVM teaching hospital for evaluation of the nonunion and surgical correction. **A,** Immediate postoperative craniocaudal view after the second surgery. Note the cancellous bone graft in the fracture gap. **B,** Immediate postoperative lateral view after the second surgery.

strate some evidence of biological healing activity when examined by intraosseous venography and nuclear scan. Biologically inactive (nonviable), avascular nonunions respond poorly to electric stimulation and must be grafted to start the healing process before electric stimulation is successful. Coincident with electric stimulation, the fracture must be stabilized. Once started, the process is carried out over at least 12 weeks.

Three devices are currently in use: (1) a semiinvasive, direct-current electrostimulator; (2) a completely implantable, direct-current stimulator; and (3) an electric current produced in bone by creating an electric field external to the affected limb. Because of the need for patient cooperation, the totally implantable system seems most suited for use in animals.[10] Some amazing results have been achieved in people, but it is difficult to isolate the effect of the electrostimulation from the overall management of these patients. Some meaningful trials must be done in animals and the cost factor decreased before this technique gains widespread acceptance in veterinary medicine.

Infected nonunions. Osteomyelitis often results from the surgeon creating an open fracture. This may cause a nonunion in a fracture that would have healed otherwise. Many fractures presented as open fractures are not handled as emergencies, and the opportunity to maintain the wound at the clean or contaminated level is lost. It is very discouraging to receive a referral of an open fracture 2 to 4 days after injury that has not been given proper wound care and has not been splinted or bandaged. Even with plate fixation, this fracture may be doomed to failure because of the ensuing osteomyelitis. The fracture may heal if stability and a good blood supply exist, but frequently an infected nonunion develops. There are two basic schools of thought:

1. Treat the infection locally first, by debridement of soft tissue and bone, and provide drainage, followed by rigid stabilization of the nonunion and cancellous bone grafting when indicated.[24,32]
2. Accomplish bony union first, and then soft tissue healing follows or is easier to achieve.[29]

The former method takes a tremendous amount of time, treatment, and patient cooperation and is very expensive. The latter approach is more applicable to the veterinary patient. The resurgence in popularity of external skeletal fixators in both human and veterinary orthopedics allows simultaneous treatment of bone and soft tissue.

The technique of *distraction osteosynthesis* with a dynamic external skeletal fixator has been used to treat infected nonunions with segmental defects.[36] This technique, based on the work of Professor Ilizarov in Russia, has been used successfully in humans and dogs.[6,46]

---

*References 8, 14, 28, 31, 35, 43.

Surgeons have a tendency to close all wounds, especially if an implant is used for fracture repair.[40] This is not always the best approach. Soft tissue wounds granulate readily over implants when proper wound care is provided, and delayed closure works very well in veterinary patients if the wound can be protected.

The following regimen is applicable for most infected nonunions.[45]

Infected nonunion without drainage. The previously discussed principles for aligned and nonaligned nonunions apply, but it is critical that dead bone be excised. A cancellous bone graft should be added if there is any concern about fragment vascularity, and decortication (Judet technique) should be done if the cortex is thick enough.

Infected nonunion with drainage. All dead bone (sequestra) should be excised, along with the draining tract and other fistulas. Saucerization should be done in areas of defect to the level of healthy bleeding bone by rongeuring and curettage to create a shallow, bowl-like area. The medullary canal should be opened with a pin or large drill bit to encourage revascularization. Stable, rigid fixation should be accomplished and cancellous bone harvested and packed generously around the fracture site.[37] Aerobic and anaerobic cultures can be submitted and sensitivity testing done. Appropriate antibiotics should be administered systemically and used locally when necessary, but antibiotics play a secondary role in chronic osteomyelitis. Although the osteomyelitic bone can be penetrated by many antibiotics, avascular bone encapsulated by fibrous tissue is penetrated poorly.[15] Indwelling irrigation/drainage systems can be used to flush the area with large volumes of sterile fluid containing antibiotics for therapeutic treatment and mechanical cleansing. The decision to close the wound should be based on the wound's condition at the end of surgery. Wound closure is preferable when possible, but the surgeon should never be reluctant to leave an open (infected) fracture open.

Chronic osteomyelitis is often caused by Gram-negative organisms, which are difficult to treat systemically. Effective handling of the nonunion and aggressive local management of the infection are paramount. Rigid stabilization of fracture fragments favors healing, and the advantages of the stabilizing implant outweigh the disadvantage of it being a foreign body. Internal fixation devices should be removed only after the fracture has healed or if the implant is loose and is part of the problem.[37] After surgery, it is advisable to use culture and sensitivity results as a guideline for appropriate antibiotic therapy for several weeks when treating chronically infected nonunions.

Metaphyseal and articular nonunions. Nonunions at the end of long bones adjacent to or involving a major joint are often difficult to treat and are a technical challenge.[16,17,39] The resulting functional disability is often profound because of limitation of motion, instability, and pain. A review of 20 patients treated for a nonunion of the distal humerus evaluated 3.6 years (average) after treatment revealed the following: only 1 patient had an excellent result; 6, good; 7, fair; and 6, poor. Patients with extraarticular supracondylar nonunion did the best, whereas those with an intraarticular component or severe soft tissue trauma did less well.[1]

Treatment of these fractures is difficult and demanding. The adjacent joint should be opened and inspected. Hypertrophic or redundant synovial membrane should be resected and loose bone or soft tissue fragments removed. A concerted effort should be made to restore normal joint alignment and congruency. Two-point fixation with pins or screws is needed in small fragments, which can often be reinforced by buttress plating. Fracture disease is a common sequela to repair of these fractures, and early return to function is essential. Physical therapy should be instituted early, and client education and cooperation are integral components of postoperative management.[7]

Postoperative management of nonunions. Without exception, patients with nonunions have varying degrees of loss of function in the affected limb before definitive treatment. Many have had several surgical procedures, and restoration of function is more difficult to achieve than bony union. The basic guideline of providing stable fixation to facilitate early return to function is critical to a satisfactory outcome. Certain nonunions demand specific treatment (i.e., antibiotics), but physical therapy, management of exercise, and encouragement of limb use under supervision are essential.[5]

Swimming is an excellent exercise for these patients to promote use of muscles and to prevent adhesions. Leash walking initially, followed by gentle play as bone healing progresses, gradually stimulates osteogenesis and increases stress and load on the healing bone in a controlled manner. Radiographic evaluation should be done regularly at sensible intervals so appropriate changes in management can be instituted at the correct time. When presented with a nonunion case, the experienced surgeon is usually more concerned about restoring function than correcting the nonunion. By understanding the biology of nonunions and the steps and principles involved in correcting nonunions, bone union can often be accomplished. This same knowledge should enable the surgeon to prevent a nonunion from developing by intervening early with the necessary ingredients for success.

REFERENCES

1. Ackerman G, Jupiter JB: Nonunion of the distal end of the humerus, *J Bone Joint Surg (Am)* 70(1):75-83, 1988.
2. Aron DN: Management of delayed union and nonunion fractures in small animals, *Compend Cont Educ Pract Vet* 1(9):697-702, 1979.
3. Atilola MAO, Sumner-Smith G: Nonunion fractures in dogs, *J Vet Orthop* 3(2):21-24, 1984.
4. Bartels KE: Nonunion, *Vet Clin North Am Small Anim Pract* 17(4):799-809, 1987.
5. Betts CW: General nursing and client education. In Betts CW, Crane SW, editors: *Manual of small animal surgical therapeutics*, New York, 1986, Churchill Livingstone.
6. Bianchi-Maiocchi A: *L'osteosintesi transossea secondo G.A. Ilizarov. A cura di*, Milan, Italy, 1985, Medi Surgical Video.
7. Binnington AG: Delayed union and nonunion. In Slatter DH, editor: *Textbook of small animal surgery*, vol 2, Philadelphia, 1985, Saunders.
8. Brighton CT, Pollack SR: Treatment of recalcitrant nonunion with a capacitively coupled electrical field, *J Bone Joint Surg (Am)* 67(4):577-585, 1985.
9. Brinker WA, Hohn RB, Prieur WD: Delayed union and nonunion. In *Manual of internal fixation in small animals*, New York, 1984, Springer-Verlag.
10. Clark DM: The use of electrical current in the treatment of nonunions, *Vet Clin North Am Small Anim Pract* 17(4):793-798, 1987.
11. Connolly JF: Common avoidable problems in nonunions, *Clin Orthop* 194:226-235, 1985.
12. Dallman MJ and others: Rotational strength of double-pinning techniques in repair of transverse fractures in femurs of dogs, *Am J Vet Res* 51:123-127, 1990.
13. Ehricht HG, Schellnack K: Treatment of noninfected and infected pseudoarthrosis by external fixation, *Reconstr Surg Traumatol* 16:32-50, 1978.
14. Esterhai JL, and others: Nonunion of the humerus: clinical, roentgenographic, scintigraphic, and response characteristics to treatment with constant direct current stimulation of osteogenesis, *Clin Orthop* (211):228-234, 1986.
15. Esterhai JL, and others: Treatment of chronic osteomyelitis complicating nonunion and segmental defects of the tibia with open cancellous bone graft, posterolateral bone graft, and soft-tissue transfer, *J Trauma* 30(1):49-54, 1990.
16. Fernandez DL: Anterior bone grafting and conventional lag screw fixation to treat scaphoid nonunions, *J Hand Surg* 15A(1):140-147, 1990.
17. Flynn JC: Nonunion of slightly displaced fractures of the lateral humeral condyle in children: an update, *J Pediatr Orthop* 9(6):691-696, 1989.
18. Foster RJ, and others: Internal fixation of fractures and nonunions of the humeral shaft, *J Bone Joint Surg (Am)* 67(6):857-864, 1985.
19. Frost HM: *An introduction to biomechanics*, Springfield, Ill, 1967, Charles C Thomas.
20. Gordon L, Chiu EJ: Treatment of infected non-unions and segmental defects of the tibia with staged microvascular muscle transplantation and bone-grafting, *J Bone Joint Surg (Am)* 70(3):377-385, 1988.
21. Green SA, Moore TA, Spohn PJ: Nonunion of the tibial shaft, *Orthopedics* 11(8):1149-1157, 1988.
22. Hohn RB: *Notes: delayed union and nonunion*, annual AO/ASIF course, Columbus, Ohio, 1984.
23. Johnson EE: Custom titanium plating for failed nonunion or delayed internal fixation of femoral fractures, *Clin Orthop* 234:195-203, 1988.
24. Johnson KD: Management of malunion and nonunion of the tibia, *Orthop Clin North Am* 18(1):157-171, 1987.
25. Jupiter JB: Complex nonunion of the humeral diaphysis: treatment with a medial approach, an anterior plate, and a vascularized fibular graft, *J Bone Joint Surg (Am)* 72(5):701-707, 1990.
26. Jupiter JB, and others: The role of external fixation in the treatment of posttraumatic osteomyelitis, *J Orthop Trauma* 2(2):79-93, 1988.
27. Mandt PR, Gershuni DH: Treatment of nonunion of fractures in the epiphyseal-metaphyseal region of the long bones, *J Orthop Trauma* 1(2):141-151, 1987.

28. Marcer M, Musatti G, Bassett CAL: Results of pulsed electromagnetic fields (PEMFs) in ununited fractures after external skeletal fixation, *Clin Orthop* 190:260-265, 1984.

29. Meister KM, Segal D, Whitelaw GP: The role of bone grafting in the treatment of delayed unions and nonunions of the tibia, *Orthop Rev* 19(3):261-271, 1990.

30. Menon J: Correction of rotary malunion of the fingers by metacarpal rotational osteotomy, *Orthopedics* 13(2):197-200, 1990.

31. Meskens MWA, Stuyck JAE, Mulier JC: Treatment of delayed union and nonunion of the tibia by pulsed electromagnetic fields: a retrospective follow-up, *Bull Hosp Joint Dis Orthop Inst* 48(2):170-175, 1988.

32. Meyer S, and others: The treatment of infected non-union of fractures of long bones, *J Bone Joint Surg (Am)* 57(6):836-842, 1975.

33. Neto FLDS, Volpon JB: Experimental nonunion in dogs, *Clin Orthop* 187:260-271, 1984.

34. Nunamaker DM, Rhinelander FW, Heppenstall RB: Delayed union, nonunion, and malunion. In Newton CD, Nunamaker DM, editors: *Textbook of small animal orthopaedics*, Philadelphia, 1985, Lippincott.

35. *Orthopaedic Review*: A conversation with Andrew C, Bassett L: Pulsed electromagnetic fields, a noninvasive therapeutic modality for fracture nonunion, 15(12):781/55-795/69, 1986.

36. Pearson RL, Perry CR: The Ilizarov technique in the treatment of infected tibial nonunions, *Orthop Rev* 17(5):609-613, 1989.

37. Rittmann WW, Perren SM: *Cortical bone healing after internal fixation and infection*, New York, 1974, Springer-Verlag.

38. Rosen H: Compression treatment of long bone pseudoarthroses, *Clin Orthop* 138:154-166, 1979.

39. Ruby LK, Stinson J, Belsky MR: The natural history of scaphoid nonunion, *J Bone Joint Surg (Am)* 67(3):428-432, 1985.

40. Russell GG, Henderson R, Arnett G: Primary or delayed closure for open tibial fractures, *J Bone Joint Surg (Br)* 72(1):125-128, 1990.

41. Schatzker J, Burgess RC, Glynn MK: The management of nonunions following high tibial osteotomies, *Clin Orthop* 193:230-233, 1985.

42. Schenk RK, and others: Nonunion of fractures. Section B. Nonunion: the histologic picture. In Sumner-Smith G, editor: *Bone in clinical orthopaedics*, Philadelphia, 1982, Saunders.

43. Sharrard WJW: A double-blind trial of pulsed electromagnetic fields for delayed union of tibial fractures, *J Bone Joint Surg (Br)* 72(3):347-355, 1990.

44. Spaulding K, Berry C: Personal communication, 1991.

45. Sumner-Smith G, Bishop, HM: Nonunions of fractures. Section A. Nonunion: pathogenesis and treatment. In Sumner-Smith G, editor: *Bone in clinical orthopaedics*, Philadelphia, 1982, Saunders.

46. Thommasini MD, Betts CW: Use of the "Ilizarov" external fixator in a dog, *VCOT* 3(4):70-76, 1991.

47. Trotter DH, Dobozi W: Nonunion of the humerus: rigid fixation, bone grafting, and adjunctive bone cement, *Clin Orthop* 204:162-168, 1986.

48. Ward WG, Goldner RD, Nunley JA: Reconstruction of tibial bone defects in tibial nonunion, *Microsurgery* 11:63-73, 1990.

49. Watson-Jones R, Coltart WD: The classic: slow union of fractures: with a study of 804 fractures of the shafts of the tibia and femur, *Clin Orthop* 168:2-16, 1982.

50. Wray RC, Glunk R: Treatment of delayed union, nonunion, and malunion of the phalanges of the hand, *Ann Plast Surg* 22(1):14-18, 1989.

13

Growth Deformities

ANN L. JOHNSON

Musculoskeletal growth deformities can result from any alteration in the normal sequence of maturation of bone and muscle. The most common growth deformities encountered in small animal orthopedic practice are a result of a premature decrease or cessation in the function of the physis. Congenital deformities of the limbs are occasionally encountered. Developmental deformities of bone and joints can occur because of abnormal forces generated by the surrounding hard and soft tissues. This chapter discusses the etiology, diagnosis, treatment, and outcome of growth deformities.

ETIOLOGY
Congenital Growth Deformities

Congenital growth deformities are conditions of the musculoskeletal system that are present when the animal is born, originating from a failure of normal development in utero. These conditions may be hereditary or caused by exposure to toxins during the first trimester.[10,11,20,25,34] Usually, only one or two animals in a litter are affected. The deformity may be unilateral or bilateral. Congenital deformities are classified as deficiencies, duplications, or

293

lack of normal articulation of joints. Congenital growth deformities seen in small animals include hemimelia, polydactyly, duplication of limbs, humeroulnar luxation, humeroradial luxation, patellar luxation, and polyarthrodysplasia.*

Developmental Growth Deformities

Certain musculoskeletal deformities are influenced by changes in the hard and soft tissues during the animal's development. Failure of normal ossification of the physeal cartilage leads to retained cartilage cores, which may affect the growth of the physis.[17,37] Abnormal pull of the musculature on the physes can result in angular and torsional deformities of the bone.[28] Abnormal pressure on cartilage results in failure of normal joint development. This can occur with a decrease of pressure, as seen in the shallow trochlear grooves associated with congenital patellar luxation.[13,28,30]

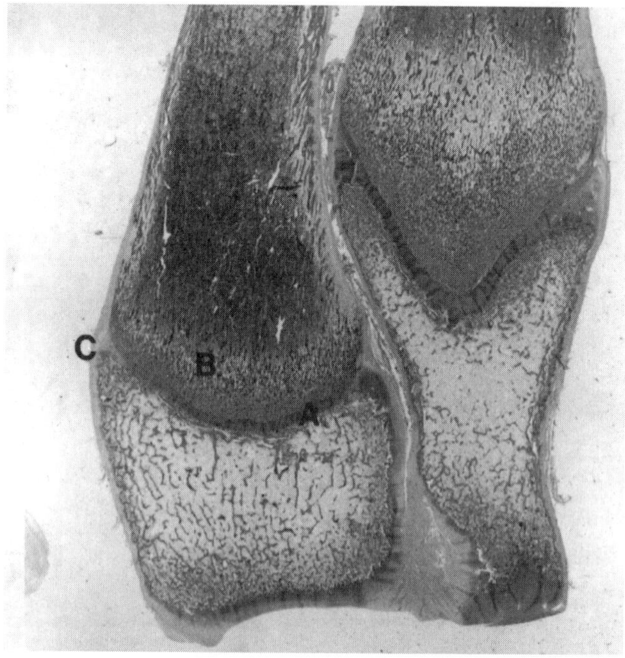

Anatomy and Physiology of the Physis

Knowledge of the anatomy, physiology, and biomechanical properties of the physis is necessary for understanding the pathophysiology of physeal trauma and determining the correct diagnosis and most appropriate surgical technique for treatment of the resultant growth deformity.

The physis consists of (1) a cartilaginous component containing four zones, (2) a bony component at the metaphysis, (3) and a fibrous component surrounding the periphery of the physis (Fig. 13-1).[3,14] In the cartilaginous physis the reserve zone is located immediately adjacent to the epiphyseal bone and consists of cartilage cells and matrix. The function of the reserve zone is unclear and may be storage for later nutritional requirements. The growth of the physis results from the division of chondrocytes located in the proliferating zone. The top cell of each cell column is the true germinal layer of the physis. The function of chondrocytes in the proliferating zone appears to be duplication and matrix production. Longitudinal growth of the physis is equal to the rate of production of new chondrocytes multiplied by the maximum size of the chondrocytes at the bottom of the hypertrophic zone. In the hypertrophic zone the chondrocytes are approximately five times the size of chondrocytes in the proliferating zone, and a corresponding decrease occurs in the amount of matrix around the cells. Biochemical changes occur that prepare the matrix for calcification. Seeding of the matrix with amorphous calcium phosphate leads to hydroxyapatite crystal formation and calcification of the longitudinal septa of the matrix in the zone of provisional

*References 6, 10, 11, 20, 24, 25, 34.

Fig. 13-1 Histological section of the distal radial physis. **A,** Cartilaginous physis. **B,** Metaphysis. **C,** Fibrous periphery. (Hematoxylin and eosin stain, ×4).
Courtesy WH Riser.

calcification. The metaphysis begins adjacent to the last intact transverse septum of each cell column. Vascularization of the longitudinal septa followed by osteogenic cell proliferation allows bone formation on the cartilaginous septa. Gradually, the calcified septa are remodeled with bone (Fig. 13-2).[3,14]

The epiphyseal and metaphyseal sides of the physis have separate blood supplies. The proliferating zone cell columns are well supplied by terminal branches of the epiphyseal vasculature. The metaphysis is supplied by the metaphyseal arteries and terminal branches of the nutrient artery, which loop just below the last intact transverse septum of the cartilage portion of the physis. The fibrous peripheral structures are supplied with blood from perichondrial arteries (Fig. 13-2).[3,14,42]

Trauma to the Physis

Trauma to the physis can result from disruption of the blood supply, with subsequent cell necrosis, or direct damage to chondrocytes. Traumatic interruption of the epiphyseal blood supply results in necrosis of the growing cells and closure of the affected portion of the physis. In contrast, damage to the metaphyseal vasculature supplying the ossifying portion of the physis results in interruption of ossification, a process that resumes when the blood supply is restored.[42]

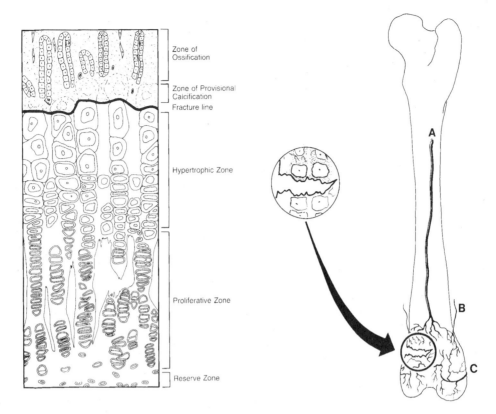

Fig. 13-2   Illustration of the distal femoral physis showing the blood supply and histological structures. **A,** Metaphyseal artery. **B,** Perichondrial artery. **C,** Epiphyseal artery. The area of the physis usually subjected to fracture is noted.

The cartilaginous physis is weaker than the surrounding bone and ligaments, making it susceptible to injury. The weakest portion of the physis is the junction of the hypertrophic zone and the zone of provisional calcification. The hypertrophic zone has a large cell-to-matrix ratio, which weakens its structure. In addition, a stress concentration is created when two areas of different mechanical properties, such as the weak hypertrophic zone and the stronger zone of provisional calcification, are located adjacent to each other. Consequently, when a cartilaginous physis is fractured, the separation usually occurs through the hypertrophic zone. A fracture in this location does not affect the proliferating cells and does not compromise potential growth (see Fig. 13-2).[21,40]

Trauma resulting in compression of the proliferating zone and destruction of the chondrocytes causes premature closure of the physis. This is seen clinically after trauma to the conically V-shaped distal ulnar physis of the dog. Because of the unusual shape of this physis, shear forces that parallel the bone's transverse plane compress the proliferating zone (Fig. 13-3).[16,41]

Fractures of the physis are classified by radiographic and histological appearance.[21,28,40] A Salter-Harris type I fracture is a separation of the physis at the hypertrophic zone. A Salter-Harris type II fracture passes through part

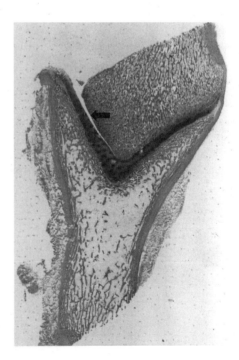

Fig. 13-3   Histological section of the cone-shaped canine distal ulnar physis after a Salter-Harris type V fracture. The physis has separated on one side (*arrow*) and has been crushed on the opposite side. (Safranin O-Fast Green stain, ×4.)

of the hypertrophic zone and then extends through a portion of the metaphysis. A Salter-Harris type III fracture is through a portion of the hypertrophic zone and then extends through the epiphysis. A Salter-Harris type IV fracture extends through the epiphysis and metaphysis, crossing the cartilaginous physis. A Salter-Harris type V fracture is a crushing of the proliferating zone. A variation on this type of fracture is the Salter-Harris type VI fracture, which is a crushing of the zone of proliferating cells in only part of the physis, resulting in asymmetrical closure of the physis (Fig. 13-4).[12,21]

The prognosis for healing of a physeal fracture is excellent. The prognosis for continued function or growth from the physis depends on the damage to the proliferating zone and the animal's age at the time of injury. A good prognosis exists for future physeal growth after a fracture that separates the cartilaginous physis at the hypertrophic zone. A poor prognosis exists for future physeal growth after trauma that crushes the physis. Fractures that cross the physis may heal with bone bridging the physis and impeding growth.[21,40] Radiographs made at the time of injury do not give information about crushing injuries to the physis or damage

to the blood supply. Therefore, it is difficult to give an accurate prognosis for growth at the time of injury. Radiographs of the injured bone and the contralateral bone should be made and compared for length 2 to 3 weeks after the injury to determine if the physis is functioning.

Effects of Fixation on the Physis

Fractures through and adjacent to the physis can be treated with external coaptation or internal fixation. External coaptation devices do not affect the function of the physis.[4,40] If internal fixation is used, one must consider its effect on physeal function. Plates and screws or external fixators that bridge the physis prevent normal bone growth and indirectly cause compression of the physis. Implants that cross the physis directly, such as pins and screws, have the potential to damage the portion of the physis invaded. The threads of a pin or screw placed across the physis do not allow continued growth. A smooth intramedullary pin or Kirschner wire crossing the physis allows the proliferating cartilage to slide along the pin.[4] Pins placed perpendicular to the physis allow growth more readily than pins placed obliquely and anchored in cortical bone, such as a cross-pinning technique. The growth potential of the individual animal also dictates the fixation used. The growth of an animal that is close to skeletal maturity is not adversely affected by fixation inhibiting physeal function.

Sequelae to Premature Physeal Closure

The sequelae to premature physeal closure include shortened limbs, angular deformities, rotational deformities, and disruption of normal joint anatomy resulting in degenerative joint disease.* Severity of the deformity depends on the animal's age when the physeal closure occurs and the location and extent of the physeal closure. The younger animal with greater growth potential is more severely affected. Physeal closure in one paired bone can interfere with the normal development of the other bone. For example, when the distal ulnar physis prematurely closes, the distance between that physis and the elbow becomes fixed. The normal radius continues to grow but becomes deformed because the ulna is no longer growing and thus acts as a restraint on radial elongation. This results not only in a shortened ulna but also in shortening, rotation, and angulation of the radius. In addition, abnormal asynchronous radius-to-ulna growth results in incongruity of the elbow and carpal joints, leading to degenerative joint disease. Symmetrical or complete physeal closure in a single bone such as the femur causes shortening of the bone. Asymmetrical or

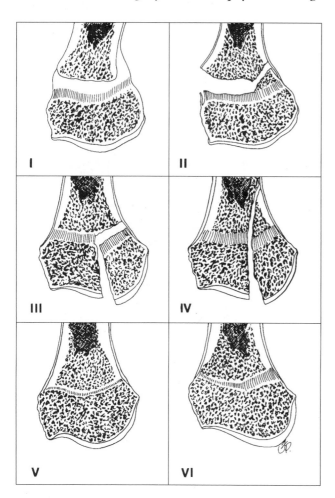

Fig. 13-4 Salter-Harris physeal fracture classification.

---

*References 5, 16, 21, 28, 29, 31, 35, 39, 41, 43, 45.

partial closure of the physis of a single or paired bone results in angular deformity of the bone and may affect the anatomy of adjacent joints, again resulting in degenerative joint disease.

Treatment of Premature Physeal Closure

Destruction of the growing cells and closure of the physis is an irreversible phenomenon. Treatment is therefore directed at reducing the severity of or correcting the sequelae to physeal closure. The goal of treating the immature animal is to allow as much growth as possible to occur to obtain maximum limb length and any natural correction of angular deformities. This is accomplished by using techniques of ostectomies or partial physeal resection and autogenous fat grafting, which are described in more detail later in this chapter.[7,16,19,44] Owners of immature animals must be informed of possible additional surgery for complete treatment of the animal after maturity. In the mature animal, treatment is aimed at correcting the deformity while preserving as much limb length as possible.*

GROWTH DEFORMITIES OF THE FORELIMB
Humerus

Growth deformities of the humerus rarely develop. Salter-Harris type IV fractures of the distal humerus are common, and the physis may close after injury and treatment. However, angular limb deformities have not been reported after complete premature closure of the distal physis. Most humeral growth is from the proximal physis, and the dog appears to compensate adequately for the small loss of length associated with premature closure of the distal physis.

Radius and Ulna
Congenital growth deformities

Hemimelia. Congenital deficiencies of the forelimb include segmental deficiencies of the radius and ulna.[20,34] Radial hemimelia, or congenital absence of the radius, is seen occasionally in dogs and cats. The affected limb or limbs are shortened with a varus deformity and are not functional for gaiting. The etiology is unknown in animals but theorized to be either hereditary or from exposure to toxins during the first trimester. Treatments have been described, with rib grafts and wiring techniques used to reestablish length to the limb and restore some function, which may be used in selected patients.[34] However, lightweight animals such as cats can learn to ambulate on the rear limbs (Fig. 13-5).

---

*References 16, 18, 26, 27, 32, 39, 43.

Ectrodactyly. Ectrodactyly, or splitting of the limb, is a failure of fusion of the embryonic precursors of the bones of the forelimb. The deformity consists of separation of the medial and lateral portions of the limb. The separation can occur between any of the metacarpal bones and extend proximally between the radius and ulna. Soft tissue separation may accompany the bone defect. Absence or hypoplasia of metacarpal and carpal bones can occur. Hypoplasia of the radius or ulna can also occur. If the deformity continues proximally, luxation of the elbow may be present.[6]

Treatment of the deformity may be feasible if most bone structure is intact and the elbow functional. Treatment is aimed at cosmetic salvage of the limb and consists of surgically uniting the segments using orthopedic wire around adjacent bones. The skin is closed on the dorsal and palmar surfaces (Fig. 13-6). Function after cosmetic repair depends on the severity of the deformity.

Congenital luxation of the elbow. The syndrome of congenital elbow luxation includes rotation of the olecranon lateral to the humerus; hypoplasia of the medial collateral and annular ligaments; hypertrophy of the lateral collateral ligament; incongruent joint surfaces with abnormal wear patterns; hypoplasia or aplasia of the

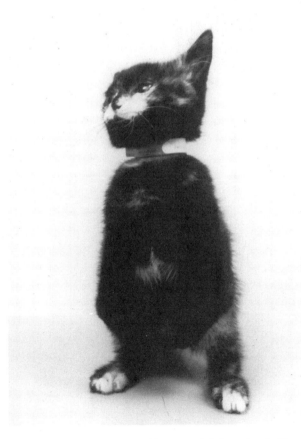

Fig. 13-5 Three-month-old kitten with bilateral radial hemimelia. The kitten balances and moves on her rear limbs.

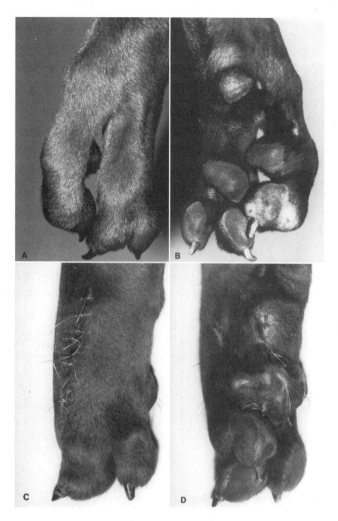

Fig. 13-6 Four-month-old Doberman with ectrodactyly. **A** and **B,** Preoperative appearance of the paw. **C** and **D,** Postoperative appearance after cosmetic repair of the paw.

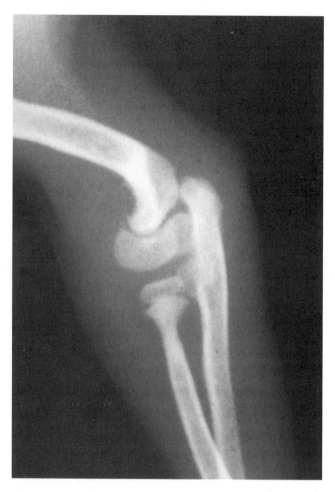

Fig. 13-7 Radiograph of a 2-month-old Lhasa Apso with congenital elbow luxation.

coronoid processes, anconeal process, trochlear notch, olecranon fossa, and humeral condyles; and skeletal muscle anomalies (Fig. 13-7). These dogs usually present at 2 to 3 months of age and are unable to walk on the affected forelimb. The condition may be unilateral or bilateral. A hereditary influence has been conjectured.[24,25]

Surgical treatment consists of reduction of the radius and ulna and internal stabilization to hold the joint in place. Stabilization includes heavy suture to plicate the medial aspect of the joint, transposition of the olecranon process to redirect the pull of the triceps muscle, and fixation with a tension-band wiring technique or a derotational osteotomy of the proximal ulna with pin and wire fixation. If surgical treatment is desired, it should be done as early as possible to restore the normal anatomy of the joint and allow for normal development of the cartilage.[24,25]

Another form of congenital elbow luxation is congenital luxation of the radial head. With this syndrome, the proximal radius is angulated laterally and the radial head is luxated laterally.[11,24] Dogs with lateral luxation of the radial head present at about 4 to 6 months with a weight-bearing forelimb lameness. Crepitance and decreased range of motion of the elbow are present. The radial head may be palpated laterally to the humerus. Treatment includes a radial osteotomy, reduction of the radial head, and fixation of the proximal portion of the radius. Results vary with the degree of joint reduction that can be attained (Fig. 13-8). Degenerative joint disease of the elbow is usually a sequela.

Developmental deformities

Retained cartilage core. Retarded endochondral ossification at the distal ulnar physis may lead to slower growth of the physis and shortening of the ulna. This causes shortening, cranial bowing, external rotation, and

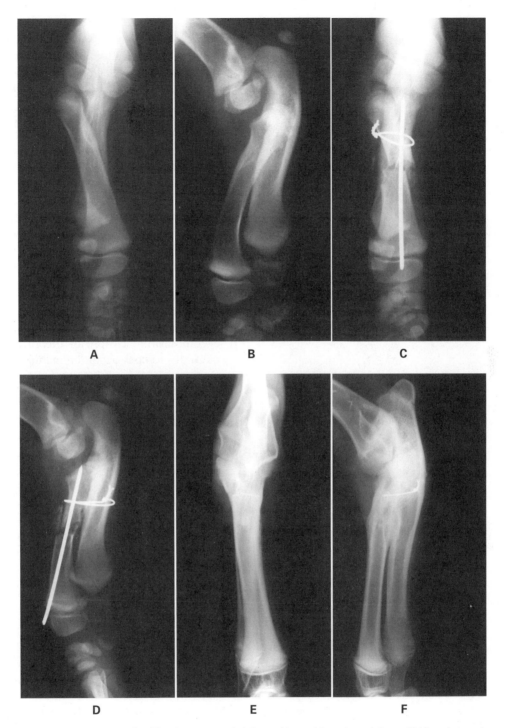

Fig. 13-8   Four-month-old Doberman with bilateral lateral luxation of the radial head. **A** and **B,** Preoperative radiographic appearance of the elbow. **C** and **D,** Postoperative radiograph of the elbow. **E** and **F,** Postoperative radiographic appearance of the elbow after 3 months.

valgus angulation of the radius.[29,37] This syndrome may be indistinguishable from traumatic premature closure of the distal ulnar physis by physical examination of the dog. Radiographic examination reveals a radiolucent cartilage core in the center of the distal ulnar physis extending into the metaphysis. Histological examination of the affected physis shows normal reserve and proliferative zones with a thickened hypertrophic zone in the center of the physis. The matrix septa in the abnormally thickened hypertrophic zone do not appear to calcify normally,

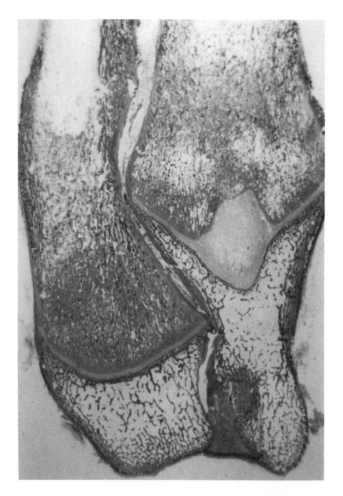

Fig. 13-9 Histological section of a canine distal ulnar physis with a retained cartilage core. (Hematoxylin and eosin stain, ×4.)

Courtesy WH Riser.

and vascularization does not occur. Therefore, bone production and remodeling are delayed (Fig. 13-9).[17,37]

Several theories describe the etiology of retained cartilage cores. The condition appears primarily in large, fast-growing dogs, and some speculate that nutrition may play a role in the development. This hypothesis is difficult to prove because the oversupplementation in the diet of many of these dogs may be done as a response to the condition. It is suggested that these dogs be fed the recommended calcium-to-phosphorus ratio and the amount of food decreased to slow the dog's overall growth.[17,37] Loss of vascularization to the central metaphysis can also result in retained cartilage core.[37] Another theory suggests that the condition is part of the generalized disease of osteochondrosis. Finally, the syndrome may result from an abnormality of the chondrocytes, which can no longer control the process of calcification of the cartilaginous septa.[17]

Treatment of the syndrome depends on the severity of the clinical signs. Dogs with mild deformities may respond to dietary limitations.[17,37] Dogs treated conservatively in this manner should be monitored weekly to determine if the deformities are correcting or progressing. If the deformities progress, an ulnar ostectomy with autogenous fat graft should be done to remove the restraint on radial growth.

Premature closure of the physis. Injury to the physis resulting in radial and ulnar deformities occurs frequently. Synchronous growth of the radius and ulna in the dog is essential for the development of a normal forelimb. The radius receives about 40% of its length from the proximal physis and about 60% from the distal physis.[31] The ulna receives about 85% of its length from the distal physis, with the proximal physis contributing only 15%, and all that growth is proximal to the radial head.[5] In most dogs, growth accelerates rapidly during the fifth to seventh month and tapers off during the ninth to tenth month.[16,29,30,39] This varies depending on the breed of dog, with smaller dogs maturing faster than larger dogs. The distal ulnar physis is most frequently injured; however, premature closure of the proximal and/or distal radial physis does occur. Premature closure of the distal ulnar physis is invariably complete and results in shortening of the ulna and cranial bowing, external rotation, and shortening of the radius. A valgus angulation to the carpus is present and there are varying amounts of elbow incongruity.* Symmetrical complete closure of the proximal or distal radial physis results in a shortened but straight radius, incongruity of the elbow, and a varus angulation of the carpus.[27,31,43] The limb deformity seen with asymmetrical or partial physeal closure of the distal radius varies depending on the location of the closure. The most common appears to be a caudal lateral closure of the physis resulting in a valgus deformity of the carpus (Fig. 13-10). The normal anatomy of the carpus may be disrupted with asymmetrical distal radial physeal closure.[43]

Diagnosis of premature closure of the radial or ulnar physis is made after physical and radiographic examination of the forelimb. Radiographs of the opposite normal limb should be made to obtain a control for determining the normal length and anatomy of the forelimb. In early cases of premature closure of the distal ulnar physis, a discrepancy in ulnar lengths may be determined before obvious deformity of the forelimb. Measurements of bone length and angular limb deformity should be made from the radiographs and on the dog to establish a preoperative standard against which the results of treatment may be compared.

Treatment of premature closure of the distal ulnar physis in the immature dog. The goals of treatment of the immature dog with premature closure of the

*References 5, 16, 28, 29, 37, 41, 45.

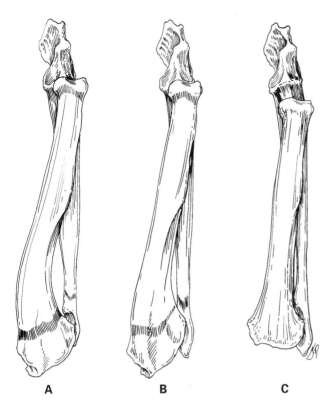

Fig. 13-10   Deformity of the radius and ulna caused by **A,** premature closure of the distal ulnar physis; **B,** asymmetrical or partial closure of the distal radial physis; and **C,** symmetrical or complete closure of the distal radial physis.

distal ulnar physis are to allow unrestricted growth of the normal physis of the radius and ulna, which results in maximum growth of the limb and in some cases correction of the angular deformity. An ulnar ostectomy is used to release the constraint placed on radial growth by the ulna and is coupled with the placement of a free autogenous fat graft to prevent union of the ulnar segments.[7,12,16]

Both the affected forelimb and the ipsilateral flank are prepared for aseptic surgery. The distal ulna is approached from the lateral side via a skin incision extending over the middle to distal ulnar area. The subcutaneous tissue is incised and the lateral digital extensor muscle separated from the extensor carpi ulnaris muscle, exposing the distal metaphyseal portion of the ulna. The area for the ostectomy is isolated by elevating the surrounding musculature and fascia, carefully ensuring that all periosteum, with its osteogenic potential, remains with the segment of bone to be resected.[9] A 1-2 cm segment of the ulna and associated periosteum is resected using bone cutters or an oscillating bone saw cooled with a saline flush (Fig. 13-11). The interosseous artery may be encountered at this time, and hemostasis should be achieved. A 2 to 3 cm skin incision is made in the ipsi-

lateral flank or axilla area, exposing the subcutaneous fat. A large single piece of fat is sharply dissected free and placed in the ostectomy gap (Fig. 13-11). Hemostasis is achieved at the donor site, and the subcutaneous tissue and skin are apposed. The transplanted fat is secured in the ostectomy gap by suturing the adjacent soft tissues. The subcutaneous tissues and skin are apposed. A soft padded bandage is placed on the limb.[16] In rare instances it is necessary to perform this procedure bilaterally. The dog is placed in dorsal recumbency, both front limbs are draped simultaneously, and the fat graft is obtained from the falciform ligament.

Postoperative radiographs are made to document the location and length of the ostectomy gap. A soft padded bandage or splint may be used to protect the limbs for 2 to 3 weeks if bilateral procedures are done. The dog is released to the owners with instructions to limit activity and to return for monthly reexaminations. Reevaluation radiographs are compared with the postoperative radiographs for growth of the radius, correction of the angular deformity, and patency of the ostectomy gap. Restoration of the normal configuration of the elbow from the release of the proximal ulna may be noted. Reevaluations are discontinued when the animal is skeletally mature. Union of the ulna while the animal is still growing is an indication for repeat surgery. A corrective osteotomy of the radius may be indicated if the angular or rotational deformity has not corrected when the dog has reached maturity.[12,16]

Treatment of premature closure of the distal ulnar physis in the mature dog. Some dogs that have premature physeal closure do not receive treatment until they have reached or are near maturity. The goals of treatment are to correct angular and rotational deformities while preserving as much limb length as possible. Procedures used include oblique or opening wedge radial and ulnar osteotomy with repositioning of the distal radial segment, cuneiform or closing wedge osteotomy, or reverse wedge osteotomy.[16,26,39] Only the oblique osteotomy preserves or increases limb length. Preoperative radiographs are studied to determine the location of the point of greatest curvature of the radius and to evaluate the anatomy of the adjacent elbow and carpus. The dog is anesthetized, and the affected forelimb and a donor site for cancellous bone, usually the proximal humerus of the same limb, are prepared for aseptic surgery.

Oblique or opening wedge osteotomy. An external fixation pin is placed in the proximal radius from the lateral aspect. The pin is parallel to the joint surface of the radial head and within the lateral transverse plane of the proximal radius. A second pin is placed in the distal radius from the lateral aspect. This pin is parallel to the distal radial joint surface and within the lateral transverse plane of the distal radius. Both pins exit on the limb's

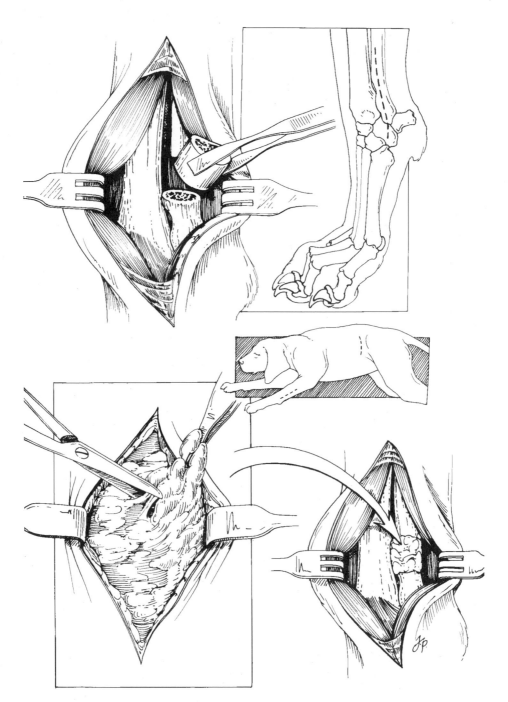

Fig. 13-11 Release ostectomy of the distal ulna for treatment of premature closure of the distal ulnar physis in the immature dog. The ostectomy site is filled with autogenous fat harvested from the flank.

medial aspect. The distal ulna is approached as described earlier and an ulnar osteotomy performed. The distal radius is approached from the medial aspect at its point of greatest curvature. The muscles and tendons are separated and the distal radius exposed. An oblique osteotomy of the radius is performed with an osteotome or an oscillating bone saw, directing the osteotomy line parallel to the distal radial joint surface. The radius and

ulnar are repositioned using the proximal and distal transfixation pins to aid in correctly aligning the limb and eliminating any angular or rotational deformity. The pins should be positioned parallel to each other and in the same lateral transverse plane. A connecting bar is placed on the lateral and medial aspect of the limb, and additional fixation pins are introduced through single clamps placed on the lateral connecting bar. At least one

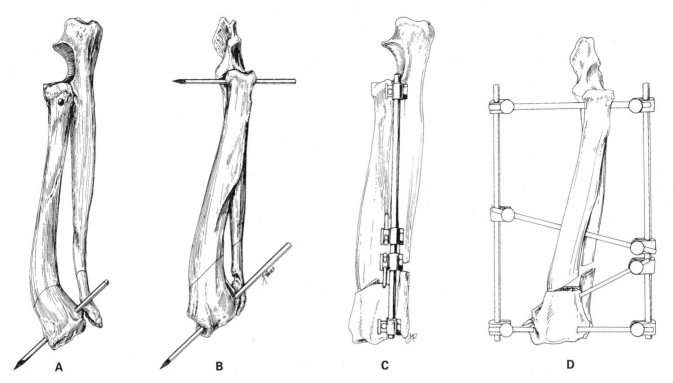

Fig. 13-12   Oblique osteotomy for correction of angular, rotational, and shortening deformities of the radius caused by premature closure of the distal ulnar physis. **A** and **B,** Placement of the proximal and distal fixation pins and the osteotomy line. **C** and **D,** Corrected alignment after osteotomy and stabilization with an external fixator.

additional pin should be placed in each radial segment (Fig. 13-12).

Autogenous cancellous bone graft may be harvested and placed at the radial osteotomy site. The surgical wounds are apposed, the clamps tightened, and the fixation pins cut to the correct length. Postoperative radiographs are made to document the correction obtained and the position of the fixation pins. The proximal and distal radial joint surfaces must be parallel and the cranial surfaces of the proximal and distal radial segments located in the same transverse plane. If they are not, some correction may be obtained by readjusting the external fixator.[16]

Cuneiform or closing wedge osteotomy. Preoperative planning for a closing wedge osteotomy includes careful estimation of the angles for the corrective osteotomy. Templates are drawn over the craniocaudal and lateral radiographs. Over the craniocaudal radiograph, a line (1) is drawn parallel to the proximal radial articular surface, and another line (4) is drawn parallel to the distal radial articular surface. A line (2) is drawn parallel to line 1 at the area of greatest radial curvature, and another line (3) is drawn parallel to line 4 at the area of greatest radial curvature. The angle formed at the radial diaphysis delineates the shape and amount of bone to be removed to correct the angular deformity. In addition, a template is made over the lateral radiograph by lines (5 and 8) per-

pendicular to the long axis of the radius proximally and distally to the area of greatest curvature. Lines (6 and 7) are drawn perpendicular to lines 5 and 8 at the area of greatest curvature and delineate the amount of bone to be removed to correct cranial bowing (Fig. 13-13).

The surgical approach is the same as described for the oblique osteotomy of the radius and ulna. An ulnar osteotomy is performed. The radial osteotomy is performed following the guidelines created on the templates. The fracture is reduced, correcting angular deformity, rotational deformity, and cranial bowing. The osteotomy is compressed and stabilized with a plate and bone screws, or stabilization is achieved with an external fixator.[26]

Reverse wedge osteotomy. Because significant loss of bone length may occur with the closing wedge osteotomy, a reverse wedge osteotomy is designed to reduce the amount of bone removed from the radius. The wedge size is predetermined by determining a wedge size as described for the closing wedge osteotomy and then dividing that wedge in half (see Fig. 13-18, *D*). The osteotomy is performed, and the wedge is rotated 180 degrees and replaced at the osteotomy site. The fracture and wedge are stabilized with a plate and bone screws.[26] Radiographs are made after surgery to record position of the bone segments, alignment of the joint surfaces, and position of the implants.

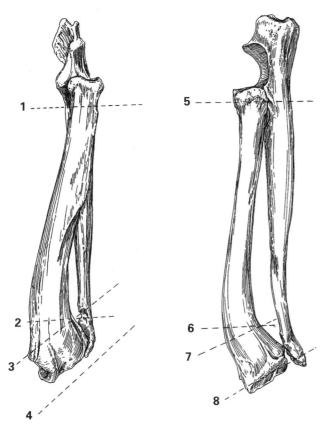

Fig. 13-13   Cuneiform or closing wedge osteotomy for treatment of angular and rotational deformity of the radius caused by premature closure of the distal ulnar physis. See text for a description of the numbered lines.

Treatment of partial premature closure of the distal radial physis in the immature dog. The goal of treatment is to allow unrestricted growth of the normal portion of the distal radial physis. Tomographic examination of the distal radial physis may be indicated to define accurately the area of the physis that is closed and bridged with bone. The animal is treated by resecting the

bone bridge area of the physis and placing a free autogenous fat graft in the defect to prevent reestablishment of the bone bridge.[43] The closed and bridged portion of the distal radial physis is surgically exposed. The limitations of the bone bridge are defined by inserting small-gauge hypodermic needles into the physis at the bone bridge–physeal cartilage junction. The cartilage of the normal physis is easily penetrated by the needle, in contrast to the resistance felt when the bone bridge or adjacent metaphyseal or epiphyseal bone is probed. The bone bridge is removed using a curette or a high-speed burr. Curettage is complete when normal physeal cartilage is observed or probed with the needle. Free autogenous fat is harvested as described previously and placed within the physeal defect (Fig. 13-14). The soft tissues and skin are closed over the transplanted fat.

Postoperative radiographs are made to document complete resection of the bone bridge and placement of the fat graft. A soft padded bandage is used to protect the limb postoperatively. The dog is released to the owners with instructions to limit exercise and return monthly for reevaluation. Reevaluation radiographs are compared with the postoperative radiographs for length of the radius, correction of angular deformity, and patency of the resected area. The goniometer is used to determine angular limb deformity, and results are compared with preoperative results for changes in severity of the deformity. Reevaluations are discontinued when the animal reaches skeletal maturity. Reestablishment of the bone bridge or worsening of the angular deformity may be indications for repeat surgery. A corrective osteotomy of the radius may be indicated if the angular deformity has not corrected when the dog has reached maturity.

Treatment of complete premature closure of the proximal or distal radial physis in the immature dog. The goals of treatment are to allow unrestricted growth of the normal physes of the radius and ulna and to restore and maintain congruity of the elbow.

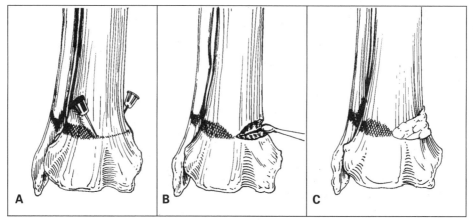

Fig. 13-14   Resection of a bone bridge of the physis. **A,** Extent of the bridge is identified with hypodermic needles. **B,** Bridge is removed with a bone curette. **C,** Space is filled with autogenous fat.

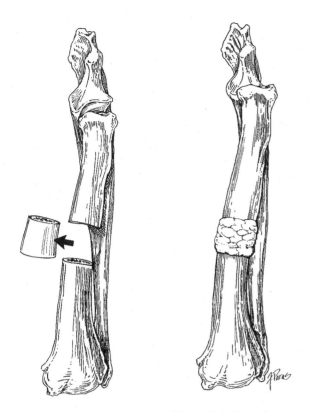

Fig. 13-15 Release ostectomy of the radius for treatment of premature closure of a radial physis in an immature animal. The gap is filled with autogenous fat to prevent premature bone union.

Radial ostectomy and free autogenous fat graft. The animal is treated with a mid-diaphyseal ostectomy of the radius coupled with the placement of a free autogenous fat graft in the defect to prevent bone union (Fig. 13-15). Release of the tension on the proximal and distal radius usually allows the adjacent joints to reestablish normal position. Postoperatively, the limb may require soft padded bandage or splint support, since the radius is the primary weight-bearing bone in the distal forelimb. For the same reasons, a second surgical procedure to reunite the radial segments by bridging the ostectomy gap with autogenous cancellous bone graft may be indicated when the dog has reached maturity[16]

Transverse radial osteotomy with continuous distraction. A mid-diaphyseal radial osteotomy is made after two bilateral external fixation pins are placed in the transverse plane proximally to the osteotomy site and two bilateral external fixation pins are placed in the transverse plane distally to the osteotomy site. A turnbuckle distractor* is attached to the transfixation pins. The apparatus is opened until the pins come under tension.

Recent literature has described the use of continuous distraction to lengthen an osteotomized or corticotomized bone and stimulate simultaneous membranous

bone formation.[15,47] Optimal distraction is at the rate of 1 mm per day starting on the fifth day after surgery. This distraction should be divided into at least two to four increments per day. The apparatus is adjusted every 12 hours by turning the bolt. Adjustments are made based on the growth rate of the contralateral limb and to keep up with the growth of the ipsilateral ulna. The fixator is removed when skeletal maturity is attained and the osteotomy is healed.[19,27,45] The same procedure can be used when both the radial physis and the distal ulnar physis are prematurely closed. An osteotomy is made in both the radius and the ulna, the distraction device is applied to the radius, and adjustments are made to distract the limb during the growth period to match the growth of the contralateral limb.[19]

Treatment of premature closure of the proximal or distal radial physis in mature dogs. The goals of treatment are to reestablish normal length to the radius, establish a congruent elbow, and improve function of the limb.

Transverse lengthening osteotomy. A transverse mid-diaphyseal radial osteotomy is performed after placement of the proximal and distal transfixation pins in the radius. The proximal and distal segments of the radius are distracted using an Inge laminectomy spreader or a Gelpi retractor until the gap is equal to the distance needed to restore the length of the radius. While the segments of the radius are distracted, the medial and lateral connecting bars are secured, and additional fixation pins are introduced into the proximal and distal segments of the radius. The osteotomy gap is filled with autogenous cancellous bone and held in place by suturing the soft tissues (Fig. 13-16). The surgical wounds are closed.

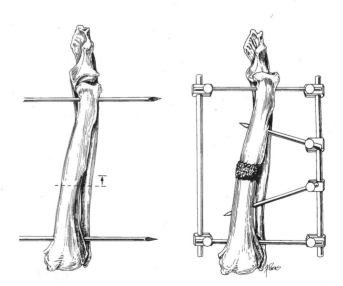

Fig. 13-16 Transverse lengthening osteotomy of the radius to reestablish humeroradial joint congruity. The osteotomy is stabilized with an external fixator. Autogenous cancellous bone is packed into the osteotomy gap.

---

*Imex Co., Longview, Texas.

Postoperative radiographs are made to document the position of the radial head and the locations of the fixation pins. If necessary, some correction of the radial segment locations can be made at this time by adjusting the external fixator. If the head of the radius does not appear to contact the capitulum of the humerus, a transverse bilateral fixation pin is placed through the olecranon proximally to the most proximal transverse pin through the radius. The external fixator clamps proximal to the radial osteotomy are loosened. The ulnar pin and the proximal radial pin are connected bilaterally with elastic bands, placing tension on the proximal radius and pulling it toward the humerus. The limb is radiographed in 24 to 48 hours, and when the articulation is correct, the elastics and the ulnar pin are removed and the clamps tightened.[16,23]

Stairstep osteotomy of the radius. A surgical approach is made to the mid-diaphysis of the radius. A stairstep osteotomy is created and the bone ends distracted with the Inge laminectomy spreader or Gelpi retractor. An approach exposing the lateral aspect of the elbow joint is necessary to determine if the radial head is contacting the humerus, since postoperative corrections cannot easily be made. Lag screws are used to compress the longitudinal portions of the stairstep created in the bone. A bone plate and screws are used to stabilize the fracture. Autogenous cancellous bone is placed in the gaps created by the distraction (Fig. 13-17).[32,43]

Care of the animal after corrective osteotomy of the forelimb includes hydrotherapy to the operated limb to aid in decreasing swelling and to keep fixator pins clean. Hydrotherapy can be done with hot compresses, placement in a whirlpool, or use of a hand-held shower massage. In some patients a soft padded bandage is useful to prevent excessive postoperative swelling. The dog is released to the owners with instructions to continue hydrotherapy if necessary, limit activity, and return for monthly reevaluations. Monthly radiographs are made to evaluate bone healing. In animals treated with the external fixator, the device is removed when bone union has occurred. Removal of plate and screws is also recommended after bone union and entails a second surgical procedure.

GROWTH DEFORMITIES OF THE REAR LIMB
Femur

Femoral head and neck. Trauma to the femoral head and neck can result in altered growth patterns of the area, leading to an incongruent hip and osteoarthritis. A Salter-Harris type I fracture of the proximal femoral physis, also called a *slipped capital physis,* is a common result of trauma to the hip in the immature animal. Because the cartilaginous growth plate is weak com-

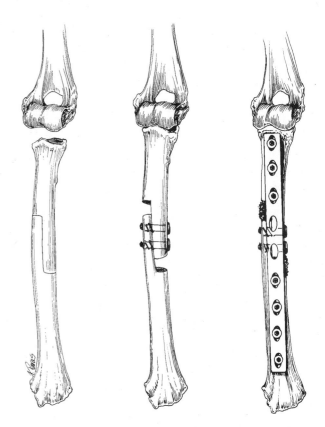

Fig. 13-17 Stairstep osteotomy for lengthening the radius to reestablish humeroradial joint congruity. The osteotomy is stabilized with plate and screws. Autogenous cancellous bone is packed into the defects.

pared with the surrounding bone and ligamentous structures, trauma that results in coxofemoral luxation in the mature animal causes physeal fracture in the immature animal. This fracture is repaired with open reduction and internal fixation.

Premature closure of the proximal femoral physis secondary to the trauma of injury and surgical repair can result in a shortened femoral neck. Although avascular necrosis of the femoral head does not usually occur after this injury,[8] flattening of the femoral head is possible. This may result from a disruption of the blood supply to portions of the articular epiphyseal cartilage complex, which is responsible for development of the secondary center of ossification that makes up the femoral head. Severe coxa vara may result in subluxation of the femoral head.[33] If the clinical signs associated with coxofemoral osteoarthritis are severe, surgical salvage procedures such as excision arthroplasty or total hip replacement may be beneficial.

Intramedullary pin fixation for diaphyseal fractures of the femur in the immature dog can occasionally cause growth deformities in the proximal femur. The changes include coxa valga, shortening and narrowing of the femoral neck and small femoral head, subluxation of the femoral head, and premature closure of the greater trochanteric physis. These changes are associated with the passage of a large intramedullary pin through the trochanteric fossa or greater trochanter. The pin may damage the blood supply to the physis or mechanically impede the growth of the physes.[2]

Premature closure of the distal femoral physis. Salter-Harris types I and II fractures of the distal femoral physis occur often in the immature animal.[22,45] Although Salter and Harris give these fractures a good prognosis for continued physeal function, it is becoming evident that many animals are affected with premature closure of the distal femoral physis after fracture and surgical repair.[1,22] Diaphyseal fractures are also associated with premature distal femoral physeal closure.[36] Asymmetrical closure of the physis causes shortening and angulation of the femur. Much more frequently, symmetrical closure of the physis results in a shortened femur. The amount of femoral shortening depends on the animal's age and growth potential at the time of fracture. In most cases the animal compensates well for loss of femoral length by extending the stifle joint. If the animal with femoral shortening caused by premature closure of the distal physis is unable to function because of the deformity, a lengthening osteotomy should be performed.

Tibia

Premature closure of the physes. Fractures of the proximal and distal physes of the tibia can result in premature closure of the affected physis. The ensuing deformity depends on whether the closure is symmetrical or asymmetrical and on the animal's age when fracture occurs. Symmetrical closure results in shortening of the tibia. A lengthening osteotomy is indicated if the deformity is severe enough to preclude compensation by extension of the adjacent joints. Angular deformities resulting from asymmetrical closure of the physis are treated with corrective osteotomy (Fig. 13-18).

Pes varus. Pes varus is a syndrome occurring in dachshunds. The deformity is a varus angulation of the distal tibia caused by asymmetrical closure of the distal tibial physis. There does not appear to be any history of traumatic incidents in these animals. A genetic etiology has been suggested but not confirmed. Clinical signs appear at 5 to 6 months but may be ignored until chronic soft tissue and bone changes cause lameness. Surgical correction is recommended to prevent severe osteoarthritis of the tarsus. An opening wedge corrective osteotomy is performed and stabilized with an external fixator. A transfixation pin is placed in the proximal tibia parallel to the proximal articular surface. A second transfixation pin is placed in the distal tibia parallel to the distal articular surface. An oblique osteotomy is made parallel to

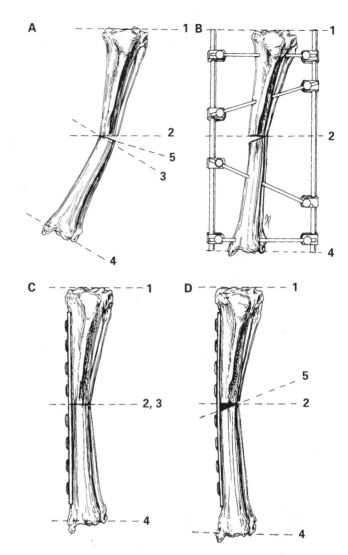

Fig. 13-18 Wedge osteotomy for correction of an angular deformity of the tibia. **A,** Angular deformity of the tibia. **B,** Opening wedge osteotomy stabilized with external skeletal fixation. **C,** Closing wedge osteotomy stabilized with internal fixation. **D,** Reverse wedge osteotomy stabilized with internal fixation. (See Chapter 5.)

the distal transfixation pin and distal articular surface through the metaphysis at the site of greatest curvature of the bone. The proximal and distal transfixation pins are aligned parallel to each other, correcting the varus deformity. A fixation pin is placed medially into the proximal segment of bone. Because the distal segment is small, a smaller pin is placed diagonally from the medial malleolus, across the fracture line, and seated into the lateral cortex of the proximal segment. Autogenous cancellous bone graft is placed at the osteotomy site. The fixation pins are held in alignment with methylmethacrylate or small external fixator bars and clamps. When bone union has occurred, the fixation device is removed.[18,28]

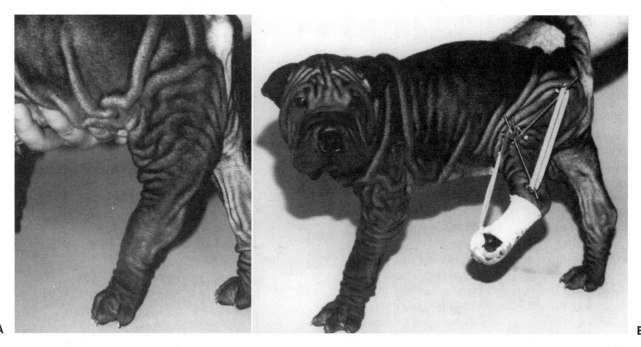

Fig. 13-19 Three-month-old Sharpei with genu recurvatum. **A,** Preoperative appearance of the dog. **B,** Postoperative appearance showing the external skeletal fixation connected with rubber bands to create flexural forces on the stifle and hock.

Stifle

Genu valgum and genu varum. Genu valgum is most often associated with lateral patellar luxation in giant-breed dogs. Genu varum is usually associated with medial patellar luxation in small-breed dogs. A complete discussion of both conditions is found in Chapter 18.

Genu recurvatum. Genu recurvatum or hyperextension syndrome is an infrequent developmental deformity. The syndrome appears in young puppies as a hyperextension of the stifle and hock. The stifle can be passively flexed, but the flexor muscles appear weak and inadequate for proper function. As the deformity progresses, the limb becomes fixed in hyperextension and held stiffly along the body. Treatment can be attempted early in the progression of the deformity, while the stifle and hock can still be easily flexed, by recreating the flexural forces on the stifle and hock. This is accomplished using external fixator pins placed through the lateral aspect of the femur and tibia. The two pins in the tibia and the two pins in the femur are each connected with single clamps and a connecting bar. Rubber bands are used to connect the external fixator frames so as to cause flexion of the stifle. A tape boot correctly fitted around the foot can also be connected to the fixation device with rubber bands to correct the hyperextension of the hock. The pressure used should be only enough to accomplish the correction. The device is left on for 1 to 2 weeks. Development of the flexor muscles can be assessed by removing the rubber bands and observing the dog using the leg. Treatment of the condition requires close monitoring of the patient and is not always successful (Fig. 13-19).[38]

REFERENCES

1. Berg RJ, and others: Evaluation of prognostic factors for growth following distal femoral physeal injuries in 17 dogs, *Vet Surg* 13:172-180, 1984.
2. Black AP, Withrow SJ: Changes in the proximal femur and coxofemoral joint following intramedullary pinning of diaphyseal fractures in young dogs, *Vet Surg* 8:19-24, 1979.
3. Brighton CT: Structure and function of the growth plate, *Clin Orthop Rel Res* 136:22-32, 1978.
4. Campbell CJ. Grisolia A, Zanconato G: The effects produced in the cartilaginous epiphyseal plate of immature dogs by experimental traumata, *J Bone Joint Surg (Am)* 41:1221-1242, 1959.
5. Carrig CB, Morgan JP, Pool RR: Effects of asynchronous growth of the radius and ulna on the canine elbow joint following experimental retardation of longitudinal growth of the ulna, *J Am Anim Hosp Assoc* 11:560-567, 1975.
6. Carrig CB, and others: Ectrodactyly (split hand deformity) in the dog, *Vet Radial* 22:123-143, 1981.
7. Craig E: Autogenous fat grafts to prevent recurrence following the surgical correction of growth deformities of the radius and ulna in the dog, *Vet Surg* 10:69-76, 1981.
8. Daly W: Femoral head and neck fractures in the dog and cat: a review of 115 cases, *Vet Surg* 7:29-38, 1978.
9. DeCamp CE, and others: Periosteum and the healing of partial ulnar ostectomy in radius curvus of dogs, *Vet Surg* 15:185-190, 1986.
10. Fox MW: Polyarthrodysplasia (congenital joint luxation) in the dog, *J Am Vet Med Assoc* 145:1204-1205, 1964.
11. Grondalen J: Malformation of the elbow joint in an Afghan hound litter, *J Small Anim Pract* 14:83-89, 1973.
12. Henney LHS, Gambardella PC: Premature closure of the ulnar physis in the dog: a retrospective study, *J Am Anim Hosp Assoc* 25:573-581, 1989.

13. Hulse DA: Medial patellar luxation in the dog. In Bojrab MJ, editor: *Pathophysiology in small animal surgery*, Philadelphia, 1981, Lea & Febiger.

14. Iannotti JP: Growth plate physiology and pathology, *Orthop Clin North Am* 21:1-17, 1990.

15. Ilizarov GA: Clinical application of the tension stress effect for limb lengthening, *Clin Orthop Rel Res* 250:8-26, 1990.

16. Johnson AL: Correction of radial and ulnar growth deformities resulting from premature physeal closure. In Bojrab MJ, editor: *Current techniques in small animal surgery*, ed 3, Philadelphia, 1990, Lea & Febiger.

17. Johnson KA: Retardation of endochondral ossification at the distal ulnar growth plate in dogs, *Aust Vet J* 57:474, 1981.

18. Johnson SG, and others: Corrective osteotomy for pes varus in the dachshund, *Vet Surg* 18:373-379, 1989.

19. Knecht CD, Bloomberg MS: Distraction with an external fixation clamp (Charnley apparatus) to maintain length in premature physeal closure, *J Am Anim Hosp Assoc* 16:873-880,1980.

20. Lewis RE, Van Sickle DC: Congenital hemimelia (agenesis) of the radius in a dog and a cat, *J Am Vet Med Assoc* 156:1892-1897, 1970.

21. Llewellyn HR: Growth plate injuries—diagnosis, prognosis and treatment, *J Am Anim Hosp Assoc* 12:77-82, 1976.

22. Marretta SM, Schrader SC: Physeal injuries in the dog: a review of 135 cases, *J Am Vet Med Assoc* 182:708-710, 1983.

23. Mason TA, Baker MJ: The surgical management of elbow joint deformity associated with premature growth plate closure in dogs, *J Small Anim Pract* 19:639-645, 1978.

24. Milton JL, Montgomery RD: Congenital elbow dislocations, *Vet Clin North Am* 17:873-888, 1987.

25. Milton JL, and others: Congenital elbow luxation in the dog, *J Am Vet Med Assoc* 175:572-582, 1979.

26. Newton CD: Surgical management of distal ulnar physeal growth disturbances in dogs, *J Am Vet Med Assoc* 164:479-487, 1974.

27. Newton CD, Nunamaker DM, Dickenson CR: Surgical management of radial physeal growth disturbance in dogs, *J Am Vet Med Assoc* 167:1011-1018, 1975.

28. O'Brien TR: Developmental deformities due to arrested epiphyseal growth, *Vet Clin North Am* 1:441-454, 1971.

29. O'Brien TR, Morgan JP, Suter PF: Epiphyseal plate injury in the dog: a radiographic study of growth disturbance in the forelimb, *J Small Anim Pract* 12:19-36, 1971.

30. Olmstead ML: Lateral luxation of the patella. In Bojrab MJ, editor: *Pathophysiology in small animal surgery*, Philadelphia, 1981, Lea & Febiger.

31. Olson NC, Carry CB, Bronker WO: Asynchronous growth of the canine radius and ulna: effects of retardation of longitudinal growth of the radius, *Am J Vet Res* 40:351-355, 1979.

32. Olson NC, and others: Asynchronous growth of the canine radius and ulna: surgical correction following experimental premature closure of the distal radial physis, *Vet Surg* 10:125-131, 1981.

33. Olsson SE, Poulos PW, Ljunggren G: Coxa plana vara and femoral capital fractures in the dog, *J Am Anim Hosp Assoc* 21:563-571, 1985.

34. Pederson NC: Surgical correction of a congenital defect of the radius and ulna of a dog, *J Am Vet Med Assoc* 153:1328-1331, 1968.

35. Ramadan RO, Vaughan LC: Premature closure of the distal ulnar growth plate in dogs: a review of 58 cases, *J Small Anim Pract* 19:647-667, 1978.

36. Ramadan RO, Vaughan LC: Disturbance in growth of the tibia and femur in dogs, *Vet Rec* 104:433-435, 1979.

37. Riser WH, Shirer JF: Normal and abnormal growth of the distal foreleg in large and giant dogs, *J Am Vet Radiol Soc* 6:50-64, 1965.

38. Rudy RL: Stifle joint. In Archibald J, editor: *Canine Surgery*, Archibald, ed 2, Santa Barbara, Calif, 1944, American Veterinary Publications.

39. Rudy RL: Corrective osteotomy of angular deformities, *Vet Clin North Am* 1:549-583, 1971.

40. Salter RB, Harris WR: Injuries involving the epiphyseal plate, *J Bone Joint Surg (Am)* 45:587-622, 1963.

41. Skaggs S, DeAngelis MP, Rosen H: Deformities due to premature closure of the distal ulna in fourteen dogs: a radiographic evaluation, *J Am Anim Hosp Assoc* 9:496-500, 1973.

42. Trueta J, Amato VP: The vascular contribution to osteogenesis. III. Changes in the growth cartilage caused by experimentally induced ischemia, *J Bone Joint Surg (Br)* 42:571-587, 1960.

43. VanDeWater AL, Olmstead ML: Premature closure of the distal radial physis: a review of 14 dogs, *Vet Surg* 12:7-12, 1983.

44. VanDeWater AL, Olmstead ML, Stevenson S: Partial ulnar ostectomy with free autogenous fat grafting for treatment of radius curvus in the dog, *Vet Surg* 11:92-99, 1982.

45. Vaughan LC: Growth plate defects in dogs, *Vet Rec* 98:185-189, 1976.

46. Wagner SD, and others: Effect of distal femoral growth plate fusion on femoral-tibial length, *Vet Surg* 16:435-439, 1987.

47. Yanoff SR, and others: Distraction osteogenesis using modified external fixation devices in five dogs, *Vet Surg* 21:480-487, 1992.

14

Fixation Failure

ERICK L. EGGER

Mechanical Fixation Failure
   Improper Fixation Selection
   Improper Fixation Application
Biological Failure

Veterinarians tend to ignore fixation failures or ascribe them to outside factors such as poor owner compliance with postoperative instructions. However, since much more can be learned from failures than successes, it is wise to examine these situations closely. Such analysis of failures can improve overall results by two mechanisms. First, for the case in question, recognition of an established or potential problem may direct preemptive treatment and preclude complete failure. More importantly, recognition of the causes of failures should help to avoid the same mistakes on future cases. It is impossible to predict all specific causes for fracture fixation failure, but Box 14-1 lists some of the more common "generic" problems that result in failure. This chapter does not attempt

---

BOX 14-1
COMMON PROBLEMS THAT RESULT IN FRACTURE FIXATION FAILURE

Implant breakage
Failure of implant attachment to bone
Implant loosening
Incorrect implant size
Incorrect implant application
Implant interference with fracture healing
Primary failure of fracture healing

---

to cover all the specific examples of fixation failure and their treaments, but rather includes examples to present a scheme the clinician can use to analyze these problems and take appropriate steps to avoid or treat failure.

Why do fracture fixations fail? There are basically two reasons: (1) the fixation device fails to provide adequate fracture immobilization for normal fracture healing to occur, and (2) if fracture healing is impeded long enough, any fixation technique eventually breaks down. Consequently, the veterinarian treating fractures must approach the problem from two viewpoints: the carpenter placing and holding the bone fragments in their proper relationship and the gardener in cultivating the regrowth of living bone. If the veterinarian is an inadequate carpenter, fixation is not achieved or not maintained. This can be considered mechanical failure. If an inadequate gardener, the fracture does not heal and the fixation eventually breaks down. This can be considered biological failure.

MECHANICAL FIXATION FAILURE

Mechanical fixation failure can result from several causes. Ultimately, the fixation device or its bone-to-implant interface does not possess the mechanical characteristics necessary to resist the disruptive forces to which it is exposed. Consequently, these forces overpower the fixation and cause its failure. In the early days of fracture treatment, "primary" implant failures under normal loading conditions could often be ascribed to poor device design, weak materials, or faulty manufacturing technique. This occurred because implants were often "invented" by surgeons and applied to patients in a trial-and-error approach without critical evaluation of their mechanical attributes.[1] For example, the original

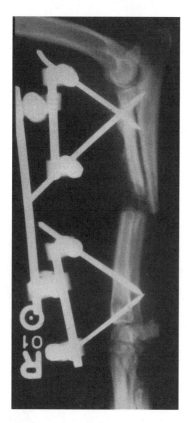

Fig. 14-1 Nonunion of a radius and ulnar fracture caused by mechanical fixation failure of the double connecting clamps of the external fixator in an 18 kg dog.

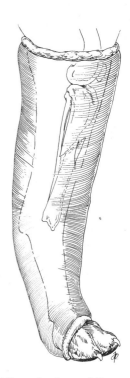

Fig. 14-2 Overriding of a long oblique tibial fracture with axial compression when treated with a cylindrical cast.

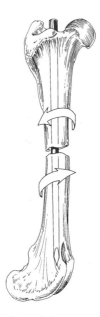

Fig. 14-3 Rotational instability around a single intramedullary pin in a transverse femoral fracture.

configuration of the Kirschner external fixator used a poorly designed connecting clamp that frequently slipped, resulting in loss of fracture reduction (Fig. 14-1). However, starting in the 1950s, engineering principles began to be applied to fixation techniques, and the discipline of fracture biomechanics developed.[2] This approach considers the orientation and magnitude of disruptive forces in the design, manufacturing, and application of implants. Additionally, advancements in implant materials have significantly enhanced the inherent strength of modern fixation devices and decreased adverse biological responses. As this work continues, "primary" fixation failures are becoming unusual and it must be recognized that most mechanical failures are caused by some other problem if their incidence is to be further decreased.

Improper Fixation Selection

Improper fixation selection results in mechanical failure because the fixation selected does not control the disruptive forces acting at the fracture. For example, a cast applied to a long oblique fracture does not control the axial compressive force that results from the gravitational effect of weight bearing and muscle contraction. Consequently, the fracture often overrides and the result-ing instability prevents fracture healing (Fig. 14-2). Likewise, a single intramedullary pin applied to a smooth transverse fracture fails to control torsional forces and the resultant rotational instability can impede fracture healing (Fig. 14-3).

Certain techniques of fixation tend to amplify disruptive forces in one orientation while they are controlling

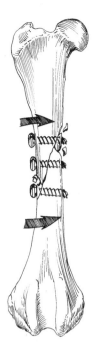

Fig. 14-4 Interfragmentary screws tend to collect bending forces and can result in additional bone fragmentation when used without fixation competent at controlling bending.

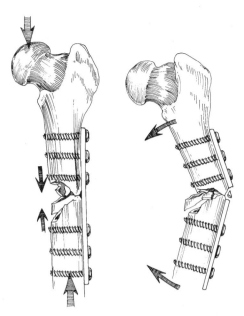

Fig. 14-5 Axial compression is converted to a bending force by the femur's anatomical configuration. Lack of adequate medial cortical bone contacts can result in cyclical fatigue failure of the fixation because of the loss of the bone's medial buttress effect.

forces in another. For example, interfragmentary screws applied to a long oblique fracture control axial and rotational forces. However, these screws tend to collect bending forces and, if used alone for fixation, often cause additional bone fragmentation, loss of fixation, and failure (Fig. 14-4).

The anatomical configuration of the bone may convert one force to another that the fixation is unable to control. For example, the offset configuration of the femoral head converts the axial compressive force resulting from weight bearing to a bending force in a comminuted shaft fracture where the medial cortex is not reconstructed. Unless a heavy buttress plate is used, the repeated implant bending generated by muscle pull and weight bearing can result in fatigue failure of the fixation (Fig. 14-5).

To avoid improper fixation selection, the fracture's stabilization requirements must be matched to the fixation device's abilities. This first requires analysis of the forces (loads) experienced in the fixation of various fractures (Table 14-1).[3] Comminuted fractures should be viewed as multiple simple fracture lines and the forces acting on each considered. In general, bending is almost always a disruptive force that must be controlled. Rotation is more of a problem with transversely oriented fractures. Axial compressive forces that result from weight bearing and muscle contraction have a more disruptive effect on longitudinally oriented fractures. Tension as a disruptive force is seen less often, except in avulsion fractures of a ligamentous or tendinous attachment. However, tension is a very potent force and requires specific techniques to

Table 14-1 Disruptive Forces That Typically Must Be Controlled with Various Simple Fracture Configurations

| Fracture configuration | Disruptive force | | | |
	Bending	Torsion	Axial compression	Axial tension
Transverse	++++	++++	---	---
Short oblique	++++	+++	+++	---
Long oblique	++++	++	++++	---
Avulsion	++	++	---	++++

++++, Most subject to disruptive force; ---, least subject to disruptive force.

control. Second, the forces that each fixation technique controls and those they do not must be recognized.[3] Table 14-2 summarizes the forces that common means of fixation control, assuming proper application technique and appropriate location.

Treatment of fixation failure resulting from improper fixation selection varies depending on the case. However, the goal of treatment can usually be considered in one of three broad categories. Since the problem stems from a mismatch of the disruptive forces acting on the fracture with the ability of the fixation to control those forces, the first approach is to obtain control of the existing forces. This might be done by changing to an entirely different form of fixation, such as removing the cast from a long oblique tibial fracture and applying a plate or type II external fixator that controls axial compression. Alternately,

Table 14-2 Disruptive Forces That Common Means of Fixation Will Control, Assuming Proper Application and Location

Fixation technique	Disruptive force			
	Bending	Torsion	Axial compression	Axial tension
External coaptation	+++	+	---	---
Intramedullary pinning	++++	---	---	---
External fixation	+++	++	+++	++
Tension-band plating	++++	+++	+++	++
Cerclage wires	----	+++	+++	--
Interfragmentary wires	----	+	+	-
Interfragmentary screws	---	+++	+++	-
Tension-band wires	-	-	-	++++

++++, Most effective at controlling disruptive force; ----, least effective at controlling disruptive force.

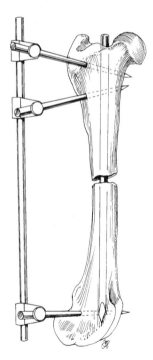

Fig. 14-6 Addition of ancillary fixation (type I external fixator) to control disruptive torsional forces that the primary fixation (intramedullary pin) did not.

often the existing fixation can be supplemented by adding ancillary fixation that controls the problem force, as illustrated by the addition of a type I external fixator to the intramedullary pin fixation of a transverse femoral fracture (Fig. 14-6).

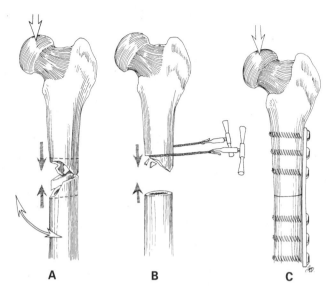

Fig. 14-7 Changing the disruptive forces of an unstable comminuted fracture (**A**) by removing small fragments and resecting oblique fragment ends (**B**). The resulting disruptive forces can now be controlled by the chosen fixation (**C**).

A second approach to the mismatch is to alter the configuration of the fracture, resulting in disruptive forces the existing fixation can control. Converting a comminuted femoral fracture to a simple transverse configuration by fragment removal and resection of oblique fracture ends is an example (Fig. 14-7). The axial compressive forces of weight bearing now result in compression and actually increase stability of the fracture fixation.

Finally, the disruptive forces can be altered by limiting their origin, which is usually weight bearing. It is very difficult to totally confine most veterinary patients; in general, attempts should be made to avoid the joint stiffness and muscle atrophy that typically result from the prolonged combination of external coaptation with surgical fracture treatment. However, when fixation potential is limited, such as in intraarticular fractures, off–weight-bearing slings can prevent or limit disruptive forces while still allowing beneficial joint motion (Fig. 14-8). Unfortunately, attempting to alter the forces once fixation has completely failed is rarely effective, and revision of the primary fixation is usually necessary.

Improper Fixation Application

Fixation failure caused by improper application can result in mechanical or biological failure. All fixation techniques or devices have principles or "rules" for their correct application. If enough of these rules are broken, any fixation technique will fail. Some devices are more sensitive to application technique than others, and attention to detail is particularly important with these devices. If an

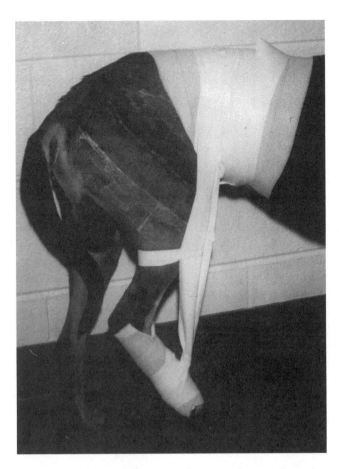

Fig. 14-8 Limiting disruptive forces with an off–weight-bearing sling may be necessary if fracture configuration cannot be changed and fixation stability is limited.

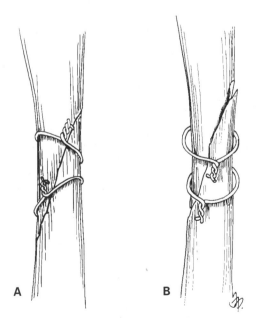

Fig. 14-9 Cerclage wires that are not applied perpendicular to the long axis of the bone (**A**) rotate and loosen, resulting in instability and bone segment collapse with axial loading (**B**).

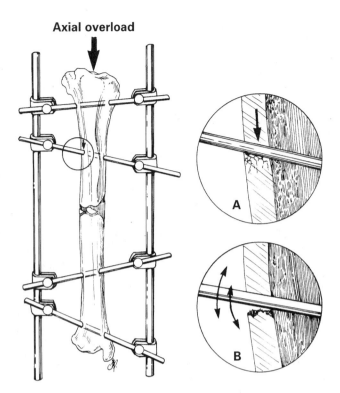

Fig. 14-10 **A,** Using too few fixation pins with an external fixator stabilizing a comminuted tibial fracture results in bone overloading and microfracture surrounding the pins. **B,** Resorption of this damaged bone then results in premature pin loosening and potential fixation failure.

inappropriately small device is used, it may not be strong enough to control the forces to which it is exposed, even if the fixation is designed for forces in that orientation. Consequently, it can be expected to fail. Likewise, cerclage wires that are not oriented perpendicular to the long axis of the bone when placed on a long oblique fracture usually rotate to that perpendicular position in the postoperative period (Fig. 14-9). The wires become loose by increasing their effective diameter. Loose wires cease to compress the fracture faces together, resulting in fracture instability and collapse with the axial compression of weight bearing. Additionally, the loose moving wires can interfere with fracture vascularity, interfering with healing and contributing to biological failure.

Often the mechanism of failure is not failure of the device itself, but failure of the implant-bone interface. The use of fewer-than-recommended fixation pins in the treatment of comminuted tibial fracture with external fixation often leads to bone resorption around the pins, loss of fixation stability, and possibly healing failure (Fig. 14-10). With too few pins, the axial compressive loads of weight bearing are concentrated on small areas of bone, exceeding its capacity and resulting in microfracture. The body responds by resorbing the damaged bone resulting in pin loosening.

Avoiding fixation failure caused by poor application technique requires not only knowledge of the methods of a particular fixation device's application but, more importantly, understanding of the principles of application. This allows successful modification of the methods to fit the individual requirements of each fracture.

Treatment of failure from improper application requires one first to determine which application principles have been broken. In some cases the same type of fixation can be correctly reapplied, as in replacing cerclage wires in the correct orientation perpendicular to the long axis of the bone. Occasionally, the existing fixation device can be augmented, as in adding more fixation pins to an external fixator to disperse the weight-bearing loads at each bone-to-pin interface to a tolerable level. However, often the fixation failure causes a change in fracture type or damage to the local biology that requires selection and correct application of another form of fixation. For example, the long oblique fracture that has collapsed because of obliquely applied cerclage wires may be best treated by resecting the avascular oblique fracture ends and applying a plate or external fixator to the resultant transverse configuration.

BIOLOGICAL FAILURE

Biological failure occurs when the fracture fails to heal within the longevity of its fixation's ability to control disruptive forces adequately. Although virtually all techniques of fixation eventually fail if they are continually loaded and no support is supplied by the healing bone, some techniques of fixation are more sensitive to biological failure than others because of differences in expected effective longevity. For example, a plaster cast can only be expected to last 4 to 6 weeks under normal circumstances, whereas a heavy buttress plate applied with many screws routinely stabilizes even an unstable, highly comminuted fracture for many months. Consequently, the shorter the expected longevity of the device used, the more rapid the fracture healing required to avoid biological failure. Conversely, the effective longevity of a given fixation technique is often directly related to the adverse biological impact of that technique. The same heavy buttress plate requires extensive soft tissue dissection for its application.

Various factors can adversely affect fracture healing rate and, if recognized, can either be avoided or lead to the choice of a fixation technique with longer effective longevity. Some of these factors, such as the patient's age, are beyond the veterinarian's control, but many are affected by his or her actions. Causing excessive soft tissue damage with resultant osseous vascular damage while applying cerclage wires (Fig. 14-11), accepting inadequate initial fracture reduction, and introducing infection to the fracture site by contamination at surgery illustrate

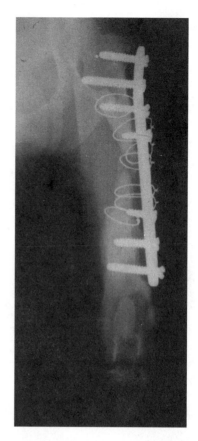

Fig. 14-11 Biological failure can result from excessive damage to osseous vascularity when applying fixation such as cerclage wires, leading to bone resorption. Without fracture healing, ultimately the fixation or its bone interface fails.

ways fracture healing can be impeded long enough for the fixation device to fail.

To avoid primary failure of fracture healing, the surgeon must balance the projected need for fixation longevity against providing, or at least not damaging, an environment conducive to fracture healing. For example, obtaining adequate fracture reduction by using open reduction if needed or incorporating a cancellous bone graft if reduction is marginal, minimizing soft tissue and vascular damage during implant application, and treating infection appropriately are all activities that promote fracture healing and decrease the incidence of biological failure.

Treatment once biological failure has occurred is often challenging, since the fracture has often lost the stimulus to heal. Consequently, simple application of another fixation device is rarely effective. Adverse factors in the fracture environment, such as infection, loose implants, and unstable, avascular bone fragments, must be removed. Adequate fracture reduction with stable fixation, such as bone plates or rigid external fixators, must be obtained to allow revascularization. Most importantly, since at this point the biological process is often stalled, the fracture must be stimulated to start healing again. This is usually achieved by packing autogenous cancellous bone graft around the fracture and into any defects remaining after reduction and fixation.

• • •

This discussion has not attempted to describe all forms of fixation failure but rather has offered a scheme (illustrated with a few examples) with which to consider the causes and to develop a logical means to avoid or treat fixation failure.

REFERENCES

1. Colton CL: The history of fracture treatment. In Browner BD, and others, editors: *Skeletal trauma*, Philadelphia, 1992, Saunders.
2. Rand JA, Davis JJ, Chao EYS: Biomechanical factors in fracture treatment, *Minn Med* 65:558-563, 1982.
3. Schwarz PD: Fracture biomechanics of the appendicular skeleton: causes and assessment. In Bojrab MJ, editor: *Disease mechanisms in small animal surgery*, Philadelphia, 1993, Lea & Febiger.

15

Fracture Disease

JEAN F. BARDET

Fracture disease is a complication of long bone fractures seen in association with various surgical treatments and immobilization methods that tend to be unstable or restrict or eliminate early active movement and controlled weight bearing. It is characterized by signs of dystrophy in the affected limb, such as pain, joint stiffness, and deterioration of soft tissues, bones, and cartilage. Immobilization of a limb can lead to many structural, biochemical, biomechanical, and metabolic changes in the affected tissues. Internal fixation combined with immobilization of periarticular fractures most often produces stiffness in the nearby joint. Stifles and elbow are particularly susceptible to posttraumatic stiffness. Quadriceps contracture, the most dramatic example of fracture disease, usually results from immobilization of distal femoral fractures by extension splints, particularly in young dogs. This chapter presents current concepts concerning the causes, clinical signs, pathophysiology, and treatment of fracture disease.

CAUSES

Prolonged immobilization and non–weight bearing are the two most common causes of fracture disease. This is most often seen after inadequate internal fixation of a fracture, nonunion, posttraumatic osteomyelitis, and periarticular and articular fracture treatment.[13] Distal femoral fracture may lead to a stiff stifle with quadriceps atrophy and contracture (Fig. 15-1). This problem occurs most often in immature animals and develops more readily when an internal fixation is supplemented by an external coaptation or an extension splint. The same condition has also been observed after treatment of pelvic and femoral fractures, condylar femoral fractures, and recurrent patellar luxation.[2,3] The initiating factor of stifle stiffness appears to be fibrous adhesions tying down the vastus intermedius muscle to the distal end of the femur. The influence of the trauma seems to be limited. Three weeks of experimental immobilization alone or with concurrent muscle trauma in growing dogs was shown

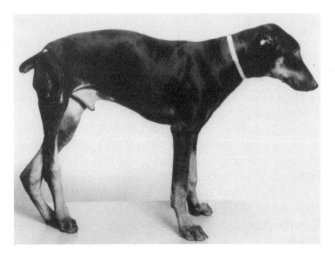

Fig. 15-1 Two-month-old Doberman puppy with a quadriceps contracture secondary to treatment of a distal femoral fracture with an intramedullary pin and extension splint for 2 weeks.

319

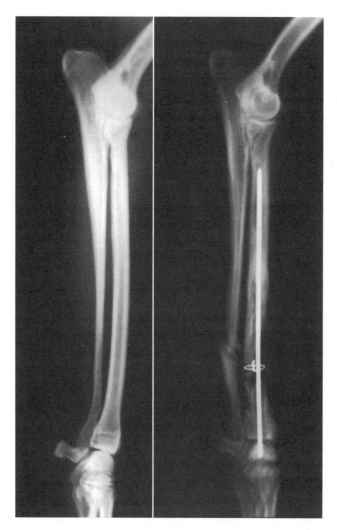

Fig. 15-2 Lateral radiographs of a 2-year-old poodle with fracture disease of the front limb (*right*) after a distal radial fracture treated by an intramedullary pin and immobilized for 3 months. Note the osteoporosis and atrophy of the bones below the fracture. The left radiograph is of the normal limb.

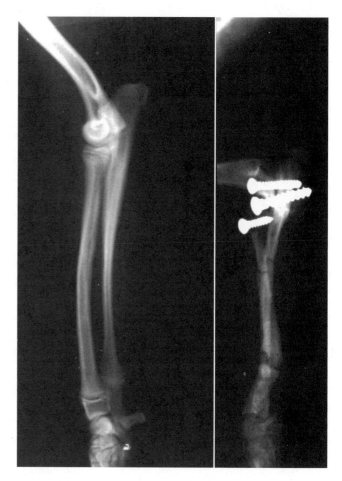

Fig. 15-3 Craniocaudal radiographs of the normal (*left*) and abnormal front limb (*right*) of a 6-month-old poodle treated for a lateral humeral condylar fracture. Notice the radial and ulnar pathological fractures, severe disuse osteoporosis, and bone hypoplasia.

not to cause joint stiffness.[14] In contrast, immobilization of distal femoral fractures treated by extension splintage resulted in a stiff stifle joint after 3 to 7 weeks.[4,14]

Long bone fractures adjacent to joints frequently produce early soft tissue swelling and later joint stiffness. The stiffness may be permanent and may cause considerable disability. Although the joint itself is not directly injured, its motion is affected by the restrictive healing response in periarticular connective tissues. Small joints, including the carpal joints, are particularly susceptible to this reaction.[13] Other joints (e.g., elbow, stifle) may also be affected after distal humeral and distal femoral fracture treatment. Prolonged immobilization or inadequate internal fixation of shaft fractures leads to fracture dis-

ease (Fig. 15-2). This may also be true for any articular fracture (Fig. 15-3) improperly treated and immobilized.

Age appears to be a factor in the development and severity of fracture disease.[4] In growing animals, the changes resulting from immobilization are much more pronounced than in adults. Because immature animals are still developing, disturbances in bone growth, joint subluxation, abnormal bone torsion, bone hypoplasia, and limb shortening can result.

CLINICAL SIGNS

The clinical signs of fracture disease depend on the duration of the condition, the tissues or structures involved, and the condition's severity. A patient that has been in a cast while a fracture heals may only exhibit mild lameness and radiographic evidence of disuse osteoporosis.

These signs resolve themselves as the animal begins weight bearing again. Patients with marked fracture disease may have severe lameness, decreased joint motion, and disuse atrophy of the affected limb. The clinical signs are most dramatic in quadriceps contracture. The affected limb is held in rigid extension and is generally not used or used only as a peg when walking. At rest, it is carried cranially relative to the nonaffected hind limb. The stifle may be bent caudally in genu recurvatum. Examination of the limb shows varying degrees of muscle atrophy and leg shortening.

With quadriceps contracture, neither the hock nor the stifle can be flexed. The stifle's range of motion varies between 0 and 30 degrees. The patella is located proximally in the trochlear groove and may be luxated medially. Palpation of the thigh muscles reveals atrophy and a hard quadriceps muscle. A careful examination of the hip joint is mandatory in younger dogs. The hip joint may be painful in full extension and in adduction. Inward and outward rotation may be limited. There may be a positive Ortolani sign.

Fracture disease after an elbow fracture or a periarticular fracture of the elbow may cause either a severe lameness with a loss of motion or a non-weight-bearing lameness because of a pathological fracture or limb shortening. The lameness associated with fracture disease after periarticular fracture of the hock or carpus is less severe; most patients can bear weight, but the joint cannot be fully flexed. The loss of flexion may be permanent.

PATHOPHYSIOLOGY

The changes after immobilization have been reproduced experimentally in different species, including rats, rabbits, monkeys, cats, and dogs. Various techniques of immobilization have been used, including casting, splinting, extension splints, extraarticular pinning, paw transection, and nerve and tendon transection. Joints have been immobilized either in full extension or in flexion. All these experiments have demonstrated changes in bones, muscles, articular cartilage, synovium, ligaments, and other periarticular structures, as well as growth disturbances.

Disuse Osteoporosis

Lack of movement and decreased muscle loading of normally loaded limb bones cause a loss of bone mass (osteoporosis) from disuse and an associated negative calcium balance. Nontraumatic immobilization of a young adult beagle's forelimb for 60 weeks produced 66% trabecular bone loss in the distal metaphysis of the third metacarpus, 50% loss in the radius, and 25% loss in the humerus. Compact bone loss in the bones of the same dog amounted to 58%, 20%, and 7%, respectively. In young adult dogs the loss is most prominent on the periosteal surface; cortical area and thickness are greatly decreased. Bone loss from the spongiosa appears to be caused by a thinning and loss of trabeculae. In older dogs the bone loss is slightly less important, and there is a marked expansion of the bone and marrow cavity and thinning within the cortex. Disuse osteoporosis is observed in dogs as early as 2 weeks after immobilization and may occur at an approximate rate of 5% loss per month. Bone loss as a result of disuse occurs at rates 5 to 20 times greater than loss caused by other metabolic disorders affecting bone.

Disuse osteoporosis is reported as a sequela of quadriceps contracture in growing dogs. Cortices may be extremely thin, with large intracortical resorption cavities appearing 10 weeks after immobilization (Fig. 15-4). Pathological fractures may be observed.

The initiating cause of disuse osteoporosis is not well understood. Lack of muscular activity, increased vascular supply to the affected limb, and absence of weight bearing, which decreases the piezoelectric action of crystals on bone cells, are important factors in inducing bone atrophy.

The reversibility of osteoporotic changes with remobilization is probably related to the severity of the changes and the length of immobilization periods. Recovery of loss may take as much as 5 to 10 times longer than the period of immobilization. However, more permanent changes occur with immobilization periods exceeding 12 weeks. Recently, disuse osteoporosis has been prevented experimentally by intracast quadriceps muscle stimulation in cast-immobilized rabbits.

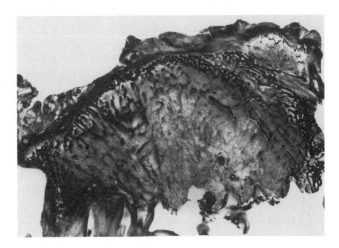

Fig. 15-4 A 200 mu section from femur of the cortex is extremely thin, with large intracortical resorption cavities. (Zesiger's stain, original magnification × 1.)

Reprinted with permission from Bardet JF, Hohn RB: Quadriceps contracture in dogs, J Am Vet Med Assoc 183:680-685, 1983.

Muscle Atrophy

Skeletal muscles atrophy when the muscle use level is decreased because of immobilization. Under such conditions, investigators have demonstrated that muscles composed mainly of type I fibers (i.e., "slow" muscles) atrophy to a greater extent than muscles composed mainly of type II fibers (i.e., "fast" muscles). Additionally, antigravity muscles atrophy to a greater extent than their antagonists.

Disuse muscle atrophy is reversible. Immobilized skeletal muscles have a good regenerative potential that is not affected by the duration of immobilization. The recovery period may be two to four times longer than the period of immobilization. Although bony and muscular atrophic changes are reversible, most articular and periarticular changes are irreversible.

Articular and Periarticular Changes

Joint immobilization results in a progressive contracture of the capsule and periarticular structure, with a subsequent degeneration of the joint (Fig. 15-5). After prolonged immobilization, fatty connective tissue envelops the cruciate ligaments and completely fills the joint cavity. Adhesions form between fibrous tissue and nonarticulating surfaces of articular cartilage. In dogs, adhesions are not observed 8 weeks after immobilization but are common at 3 months. Other changes are observed in the articular cartilage, synovium, ligaments, and periarticular structures.

Articular Cartilage Changes

Joint immobilization results in morphological, biochemical, and metabolic changes within a few days. Rigid, sustained pressure on the articular cartilage of rabbit knee joints causes chondrocytic death. In the noncontact areas of articular cartilage, the interface between fibrous tissue and hyaline cartilage is initially distinct, but within 2 weeks, this interface is replaced by pannus, which matures to fibrous tissue (Fig. 15-6). When articular cartilage surfaces are in apposition, microscopic changes are observed as early as 4 days after immobilization. With time, various cartilaginous changes are observed, including fibrillation, deep erosion, fibrous ankylosis, and sometimes cartilaginous or bony ankylosis (Fig. 15-7). Only after months of immobilization are the late changes of cartilaginous and bony ankylosis observed. Immobilization of joints for as little as 6 days can result in a massive reduction of cartilage proteoglycans synthesis and content with subsequent cartilage softening.

These morphological, metabolic, and biochemical changes appear to result from reduced joint motion and loading. Intermittent joint loading stimulates the formation and circulation of synovial and interstitial fluids that

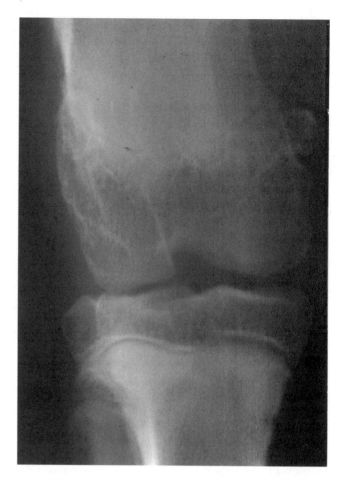

Fig. 15-5 Craniocaudal radiograph of a right stifle from dog in Fig. 15-1. The joint space is greatly decreased, and degenerative joint disease is evident.

Reprinted with permission from Bardet JF, Hohn RB: Quadriceps contracture in dogs, J Am Vet Med Assoc 183:680-685, 1983.

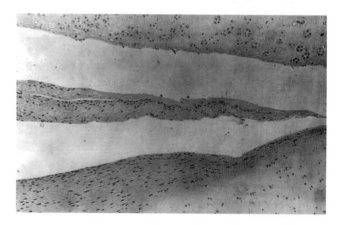

Fig. 15-6 Photomicrograph of a specimen of the right stifle from dog in Figs. 15-1 and 15-5 shows the adjacent articular surfaces of the femur (*top*) and tibia. The articular cartilage of the tibia is overlaid and invaded by fibrous tissue. Note the large flap of dense fibrous tissue in the center. Marked degeneration of the femoral articular surface is demonstrated by the formation of aggregates of chondrocytes. (Hematoxylin and eosin stain, × 5.)

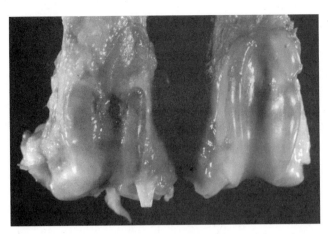

Fig. 15-7 Cranial view of the femoral condyles after 5 months of immobilization on the left. Normal femoral condyles are on the right. Note the flattening of the condyles and the medial ridge of the trochlear groove and the erosion of the articular cartilage of the immobilized limb.

Reprinted with permission from Bardet JF: Quadriceps contracture and fracture disease, *Vet Clin* 17:957-973, 1987.

nourish and lubricate the cartilage. Joint immobilization may compromise the metabolic exchange needed for proper structure and function of the articular cartilage. Recent experiments suggest that joint motion alone is not sufficient to maintain cartilage health. Degenerative changes occur in stifle joints of dogs even in the presence of joint motion if the joint remains unloaded. Joint motion without joint loading during the immobilization period does not prevent deterioration of the articular cartilage.

The reversibility of articular cartilage changes depends on the length of immobilization and the extent to which movement is really restricted during immobilization. Morphological and biochemical cartilage changes are fully reversible if the immobilization period is less than 4 weeks. The time required for cartilage to recover may be many times longer than the initial immobilization period. After 7 weeks of immobilization, the articular cartilage defects may be permanent and may continue to progress, even on remobilization. Articular cartilage changes have been prevented in short-term cast immobilization by intercast muscle stimulation and intraarticular injection of hyaluronic acid.

Synovial, Ligamentous, and Periarticular Connective Tissue Changes

The metabolic activity in the joint capsule increases greatly as early as 4 days after immobilization. Thickening of the joint capsule is one of the first microscopic changes. There is a nonspecific fibrous hyperplasia of the joint capsule and proliferation of the type B synoviocytes in the synovial membrane.

The biochemical changes of periarticular connective tissue after stress deprivation can be summarized as follows: small losses of collagen mass, loss of water content in the matrix, loss of content of glycosaminoglycans (GAGs), a large increase of reductible chemical cross-linkages, and a large increase in collagen turnover. The resorption rate of collagen exceeds the synthesis rate, gradually producing losses of mass.

Stress deprivation weakens articular ligaments. The cranial cruciate ligament shows a disorganization of its matrix after several weeks of immobilization. Furthermore, ligament attachment sites are subject to significant weakening from localized osteoporosis. Structural properties of the ligament-bone complex are reduced to the level ranging from one-half to about one-third those in normal joints. There is a stress dependence of connective tissue. Wolff's law of bone may be expanded to a broader concept embracing fibrous connective tissue and other specialized connective tissues of joints.

A brief review of anatomical biochemical interaction is necessary to understand the fundamental changes operating in soft tissues associated with joint contracture and stiffness after immobilization. The soft tissue support structures about joints have a uniform biochemical composition despite dissimilar functions. The two components are collagen and ground substance. The collagen can provide both resistance to high-tensile forces and the flexibility that synovial joints require. The collagen fiber patterns about joints fall into two categories: a relatively straight, parallel wave form seen in tendon and ligament and a matrix form, typically called a "nylon hose pattern," seen in flexible structures such as capsule, synovium, and skin. The elasticity of individual fibers to stretch is relatively small, but the pattern of a wave creates elasticity in the composite. The ability of this structure to lengthen is many times greater than the stretching capacity of individual fibers. Crucial to this change in shape of the fiber mesh is the fiber's ability to glide past one another at intercept points. If the intercept points are locked, the mesh loses its ability to stretch, and the structure no longer adapts to functional demands that require a change in shape. Stiffness of soft tissue structures about the joint after immobilization is described as a disturbance of free gliding in the fiber mesh system. The process probably results from chemical bonding between fibers at intercept points. The changes appear time dependent, but are reversible by remodeling if the new fibers are not too numerous.

Osteoarthritis of immobilized synovial joints is the result of capsular and periarticular connective tissue contracture. The severity of degenerative joint disease is directly related to the duration of immobilization. The increased intraarticular pressure in the stifle seems to be caused by contracture of periarticular tissues and muscle contraction in the shortened position, causing static compression of the articular cartilage. Pressure necrosis of the articular cartilage occurs. The position in extension of the immobilized joint appears important, since only a few cases of osteoarthritis are observed when rabbits' knees are immobilized in flexion.

Joint stiffness after immobilization may be decreased or prevented by hyaluronic acid, dimethyl sulfoxide (DMSO), and dexamethasone. Joint stiffness from immobilization is inhibited by intraarticular hyaluronic acid injection in experimental joint contracture in rabbits. Injected hyaluronic acid appears to have a significant protective effect on the immobilized tissue by stimulating hyaluronic acid synthesis by fibrous connective tissue, by minimizing the loss of GAGs, and by reducing joint stiffness. DMSO has reduced postinjury experimental ankle stiffness by 41%. Postulated mechanisms of decreased joint stiffness include oxygen-free radical scavenging and inhibition of fibroblast proliferation. Dexamethasone produces a significant dose-dependent decrease of ankle stiffness. Likely explanations for the diminished stiffness are corticosteroids' effect of blocking inflammatory mediators and decreasing collagen production and cross-linking.

In an experimental model of intraarticular fracture in rabbits, joint stiffness was increased 2.6 times the preinjury levels in limbs that were immobilized for 3 weeks. Stiffness in the joint treated did not increase with passive motion. On the other hand, pressurization and two nonsteroidal antiinflammatory drugs (NSAIDs) did not influence joint stiffness. Intermittent passive exercise increases joint stiffness after periarticular fractures. It is suggested that passive exercise additionally injures tissue surrounding the fracture.

Growth Disturbances

The influence of immobilization in growing dogs with quadriceps contracture is observed clinically and in experimental studies. Immobilization of the stifle in dogs younger than 3 months of age induces multiple changes, including hip subluxation, bone hypoplasia, and increased femoral torsion. Hip subluxation is constituently evident after 8 to 10 weeks of stifle hyperextension because of cast immobilization. Stifle immobilization in extension with intact hamstring muscles results in an unresisted pull of the muscle groups across the hip joint and subsequent hip subluxation or dislocation. Other coxofemoral changes are also found, including hypertrophy of the ligament of the femoral head, significant decrease in blood flow of the femoral head, and progressive degenerative changes developing in the dislocated hip.

Bone hypoplasia is more severe in bones distal to the fracture. Absence of mechanical stimulation from normal weight bearing decreases osteoblastic activity and epi-

physeal growth. As a result, changes resulting from immobilization of a limb in very young dogs are more pronounced than in adults.

TREATMENT

Patients with mild fracture disease are easily treated. An example of mild changes is the muscle atrophy, osteoporosis, and joint stiffness observed with even a properly applied and managed cast. Generally, the changes reverse themselves when the animal begins to bear weight normally on the involved limb.

Severe fracture disease most often leads to a functional deficit despite adequate fracture union. The soft tissue lesions are often permanent and frequently cause more disability than the original bone injury. Loss of function of carpal and tarsal joints is most often well tolerated by canine patients. Because quadriceps contracture is the most clinically disabling form of fracture disease, the description of treatment is limited to this syndrome.

Quadriceps contracture cases should not be considered only as a stifle problem, and the entire affected leg should be evaluated before any treatment is started. Passive physical therapy can have disastrous results. Attempts to increase range of motion in the stifle by forced bending of the joint often result in fracture of the tibia. Most treatments are surgical, but even they have limited success rates. Treatment is directed at restoring movement to the stifle by:

1. Freeing the adhesions between the vastus intermedius and the distal femur
2. Lengthening the quadriceps femoris mechanism
3. Releasing the periarticular connective tissue contracture
4. Positioning the stifle in a physiological weight bearing position

The two major contradictions for surgical treatment are (1) major limb shortening and (2) combination of limb shortening, hip subluxation, and severe disuse osteoporosis in young dogs. Several surgical techniques have been described:

1. Z-plasty of the quadriceps muscles
2. Quadriceps plasty, using plastic sheeting
3. Sliding myoplasty
4. Vastus intermedius excision
5. Quadriceps insertions relocation
6. Stifle arthrodesis
7. Limb amputation

Currently, I use only the last four procedures. When the changes are severe, it is not unreasonable to do nothing and allow the animal to use the limb as a peg when walking, provided the limb is not painful and does not greatly interfere with locomotion.

A review of the surgical anatomy is needed to understand the following discussion. The quadriceps muscle extends between the pelvis and femur proximally and the patella and tibial tuberosity distally. This muscle covers the femur cranially, laterally, and medially. Distally, the quadriceps muscle forms a tendon that includes the patella and ends on the tibial tuberosity. The quadriceps muscle is covered medially and cranially by both heads of the sartorius muscle. The quadriceps femoris muscle consists of the rectus femoris, the vastus lateralis, the vastus medialis, and vastus intermedius. The rectus femoris muscle is enclosed between the vasti (Fig. 15-8). The vastus lateralis is united with the rectus femoris and its terminal tendon except proximally. The vastus medialis extends from the proximal femur medially and covers the distal portion of the rectus femoris medially. Above the patella, its tendinous elements fuse with those of the rectus femoris. The vastus intermedius muscle is the weakest portion of the quadriceps muscle and covers the medial, cranial, and lateral aspect of the femur, lying just under the rectus femoris. The vastus intermedius muscle is separated from the femur by a very loose, thin connective tissue.

The vastus intermedius excision procedure is used only in the first few days of quadriceps contracture before the appearance of irreversible cartilage changes. The patient is positioned in dorsal recumbency. A craniomedial approach to the femur and stifle joint is used. The skin incision is made on the craniomedial aspect of the thigh from the proximal third of the femur and ends distally over the medial aspect of the tibial tuberosity. The subcutaneous fat and facia are incised and cleared from the area so that the separation between the cranial and caudal parts of the sartorius muscle can be clearly visualized. The fascia between these two parts is incised. The cranial part of the sartorius muscle is reflected laterally and the caudal part medially (Fig. 15-9). The rectus

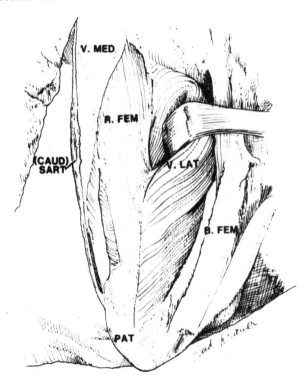

Fig. 15-8 Cranial aspect of the left thigh muscles. The cranial part of the sartorius muscle has been removed to expose the underlying musculature. The rectus femoris muscle (**R FEM**) appears between the vastus lateralis muscle (**V LAT**) and the vastus medialis muscle (**V MED**). The biceps femoris muscle (**B FEM**) is seen retracted laterally on the right, and the patella (**PAT**) appears on the bottom. Note the decussation of the muscle fibers between rectus femoris and vastus lateralis muscles below the retractor.

Reprinted with permission from Bardet JF: Quadriceps contracture and fracture disease, *Vet Clin* 17:957-973, 1987.

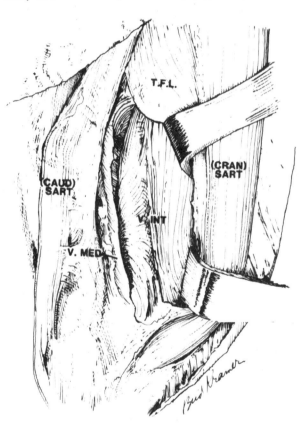

Fig. 15-9 Same view as Fig. 15-8. The cranial part of the sartorius muscle has been retracted laterally on the right. The underlying vastus intermedius muscle appears between the retracted muscle laterally and the vastus medialis muscle. It covers the cranial, medial, and lateral aspects of the femur. The cranial part (**CRAN SART**) of the sartorius muscle and the tensor facia lata muscle (**TFL**) cover the quadriceps muscle. The caudal part (**CAUD SART**) appears medially on the left.

Reprinted with permission from Bardet JF: Quadriceps contracture and fracture disease, *Vet Clin* 17:957-973, 1987.

femoris and vastus medialis muscles are separated by incising the tendinous elements of the vastus medialis where it fuses distally with those of the rectus femoris. The incision may be extended distally in the medial retinaculum, exposing the medial joint capsule. The cranial and medial aspects of the vastus intermedius muscle are visualized with medial retraction of the vastus medialis muscle and lateral retraction of the rectus femoris muscle. The excision of the vastus intermedius starts just above the joint capsule and extends dorsally on the cranial, lateral, and medial aspects of the femur. The strong adhesions are excised, exposing the femoral callus. The excision of the lateral part of the vastus intermedius may be facilitated by a medial arthrotomy and lateral luxation of the patella (Fig. 15-10).

The stifle may now be flexed 45 to 60 degrees. Further flexion may be facilitated by a release incision in the lateral retinaculum. In immature animals, care must be taken to avoid avulsion of the tibial tuberosity. Excess callus is removed using rongeurs and bone rasps. After a joint lavage using lactated Ringer's solution, the patella is relocated in its femoral trochlear groove. The surgical site is closed in layers. A half-splint external fixator is then applied on the lateral aspect of the femur (Fig. 15-11). A second half-splint external skeletal fixation is secured distally with the proximal pin in the body of the calcaneum and the distal pin in the base of the metatarsus. The stifle joint is fixed in maximum flexion with a connecting bar. Postoperatively, the connecting bar is removed the fourth day after surgery for physical therapy, with full range of motion twice a day for 10 minutes. The stifle is maintained in full flexion for 3 weeks; otherwise, most of the range of motion is lost in only a few days.

The quadriceps insertion relocation may be used in every patient with quadriceps contracture. This allows better flexion of the stifle joint and gives a better clinical outcome than the excision of the vastus intermedius muscle. It can be used months after the appearance of the quadriceps contracture and in patients with severe changes (Fig. 15-12 and 15-13). The skin incision is made along the cranial border of the femoral shaft from the level of the greater trochanter to the level of the tibial tuberosity. The facia lata is incised along the cranial border of the biceps femoris muscle. The incision is extended distally through the lateral retinaculum. The biceps femoris is retracted caudally, and cranial retraction of the vastus lateralis muscle exposes the femoral shaft. A parapatellar incision is made through the joint capsule. Dissection is carried out on the cranial aspect of the distal femur, where most of the adhesions between the vastus intermedius and the femur are located (Fig. 15-14). After freeing quadriceps muscle from adhesions, the insertions of the vastus lateralis and vastus medialis are transsected from the proximal femoral metaphysis.

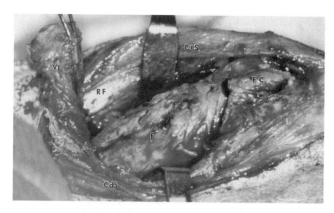

Fig. 15-10 Craniomedial view of the distal femur and stifle joint after excision of the vastus intermedius muscle. The vastus intermedius muscle (**VI**) is retracted dorsally, exposing the distal femoral callus (**F**). A medial arthrotomy allows lateral luxation of the patella and exposure of the femoral condyles (**FC**). Retracted rectus femoris muscle (**RF**) and the caudal part of the sartorius muscle (**CdS**). The cranial part of the sartorius muscle (**CrS**) is retracted.

Reprinted with permission from Bardet JF: Quadriceps contracture and fracture disease, *Vet Clin* 17:957-973, 1987.

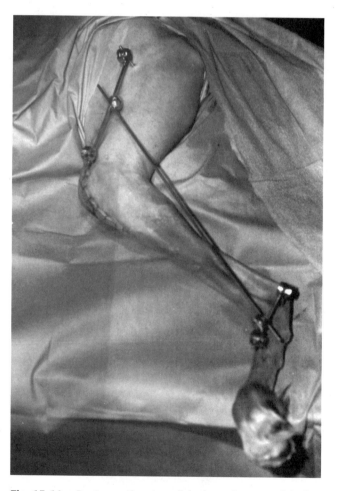

Fig. 15-11 Postoperative view of the lateral aspect of the left hind limb in flexion with the external skeletal fixation device.

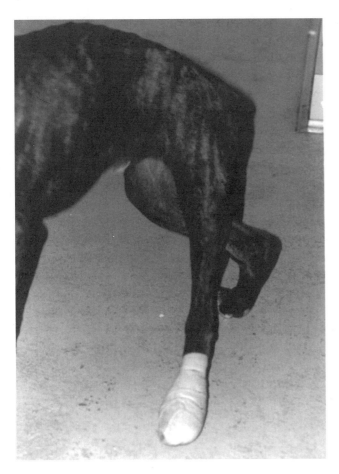

Fig. 15-12 Lateral view of a 6-month-old boxer with quadriceps contracture of the left hind limb after a distal femoral fracture.

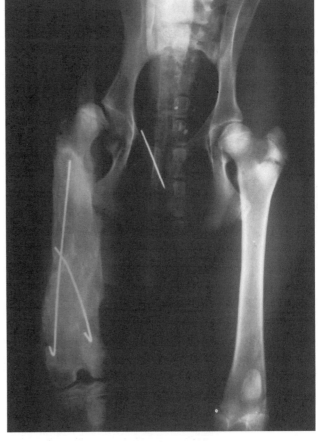

Fig. 15-13 Ventrodorsal view of dog in Fig. 15-12. Note the marked subluxation of the coxofemoral hip joint.

The stifle joint is flexed at this stage. If flexion is not completed, the strong tendon of insertion of the rectus femoris muscle is detached from the iliopubic eminence cranial to the acetabulum. Careful forced flexion may be needed to liberate the intraarticular adhesions (Fig. 15-15). The quadriceps muscle is anchored through a drill hole in the femur with nonabsorbable suture while the stifle is flexed 90 degrees (Fig. 15-16). The facia lata and the lateral retinaculum are sutured in a routine manner using absorbable suture. Postoperatively, an external skeletal fixation device is implanted as previously described, and the same physical therapy regimen is conducted. The hip subluxation should be treated if present (Fig. 15-17). The involved stifle joint does not recover a full range of motion, but its flexed position (Fig. 15-18) allows a satisfactory clinical outcome.

Indications for stifle arthrodesis are failure of the aforementioned surgical procedures, advanced stage of osteoarthritis of the stifle, osteomyelitis of the distal femur, and septic arthritis of the stifle. Chapter 23 describes the surgical technique for arthrodesis of the stifle.

Amputation is recommended in advanced stages of quadriceps contracture such as in very young dogs when multiple problems are present, as with a stiff stifle associated with hip subluxation, short bones, and pathological fractures.

All the pathophysiological changes occurring in bones, muscles, and joints after limb immobilization or fracture repair should be kept in mind. Because the changes associated with fracture disease can be devastating, the clinician should adhere to well-established principles of fracture repair and consider recent investigations to help prevent or minimize the effects of this condition. Stable fixation of fractures allows an early return to functional weight bearing without immobilization. When an external support is used, the leg should be fixed in a flexed walking position. Intraarticular hyaluronic acid injection may be a useful therapeutic approach to prevent joint contractures. Fortunately, most forms of fracture disease are reversible, and the severe manifestations can be avoided with proper fracture management.

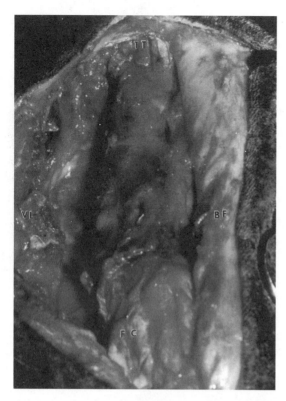

Fig. 15-14 Lateral view of the left femur and stifle joint of dog in Fig. 15-12 after freeing the quadriceps muscle and section of its proximal insertions. The vastus lateralis muscle (**VL**), femoral condyles (**FC**), biceps femoris muscle (**BF**), and the third trochanter (**TT**) are identified.

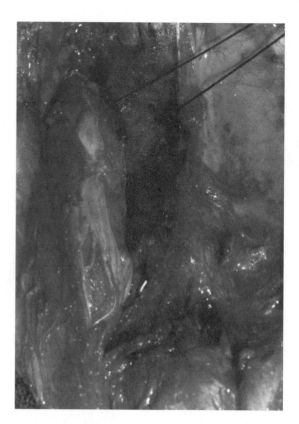

Fig. 15-16 Lateral view of the left femur and quadriceps muscle of dog in Fig. 15-12. The quadriceps muscle is anchored through a drill hole in the femur with nonabsorbable suture.

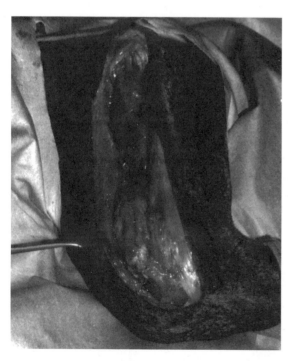

Fig. 15-15 Lateral view of the left hind limb in flexion of dog in Fig. 15-12 after freeing the quadriceps muscle of its proximal insertions.

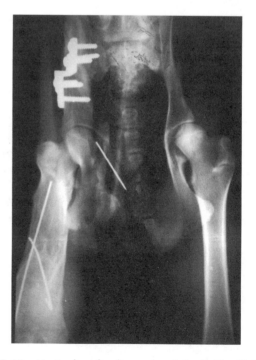

Fig. 15-17 Ventrodorsal radiographs of dog in Fig. 15-12, 12 weeks postoperatively. Note the reduction of the left hip subluxation. A triple pelvic osteotomy was performed on the left hip 4 weeks after freeing the quadriceps muscles.

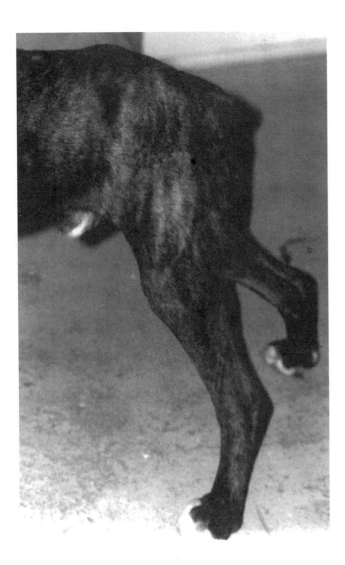

Fig. 15-18 Lateral view of the left hind limb of dog in Fig. 15-12, 10 weeks postoperatively.

REFERENCES

1. Akeson WH, Amiel D, Woo SLY: Immobilization versus continuous passive motion. In Lane JM, editor: *Fracture healing*, New York, 1987, Churchill Livingstone.
2. Bardet JF: Quadriceps contracture and fracture disease, *Vet Clin* 17:957-973, 1987.
3. Bardet JF, Hohn RB: Quadriceps contracture in dogs, *J Am Vet Med Assoc* 183:680-685, 1983.
4. Bardet JF, Hohn RB: Subluxation of the hip joint and bone hypoplasia associated with quadriceps contracture in young dogs, *J Am Anim Hosp Assoc* 20:421, 1984.
5. Braund KJ, Shires PK, Mikeal RL: Type I fiber atrophy in the vastus lateralis in dogs with femoral fractures treated by hyperextension, *Vet Path* 17:166-177, 1986.
6. Grauer JD, and others: The effects of intermittent passive exercise on joint stiffness following periarticular fracture in rabbits, *Clin Orthop* 220:259-265, 1987.
7. Grauer JD, and others: The effects of dexamethasone on periarticular swelling and joint stiffness following fracture in rabbit hind limb model, *Clin Orthop* 42:78-84, 1989.
8. Jurvelin J, and others: Partial restoration of immobilization induced softening of canine articular cartilage after remobilization of the stifle joint, *J Orthop Res* 7:352-358, 1989.
9. Lieber RL, McKee-Woodburn T, Gershuni DM: Recovery of the dog quadriceps after two weeks of immobilization followed by 4 weeks of remobilization, *J Orthop Res* 7:408-418, 1989.
10. More RC, and others: The effects of dimethyl sulfoxide on post traumatic limb swelling on joint stiffness, *Clin Orthop* 233:304-310, 1988.
11. More RC, and others: The effects of two nonsteroidal anti-inflammatory drugs on limb swelling, joint stiffness and bone torsional strength following fracture in a rabbit model, *Clin Orthop* 247:306-312, 1989.
12. Namba RS, and others: Continuous passive motion versus immobilization: the effect on post-traumatic joint stiffness, *Clin Orthop* 267:218-223, 1991.
13. Ouzounian TJ, and others: The effect of pressurization on fracture swelling and joint stiffness in the rabbit hind limb, *Clin Orthop* 210:252-257, 1986.
14. Shires PK, Braund KG, Milton JL: Effect of localized trauma and temporary splinting on immature skeletal muscle and mobility of the femorotibial joint in the dog, *Am J Vet Res* 43:454, 1982.
15. Uhthoff HK, Jaworski ZFG: Bone loss in response to long term immobilization, *J Bone Joint Surg (Am)* 60:420-429, 1978.
16. Uhthoff HK, Sékaly G, Jaworski ZFG: Effects of long term immobilization on metaphyseal spongiosa in young adult beagle dogs, *Clin Orthop* 192:278-283, 1985.

IV

NONFRACTURE RELATED ORTHOPEDIC PROBLEMS

16

Dislocations

CHARLES E. DECAMP

Dislocation of a joint is the disruption of normal dynamic anatomical relationships between two or more bones. Synovial joints are complex structures of bone, cartilage, fibrous capsule, synovium, and neuromuscular and ligamentous support that must work synergistically to allow normal joint movement. When a joint luxation occurs, any of these structures may be injured. Irreversible changes in a joint's anatomical structure and biomechanical function develop within the context of healing and from degenerative joint disease (DJD). Whereas a fracture may heal and remodel to become indistinguishable from normal bone, an injured joint has no such certain future. Future function of a luxated joint depends on the extent of the original injury and on the quality of the healing process.

CLINICAL TERMINOLOGY

Normal joint movement is defined and limited by bone structure, ligamentous and capsular restraints, and neuromuscular interactions. Ligaments are generally considered to be the primary restraints of joint anatomy. When a partial or complete dislocation develops, ligament damage is usually present. A *sprain* is a traumatic rupture of a ligament. A *mild sprain* is partial disruption of the ligament. Although displacement may have occurred at the time of the traumatic incident, little or no displacement of the joint may be evident on clinical examination. The amount of joint displacement worsens with more severe injuries, and more anatomical structures of the joint are involved. A *severe sprain* denotes that the articular surfaces of the joint may be displaced with palpation in clinical examination. The ligament injury may be partial or complete, and disruption of the joint capsule and other structures is often present. The terminology used to describe ligament sprain somewhat overlaps the terminology used to describe dislocation.

Abnormal laxity and displacement of a joint, without complete loss of continuity of the joint surfaces, are described clinically as *subluxation* (Fig. 16-1). Subluxation develops from partial injury to a joint's supporting structures. It is also frequently seen in congenital deformity in which bone and ligaments are improperly formed. A *complete luxation* indicates that a joint's articular surfaces are severely displaced and have no continuity. Complete luxation develops if the ligamentous and joint capsular support of a joint are badly disrupted and may also denote serious injury to surrounding tissues. For example, it is not unusual for severe damage of the gluteal, internal obturator, and gemellus muscles to accompany coxofemoral luxation in the dog or cat. Joints that are highly unstable from multiple ligament and muscle injuries are less likely to return to normal function, even if adequate care is provided.

The clinical terminology used to describe ligament injury is widely used and accepted, but the language tends to downplay the injury's seriousness. "Don't worry, it's only a sprain" is a typically used refrain that indicates to a client that everything will turn out well. It

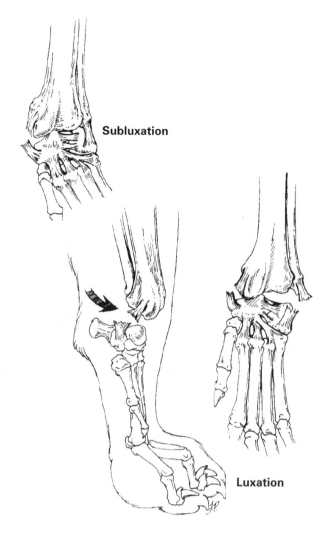

Fig. 16-1 Luxation of a joint results in more severe displacement and tissue damage than subluxation. The prognosis for return to full function is always more guarded with luxation.

should be recognized that damage to a ligament of a joint is always a serious injury, with long-term implications in joint mobility, DJD, and pain. Only careful appreciation of the injury's extent, appropriate stabilization, and meticulous follow-up care ensure the best recovery possible.

BIOMECHANICS OF LIGAMENT FAILURE

Ligaments placed under progressively greater tensile loading demonstrate complex biomechanical behavior. The events that develop and lead to ultimate failure of the ligament are critical to an understanding of clinical assessment of ligament failure and luxation. When a ligament is placed under a tensile load, the ligament substance begins to deform via elongation (strain). Under low-force loads, the undulating pattern of the collagen and matrix (the *crimp*) begins to straighten, allowing elongation, without damage to the fibers of collagen. As the stress to the ligament increases, more collagen fibers come into tension until virtually all the fibers are loaded. As the crimp of the ligament straightens, the rate of elongation slows and becomes almost constant until failure occurs.

Before failure of the ligament substance develops, two important phenomena should be noted. Ligaments subjected mechanically to a faster rate of elongation (strain) fail at a higher load and greater elongation.[35] This means that ligaments respond to rapid movements of the joint by being stronger and allowing more stretch before failure. The second phenomenon is that before individual fibers begin to fail within the ligament, tremendous elongation of the ligament substance develops.[35] The clinical significance of this elongation is readily apparent. If *mild subluxation* or a partial ligament rupture is diagnosed, severe deformation and internal derangement of the ligament have already taken place. *Mild instability* denotes a very severe injury to the ligamentous structure, even if complete failure has not yet developed.

Visual inspection of a ligament at the time of exploratory surgery may be an important determining factor in choosing treatment but may be inadequate to judge the extent of ligament disruption, residual elongation, or damage to the blood supply. Such factors may contribute to an unsatisfactory result in patients with partial ligament disruption.[35]

CHRONIC CHANGES AFTER DISLOCATION

When joint luxation becomes chronic without treatment, numerous changes develop that may affect the success of subsequent surgical repair (Fig. 16-2). When a joint is not properly reduced, the processes of internal wound healing proceed despite joint displacement. Scar tissue is laid down within the joint cavity and periarticular tissues. A mass of scar tissue develops over time and physically obstructs reduction of articular surfaces. Muscular contraction and fibrosis of periarticular muscles develop in response to the trauma and the abnormal position of the joint. Such contraction may impede or prevent manual reduction. Movement of the luxated joint or partial weight bearing on the limb does further damage to local tissues. Joint capsule and ligaments torn in the trauma may be macerated beyond recognition as the tissue is crushed between abnormal bony surfaces. Cartilage and bone are severely damaged from abnormal wear to the articular surface. If an immature growing animal has chronic joint luxation, the articular surfaces may grow with abnormal shape because of the lack of normal articular conformation and weight bearing. DJD develops from damage to the joint in the initial trauma and from secondary effects of chronic luxation. When DJD progresses too far, the animal remains lame, even if joint

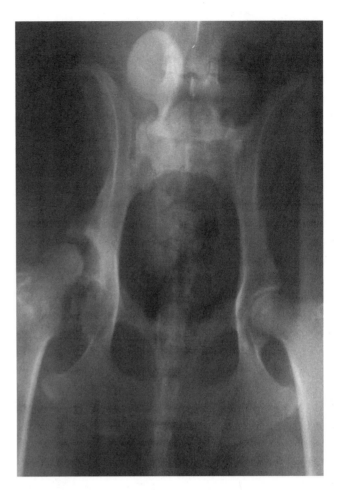

Fig. 16-2 Severe secondary degenerative changes have developed in chronic coxofemoral luxation.

reduction is successful at a later date. The sooner a luxation is reduced and properly stabilized, the fewer long-term sequelae develop.

JOINT DISLOCATIONS
Dislocation of the Shoulder

Luxation of the shoulder occurs infrequently relative to other luxations in the dog or cat (Fig. 16-3). Trauma is the most common cause of shoulder luxation and accounts for approximately two thirds of the luxations reported in the literature.[12,41] Spontaneous or congenital luxations make up the remaining one third. Traumatic luxations may affect any breed or age of animal. Toy breeds of dogs, particularly the toy poodle, account for most nontraumatic luxations. Many toy-breed dogs have congenital shoulder luxation in the first months of life (Fig. 16-4). However, it is not unusual for a toy-breed dog to have nontraumatic shoulder luxation at 5 to 8 years of age.[12,41] A congenital predisposition is suggested in these older dogs but unproved.[12,41,43] As with congenital malformation of other joints, shoulder conformation may

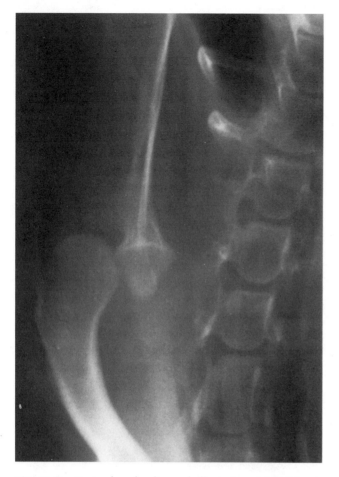

Fig. 16-3 Ventrodorsal radiograph illustrates a lateral shoulder luxation in the dog. Medial shoulder luxations occur more often.

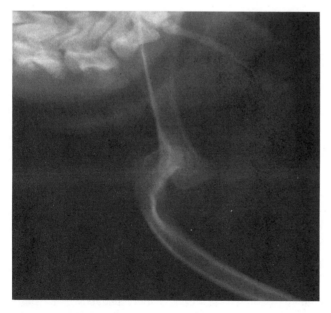

Fig. 16-4 Lateral radiograph indicates that the articular surfaces are abnormal in congenital shoulder luxations. The glenoid is shallow or sometimes rounded.

vary from dog to dog and therefore account for the different ages seen at presentation.

The humeral head luxates medial to the scapula in about two thirds of all shoulder dislocations in both traumatic and congenital luxations.[12,26,41] Most remaining luxations of the humeral head are lateral relative to the scapula and traumatic in origin. Cranial and caudal luxations have been reported but are extremely rare.[11,12,18,26]

Anatomy of shoulder luxation. The shoulder is a synovial joint consisting of the broad surface of the humeral head, which articulates with the smaller concave surface of the scapular glenoid. The glenoid surface is extended somewhat by a cartilaginous labrum. Unlike distal joints of the extremities, the shoulder joint does not have true collateral ligaments. The joint capsule is distinctly thickened medially and laterally to form the medial and lateral glenohumeral ligaments (Fig. 16-5).

The absence of true collateral ligaments has led many authors to suggest that basic support of the shoulder joint is from the musculotendinous insertions of four "cuff" muscles, as described in the human orthopedic literature.[18,26] Others dispute this claim and suggest that the primary restraints to the shoulder joint are the joint capsule and glenohumeral ligaments.[16,42] In vitro studies suggest that luxation is not possible without injury to the joint capsule.[16,42] As with all joints, stability of the shoulder is likely a result of complex interactions of bony anatomy, ligaments, capsular, and neuromuscular support. Such interactions are readily apparent when examining the defects present in dogs with congenital shoulder deformity.

Dogs with congenital shoulder luxation have numerous anatomical abnormalities that predispose them to luxation (see Fig. 16-4). The glenoid surface is shallow and flattened and corresponds to a flattened humeral head. On rare occasion the glenoid surface is convex rather than concave in shape.[43] Loss of bone and cartilage from the glenoid labrum is a common finding and may be caused by rubbing on the humeral head. It is uncertain whether the erosion of the labrum results from congenital deformity or the chronicity of recurrent luxation. The supporting "cuff" tendons of the shoulder joint may be severely stretched or ruptured in congenital luxations. The joint capsule may be ruptured but more often is intact and extremely lax. Intracapsular luxation may be evident on exploratory surgery in such patients.

Clinical presentation and diagnosis. Patients with shoulder luxations usually have a history of acute lameness after a traumatic incident. The animal is non–weight bearing on the affected limb, with elbow flexed and adducted. In a typical medial luxation, the greater tubercle of the humerus is found to be depressed medially in relation to the scapular acromion. A scapular neck

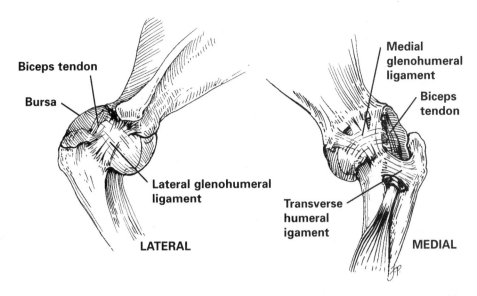

Fig. 16-5   Primary restraints of the shoulder joint are the joint capsule and glenohumeral ligaments.

fracture may have a similar presentation, so radiography must be used to confirm the diagnosis. An acute luxation is especially painful, and manipulation of the limb to determine the degree of laxity may not be possible without sedation or anesthesia. A typical lateral shoulder luxation presents similarly, except that the greater tubercle is prominent on examination, and it may be difficult to palpate the acromion process.

A dog with congenital shoulder luxation may be a puppy or an adult with chronic weight-bearing or non-weight-bearing lameness. Atrophy of the shoulder and forelimb often is evident. There may be less pain in the chronic condition, so that application of traction, abduction, and adduction may allow reduction, if only temporarily. In some dogs the joint is "fixed" in a luxated position, and reduction is not possible without surgical intervention.

Conservative care. A dog with a traumatic luxation should be anesthetized as soon as it is safe to do so. The shoulder is reduced by direct manipulation of the upper arm and digital pressure on the acromiom process and humeral head. If the shoulder joint is extremely lax and easily reduced, it is not likely that the joint will remain reduced with conservative care. Surgical stabilization should then be recommended. If the luxation requires considerable effort to reduce and seems stable after reduction, the supporting structures of the joint may maintain joint reduction. With medial luxations, a Velpeau sling is constructed and maintained for 2 to 3 weeks. Exercise is limited for several months thereafter. Lateral luxations are more amenable to treatment by conservative means than medial luxations because they seem to be more stable after reduction. A spica splint is used as external coaptation for lateral luxation, since

this rotates the proximal humerus in a slightly outward direction.[11]

Closed reduction may sometimes be easy to achieve in dogs with congenital shoulder luxation, but the prognosis for maintaining reduction is always poor. Surgery is indicated if lameness is present.

Surgical stabilization of medial luxation. Imbrication and prosthetic ligament techniques have been described for internal stabilization of medial luxation but are not as successful as transposition of the biceps brachii tendon.[11,26] Biceps tendon transposition effectively supports the joint's medial side. Two studies indicate that reduction is maintained in more than 90% of the dogs undergoing this surgery.[26,41] Although the tendon transposition maintains reduction of the luxated joint, 42% of dogs of one report remained lame when followed long term after surgery. Caution should be exercised in case selection for this procedure. Dogs with congenital luxation may have a glenoid surface that is small in size and convex in shape. It is unlikely that tendon transposition will be effective in such patients that have severe congenital deformity.

The technique for medial transposition of the biceps brachii tendon is adapted directly from the procedure described by Hohn and others.[26] The medial aspect of the shoulder joint is exposed by craniomedial approach.[39] The tendon of the coracobrachialis muscle is retracted with the insertion of the subscapularis muscle, which has been elevated to expose the lesser tubercle. The joint capsule and glenohumeral ligament are incised along the glenoid's edge. The luxation is reduced and the joint inspected. The fascia, transverse humeral ligament, and joint capsule over the bicipital groove are incised to mobilize the bicipital tendon. An osteotome is used to cut a flap of bone and periosteum in the lesser tubercle. The periosteal base of the flap is hinged cranially. A rongeur is used to deepen the osteotomy site by removing cancellous bone. The biceps tendon is lifted from the bicipital groove and placed into the osteotomy site. The bone flap is fixed over the tendon, with two small Kirschner wires placed through the flap into the humerus (Fig. 16-6).

The joint capsule is closed and imbricated with nonabsorbable sutures in a Lembert or mattress pattern. The subscapularis muscle is sutured as cranially on the greater tubercle as possible. The deep and superficial pectoral muscles are stretched across the greater tubercle and individually sutured to the fascia of its lateral surface. The remaining layers are closed routinely. A Velpeau bandage is placed postoperatively and main-

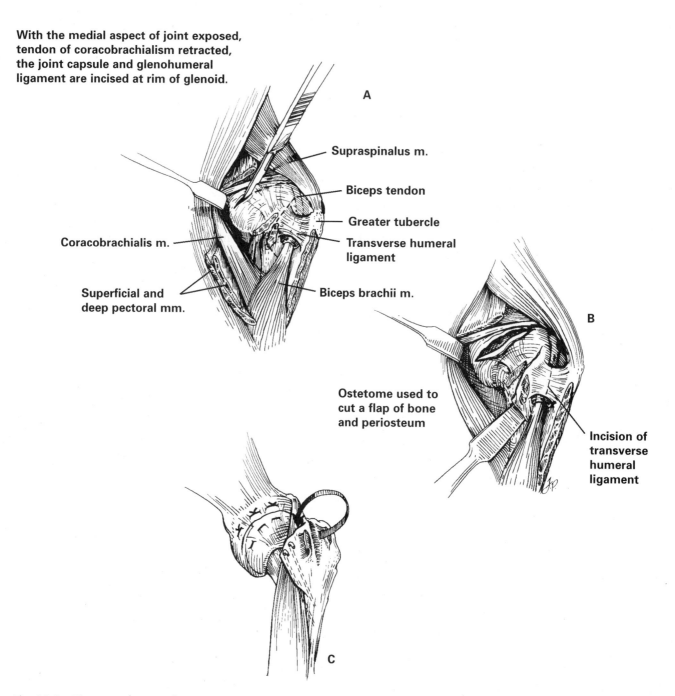

With the medial aspect of joint exposed, tendon of coracobrachialism retracted, the joint capsule and glenohumeral ligament are incised at rim of glenoid.

A

Supraspinalus m.

Biceps tendon

Greater tubercle

Transverse humeral ligament

Coracobrachialis m.

Biceps brachii m.

Superficial and deep pectoral mm.

B

Ostetome used to cut a flap of bone and periosteum

Incision of transverse humeral ligament

C

Fig. 16-6 Biceps tendon translocation is an effective treatment for shoulder dislocation.[26] **A,** Joint capsule is incised for inspection of the joint and reduction. **B,** Bone flap is raised with osteotome. **C,** Biceps tendon is transposed.

tained for 2 weeks. Exercise is limited for 2 months after the procedure.

Surgical stabilization of lateral luxation. Fewer cases of lateral shoulder luxation are reported compared with medial luxation, but surgical stabilization with tendon transposition seems to be highly effective.[26,41] Joint stability is excellent after the procedure, and dogs do not have lameness when followed long term after surgery.[41]

The technique for lateral transposition of the biceps brachii tendon is adapted directly from the procedure described by Hohn and others.[26] A cranial surgical approach with osteotomy of the greater tubercle is used to expose the region of the intertubercular groove.[29] The transverse humeral ligament and the joint capsule are incised to mobilize the tendon of the biceps brachii. A rongeur is used to cut a shallow groove at or just proximal to the osteotomy site. The biceps tendon is lifted out of the intertubercular groove and moved laterally to the prepared site. The osteotomized greater tubercle is replaced and fixed to the humerus with two or three small Kirschner wires. The joint capsule is closed with simple interrupted sutures. Several sutures are placed to fix the biceps tendon to the tendinous insertions of the supraspinatus, infraspinatus, and teres minor muscles. The remaining layers are closed in a routine manner. A spica splint may be used as external coaptation after surgery for 14 days but is usually not needed.

Salvage procedures for shoulder dislocation. When severe deformity or loss of the glenoid labrum is present, reduction and fixation of a shoulder luxation may not yield satisfactory results. Two salvage procedures are described that may yield satisfactory functional results. Arthrodesis of the shoulder (see Chapter 23) is highly recommended for recurrent shoulder luxation. A dog with a healed shoulder arthrodesis may walk and run with minimal gait disturbance or lameness. Another salvage procedure for intractable shoulder luxation is excision arthroplasty of the glenoid and humeral head,[11] which provides very good results, especially in smaller dogs.

Dislocation of the Elbow

Dislocation of the elbow occurs more often than shoulder dislocation in the dog and is usually caused by trauma.[13,25] The proximal radius and ulna are usually displaced in a proximal and lateral direction (Fig. 16-7). Precise and timely management is required if a successful outcome is to be achieved. Congenital and developmental elbow luxations are also seen in dogs.[7,24] Developmental luxations of the elbow joint occur from abnormal physeal growth of the radius and ulna and are often associated with angular deformity. Subluxation and

incongruency of the articular surfaces, rather than complete luxation, most often occur with developmental conditions. Chapters 13 and 21 discuss developmental conditions secondary to abnormal physeal growth. Whereas developmental conditions of the elbow appear at 4 to 10 months of age, congenital elbow dislocation is present at birth but may not be diagnosed until the first 3 to 6 weeks of life. Complete luxations of the humeroulnar or humeroradial joints are the most common congenital luxations. Except for displacement of the bones, the radiographic anatomy of the elbow appears normal at first presentation. As congenital luxation becomes more chronic, secondary growth abnormalities develop.

Anatomy of the elbow. The elbow is a compound synovial joint that is classified as a ginglymus, or hinge, joint. There are three articulations: humeroradial, humeroulnar, and proximal radioulnar. The humeroradial joint provides the joint's major weight-bearing surface.[23] The humeroulnar articulation acts to limit movement in a sagittal plane and enhances joint stability.[23,32] The elbow flexes, extends, and allows some rotation. The collateral

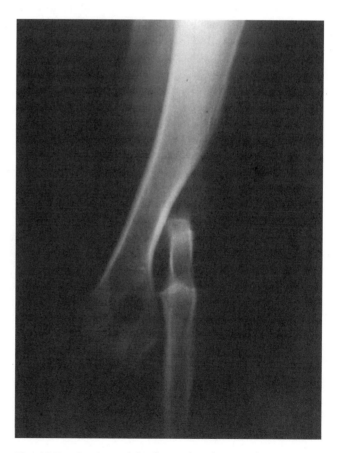

Fig. 16-7 Craniocaudal radiograph indicating that traumatic elbow luxation results in lateral and proximal displacement of the ulna and radius.

ligaments limit lateral (valgus) and medial (varus) displacements of the joint (Fig. 16-8). The lateral collateral ligament extends from the lateral epicondyle of the humerus and divides distally to attach to the proximal radius and ulna. The smaller medial collateral ligament extends from the medial epicondyle and divides distally into two crura. The cranial crus attaches to the radial tuberosity, and the caudal crus passes through the interosseous space and attaches to the radius and ulna.[23] A thick annular ligament supports the radioulnar joint by forming a restricting band around the proximal radius.

Traumatic dislocation of the elbow joint. The proximal radius and ulna are almost always displaced lateral and slightly proximal to the humeral condyles in elbow dislocation. Apparently, the large medial epicondyle of the humerus helps to prevent luxation in a medial direction. Luxation of the elbow may develop with or without disruption of the collateral ligaments.[13] Relative to other joints, the elbow joint is quite stable despite collateral ligament injury. The interlocking nature of the bones (hinge joint) contributes to stability after closed or open reduction. If the collateral ligaments are intact, an elbow luxation may be difficult to reduce but is quite stable when anatomically replaced. If collateral ligament and severe joint capsule disruption is present, instability of the joint sometimes requires reconstruction of the collateral ligaments.

Traumatic elbow luxations develop in adult dogs of either gender. It is unusual to see this injury in an immature animal. A dog with elbow luxation presents with a non-weight-bearing lameness with the elbow held in a flexed, pronated, and slightly abducted position. Joint palpation is characterized by firm swelling laterally and inability to locate the lateral epicondyle of the humerus. Severe pain and crepitus are evident with joint movement.

Closed reduction of traumatic elbow dislocation. General anesthesia is required for reduction of elbow dislocation. Closed reduction is appropriate for most acute traumatic dislocations and may be attempted up to 7 to 10 days after injury. The best results are achieved when reduction is completed very soon after the trauma. The dog is placed in lateral recumbency and the joint flexed and rotated in an outward direction. This allows the ulnar anconeus to clear the edge of the lateral condyle. As the joint is extended, the forearm is forcibly rotated inward, allowing the anconeal process to catch the lateral condyle's inner surface. As the anconeal process "catches" the lateral condyle, the joint is put through a range of motion, which further reduces the joint. This manipulation can require considerable force to accomplish and can damage the joint's articular surfaces. Exploratory surgery and open reduction may be less traumatic to the joint than forcible closed reduction in some patients.

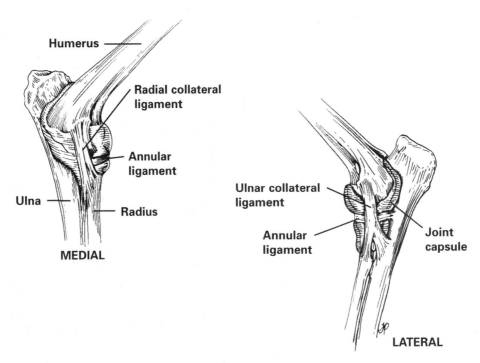

Fig. 16-8 Primary restraints of the elbow joint are the collateral and annular ligaments and the joint capsule.

Radiographs should be taken after closed reduction to ensure adequate replacement. Slight internal displacement is not unusual after closed reduction and generally disappears in several weeks. If the radial head is not seen to be well seated under the humeral condyle, further closed manipulation or open reduction is indicated. An extension splint is advised for 1 to 2 weeks to help maintain reduction (Fig. 16-9). A splint is constructed by reinforcing a soft, padded bandage on its cranial surface with cast material or a splint rod with the joint in full extension.

Surgical reduction of traumatic elbow dislocation. Within 10 days of traumatic elbow luxation, closed reduction may no longer be possible. If no treatment is performed, the luxation becomes firmly fixed in malreduction by fibrous adhesions and muscular contracture. Damage to the articular cartilage of the lateral condyle develops from abnormal wear. The joint cavity is gradually filled with fibrous scar tissue. DJD progresses, and lameness is quite severe. Open reduction is most effective if achieved before severe chronic changes develop.

A simple caudolateral surgical approach provides sufficient exposure to effect reduction in luxations up to 10 to 14 days after injury. After several weeks, a transolecranon approach may be required to remove or incise scar tissue restraints to reduction.

Caudolateral surgical approach. The elbow is exposed by an approach to the joint's caudolateral compartments.[39] The incision in the anconeal muscle may be extended cranially to allow full access to the ulnar trochlear notch. Blood clots, fibrin, and other debris are removed from the joint. The joint is manipulated as described for closed reduction. If reduction is difficult, the manipulation is repeated, but a pair of blunt, closed scissors or other smooth instrument is placed into the trochlear notch and used to lever the humeral condyles back onto the radial head (Fig. 16-10). Once replaced, the joint is passively flexed and extended. Collateral instability should be assessed. If the reduction

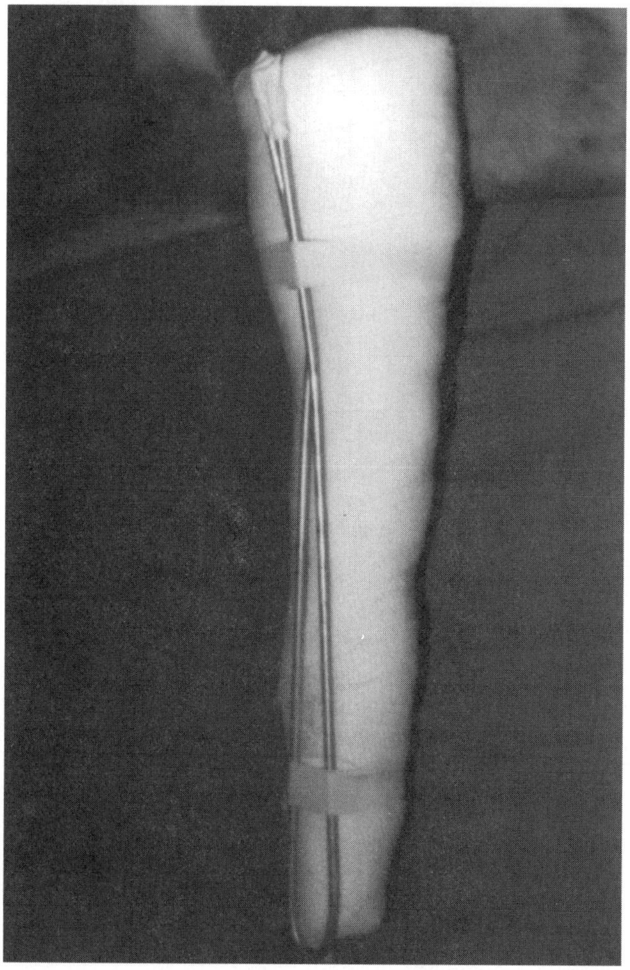

Fig. 16-9 Extension splint prevents reluxation after reduction of an elbow luxation.

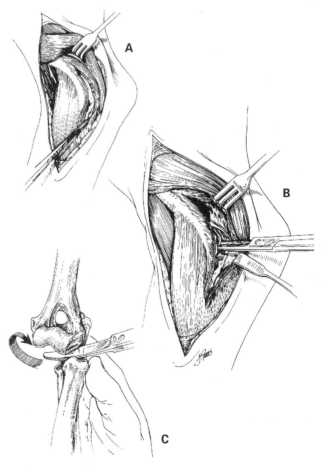

Fig. 16-10 **A,** Caudolateral approach may be used to reduce acute elbow luxation if closed reduction fails. The joint capsule is incised beneath the anconeus muscle. **B,** Curved scissors may be introduced to aid reduction. **C,** Considerable force may be required. Digital pressure on the radial head is helpful.

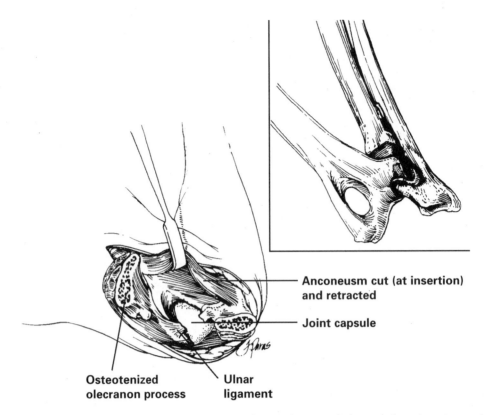

Anconeusm cut (at insertion) and retracted

Joint capsule

Osteotenized olecranon process   **Ulnar ligament**

Fig. 16-11 Transolecranon approach is used for reduction of chronic elbow luxation and allows access to the caudal aspect of the joint for removal of fibrous scar tissue.

is extremely unstable, the collateral ligaments should be primarily repaired or augmented with screw and suture fixation.

Transolecranon surgical approach. A transolecranon approach provides excellent visibility of the elbow joint to excise chronic scar tissue that is limiting reduction.[39] Care must be taken during the surgical exposure to preserve the joint capsule and collateral ligaments (Fig. 16-11). Once a chronic luxation is reduced, the elbow joint is frequently unstable. Primary repair of the collateral ligaments may be difficult to achieve if they are engulfed in the fibrous scar of chronic luxation. Augmentation of collateral ligament stability (Fig. 16-12) may be achieved with screw, washer, and suture fixation.

After open reduction, care for the animal is similar to that after closed reduction. An extension splint may be used to support the limb for 2 weeks. Passive flexion and extension exercise, as well as non-weight-bearing activity such as swimming, are advised after splint removal to help maintain a range of motion.

Congenital elbow dislocation. Congenital elbow dislocations in puppies are infrequently seen. The puppies sometimes may appear affected as early as 3 to 6 weeks of age with varying degrees of lameness and deformity. Some have no lameness, but owners have noticed a firm swelling over the elbow joint's lateral

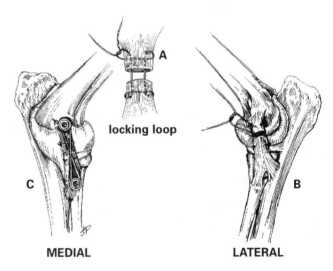

locking loop

MEDIAL   **LATERAL**

Fig. 16-12 Elbow luxation may require repair of the collateral ligaments. **A,** Collateral ligaments may be primarily sutured with a locking loop pattern. **B,** Ligament tears may be difficult to appose. **C,** Collateral ligament repair strength may be augmented with screw, washer, and figure-eight suture or wire.

side. Other puppies are lame or completely non–weight bearing on the affected limbs. The condition is usually bilateral. The limbs typically deviate medially, below the level of the elbow joint, to cause a bowlegged stance. Congenital luxation is most frequently described in

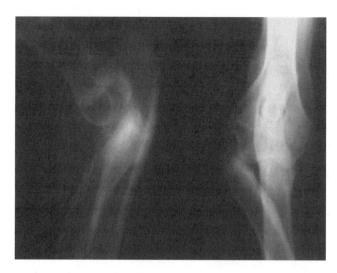

Fig. 16-13 Lateral and craniocaudal radiographs indicating luxation of the proximal radius that developed during growth. Note the abnormal rounded shape of the articular surface of the radial head.

smaller breeds, such as Pekingese, Shetland sheepdog, dachshund, and Yorkshire terrier.[40] Larger breeds are also affected and include bulldogs, basset hounds, Akitas, and German shepherds.[22,40] Males seem to be affected more often than females.[32]

The cause of congenital elbow luxation is unknown. Bingel and Riser[7] suggest that the primary defect consists of hypoplagia or aplasia of the collateral ligaments of the elbow. A hereditary predisposition is suggested by the presentation, a bilateral condition that develops in specific dog breeds. An inherited predisposition for elbow luxation has not been proved.

Congenital elbow dislocation is classified by radiographic appearance into three types.[30] In a type I luxation the proximal radius is displaced caudally and laterally and does not articulate with the humeral condyle. Type I luxation is also described as *humeroradial luxation* (Fig. 16-13). In the early stages the radius and ulna have a normal radiographic appearance, except for joint displacement. As the condition becomes chronic, numerous changes develop. The proximal radial epiphysis is underdeveloped and shows a convex outline. There may be cranial curvature of the proximal ulna and lateral curvature to the proximal radius. The radial head's articular surface becomes rounded and irregular in shape. The anconeal and coronoid processes may be small, and the trochlear notch is shallow. In type II elbow luxation the ulna is displaced laterally and does not articulate with the humerus.[30]

Type II luxation is also described as *humeroulnar luxation* (Fig. 16-14). The proximal radius maintains a normal relationship with the humerus, but the ulna rotates away from its normal articulation. The anconeal and coronoid processes may be small or absent, and the

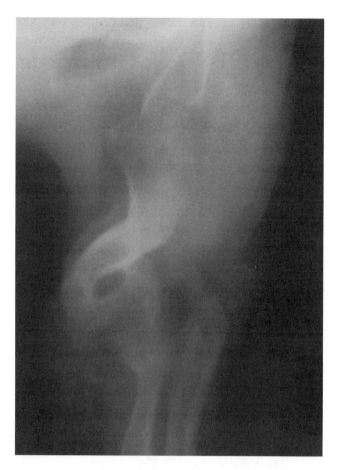

Fig. 16-14 Craniocaudal radiograph indicating that the proximal ulna is displaced laterally in humeroulnar luxations. Note the abnormal articular surfaces in this growing dog.

ulnar trochlear notch appears shallow. The proximal radial physis and epiphysis appear normal.

In type III elbow dislocation, also known as *humeroulnar and radioulnar luxation*, both radius and ulna are displaced laterally to the humeral condyle and rotated by about 90 degrees.[30] The anconeal process is not developed, and the medial coronoid process is small. The ulnar trochlear notch may be very shallow.

Treatment. Treatment of dogs with congenital elbow luxation depends on the type and severity of luxation present, the age of animal, and the degree of secondary growth and degenerative change present. As a general principle, aggressive treatment should be begun by 3 to 4 months of age in the growing animal to reduce the problems from secondary growth abnormality. If treatment is delayed until the animal is mature, the resultant joint incongruity results in severe secondary degenerative change that affects the functional outcome.

Congenital humeroradial luxation (type I). Conservative management of congenital radial head luxation is not effective. Although reduction may sometimes be accomplished with anesthesia and manipulation of the limb, there are no reported cases with a successful outcome. Surgical correction of humeroradial luxation achieves the best results if completed between 3 and 6 months of age and is accomplished with wedge osteotomy and fixation of the radius. In a limited series of patients, one third of the elbows reluxated after internal repair. Secondary degenerative changes and lameness possibly occurred, despite maintaining reduction of the humeroradial joint.[22] The prognosis for normal function after internal repair therefore is guarded.

Reduction of humeroradial luxation is accomplished through a lateral surgical approach to the proximal radius.[39] Care is taken to preserve the deep branch of the radial nerve as it courses beneath the supinator muscle. An oscillating saw is used to remove a wedge of bone from the proximal radius so as to reduce the proximal radius to the articular surface of the lateral humeral condyle. Fixation for the osteotomy is accomplished with several small pins or a bone plate, depending on the patient's size (Fig. 16-15). The pins are placed from proximal to distal, avoiding the articular surface of the proximal radius. If the lateral collateral ligament is absent, or

if significant collateral instability remains, a prosthetic collateral ligament is constructed with two screws, washers, and nonabsorbable suture material.[22] The surgical incision is closed in a routine manner. Postoperative care consists of a soft, padded bandage for 2 to 3 weeks. The dog's activity should be limited for several months or until the elbow has proved stable.

Congenital humeroulnar luxation (type II). Closed reduction of humeroulnar luxation may be attempted under general anesthesia in puppies less than 3 to 4 months of age.[32] Reduction is achieved by flexion of the elbow, rotating and digitally forcing the ulna medial in relation to the humeral condyle. The joint is then extended to seat the anconeus muscle in the humeral condyles. Reduction is best maintained in a small puppy with transarticular pinning.[44] As the joint is placed in a standing position, one or two small Kirschner wires (0.035 to 0.062 inch) are driven through the caudal aspect of the olecranon into and through the humeral condyles. The pins are cut off below the skin surface, leaving sufficient length for pin removal. The puppy should have cage rest until the pins are removed. The limb may be lightly bandaged. The pins are left for 2 to 3 weeks and then removed. The prognosis for maintaining elbow reduction with transarticular pinning is always guarded because premature loosening of the pins may occur.

Transarticular pinning for elbow luxation is generally reserved for small puppies. Older puppies or dogs with more severe deformity require open reduction and fixation. Surgery varies depending on the deformity's severity. The luxation is surgically exposed through a caudomedial or transolecranon approach.[11,33] Reduction is accomplished by flexing the elbow and rotating the ulna medially to position the ulnar trochlear notch into the humeral trochlea. The joint is inspected and revision of the trochlear notch completed, if necessary, by deepening the notch with a scalpel blade until a more congruent fit is achieved. The reduction is maintained by a combination of imbrication of the medial joint capsule, transposition of the olecranon distally on the ulna, and transfixation of the ulna to the proximal radius with a small pin.[33] This transfixation should not be performed in the rapidly growing animal (4 to 8 months of age). A light bandage may be placed on the limb after surgery, and exercise should be restricted for several months. A guarded prognosis should be given for return to normal function.

Congenital humeroulnar and radioulnar luxation (type III). Complete congenital luxation of the elbow is less common than type I or type II luxation. Continuity of the humeroulnar and radioulnar joints is lost, and bony deformity is often severe. The combined humeroulnar and radioulnar luxation may be treated as described for humeroulnar luxation but carries a more guarded prognosis.

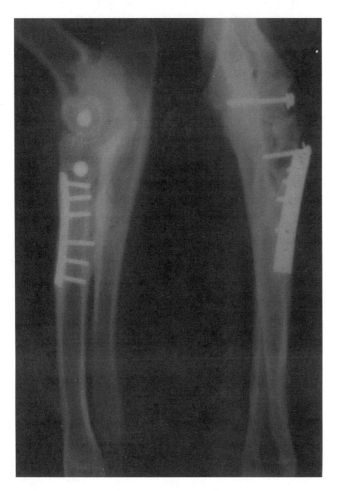

Fig. 16-15 Lateral and craniocaudal radiographs taken several months after surgical correction for humeroradial luxation in the animal from Fig. 16-13. The joint congruity is improved.

Dislocation of the Carpus

Dislocation of the carpus is a frequent injury in the dog and most often caused by a traumatic incident (Fig. 16-16). A genetic and congenital predisposition to carpal luxation is described in the dog but is extremely rare.[38] Automobile trauma and jumping or falling from a height are the most frequent causes of carpal injury and typically result in fractures and/or dislocation. The anatomy of the carpus is complex, and numerous complex bone and ligament injuries are seen. This section describes only the most commonly seen dislocations of the carpus. Chapter 8 describes fractures of the carpus.

Anatomy of the carpus. The carpus has seven bones that articulate with the radius proximally and the metacarpus distally. The three bones in the proximal row are the radial, ulnar, and accessory carpal bones. The distal row are numbered carpal bones 1 to 4. There are three main carpal joints: the proximal, middle and distal. The ligamentous anatomy of the carpus is complex but may be described in terms of three supporting groups. The collateral ligaments support the medial and lateral surfaces of the carpus (Fig. 16-17). They consist of two short radial collateral ligaments that connect the styloid of the radius to the radial carpal bone and one short ulnar collateral ligament from the styloid of the ulna to the ulnar carpal bone. No continuous collateral ligament supports all three joint levels.[11] A second supporting group of ligaments consists of numerous small intercarpal ligaments that connect and support individual carpal bones. A third group of carpal ligaments supports the palmar surface of the carpus and prevents hyperextension during weight bearing. There are four ligaments

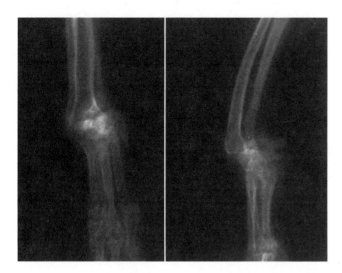

Fig. 16-16 Note the chronic changes seen on the craniocaudal and lateral radiographs that have developed with carpal luxation in a small poodle. Displacement of carpal bones indicates severe ligamentous injury.

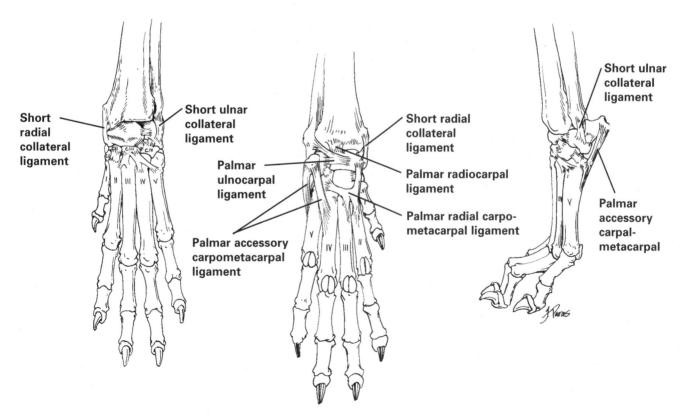

Fig. 16-17 Collateral and palmar ligaments and the joint capsule are the main restraints of the carpus.

in this group: the palmar radiocarpal, the palmar accessory carpometacarpal, the palmar ulnocarpal, and the palmar radial carpometacarpal ligaments. In addition to the ligamentous support, a well-developed joint capsule and palmar carpal fibercartilage also support the palmar surface of the carpus.

Clinical presentation and diagnosis. Most carpal injuries are quite painful, and the animal is non–weight bearing or severely lame. Moderate to severe swelling may extend from the carpus and in some patients extends distally to involve the foot. Palpation of the carpal joint may demonstrate valgus or varus instability, excessive rotation, or hyperextension. Craniocaudal and lateral radiographic views are usually sufficient for diagnosis. Oblique or stress radiographic views are necessary to diagnose subtle fractures or instability.

Subluxation of the antebrachiocarpal joint. The radial collateral ligaments are frequently ruptured as an isolated injury or in combination with shear wounds of the carpus. Subluxation of the antebrachiocarpal joint develops from medial instability. The foot is held in a valgus position below the level of the carpus. Conservative care of this injury is not effective treatment because of continual stress during weight bearing. Since the dog normally stands with the foot slightly in a valgus position, the medial ligaments are always under tension.[11]

The collateral ligament is repaired through a medial approach. The skin, subcutaneous tissue, and deep fascia are incised directly over the ligament. The ligaments are inspected and appropriately sutured (see Chapter 22). The joint capsule and periarticular fascia are imbricated with nonabsorbable sutures in a mattress or Lembert pattern. The strength of the sutured ligaments may be augmented with one of two techniques. Screw and suture technique may be used by placing a small bone screw and washer in both the styloid of the radius and the radial carpal bone (Fig. 16-18). Nonabsorbable suture is used in a figure-eight pattern around the screws and under the washers. If a shear wound to the carpus is present, stainless steel orthopedic wire is substituted for nonabsorbable suture. An alternate technique is to drill bony tunnels in the radius and radial carpal bone.[11] Nonabsorbable suture is passed through the tunnels and tied to mimic the action of the collateral ligaments until ligament healing progresses.

After surgery the limb is placed in a well-padded palmar splint for 6 weeks. A padded bandage may be used for another 2 to 3 weeks, when normal activity may be gradually resumed. If orthopedic wire was used in the reconstruction, it should be removed after 2 to 3 months to prevent irritation from broken strands. The prognosis for an isolated collateral injury to the carpus is very good.

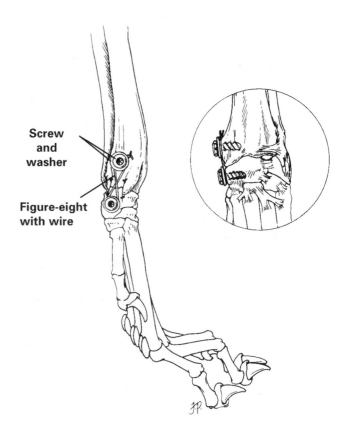

Screw and washer

Figure-eight with wire

Fig. 16-18 Screws, washers, and figure-eight suture or wire may be used to augment collateral ligament repair of the carpus.

Complete luxation of the carpus. Complete luxation of the antebrachiocarpal joint is less common than subluxation. In this injury the collateral ligaments and much of the palmar ligamentous support are disrupted. Severe instability of the antebrachiocarpal joint results and is accompanied by severe pain and swelling. Conservative care by coaptation or reconstruction by ligamentous repair is not appropriate for this injury.[11,34] Pancarpal arthrodesis is the best choice for treatment of complete antebrachiocarpal luxation. Chapter 23 discusses details of the surgical technique of arthrodesis.

Hyperextension of the carpus. Injury to the palmar supporting ligaments typically results in subluxation with hyperextension of the carpus. Any joint level may be involved, and the following distribution has been reported[11]:

Antebrachiocarpal	10%
Middle carpal	50%
Carpometacarpal	40%

The carpus may extend 30 degrees beyond normal in a typical hyperextension injury, but in some the animal walks on the palmar surface of the carpus and the carpal pad. Associated fractures and complex ligament injuries are common. In dogs with mild displacement, the clinical signs of lameness and swelling may be minimal.[11] In dogs with fractures or severe displacement, severe swelling and pain are frequently evident.

Surgical repair of hyperextension injury. Stabilization of carpal hyperextension is somewhat controversial. Reconstruction of the palmar ligaments with autogenous tissue and wire support has been reported but not widely practiced.[20] Partial or pancarpal arthrodesis are the most widely used techniques to treat dogs with hyperextension injuries. Limb function after healing of carpal arthrodesis is excellent for pet dogs. Pancarpal arthrodesis may be used for hyperextension injury at any level of the carpus. Partial arthrodesis may be used for injuries of the middle and carpometacarpal joints. Caution should be exercised in performing arthrodesis in dogs with acute, severely displaced luxations. These animals often have severe swelling of the carpus and foot because of the injury and are likely to have vascular compromise. It is appropriate to support the foot and carpus in such patients with a well-padded splint for 7 to 10 days before performing arthrodesis. This allows some inflammation of the traumatic episode to subside before surgical intervention. (For details of the surgical technique for carpal arthrodesis, see Chapter 23).

Dislocation of the Coxofemoral Joint

The coxofemoral joint is more frequently dislocated than any other joint in the dog and cat, accounting for approximately 50% of all joint luxations.[11] Dislocation most frequently affects adult animals, but immature dogs and cats are also affected.[5,8] Traumatic injury is the most prevalent cause of hip dislocation, but luxation may also develop from severe hip dysplasia. Hip dysplasia typically alters the treatment plan and prognosis for a dog with hip luxation and so must be carefully addressed.

Anatomy of coxofemoral luxation. No collateral ligaments exist in the coxofemoral joint. Dislocation of the joint develops when the joint capsule and round ligament are torn and the femoral head is displaced from the acetabulum. The joint capsule may be torn in several locations. It may be avulsed from the dorsal acetabular rim or torn in the middle of the capsule. Less often, the joint capsule is avulsed from the femoral neck. The muscular support of the hip joint, particularly the gluteal, internal obturator, and gemellus muscles, may also be damaged in luxation. Although severe muscular rupture does not frequently accompany dislocation, it results in severe joint instability when present.

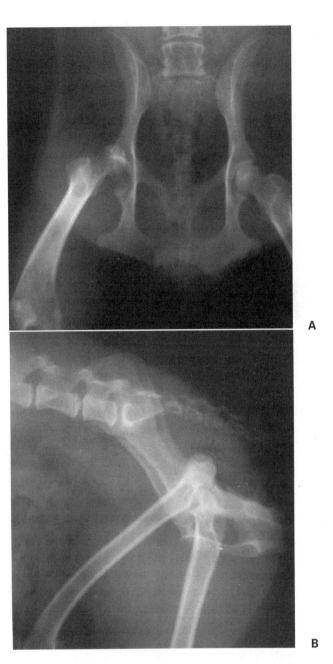

Fig. 16-19 **A** and **B,** Ventrodorsal and lateral radiographs are required to determine the direction of luxation, as seen in this craniodorsal coxofemoral luxation.

Displacement of the femoral head is usually craniodorsal to the acetabulum (Fig. 16-19) and accounts for 95% of coxofemoral luxations seen.[8] Caudoventral and cranioventral displacements are recognized, but far less frequently (Fig. 16-20). Medial luxation of the coxofemoral joint is described but only develops with acetabular fracture. Acetabular rim fractures must be repaired if stability of the coxofemoral joint is to be achieved but are not discussed in this chapter. Avulsion

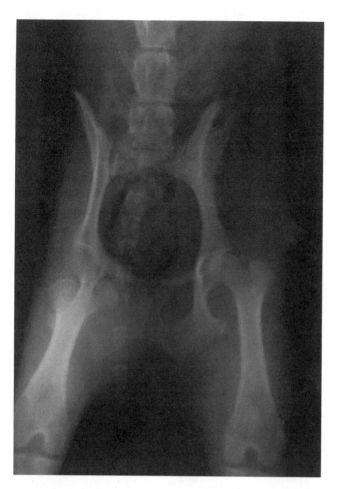

Fig. 16-20 Ventrodorsal radiograph indicating caudoventral displacement in coxofemoral luxation. The femoral head is often displaced and "locked" into the obturator foramen.

fractures of the femoral head, with a fragment attached to the round ligament, are also frequently seen. If the fragment is large, it may necessitate removal or fixation to allow joint reduction.

Hip dysplasia and coxofemoral luxation. Hip dysplasia is a genetic and developmental abnormality of coxofemoral joint conformation. The coxofemoral joint is predisposed to dislocation in dogs with hip dysplasia. Luxation may develop with a traumatic incident or may develop spontaneously because of inherent joint instability during normal running and playing. Reduction of the hip joint is not difficult in dysplastic dogs; however, because of anatomical abnormalities, maintaining reduction is almost impossible whether a closed technique or surgical reduction is chosen (see Chapter 17).

Clinical signs and diagnosis. Acute hip dislocation results in a severe non-weight-bearing lameness in the affected limb. As the condition becomes chronic over a period of weeks, the animal may begin to bear weight on

the limb, but lameness usually persists. In a typical luxation with craniodorsal displacement, the limb is held with the stifle externally rotated and slightly flexed. The pelvic region may be swollen, and the greater trochanter is palpated dorsal and somewhat cranial to its normal position below a line drawn between the iliac crest and the ischium. If limb length is compared with the opposite normal limb, the luxated limb appears shorter because of the dorsal shift of the femur. Measurement of limb length may be accomplished in the small dog by lifting both rear legs from the ground and examining the comparable foot position. Limb length may be difficult to perceive in larger dogs because no easy clinical method is available. The physical signs of hip luxation, although useful for a clinical diagnosis, are not pathognomonic for hip luxation. Fractures of the pelvis or femoral head and neck may mimic the clinical signs of luxation. Standard ventrodorsal and lateral radiographic views should always be taken to establish the diagnosis and look for avulsed bone chips from the femoral head. The chips are seen in the acetabular cup because they are attached to the ligament of the femoral head. Presence of these chips is a definite indication for open reduction to allow removal of all bone fragments.

The physical signs of luxation vary somewhat with the direction of femoral head displacement. When a caudoventral or medial luxation is present, the greater trochanter may be difficult to locate by palpation or may be detected much deeper in a medial sagittal plane. The limb is usually non–weight bearing, with the lower limb held in an adducted position.

Treatment of craniodorsal luxation. Treatment of coxofemoral luxation is generally successful and yields good limb function after repair. Recurrence of luxation is the major complication and is related to numerous factors of the trauma and its treatment. Closed reduction under general anesthesia is the accepted initial treatment for acute traumatic hip luxation but yields a 50% to 60% rate of recurrence. The rate of reluxation is reduced to approximately 10% to 20% when an open surgical technique is used.[5,8] Lameness sometimes persists after successful reduction of a hip luxation. Long-term radiographic changes of the hip joint include periosteal reactions of the ilium, subluxation of the femoral head, partial resorption of the femoral head and neck, periarticular osteophytes, and subchondral bone erosion.[8] Persistent lameness is present in 30% to 35% of dogs after successful reduction of recurrent or chronic luxation.[8,29]

No long-term studies have been completed on dysplastic dogs with coxofemoral luxation, but clinical experience indicates that the rate of reluxation after closed or open reduction is very high. Unless an animal has a very mild dysplastic condition, a salvage procedure such as femoral head and neck excision or total hip replacement should be used to treat coxofemoral luxation when dysplasia is present.[11]

Closed-reduction technique. Closed reduction is the initial treatment of choice for acute uncomplicated hip luxation in the dog or cat.[5,8,11] It may be easily accomplished in the first 10 to 14 days after the traumatic incident. However, the sooner the hip is reduced, the better. As long as the hip is dislocated, damage to the joint capsule and dorsal acetabular rim from femoral head motion continues. If subsequent surgical reduction is required, having attempted closed reduction does not increase the subsequent rate of reluxation.[8] As hip luxation becomes more chronic, numerous changes may make closed reduction unlikely to succeed. Maceration of the joint capsule, fibrous scar tissue growth into the joint cavity, hypertrophy of the round ligament, and contracture of gluteal musculature can make closed reduction impossible to achieve or maintain.

Closed reduction is completed under general anesthesia with the animal positioned in lateral recumbency and the affected limb up. A length of doubled-over gauze is placed between the legs and used by an assistant to pull in a dorsal direction. The stifle is grasped and rotated externally to free the femoral head from the ilial wing. Substantial force is now used, counteracted by the assistant pulling dorsally, to exert traction on the limb in a distal direction. While traction continues, the stifle is rotated internally, and digital pressure is applied to the greater trochanter to push the femoral head toward the acetabulum. Several attempts may be required before the femoral head is felt to "pop" into the joint. With the stifle held in an adducted position, the hip joint is flexed and extended vigorously to displace soft tissue and debris from the joint. Slight lateral pressure (Bardens maneuver) may be applied to assess the luxation's stability.[15] If gross instability is present, closed reduction is not likely to be successful, and internal repair may be considered. After closed reduction, an Ehmer sling is used to prevent weight bearing and to hold the joint in a slightly internally rotated position (Fig. 16-21). The sling is maintained for 14 days and exercise carefully restricted for another 6 weeks.

Open reduction for craniodorsal luxation. Surgical repair of a luxated coxofemoral joint is indicated when conservative treatment fails to maintain reduction or when preexisting conditions make closed treatment less likely to succeed. Open reduction is advised if bilateral coxofemoral luxations are present or if multiple orthopedic injuries mandate earlier weight bearing on the affected limb. If a dog has a severe fracture in one hind limb and a hip luxation in the other, open reduction of the coxofemoral luxation ensures earlier use of both limbs and a stronger coxofemoral repair. If acetabular fracture is associated with the coxofemoral luxation,

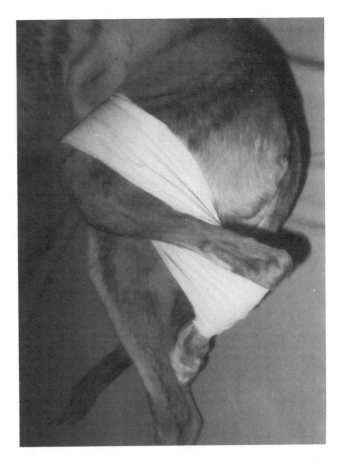

Fig. 16-21 Ehmer slings help maintain stability of the hip joint after reduction of craniodorsal luxation.

surgical reduction and fixation of the fracture precede open treatment of the luxation. If an avulsion fracture of the femoral head is present, large bone fragments must be either surgically removed or stabilized before the luxation is repaired.

Numerous techniques have been described for open reduction of hip luxation and include capsulorrhaphy,[5,8,9] transarticular pinning,[6] ischial-ilial pinning,[19] translocation of the greater trochanter,[17] toggle techniques,[11,31] and the prosthetic joint capsule technique.[29] The capsulorrhaphy, prosthetic capsule, and toggle techniques are described in this section. They are chosen for proven effectiveness and minimal disruption to existing joint structures. Each technique may be useful under different circumstances.

Capsulorrhaphy technique. Surgical reduction of the coxofemoral joint and closure of the joint capsule with interrupted sutures are described as the capsulorrhaphy technique (Fig. 16-22).[5,8,9] This technique provides strong closure and maintenance of hip reduction. It is the procedure of choice for open reduction of hip dislocation, as long as sufficient quantity and quality of joint capsule remain for closure. If the joint capsule has

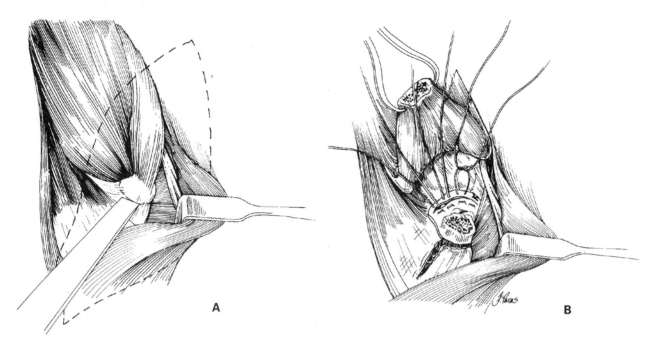

Fig. 16-22 Open reduction and repair of the joint capsule is indicated for recurrent coxofemoral luxation. **A,** Trochanter osteotomy may be performed to enhance visibility of the joint capsule tear but is not always needed. **B,** Primary closure of the joint capsule gives adequate strength to maintain reduction of coxofemoral luxation.

been macerated because of longstanding luxation, a prosthetic capsule or toggle technique is chosen.

A dorsal approach to the coxofemoral joint with osteotomy of the greater trochanter provides ample exposure for capsulorrhaphy.[39] This can also be completed through a craniolateral approach, but the exposure is more limited. Care is taken to preserve the joint capsule as the deep gluteal muscle is elevated from the joint's dorsal aspect. Rough tissue handling further damages the joint capsule and so weakens the closure. When the joint is exposed, the acetabulum and femoral head are carefully inspected. Blood clots and fibrin debris are removed from the joint. The swollen remnants of the round ligament are excised from the femoral head and acetabulum. Avulsion fragments from the femoral head, if present, are found attached to the ligament of the head of the femur deep in the medial aspect of acetabulum and are removed.

If the luxation is chronic, sharp dissection may be required to excise fibrous tissue from the joint. When the joint is clear of obstructions, the femoral head is reduced. A bone-holding forceps is applied at the base of the greater trochanter to use for manipulation of the femur during reduction. The joint capsule is now carefully inspected to reveal the location and extent of the tear and whether tissue loss has occurred. If the capsule cannot be closed without tension, a prosthetic capsule or toggle technique should be used to strengthen the repair. If the joint capsule is easily apposed, simple interrupted or horizontal mattress sutures are preplaced in

the capsule. Three to five sutures are usually sufficient for closure. After all sutures are preplaced, they are tied. The joint is stressed in dorsal and lateral directions to examine the suture line for gaps or weakness. If no gaps are present, the remaining closure is routine.

Prosthetic capsule technique. This technique is used to stabilize hip luxation when insufficient joint capsule is present for primary closure.[10,29] This method uses heavy nonabsorbable suture material to replace the function of the absent joint capsule (Fig. 16-23). The

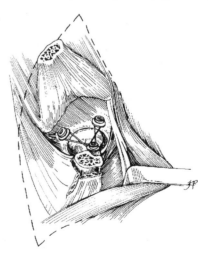

Fig. 16-23 Prosthetic capsule constructed of screws, washers, and heavy suture may be used to stabilize coxofemoral reduction if the joint capsule is badly damaged and cannot be sutured.

suture is woven between screws placed in the acetabular rim and the proximal femur. Although the suture material is expected eventually to fatigue and fail, the absent capsule is replaced with fibrous scar tissue and new synovium after sufficient time elapses.

A dorsal approach with osteotomy of the greater trochanter provides adequate exposure to the hip joint.[39] The deep gluteal muscle is elevated by subperiosteal dissection to expose the complete dorsal aspect of the acetabulum. Joint debris and bone fragments are removed as described in the capsulorrhaphy technique. The joint is reduced and the joint capsule inspected. Interrupted sutures are placed in the joint capsule to close as much of the capsule as possible without excessive tension on the sutures. Selection of screw size is based on the animal's size. Cortical screws (2.7 or 3.5 mm)* are generally selected for the acetabular rim and a cancellous screw (4.0 or 6.5 mm)* for the intertrochanteric space. Two bone screws with washers are placed in the acetabular rim, dorsal and cranial to the joint, separated approximately by the width of the femoral head. A third screw and washer are placed into the intertrochanteric fossa of the femur. All the screws are left sufficiently loose to allow placement of suture beneath the washers. Heavy nonabsorbable suture material is placed in figure-eight fashion from each of the acetabular screws to the femoral screw. Suture size, depending on the dog's size, may range from 2-0 to no. 8. As the sutures are tightened, the hip is held in a slightly abducted position. After the sutures are tied, the screws are tightened. The hip joint is tested for stability and adequate range of motion. The remaining tissue closure is routine.

Toggle pin technique. Toggle pin fixation (Fig. 16-24) of a luxated hip has similar indications as the prosthetic capsule technique but replaces the ligament of the femoral head, rather than the joint capsule, with heavy suture.[11,31] The suture used to replace the ligament is expected to fatigue and eventually fail, as with the prosthetic capsule sutures. However, the joint capsule is expected to reform with scar tissue and heal with sufficient strength to maintain reduction before the sutures fail.

A dorsal approach with osteotomy of the greater trochanter is completed to expose the acetabulum.[39] This technique can also be completed through a caudal approach to the hip. A hole is drilled through the femoral head and neck, beginning at the fovea capitis and following the angle of the neck toward the femoral shaft. The hole exits the lateral surface of the femur distal to the trochanters. The joint is reduced and maintained in approximation of a standing position. The drill is introduced into the femoral hole from the lateral side, and a hole is drilled through the acetabulum. Two heavy

*Synthes, Ltd., 983 Old Eagle School Rd., Wayne, PA 19087.

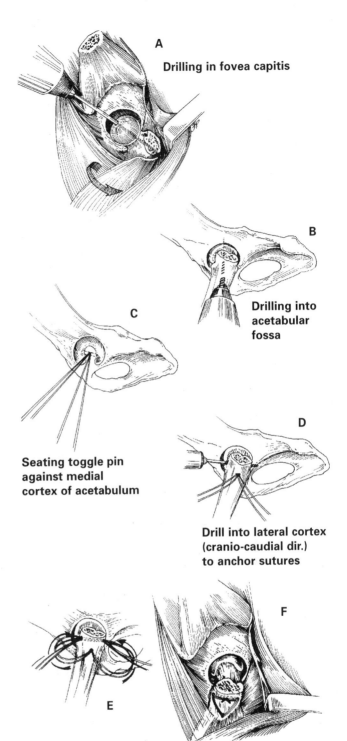

A Drilling in fovea capitis

B Drilling into acetabular fossa

C Seating toggle pin against medial cortex of acetabulum

D Drill into lateral cortex (cranio-caudal dir.) to anchor sutures

E

F

Fig. 16-24 Toggle suture technique may be used for added stability in coxofemoral luxation if the joint capsule cannot be sutured. **A,** Hole is drilled through the femoral head and neck, exiting the trochanter's lateral surface. **B,** Corresponding hole is drilled through the medial wall of the acetabulum. **C,** Toggle, with doubled heavy suture attached, is placed through the hole in the acetabulum. **D,** Suture is threaded through the femoral hole, and a second hole is drilled in the trochanter in a craniocaudal direction. **E** and **F,** Suture is threaded through the second femoral hole and tied on the lateral surface of the femoral trochanter.

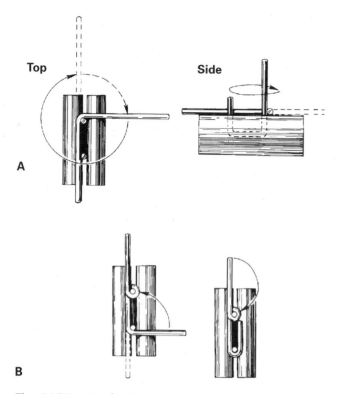

Top   **Side**

A

B

Fig. 16-25. Toggle pins may be constructed with simple tools and stiff wire.[11] **A,** Vise is used to firmly grasp a bent pin, which is used to provide proper length and pivot for bending the toggle. A central "eye" is constructed first. **B,** Ends of the toggle are bent back to the central eye.

nonabsorbable sutures are passed through a toggle pin (Fig. 16-25). The joint is dislocated, and with the femoral head held somewhat caudal and ventral, the toggle pin with the sutures is passed into the acetabular hole to the medial aspect of the pelvis. The toggle pin is rotated by 90 degrees and secured to the joint by pulling on the sutures. A fine wire loop is passed from lateral to medial in the femoral hole and used to retrieve the toggle sutures through the femoral hole. The joint is reduced, and the toggle sutures are pulled taught. An additional hole is drilled in the femur, from cranial to caudal, above the exit hole of the toggle sutures.[11] The toggle suture strands are divided and are passed in opposite directions through this hole and tied on the lateral surface of the femur.[11] Interrupted sutures are placed in the joint capsule to close as much of the capsule as possible without excessive tension on the sutures. The joint is checked for laxity, and the remaining tissue closure is routine.

Aftercare for open reduction. The limb is placed in an Ehmer sling before anesthetic recovery. The sling is maintained for 10 to 14 days. Care is taken to observe the limb daily for abrasion and vascular compromise caused by the sling. The animal's activity is restricted to

short leash walks for 6 to 8 weeks after surgery to allow the soft tissues of the hip joint to heal before being subjected to excessive stress. Dogs with bilateral luxation are not placed in a sling, but cage rest is enforced for 14 days, followed by 6 to 8 weeks of restricted activity.

Salvage techniques for hip luxation. Femoral head and neck excision or total hip replacement may be used to salvage limb function in patients with hip dislocation that no longer have hope of normal function. Recurrent luxation, preexisting hip dysplasia, aseptic necrosis of the femoral neck, or severe trauma to femoral head and acetabulum are indications for performing a salvage procedure. (See Chapter 17 for descriptions of these techniques.)

Treatment of caudoventral dislocation

Closed reduction. Under general anesthesia the animal is placed in lateral recumbency with the affected side up. The limb is grasped at the stifle and abducted to free the femoral head from the obturator foramen. The limb is externally rotated and pushed in a dorsal direction, and simultaneous digital pressure is applied to force the proximal femur in a cranial direction. The limb is then internally rotated to reduce the luxation.

Surgical reduction of caudoventral luxation. Surgical reduction of caudoventral coxofemoral luxation is used when closed reduction and conservative care are ineffective at maintaining reduction. A craniolateral approach to the hip joint is used to expose the acetabulum.[39] Care is taken to preserve the sciatic nerve, which is encroached on by the caudal displacement of the femur. The joint capsule is usually not torn dorsally but may be opened to remove debris from the joint. A bone-holding forceps is placed on the proximal femur. The stifle is abducted to free the femoral head from the obturator foramen. The joint is externally rotated, and the forceps is used to force the femoral head in a dorsal and cranial direction. The hip is then internally rotated to complete the reduction. When reduced, the hip is tested for stability. Any visible tears or incisions into the capsule are sutured. If gross instability of the joint is present, a screw or washer is placed in the cranial acetabular rim and another placed at the junction of the femoral neck and the femur on the cranial surface. A heavy nonabsorbable suture is placed between the two screws in figure-eight fashion beneath the washers, and the screws are tightened (Fig. 16-26). This extracapsular suture prevents caudal displacement of the femoral head, but not ventral displacement. The remaining closure is routine.

Aftercare for caudoventral luxation. Whether closed reduction or surgical management of caudoventral luxation is used, stifle hobbles are constructed before anesthetic recovery (Fig. 16-27). Stifle hobbles prevent abduction of the limb at the level of the stifle joint and prevent ventral displacement of the femoral head as long

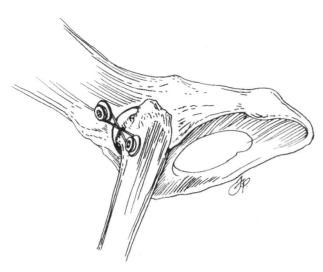

Fig. 16-26 Extracapsular screws, washers, and figure-eight suture placed craniocaudally help prevent caudal displacement after reduction of chronic caudoventral luxation. Stifle hobbles must also be used with this fixation.

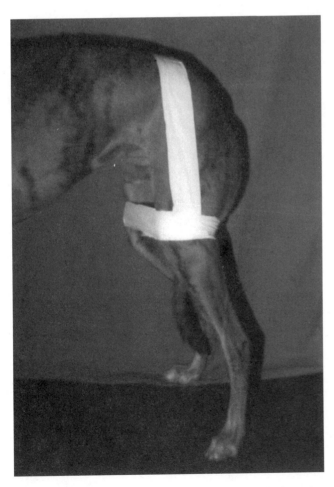

Fig. 16-27 Stifle hobbles prevent abduction of the hip joint and help maintain stability after reduction of caudoventral hip luxation.

as the ventral labrum of the acetabulum is intact. Tarsal hobbles do not prevent stifle abduction and thus are ineffective for this injury. Stifle hobbles are maintained for 2 to 3 weeks, and exercise is limited to short leash walks for 6 to 8 weeks after repair.

Dislocation of the Stifle

Although isolated cruciate ligament ruptures of the stifle constitute one of the most common orthopedic conditions seen in dogs, stifle dislocation with multiple ligament injury and articular displacement is quite rare (Fig. 16-28). Some authors report that complete traumatic stifle dislocation occurs more frequently in the cat than the dog, but actual numbers of cases are so low that literature reports are inconsistent.[2,11,37]

Anatomy of dislocation. Numerous ligaments are injured in stifle dislocation and may result in subluxation or complete luxation of the stifle joint. The most frequent combination of ligament injuries is rupture of both cruciate and medial collateral ligaments.[2] Other combinations may include both cruciate and both collateral ligaments, individual cranial or caudal cruciate ligaments and the medial collateral ligament, both cruciate and lateral collateral ligaments, and both cruciate ligaments with no collateral ligament injury. Infrequently,

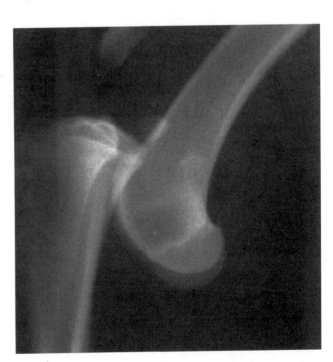

Fig. 16-28 Lateral radiograph indicating luxation of the stifle. Displacement of the femur and tibia on radiographs usually indicates severe damage to the cruciate and collateral ligaments, menisci, and joint capsule.

the long digital extensor tendon and the popliteal muscle or tendon may be torn with the associated ligament injures. The medial and lateral menisci are often ruptured in stifle dislocation or torn free of joint capsule attachment. Joint capsule injury is variable with stifle dislocation but may be quite severe with severe displacement. Vascular and nerve injuries, although common in humans with knee dislocations, have not been reported in animals.[2]

Clinical presentation and diagnosis. Dogs or cats with stifle dislocation have a history of trauma. They are non–weight bearing on the affected limb, and other soft tissue injuries or fractures may be present. Although the joint is generally swollen and painful, gentle palpation in the awake animal may reveal gross cranial and caudal drawer sign, indicating cruciate ligament insufficiency. The joint opens with palpation on the medial or lateral sides, indicating collateral ligament instability. With gross displacement, the joint may be extremely lax, or palpation may indicate the femoral condyles firmly lodged behind the tibial plateau. Radiographs taken with the animal under heavy sedation or general anesthesia are necessary to ensure that no fractures are present. Stress views are useful to assess individual ligaments. After the diagnosis is established, the limb should be stabilized in a reduced position with a Robert Jones bandage until surgical repair may be completed.

Treatment of stifle dislocation. Conservative care with closed reduction and stabilization with external coaptation has been reported in the dog.[34] The joint is reduced under general anesthesia and immobilized for 4 to 8 weeks in a lateral plaster spica or Schroeder-Thomas splint. This method is not recommended because results are quite variable.[34] More consistent functional results may be achieved with reduction and surgical stabilization of the ligament injuries. Clinical reports indicate that lameness is minimal on long-term evaluation after surgical repair of stifle dislocation.[2,28,37] Although functional results are gratifying, DJD and a loss of 10 to 40 degrees in range of motion develop after repair.[2,28] Caution should be exercised in giving a favorable prognosis. The extent of injury is highly variable, and a clinical course of an individual animal may not follow that of the few cases reported in the literature.

Surgical reconstruction. A medial stifle arthrotomy is performed.[39] The joint is thoroughly inspected for the extent of ligament and meniscus injury. Most stifle dislocations have sufficient ligament damage and displacement to allow direct access to the periphery of the meniscus without requiring further surgical exposure. If either meniscus is badly ruptured, a meniscectomy is performed. If the meniscus is intact but torn from its capsular attachments, it may be carefully sutured to the

capsule with a simple interrupted pattern using absorbable suture material. Any exposed tears in the joint capsule are sutured with simple interrupted or mattress sutures.

Collateral ligament injury. The collateral ligaments are repaired before cruciate ligament stabilization. Surgical exposure to the medial and/or lateral collateral ligament is performed through the same skin incision as for the arthrotomy.[39] The torn ligament is exposed and inspected for the site and extent of injury. If the ligament is torn in the midportion of its length, it may be sutured using nonabsorbable sutures in a locking loop or three-loop-pulley ligament suture pattern. Care must be taken to reduce the stifle joint to its proper position before tightening the sutures, or a loose ligament repair and subsequent displacement may result. The ligament repair is augmented by placing a screw and washer at the origin and insertion of the ligament. The screw size appropriate for most dogs is 2.7 or 3.5 mm.* Heavy, nonabsorbable suture or orthopedic wire is placed in a figure-eight pattern around the screws and washers and over the ligament repair. After the suture is placed, the screws are tightened (Fig. 16-29). Joint reduction and the range of motion of the stifle joint are examined after each stage of repair to ensure adequate placement of the figure-eight suture. If the screws are not properly positioned, or if the figure-eight suture (especially wire) is placed too tightly, the range of motion is adversely affected. (For further details of collateral ligament repair, see Chapters 18 and 22.)

Cruciate ligament injury. Cruciate ligament stabilization is completed after repair of the collateral ligaments. Since both cruciate ligaments are usually ruptured with dislocation of the stifle, a combined cranial and caudal cruciate stabilization must be performed (Fig. 16-29). Extracapsular stabilization of combined cruciate injury is recommended.[2,11] For cranial cruciate stabilization, a heavy, nonabsorbable suture is placed from each fabella to a small hole drilled into the proximal portion of the tibial tubercle. Caudal cruciate stabilization is completed with sutures placed from holes drilled in both the proximal fibular head laterally and the caudomedial aspect of the tibial plateau, to the proximal aspect of the patellar ligament. All cruciate stabilization sutures are preplaced in the procedure after appropriate reduction is achieved. As an assistant holds the stifle in reduction, the sutures are alternately tightened until stabilization is complete. Inappropriate tension on any single suture may displace the joint. With appropriate suture placement and tension, drawer movement is eliminated. (For further details of cruciate ligament stabilization techniques, see Chapter 18.)

---

*Synthes, Ltd., 983 Old Eagle School Rd., Wayne, PA 19087.

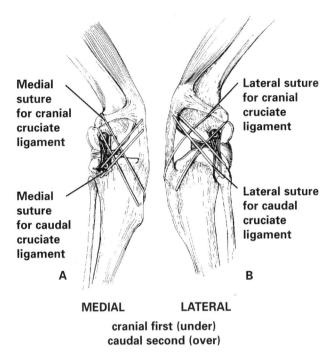

Medial suture for cranial cruciate ligament

Medial suture for caudal cruciate ligament

Lateral suture for cranial cruciate ligament

Lateral suture for caudal cruciate ligament

A   B

MEDIAL   LATERAL

cranial first (under)
caudal second (over)

Fig. 16-29 Stability is achieved in stifle luxation by repair of the collateral and cruciate ligaments. **A,** Medial view of stifle luxation repair. Collateral ligament repair strength has been augmented with screws, washers, and figure-eight suture or wire. Extracapsular cruciate repair has been used for cranial and caudal cruciate ligament rupture. **B,** Lateral view of stifle luxation repair. Collateral ligament repair strength has been augmented with figure-eight suture or wire technique, using one screw and washer and fibular head as anchor points.

Aftercare for stifle dislocation. Small dogs and cats are placed in a light Robert Jones bandage after surgery. A Robert Jones bandage is also used for larger dogs, but is reinforced at the stifle with one or two rolls of fiberglass cast material. Care should be taken to hold the stifle and hock joints in a standing position while the bandage is placed. The bandage is maintained for 3 weeks after surgery. If excessive looseness develops, it should be changed. Exercise is limited to short leash walks for 3 months after surgical repair. If the range of motion of the stifle joint is compromised, passive flexion and extension exercises and swimming may be used as physical therapy.

Salvage technique for stifle dislocation. When stifle dislocation is chronic, severe DJD is usually present. Ligament reconstruction is not likely to yield a functional pain-free gait. If DJD is too severe to allow reconstruction of the dislocation, a stifle arthrodesis may be performed to salvage use of the limb. Stifle arthrodesis yields a non-painful and useful limb, but the animal's gait remains abnormal. (For details of stifle arthrodesis, see Chapter 23.)

Dislocation of the Tarsus

Tarsal dislocation is a common traumatic injury in dogs and cats and highly variable because of the complex nature of tarsal anatomy. Only the most common injuries are discussed in this section. In athletic and older obese dogs, tarsal injuries may be caused by relatively mild trauma that overstresses the joints rather than by external traumatic forces.[11] Running and jumping movements are sufficient trauma to cause subluxation or complete dislocation at various levels of the tarsus. Severe trauma may result in dislocation and shear injuries of the tarsus. A shear injury develops when the animal's limb is dragged along the abrasive surface of a road by an automobile or becomes trapped between the vehicle and the road surface as the brakes are applied. Shear wounds with tarsal dislocation are complicated by severe loss of bone and ligament tissue, as well as superficial structures.

Traumatic injury is the most common cause of tarsal dislocation, but luxation may also develop secondary to degenerative or immunological processes of the joints, such as rheumatoid arthritis.[36] When tarsal dislocation is secondary to an immunological condition, other joints must be fully assessed before a long-term treatment plan is undertaken.

Tarsal anatomy. The canine tarsus is composed of seven bones between the tibia and metatarsus. The tibiotarsal bone (talus) articulates with the tibia to form the tarsocrural joint. The tarsocrural joint provides most of the motion in the tarsal joint. The tibiotarsal bone is paired with the fibulotarsal bone (calcaneus). Although lacking direct articulation with the tibia, the fibulotarsal bone has a large calcaneal tuber, which serves to direct the major flexor tendons across the tarsus to the lower limb. The five more tarsal bones include the central tarsal bone and the four numbered tarsal bones (1 to 4). These bones articulate with each other and the tibia and fibulotarsal bones to form the proximal and distal intertarsal joints. Little motion occurs at normal intertarsal joints, but serious disability develops if these joints are injured. The numbered tarsal bones (1 to 4) articulate distally with the metatarsal bones to form the tarsometatarsal joints. The tarsometatarsal joints also have very limited motion in the normal tarsus but may cause serious disability if injured.

The ligamentous support of the tarsus may be functionally divided into three groups of ligaments: the collateral, intertarsal, and plantar (Fig. 16-30).

The collateral ligaments provide the medial and lateral support to the tarsocrural joint. The medial and lateral collateral ligaments work synchronously with the joint capsule and the malleoli of the distal tibia to stabilize and define the motion of the tarsocrural joint.[3] The medial

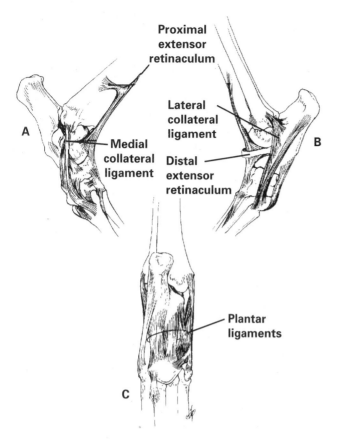

Fig. 16-30 Collateral and plantar ligaments and the joint capsule are the primary restraints of the tarsus. **A,** Medial view of the tarsus. **B,** Lateral view of the tarsus. **C,** Plantar view of the tarsus.

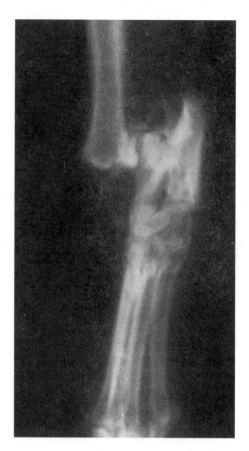

Fig. 16-31 Radiograph indicating tarsal luxation. Malleolar fractures frequently occur with tarsal luxation in the dog.

and lateral collateral ligaments are divided into long and short components. The long components stabilize the joint in extension, and the short components stabilize the joint in flexion and extension.[3] Luxation of the tarsocrural joint does not develop with injury to the collateral ligaments unless the joint capsule or malleoli is also affected.[3]

The intertarsal ligaments are multiple short ligaments that provide stability between the seven individual tarsal bones. The intertarsal ligaments restrict motion at the proximal and distal intertarsal joints. When ruptured, subluxation or dislocation of the intertarsal joints may develop and cause serious disability.

The plantar ligaments and the tarsal fibrocartilage provide major support to the caudal (or plantar) surface of the tarsus. The plantar ligaments are multiple stout ligaments that connect the tibial and fibular tarsal bones to the remaining tarsal bones and metatarsus. They prevent hyperextension of the intertarsal joints during weight bearing and are critical to normal function. If the plantar ligaments and tarsal fibrocartilage are ruptured, the intertarsal joints subluxate in hyperextension, causing the animal to walk plantigrade on the caudal aspect of the metatarsus and foot.

Clinical presentation and diagnosis. A dog or cat with dislocation of the tarsus has a history or physical evidence of major trauma. The physical examination findings vary greatly with the injury's extent. Lameness is always evident, but the animal may or may not bear some weight on the limb. When mild ligament damage is present, the tarsus is swollen, but only careful palpation demonstrates specific joint instability. When severe injury is present, gross instability of the tarsal joints is palpated, and valgus or varus angulation of the foot is present. The tarsus may be externally or internally rotated by up to 90 degrees.

Fractures of the tarsus and malleoli of the tibia or fibula are common with dislocation of the tarsus. Lateral and craniocaudal radiographs demonstrate most tarsal pathology. Oblique radiographic views may be needed to demonstrate subtle tarsal fractures. Stress views are needed to demonstrate joint laxity caused by ligament injury with mild displacement.

Tarsocrural dislocation. Fractures of the malleoli of the distal tibia and fibula frequently accompany traumatic dislocation of the tarsocrural joint (Fig. 16-31). Rupture of the collateral ligaments does not result in dislocation of the tarsocrural joint unless the joint capsule or malleoli are also injured.[3] If fractures are present, they must be repaired to achieve stability of the tarsocrural joint. (For treatment of fractures of the tarsus, see Chapter 9.) If the collateral ligaments and joint capsule are badly injured in tarsal dislocation, they must be surgically repaired to achieve joint stability.

Closed reduction. Joint instability may be relatively minor if ligament damage is partial (i.e., mild sprain) or if the ligament injury is localized to either the long or the short components of the collateral ligaments. When minor instability is present, external coaptation with a splint or cast may be applied and maintained for 6 weeks. A soft, padded bandage may be used for 2 to 4 more weeks after splint removal as additional support. Severe instability or complete dislocation of the tarsocrural joint indicates severe ligament, bone, and capsular injury. Although closed-reduction techniques with external coaptation are described for complete dislocation, surgical stabilization provides more consistent results.[1,11,21,27]

Surgical stabilization. The animal is placed under general anesthesia, and the dislocation is reduced. The joint is palpated for medial and lateral laxity. If it is determined that both medial and lateral collateral ligaments are injured, a separate surgical approach is made to each side of the joint.[39] The collateral ligaments and joint capsule are carefully inspected. Joint capsule tears are sutured with simple interrupted or horizontal mattress sutures. If a long component of the collateral ligament is ruptured, its ends may be apposed with nonabsorbable suture in a locking loop or three-loop-pulley ligament suture pattern. (For details of ligament sutures, see Chapter 22.) Short components of the collateral ligaments are also frequently ruptured but cannot be directly sutured because of insufficient length. In cats and small dogs, joint capsule and ligament repair are usually sufficiently stable to allow healing if external coaptation is applied after surgery. In larger dogs or when ligament reconstruction is not possible, prosthetic ligaments may be constructed for additional stability.[4] Prosthetic ligaments are constructed with screws, washers, and nonabsorbable suture or orthopedic wire (Fig. 16-32). The purpose of a prosthetic ligament technique is to provide stability and adequate range of motion to a joint, until fibrous scar tissue of the joint capsule and ligament are of sufficient strength to prevent reluxation.

Medial prosthetic ligaments. The medial collateral ligaments and the joint capsule are inspected and repaired as previously described. Screw size for the prosthetic technique is based on the dog's size. Cancellous screws (4.0 mm)* are selected for most dogs and are advantageous because they lack screw threads near the head of the screw, which could cut suture material.

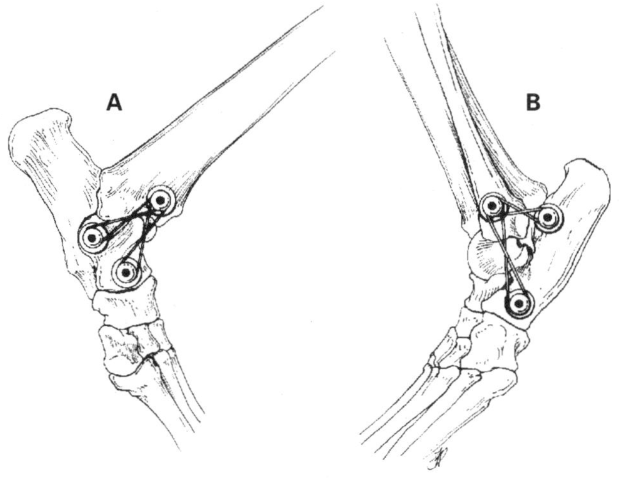

Fig. 16-32 Screws, washers, and figure-eight suture or wire may be used to augment collateral ligament repair strength in tarsal luxation. Short and long components of the ligaments are reconstructed on medial (**A**) and lateral (**B**) sides.

Smaller cortical screws may be selected for smaller patients. Three screws and washers are placed in the tarsus. The proximal screw is placed into the medial malleolus of the tibia just proximal to the concave articular surface. A second screw and washer are placed through the center of the body of the talus.[4] A suture from the tibial screw to the proximal talus screw mimics the short collateral components. A third screw is placed in the head of the talus.[4] A suture from the distal talus screw to the tibial screw mimics the long collateral ligament component. Washers are placed on each screw to prevent slippage of the sutures. A heavy, nonabsorbable suture is placed in a figure-eight pattern from the tibial screw to each of the other screws. The screws are tightened after suture placement (Fig. 16-32). The joint is tested for stability and adequate range of motion. The remaining surgical closure is routine.

Lateral prosthetic ligaments. Lateral prosthetic ligaments are constructed similar to medial ligaments, except that the anatomy of screw placement differs. The proximal screw is placed in the fibular malleolus, proximal to the articular surface. The two distal screws are placed in the coracoid process and the base of the calcaneus to mimic the short and long components of the lateral collateral ligaments[11] (Fig. 16-32).

Shear injuries of tarsus. Shear injuries of the tarsus sometimes result in dislocation of the tarsocrural joint, with severe tissue loss on the joint's medial or lateral surface. Complete loss of the medial or lateral collateral ligaments may occur in a shear injury. Meticulous wound care should include debridement, lavage, and proper bandage technique to control local inflammation and infection. Prosthetic ligament replacement is used for reconstruction of the collateral ligaments; however,

---

*Synthes, Ltd., 983 Old Eagle School Rd, Wayne, PA 19087.

orthopedic wire (18 to 22 gauge) is used rather than a braided, nonabsorbable suture. Braided suture may become chronically infected if placed in a surgical site contaminated with bacteria, such as a shearing wound.[4,11] Infection at a prosthetic suture site may contribute to joint sepsis and thus should be avoided. Although orthopedic wire is not as flexible as suture material, it is much less likely to serve as a nidus for local infection.

Aftercare of tarsocrural dislocation. External coaptation, with a well-padded splint or bivalved cast, is maintained for 6 weeks after repair. The splint is changed, as appropriate, for local wound care. Radiographs are taken at 6 weeks after repair and again after several more months. Screws may loosen or, if orthopedic wire is used, the wire may eventually break. The orthopedic hardware may be removed after stabilization of the joint with fibrosis is complete.

Proximal Intertarsal Subluxation or Dislocation

Hyperextension of the tarsus at the distal aspect of the tibial and fibular tarsal bones results in rupture of the plantar ligaments and subluxation or dislocation of the proximal intertarsal joint (Fig. 16-33). The Shetland sheepdog and collie are predisposed to this injury; however, all dog breeds may be affected.[11,14] Trauma frequently causes this injury, but proximal intertarsal luxation may also be seen in older obese dogs without sign of trauma or in animals with immunological joint conditions. The plantar lig-

ament is usually torn or avulsed between the calcaneus and the fourth tarsal bone, resulting in the animal walking in a partial or complete plantigrade stance.[11] Radiographic evaluation with plain and stress views is diagnostic.

Treatment of proximal intertarsal dislocation with external coaptation is not effective. Healing of the plantar ligaments with scar tissue does not provide sufficient strength for weight bearing. Arthrodesis is the treatment of choice for proximal intertarsal subluxation or dislocation. Arthrodesis is accomplished by removing the articular cartilage from the joint and using an autogenous cancellous graft to stimulate bone healing. Fixation with pins and figure-eight wire or with a bone plate along the lateral surface of the tarsus provides stability during healing. (For details of proximal intertarsal arthrodesis, see Chapter 23.)

Tarsometatarsal Subluxation or Dislocation

Hyperextension of the tarsometatarsal joints is a frequent traumatic injury in dogs (Fig. 16-34). The distal

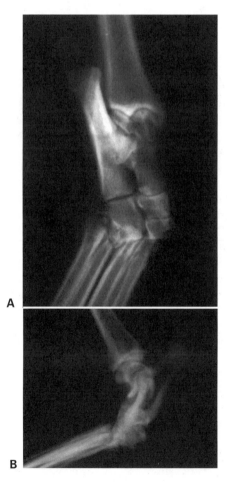

Fig. 16-34 **A** and **B,** Craniocaudal and lateral radiographs illustrate tarsometatarsal joint luxation. Note the plantigrade stance on the lateral radiograph.

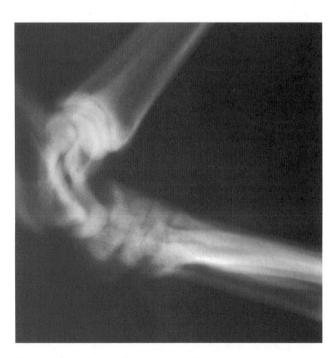

Fig. 16-33 Proximal intertarsal dislocations are frequently seen in Shetland sheepdogs and collies.

portion of the plantar ligaments, plantar fibrocartilage, and joint capsule of the tarsometatarsal joints are injured. Fractures of the distal tarsal or metatarsal bones also frequently accompany this injury. These dogs may or may not have extreme pain in the affected limb. As the animal bears weight on the limb, it may walk in a plantigrade stance. Radiographic evaluation with plain and stress views is diagnostic.

As with dislocation of the proximal intertarsal joint, external coaptation is not effective as treatment for tarsometatarsal luxation. Arthrodesis is the treatment of choice and may be accomplished by removing the articular cartilage of the joints and using an autogenous cancellous bone graft to stimulate bone healing. Fixation with pins and figure-eight wire or with a bone plate provides stability during healing. (For details of tarsometatarsal arthrodesis, see Chapter 23.)

REFERENCES

1. Aron DN: Prosthetic ligament replacement for severe tarsocrural joint instability, *J Am Anim Hosp Assoc* 23:41-55, 1987.
2. Aron DN: Traumatic dislocation of the stifle joint: treatment of 12 dogs and one cat, *J Am Anim Hosp Assoc* 24:333-340, 1988.
3. Aron DN, Purinton PT: Collateral ligaments of the tarsocrural joint: an anatomical and functional study, *Vet Surg* 14:173-177, 1985.
4. Aron DN, Purinton PT: Replacement of the collateral ligaments of the canine tarsocrural joint: a proposed technique, *Vet Surg* 14:178-184, 1985.
5. Basher WP, Walter MC, Newton CD: Coxofemoral luxation in the dog and cat, *Vet Surg* 15:356-362, 1986.
6. Bennett D, Duff SR: Transarticular pinning as a treatment for hip luxation in the dog and cat, *J Small Anim Pract* 21:373-379, 1980.
7. Bingel SA, Riser WH: Congenital elbow luxation in the dog, *J Small Anim Pract* 18:445-456, 1977.
8. Bone DL, Walker M, Cantwell HD: Traumatic coxofemoral luxation in dogs: results of repair, *Vet Surg* 13:263-270, 1984.
9. Bottareli A: *Clin Vet* 61:407, 1938.
10. Braden TD, Johnson ME: Technique and indications of a prosthetic capsule for repair of recurrent and chronic coxofemoral luxations, *Vet Comp Orth Traum* 1:26-29, 1988.
11. Brinker WO, Piermattei DL, Flo GL: *Handbook of small animal orthopedics and fracture treatment*, Philadelphia, 1983, Saunders.
12. Campbell JR: Shoulder lameness in the dog, *J Small Anim Pract* 9:189-198, 1968.
13. Campbell JR: Nonfracture injuries to the canine elbow, *J Am Vet Med Assoc* 155:735-744, 1969.
14. Campbell JR, Bennett D, Lee R: Intertarsal and tarso-metatarsal subluxation in the dog, *J Small Anim Pract* 17:427, 1976.
15. Chalman JA, Butler HC: Coxofemoral joint laxity and the Ortlani sign, *J Am Anim Hosp Assoc* 21:671-676, 1985.
16. Craig E, Hohn RB, Anderson WD: Surgical stabilization of traumatic medial shoulder dislocation, *J Am Anim Hosp Assoc* 16:93-102, 1980.
17. DeAngelis M, Prata R: Surgical repair of coxofemoral luxation in the dog, *J Am Anim Hosp Assoc* 9:175-182, 1973.
18. DeAngelis M, Schwartz A: Surgical correction of cranial dislocation of the scapulohumeral joint in a dog, *J Am Vet Med Assoc* 156:435-438, 1970.
19. DeVita J: A method of pinning for chronic dislocation of the hip joint. In *Proceedings of the 89th Annual Meeting of the American Veterinary Association*, 1952.
20. Early T: Canine carpal ligament injuries, *Vet Clin North Am* 8:183-199, 1978.
21. Early TD, Dee JF: Trauma to the carpus, tarsus, and phalanges of dogs and cats, *Vet Clin North Am* 10:717-747, 1980.
22. Flo GL, DeCamp CE: Surgical correction of congenital radial luxations. In *Proceedings of the 17th Annual Conference of the Veterinary Orthopedic Society*, Jackson hole, Wyo., 1990.
23. Fox SM, Bloomberg MS, Bright RM: Developmental anomalies of the canine elbow, *J Am Anim Hosp Assoc* 19:605-615, 1983.
24. Gurevitch R, Hohn R: Surgical management of lateral luxation and subluxation of the canine radial head, *Vet Surg* 9:49-57, 1980.
25. Hayes HM, and others: Epidemiologic observations of canine elbow disease (emphasis on dysplagia), *J Am Anim Hosp Assoc* 15:449-453, 1979.
26. Hohn RB, and others: Surgical stabilization of recurrent shoulder luxation, *Vet Clin North Am* 1:537-548, 1971.
27. Holt PE: Ligamentous injuries to the canine hock, *J Small Anim Pract* 15:457-474, 1974.
28. Hulse DA, Shires P: Multiple ligament injury of the stifle joint in the dog, *J Am Anim Hosp Assoc* 22:105-110, 1986.
29. Johnson ME, Braden TD: A retrospective study of prosthetic capsule technique for treatment of problem cases of dislocated hips, *Vet Surg* 16:346-351, 1987.
30. Kene ROC, Lee R, Bennett D: The radiographic features of congenital elbow luxation/subluxation in the dog, *J Small Anim Pract* 23:621-630, 1982.
31. Knowles AT, Knowles JO, Knowles RP: An operation to preserve the continuity of the hip joint, *J Am Vet Med Assoc* 123:508-515, 1953.
32. Milton JL, Montgomery RD: Congenital elbow dislocations, *Vet Clin North Am* 17:873-888, 1987.
33. Milton JL and others: Congenital elbow luxation in the dog, *J Am Vet Med Assoc* 175:572-581, 1979.
34. Newton CD, Nunamaker DM: *Textbook of small animal orthopaedics*, Philadelphia, 1985, Lippincott.
35. Noyes FR, and others: Biomechanics of anterior cruciate ligament failure: an analysis of strain-rate sensitivity and mechanisms of failure in primates, *J Bone Joint Surg (Am)* 56:236-253, 1974.
36. Pederson NC, and others: Noninfectious canine arthritis: rheumatoid arthritis, *J Am Vet Med Assoc* 169:295-302, 1976.
37. Phillips IR: Dislocation of the stifle joint in the cat, *J Small Anim Pract* 23:217-221, 1982.
38. Pick JR, and others: Subluxation of the carpus in dogs, an X chromosomal defect closely linked with the locus for hemophilia A, *Lab Invest* 17:243-248, 1967.
39. Piermattei DL, Greeley RG: *An atlas of surgical approaches to the bones of the dog and cat*, ed 2, Philadelphia, 1982, Saunders.
40. Stevens DR, Sande RD: An elbow dysplasia syndrome in the dog, *J Am Vet Med Assoc* 165:1065-1069, 1974.
41. Vasseur PB: Clinical results of surgical correction of shoulder luxation in dogs, *J Am Vet Med Assoc* 182:503-505, 1983.
42. Vasseur PB, Pool RR, Klein K: Effects of tendon transfer on the canine scapulohumeral joint, *Am J Vet Res* 44:811-815, 1983.
43. Vaughan LC, Jones DGC: Congenital dislocation of the shoulder joint in the dog, *J Small Anim Pract* 10:1-3, 1969.
44. Withrow SJ: Management of a congenital elbow luxation by temporary transarticular pinning, *Vet Med Small Anim Clin* 72:1597-1602, 1977.

17

Disabling Conditions of the Canine Coxofemoral Joint

LARRY J. WALLACE
MARVIN L. OLMSTEAD

The canine hip joint is subject to a wide variety of disorders with traumatic, congenital, inherited, neoplastic, infectious, or degenerative etiologies. This chapter covers Legg-Calvé-Perthes disease and canine hip dysplasia. The other disorders are covered elsewhere in this book.

361

LEGG-CALVÉ-PERTHES DISEASE

In 1910, Legg, Calvé, and Perthes independently described a disease condition of the hip joint in children that since then has been known as Legg-Calvé-Perthes disease (LCPD).[41] The disease in young children was characterized radiographically by flattening of the femoral head (coxa plana). Of the three authors, only Legg believed that the condition was caused by an impairment of the blood supply to the femoral head, which is still the most accepted pathogenesis of LCPD.[1,75] Perthes believed the condition was related in some way to a noninfective degenerative arthritis, while Calvé thought the condition was related to rickets.[22,122] Until 1910, ischemic necrosis of the superior femoral epiphysis was confused with other diseases of the hip joint, principally tuberculosis.[1] Although LCPD was named after the authors who first reported it, over the years it has also been referred to by various names related to the femoral head, including aseptic necrosis, epiphyseal aseptic necrosis, avascular necrosis, osteonecrosis, ischemic necrosis, coxa plana, osteochondrosis, and osteochondritis deformans juvenilis. Regardless of the name, the disease is characterized by necrosis of the femoral head.

The disease condition that affects the femoral head of young, predominantly small breeds of dogs was first described by Schnelle in 1937.[151] Schnelle reported 12 cases, all in wire-haired fox terriers. It was concluded that no essential difference existed between coxa plana of children and that seen in dogs. From that time until present, the disease in dogs has been known as LCPD. In 1938, Moltzen-Nielsen described the disease in 19 young, small dogs that included breeds other than wire-haired fox terriers.[103]

In the canine, LCPD is an avascular necrosis of the femoral head predominantly seen in the toy, terrier, and other small breeds. The most frequently affected breeds include, but are not limited to, the wire-haired fox terrier, miniature pinscher, miniature poodle, Lakeland terrier, West Highland white terrier, cairn terrier, and toy poodle. Regardless of breed, it occurs most frequently in dogs weighing less than 12 kg (26½ pounds). In the canine, there is no sex predilection. This is in sharp contrast to what is reported in children: LCPD affects males more than females in a proportion of about 4:1.[1] In dogs, LCPD is generally unilateral, which is also true in children. In two different reports, one with 161[84] and the other with 118 patients,[8] the right and left femoral heads were equally involved. Bilateral hip involvement was only seen in 12% of patients in one report[84] and 16.5% in the other report.[74] Similarly, in children, bilateral femoral head involvement only occurs in about 10% of patients.[1] The age range for LCPD in the dog is 3 to 13 months, with a peak incidence at about 7 months.

Pathogenesis

For years it has been a well-accepted fact that the pathological process in the femoral head is an avascular necrosis.[1,108] The exact etiology causing the avascular necrosis remains a subject of debate.

Normal Blood Supply

A brief review of the normal blood supply to the proximal femoral epiphysis is helpful to this discussion. The main blood supply to the femoral epiphysis comes from the lateral circumflex femoral artery, medial circumflex femoral artery, and a branch of the cranial and caudal gluteal arteries. All these vessels develop into a retinaculum that penetrates through various aspects of the joint capsule, supplying blood to the femoral head and neck.[110] These retinacular vessels form an arcade within the joint capsule and synovial membrane and send branches into the femoral epiphysis. The dorsal retinacular arteries supply about 70% of the blood to the epiphysis. The blood supply to the remaining 30% of the epiphysis comes from the ventral and, when present, the cranial retinacular arteries. The blood supply to the proximal femoral epiphysis has been described in mongrel puppies ranging in age from 1½ to 3 months.[11] The proximal femoral physeal blood supply is separate from the supply of the femoral neck in the growing dog with an open physis. Blood vessels from the femoral neck do not penetrate through the open physis. Once the physis closes, an anastomosis develops between the epiphyseal and metaphyseal arteries.

Pathology

Before the classical radiographic signs are observed in the femoral head, synovitis and synovial effusion are present in the affected hip joint.[1] Hip joint laxity would be the only radiographic sign present at this time. Initially, there is a loss of blood supply to the dorsal area of the proximal femoral epiphysis. The avascular incident leaves a region of subchondral bone without a blood supply, which becomes necrotic.

In the next phase, revascularization of the necrotic bone occurs, and deltas of new arterioles and capillaries bring in sufficient blood to demineralize partially the subchondral bone and weaken its supportive strength.[1] The bone collapses into the defect and becomes condensed because of stress or loading pressure on it. The characteristic radiographic change of lucent areas and a flattened femoral head are now apparent. The base of the defect reveals granulation tissue coming from the persisting mesenchymal cells and the new blood supply. Osteoclasts are seen removing the necrotic bone while new bone and cartilage are being laid down in an attempt to heal the defect.

The articular cartilage remains viable as it is nourished by the synovial fluid. However, when the subchondral bone collapses, the articular cartilage over the area also collapses into the defect and has a cracked appearance. Eventually, the debris of dead bone and cartilage is replaced by new bone or by densely organized collagenized fibrous tissue.[1] Once the subchondral bone of the femoral head collapses, the congruity between the femoral head and acetabulum is lost, and degenerative osteoarthritis involving both the femoral head and acetabulum progresses. The femoral neck also has a thickened appearance.

Etiology

Many theories have been put forth over the years as to the cause of the avascular event, including trauma, heredity, endocrine disturbances, metabolic imbalances, fat embolism, and infection. Heredity as an etiology has not been proved on repeat breeding with the same parents of affected offspring. In addition, heredity does not explain why only one hip is involved in most patients. Based on all the data available today, it appears that no genetic basis can explain the cause of the ischemic event that leads to necrosis of the femoral head in LCPD.

The endocrine theory was put forth from studies showing that osteonecrosis occurred from a high dose of either estrogens or testosterone.[85] The endocrine theory was also predicated on the basis that the morphological changes in LCPD in the dog were manifestations of precocious sexual maturity. However, the endocrine theory does not explain the predominant unilateral occurrence of LCPD or its overall low incidence in breed populations that are characterized by precocious sexual maturity.[108] In addition, affected dogs do not show other systemic or musculoskeletal signs of endocrine abnormalities.

The metabolic theory also does not seem likely as a cause for the localized ischemic event for the same reasons just stated for the endocrine theory. Infection as a cause is unacceptable because histologically the lesions are not characteristic of an infectious process. Although fat emboli have been used in experimental studies to produce ischemia of the femoral head, they have not been reported in clinical cases in the dog. The ischemic event may have occurred from a thrombosed vessel because of trauma; however, histological studies have failed to reveal any evidence of thrombi in the vessels of the femoral epiphysis.

Experimentally, the dorsal retinacular artery in puppies can be totally occluded when the intraarticular pressure reaches 40 mm Hg. Induced intraarticular tamponade of the hip joints of breed-susceptible puppies produces radiographic and histological changes similar to those in naturally occurring LCPD in the dog.[41]

Trauma of some type, perhaps of a chronic repetitive nature affecting the dorsal retinacular blood supply, seems the most likely cause of the localized ischemia to the proximal femoral epiphysis. The traumatic insult may occur from these small breeds of dogs jumping excessively on their rear legs, thus damaging the dorsal retinacular blood vessels. The affected area of the femoral head is dorsal. Since the retinacular vessels to the femoral epiphysis course under the joint capsule and synovial membrane, they would be susceptible to trauma when the dog jumps.

Radiology

The diagnosis of LCPD is confirmed on radiographic examination of the affected hip joint(s). Standard lateral and ventrodorsal (with rear legs extended) radiographic views are recommended. The ventrodorsal view with rear legs extended reveals the changes in the femoral head and allows diagnosis of the LCPD. If one were fortunate enough to see the radiograph of a patient in the very earliest stage of the disease, only a lucent area would be present in the dorsal aspect of the femoral head because of resorption of the dead subchondral bone trabecula. In clinical practice, however, by the time the patient is presented to the clinician, the most common radiographic finding is a slight, mild, or severe flattening of the femoral head's dorsal aspect (Fig. 17-1). This results from collapse of the cartilage and underlying adjacent trabecular subchondral bone into the affected area of the femoral head. Radiolucent areas also are present in the femoral head. The femoral head is flattened and irregular in shape and in some patients may appear fragmented. Joint laxity also is apparent. With time, osteoarthritis becomes apparent, with osteophyte formation around the femoral head and the acetabulum. The femoral neck appears thickened as LCPD progresses.

Treatment

Both nonsurgical and surgical treatments for LCPD in the dog have been described. Most patients with the diagnosis of LCPD are not candidates for nonsurgical treatment. In clinical practice, most patients already have some change in the contour of the affected femoral head at the time they are examined for the rear limb lameness.

Nonsurgical. If a patient is to be treated nonsurgically for LCPD, the diagnosis must be made early before there is radiographic evidence of any change in normal contour of the femoral head or acetabulum. During the treatment period, it is essential that the affected joint be

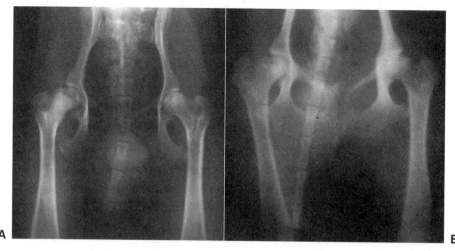

Fig. 17-1 Ventrodorsal radiographs of two dogs with avascular necrosis of their right femoral heads. The left femoral head is normal in both dogs. **A,** Changes seen in the femoral head of 11-month-old male toy poodle are primarily subchondral bone cavitation and slight flattening of the head. **B,** Collapse of the dorsal femoral head and subchondral cavitation are the prominent features seen in the femoral head of the female toy poodle.

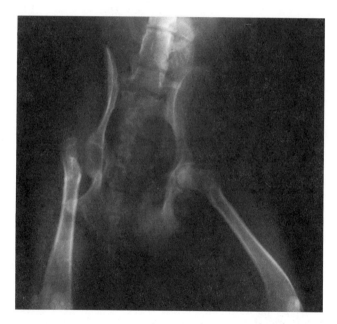

Fig. 17-2 Excision arthroplasty of the head and neck is the most common surgical treatment for avascular necrosis of the femoral head when it occurs in small dogs. Total hip replacement is also an option if the dog is large enough. The immediate postoperative radiographs of the poodle in Fig. 17-1, A, are shown here.

rested. One method is to confine the patient to a small cage until the radiolucent changes in the femoral head are completely resolved.[74] During the enforced period of rest, the patient is only allowed out of its cage for urination and defecation. The patient must be carried to and from its cage and kept on a short hand-held leash during elimination.

Monthly radiographs are taken to follow progression of the disease. It generally takes up to 4 to 6 months before the femoral head heals sufficiently to permit unrestricted weight bearing. Using this method, it is possible to have a patient's femoral head heal with a nearly normal radiographic appearance and to return to pain-free motion and normal gait.[74] If collapse of the femoral head occurs during nonsurgical treatment, surgery is done.

Major disadvantages of nonsurgical management are (1) strict adherence to a long confinement period for the patient and (2) the patient not becoming socially adjusted to a normal everyday life with the owners for several months.

One should not attempt resting the affected joint by placing the limb in a non-weight-bearing sling such as an Ehmer sling for such a long time. This would result in severe disuse atrophy of the affected limb's muscles and flexion contracture of the stifle. In addition, studies by author Wallace have shown that a limb placed in an Ehmer sling continuously for 6 weeks will initiate early degenerative changes in the articular cartilage of the distal femur. These changes occur from complete immobilization of the stifle and thus interference with normal physiology and nutrition of the articular cartilage.

Surgical. The surgical treatment consists of excision of the femoral head and neck (Fig. 17-2). The surgical procedure is discussed in the section on hip dysplasia. Reported results clearly indicate this is the treatment of choice in canine patients with LCPD.[74,108] If left untreated, progressive osteoarthritis in the affected hip will occur, along with pain, lameness, and muscle atrophy. For faster recovery, the surgery should be done early in the disease course. Because of the small size of patients with LCPD, they generally regain very good function of their hip after excision arthroplasty. If the dog is large enough to accept a hip prosthesis, total hip replacement is another treatment option.

Physical therapy is done morning and night on the affected hip. The physical therapy program recommended consists of 35 slow flexion and extension movements of the hip joint at each session. The therapy starts on the second postoperative day and continues until the patient is bearing weight on the affected limb and has a good range of motion (ROM) in the hip. Some patients required the physical therapy for 4 to 6 weeks after surgery. Patients with advanced osteoarthritis and severe muscle atrophy may show progressive improvement for up to 12 months after surgery. If the surgical procedure is done correctly and the physical therapy properly performed, a good functional result can usually be expected within 8 to 12 weeks. If the patient is affected in both femoral heads, the one that is most painful should be operated on first. The second hip can be treated surgically when the patient is weight bearing after the first surgery on the opposite hip.

We recommend surgical treatment for all canine patients with LCPD for the following reasons:

1. The success rate is high.
2. The patient does not have to be confined to a small cage.
3. The patient is free to move about the home and develop socially with the owners.
4. The patient will be weight bearing and have unrestricted activity much more quickly than if treated nonsurgically.

CANINE HIP DYSPLASIA

Hip dysplasia is a common musculoskeletal disease that affects humans and most domestic animals. The first reports of this disease in dogs were by Schnelle in 1935[148] and 1937.[149,150] Interestingly, hip dysplasia was first described in humans by Hippocrates more than 2000 years ago.[49] Hip dysplasia has been diagnosed in almost all breeds of dogs. The incidence is high in the giant, large, and medium breeds and low in the smaller breeds.[31,126] Over the years, an enormous number of clinical and research papers has been published on this disease. This section provides a general review on canine hip dysplasia with specific reference to its etiology, pathogenesis, history, clinical signs, diagnosis, and treatment.

Etiology

It has been known for many years that hip dysplasia is inherited. Although initially the mode of inheritance was

uncertain, it was established in the 1950s and 1960s that progression of the disease was influenced by various environmental factors.[56,137,146,147,164] Additional studies, while confirming the inherited nature of the disease, clarified the mode of inheritance to be polygenetic.[63,67]

Several factors besides inheritance have been proposed as being related to the development of hip dysplasia. The coxofemoral joints of pups that eventually develop hip dysplasia are structurally and functionally normal at birth.[136]

Estrogens. The effects of estrogens in the development of hip dysplasia have been studied.[48,123] Experimentally, it is possible to induce hip dysplasia in young dogs using estrogens. However, no evidence indicates that estrogen levels within the normal biological range have any relationship to the incidence of hip dysplasia in dogs.[123,136,139] Also, it seems more likely that a hormone-induced disease would exert a systemic effect, causing several joints to be abnormal.[91]

Body size and growth. Body size, body type, and growth patterns all are secondary influences in the development of hip dysplasia. As stated earlier, the incidence of the disease is lowest in the smaller breeds and highest in the giant, large, and medium breeds of dogs. Breeds with the highest incidence of hip dysplasia grow and mature more rapidly than those in the low-risk group. Starting at birth, pups of the high-incidence breeds have rapid weight gains. The pups of these breeds are aggressive eaters, both while nursing and consuming supplemental food.[139]

Nutrition. In a study involving 222 German shepherd dogs, 63% weighing more than the mean weight of all the dogs at age 60 days were dysplastic at age 1 year, whereas only 37% of those less than the mean weight became dysplastic. The same rapid rise in weight in other breeds with a high incidence of hip dysplasia has been observed.[140]

The influence of nutrition on the incidence and severity of hip dysplasia has been investigated.[54,71,90] During the growth period in puppies with a genotype for hip dysplasia, it was shown a high-calorie diet increased the incidence and severity of the disease.[33] In another study, when at least one parent was dysplastic, the course of hip dysplasia in the offspring was found not to be influenced by overfeeding the pups, by restricting their dietary intake, by putting them on a selected exercise schedule, or by restricting their movement.[90] Overfeeding a group of Great Dane puppies during their period of fast growth influenced the onset of hip dysplasia as well as other skeletal diseases.[54]

To offset the possibility of an increased incidence of hip dysplasia and other skeletal diseases in fast-growing dogs, it has been suggested that a restrictive feeding program is important for their normal development.[116] Dogs that develop normal hip joints despite being overfed when they are puppies may have stable hip joints and a better genotype than those that develop hip dysplasia.

Nutrition has a secondary effect on the incidence and progression of hip dysplasia. The level of nutrition is responsible for the increased weight gains observed in large, fast-growing puppies. The pup's increased weight exerts an extra mechanical stress on the hip joint.[136] If hip instability is already present, the added mechanical loading force on the hip will enhance both the incidence and the progression of the disease.

Pelvic muscle mass. Studies of the pelvic muscle mass of 95 dogs in three breeds (greyhound, German shepherd, July foxhound) have indicated a correlation between the amount of pelvic muscle and the prevalence of hip dysplasia.[136,138] These dogs had an age range of 5 months to 10 years when their muscles were examined. A statistical analysis indicated that the soundness of the hip joints was closely correlated with the index of pelvic muscle mass; that is, the greater the pelvic muscle mass index, the lower the incidence of hip dysplasia. The occurrence of hip dysplasia could be predicted with cut-off points on the pelvic muscle mass index scale. This allowed for determining the probability of hip dysplasia and the degree of involvement expected. It is unclear if the decrease in pelvic muscle mass in dysplastic dogs is an inherited factor or a secondary change related to the disease, or perhaps both. A lower pelvic muscle mass in dysplastic dogs may be a secondary change caused by disuse muscle atrophy in response to the lameness or hip pain associated with hip dysplasia.

Biomechanical loads. The biomechanical loads acting on the canine hip joint have been studied.[5,127] These studies revealed how different positions of the limb as well as subluxation affect development and function of the entire hip joint. Strong, well-balanced muscle support is essential to maintain proper joint congruity. If there is a generalized weakness of all hip muscles or of a particular group of muscles, the balanced support is lost, which can lead to adverse changes in the hip joints of young, growing dogs.

Protein synthesis. Studies on the rate of protein synthesis of pelvic muscles from normal and dysplastic dogs have been reported. Pelvic muscle protein synthesis occurred at about equivalent rates for approximately 3 months in dogs coming from both normal and dysplastic matings. After 3 months, the potentially dysplastic pups formed less protein in hip joint muscle tissue. It was concluded that the decreased rate of pelvic muscle protein formation observed may be a manifestation of secondary factors associated with hip dysplasia.[92]

In the adult dog, individual pelvic muscles associated with hip joint motion were examined histologically.

Evidence of muscle disease was not observed. In dogs with advanced hip dysplasia and osteoarthritis, atrophy of the pelvic muscles was present, but changes such as muscle necrosis, inflammation, and extensive fibrosis were not found on routine histological examinations.[138]

Pectineus muscle. The pectineus muscle has been a controversial subject in its relation to hip dysplasia since it was first reported in 1968 to play a role in the development of hip dysplasia.[8] That report theorized that spasm or shortening of the pectineus muscle may cause the osseous changes in the hip joint, observed radiographically, in 6- to 12-month-old dogs with hip dysplasia. Since that original report, several studies have evaluated histochemical, histological, neurophysiological, and biochemical properties of the pectineus muscle from dysplastic and normal dogs of various ages.[*]

The pectineus muscle is an adductor of the rear leg that originates on the iliopectineal eminence of the pubic bone and inserts distally on the popliteal surface of the femur. If growth and development of the pectineus muscle do not coincide with the same growth rate as the femur, extra stress is applied to the hip joint. This increased stress on the hip joint could induce changes in the acetabulum because of the upward loads on it from the femoral head. The acetabulum is most susceptible to remodeling loads from birth to approximately age 6 months.[136] In addition, this extra stress on the hip joint could initiate or facilitate the development of hip joint laxity during the first several weeks of life. Such a cause-and-effect relationship between the pectineus muscle and development of the dysplastic hip joint has not been proven.

A developmental myopathy with type II fiber hypotrophy was identified in the pectineus muscles of German shepherd puppies.[26] The histologic features observed most frequently in the pectineus muscles more closely approximated those described for neurogenic diseases of muscle. However, the lesions observed differed in that the small fibers did not always occur in groups and were rounded rather than angulated. The pectineus muscles from affected pups were smaller than those from normal pups. Individual muscles and their respective myofibers were evaluated in a histological study of the pectineus muscles from pure-bred, 2-month-old German shepherd dogs.[64] The pectineus muscles of dogs that developed normal hips contained larger relative and absolute myofiber components and smaller nonmyofiber components. Although similar differences may also be present in other hip muscles, this has not been reported.

The potential effects of the difference in composition of normal and hypotrophic pectineus muscles could be twofold. First, the smaller myofiber size in muscles of pre-dysplastic pups may result in a diminished capacity for the muscles to develop active tension. Second, the larger non-

---

*References 16, 24, 26, 64, 92, 93, 136, 138.

myofiber component in pectineus muscles of dysplastic dogs might result in diminished muscle elasticity if the increased size is caused by increased collagenous connective tissues. In support of the first consideration, the contractile properties of normal and hypotrophic pectineus muscles from 2-month-old dogs revealed that the maximum isometric twitch tensions and tetanic tensions were directly proportional to mean myofiber size.[24] Therefore, hypotrophic muscles were weaker and had a slower reaction time than normal pectineus muscles. The motor unit potential complexes recorded from muscles associated with dysplastic coxofemoral joints were longer in duration and lower in amplitude than those for muscles associated with normal coxofemoral joints. In support of the second consideration, at least one other study has reported that the fibrous component may be increased in pectineus muscles of dysplastic dogs.[87] It is not clear how or if this decrease in active tension capability, decreased elasticity, and type II fiber myopathy of pectineus muscles in 2-month-old dogs is associated with the development of dysplastic hips.

Muscle loads. Data published on the pectineus muscle and pelvic muscle mass emphasize the biomechanical influence that all these muscles have on hip joint stability. If the proper balance of muscle loads acting about the hip is not maintained, a disparity exists between the primary muscle mass and skeletal growth. A disparity of loads on the hip joint could definitely influence the progression of hip dysplasia. Based on reported data, since hip dysplasia is associated with reduced pelvic muscle mass, it may develop as a sequela to alterations in the function of pelvic muscles. It may be process mediated by neuronal dysfunction, myofiber dysfunction, and connective tissue dysplasia.

Angle of inclination and anteversion. Changes in the angles of inclination and anteversion have a direct effect on the loads created by the femoral head within the acetabulum.[5,127] Increased angles of inclination and anteversion are seen in dogs with hip dysplasia[53,137] (Fig. 17-3). Abnormal angles of inclination and anteversion

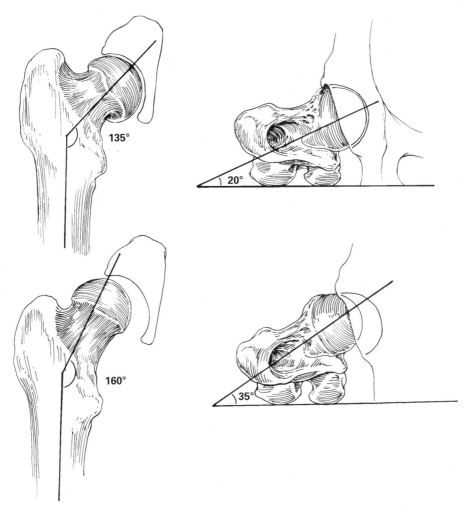

Fig. 17-3 Normal angles of inclination (135 to 145 degrees) and anteversion (20 to 25 degrees) in the dog place the femoral head in the proper position to be adequately covered by the acetabulum. Abnormal increases in inclination, and/or anteversion, promote decreased coverage of the femoral head by the acetabulum.

may be observed in dysplastic hips; however, their presence is not a consistent finding.

Pathogenesis

The main feature in the pathogenesis of hip dysplasia is *joint laxity*.[56] Regardless of the controversy that exists about nutrition, hormones, various muscles, and so forth, joint laxity is the initial change that initiates the dysplastic process in the hip joint. To determine specifically what causes hip joint laxity would be a major advance toward understanding the mechanism responsible for the dysplastic hip. Joint laxity can be identified in some patients with palpation of the hips and defined on a radiograph as subluxation or luxation. However, despite all the research that has been done, the cause of joint laxity has not been specifically defined.

An increase in synovial fluid volume and in the size of the ligament of the femoral head within the coxofemoral joint of young dogs genetically predisposed to hip dysplasia has been implicated in the development of hip joint laxity.[89,94] It would seem more likely that joint laxity would be the initiating factor for developing a synovitis, synovial fluid effusion, and other changes.[88]

The chronological radiographic and histological changes seen in the dysplastic hip joint from birth to maturity are well documented.[67] Remodeling changes that constitute the dysplasia occur sometime between 2 weeks after birth and about 4½ months of age, when acetabular growth is about completed.[134] At birth the hip joint is normal in dogs genetically predisposed to become dysplastic. The hip joint remains quite stable during the first 10 to 14 days of life.[137] After that, depending on the individual animal and the factors responsible, joint laxity develops and progresses at a variable rate to subluxation or in severe cases to eventual joint luxation. Once joint laxity has become excessive, the congruous well-balanced fit between the femoral head and the acetabulum is not maintained. Early changes include synovitis, synovial fluid effusion, thickening and eventual fraying of the femoral head ligament, and thickening of the joint capsule.

Because of the subluxation of the femoral head, abnormal wear and erosion of the articular cartilage occur on its dorsal surface. In addition, the upward load of the subluxated femoral head exerts an abnormal stress on the dorsal brim of the acetabulum, thereby interfering with its endochondral ossification. Fractures of the acetabulum's dorsal brim may occur in the young, growing dog from the increased upward stress placed on it by the subluxated femoral head.[123] This may cause pain and lameness until the fracture heals. Remodeling changes occur in the acetabulum and femoral head because of the abnormal loads acting on them. Eventually, the femoral head ligament ruptures and atrophies. The ligament may become completely covered as bone fills in the acetabular cup. Osteophytes develop around the femoral head and acetabulum. Remodeling changes continue on the femoral head and neck and within the acetabulum as the secondary degenerative osteoarthritis of hip dysplasia progresses with increasing severity over months and years.

History

The clinical signs of hip dysplasia in the dog are generally first observed between ages 4 and 12 months. However, in some dogs the rear limb lameness is not observed until after age 12 months. Some dogs, even with severe arthritis, never exhibit signs of dysplasia. As affected dogs age, the history is more of a persistent lameness associated with degenerative osteoarthritis of the hips. The history obtained on a dysplastic dog may include one or more of the following observations by the owner:

1. Decreased exercise tolerance
2. Inability or reluctance to go up and down stairs or to get in or out of a motor vehicle
3. Audible click in young dogs coming from one or both hip joints as they subluxate during walking
4. Difficulty or slowness when lying down or rising
5. Running with both hind limbs together ("bunny hopping" gait)
6. Change of disposition (aggressiveness) because of painful hips
7. Inability to clear objects with a jump
8. Lameness after strenuous exercise
9. Nonneurological, wobbly gait in the rear limbs
10. Flat hind end with wide hips

Clinical Signs

The clinical signs of hip dysplasia vary widely, from slight discomfort to severe acute or chronic pain to crippling effects of degenerative osteoarthritis. The severity of clinical signs and radiographic changes may not correlate. Some dysplastic dogs are examined and have no current lameness but were lame 2 or 3 days earlier. The lameness may be unilateral or bilateral and is caused by a painful hip joint(s). Younger dogs with subluxating hip joints may have a nonneurological, wobbly or unsteady gait, which is best observed as the patient walks away from the clinician. Some dogs stand with an arched back as they try to shift weight from the rear legs to the front legs. Disuse atrophy of the pelvic and rear leg muscles may be present depending on the duration of the lameness. Some dogs stand with the rear legs close together and the paws rotated outward.

Orthopedic Examination

Range of motion. Although the following discussion is limited to the orthopedic examination, it is very important that each patient receive a thorough physical examination to detect any other disease problem. Manipulation of the hip joints may reveal mild to severe pain in one or more ranges of motion, that is, flexion, extension, internal and external rotation, and abduction. In a dysplastic dog, it is unusual to elicit a pain response when flexing the hip, but pain on extension is common. During these manipulations, a decreased ROM may also be found, especially with abduction and extension. Advanced degenerative osteoarthritis can be seen in dogs less than 1 year old. The restricted ROM in abduction may result from not only pain, but also tight pectineus muscles. To evaluate the degree of restricted abduction, the patient can be placed in lateral or dorsal recumbency. Performing the examination in dorsal recumbency with the patient relaxed allows both legs to be evaluated at the same time. If excited or apprehensive, the patient must be sedated to evaluate properly the degree of abduction that is restricted. Sedation is not administered until a complete orthopedic evaluation has been performed.

The pain elicited on physical examination is related to the arthritic hip joints. Restricted ROM of the hip joints, in addition to pain, can also be caused by a very thick joint capsule, remodeling changes of the femoral head and acetabulum, and periarticular osteophyte formation. Crepitus may be detected on palpation of hips with advanced degenerative osteoarthritis.

Joint laxity. In all patients the hip joints should be palpated for the presence or absence of joint laxity and an Ortolani sign. Techniques for hip palpation in both puppies and older dogs have been published.[8,133] Additional information on examining dogs to detect the Ortolani sign is presented in Chapter 1. Not all dogs have enough joint laxity to permit the degree of subluxation needed to produce an Ortolani sign. In other dogs the Ortolani sign is present at examination and later disappears. This occurs because of thickening of the joint capsule, remodeling of the dorsal rim of the acetabulum and femoral head, progressive filling of the acetabulum with bone, and periarticular osteophyte production as the degenerative osteoarthritis develops.

Unless the patient has excessive hip pain or is unruly and excited, hip palpation to check for an Ortolani sign can be done without sedation in the examination room. If not completely relaxed and properly positioned, there may be a negative finding in a patient that would otherwise have a positive Ortolani sign. Since radiographs will be taken as well, the patient is sedated or lightly anesthetized. During this time the patient should be repalpated.

Lameness. On rare occasions a dog with hip dysplasia may be presented for examination because of a front limb lameness that develops after strenuous exercise, with no history of rear leg lameness. If no physical or radiographic abnormalities are found in the affected front limb, the rear limb should be carefully examined for hip dysplasia. The front limb lameness in such patients is thought to be caused by the extra stress put on the front limb articulations from the dog shifting its weight forward.

In any dog, especially in breeds with a high risk and incidence of hip dysplasia, one must never allow the diagnosis of hip dysplasia to stand as the sole cause of rear limb lameness without examining for other conditions. Dogs with rear limb lameness must be examined thoroughly from their toes to lumbosacral levels for any problems. Examples of such problems include, but are not limited to, (1) infections, (2) luxations, (3) fractures, (4) panosteitis, (5) ligament injuries, (6) osteochondritis dissecans, (7) tendon or muscle injuries, (8) vertebral arthritis, (9) lumbosacral stenosis, (10) neoplasia, and (11) neurological disease. The presence of any of these problems has an important influence on selecting the proper method of treatment for the patient who also has hip dysplasia.

Diagnosis

Radiography. The diagnosis of hip dysplasia in dogs is made by finding the changes associated with dysplasia from a ventrodorsal radiographic view of the pelvis. It is essential that the dog be properly positioned on its back to avoid an asymmetrical view of the pelvis. The dog should usually be sedated or lightly anesthetized to ensure proper positioning without movement for diagnostic films. The standard method for obtaining the ventrodorsal pelvic radiograph is to have the rear limbs extended, femurs parallel to each other and to the spine, patellas centered in the trochlear groove of the femurs, and pelvis positioned symmetrically (Fig. 17-4). This radiographic view and positioning of the dog are the currently recommended approaches.[105,133,136,181]

The Orthopedic Foundation for Animals (OFA) requires quality films with proper positioning before certifying the animal as normal or dysplastic. The radiographic appearance of the different stages of hip dysplasia and methods for measuring various angles of the hip joint have been described.* Normal hip joints have well-formed femoral heads that fit congruently and deeply into the acetabula. The animal is dysplastic when the femoral head conforms

---

*References 9, 36, 52, 53, 105, 131, 136, 139.

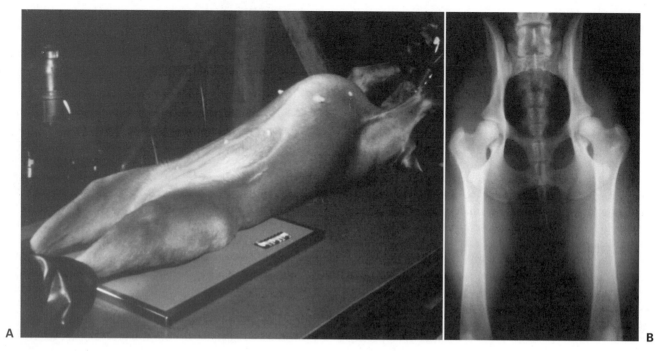

Fig. 17-4 **A,** Proper positioning for ventrodorsal radiographs of the hips requires the dog's body to be aligned in ventral recumbency and the hind limbs pulled straight in full extension. Internal rotation of the hock joints helps align the femurs properly. **B,** These radiographs show the dog was properly positioned and has normal hips.

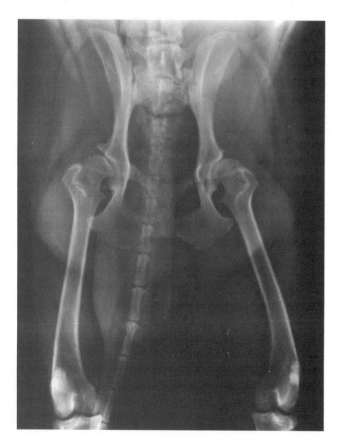

Fig. 17-5 Ventrodorsal radiographs of a 31-month-old female German shepherd with hip dysplasia and severe secondary osteoarthritis. This dog exhibited lameness and pain on full extension of both coxofemoral joints.

poorly within the acetabulum, with or without evidence of osteoarthritis. In the young animal, generally the first radiographic indication of hip dysplasia is slight to severe subluxation or, in extreme cases, luxation of the hip joint(s). The classical features of secondary degenerative osteoarthritis soon become evident if the hip joint instability is not corrected[25,136] (Fig. 17-5).

The methods of positioning animals to obtain a ventrodorsal radiographic view for making a diagnosis of hip dysplasia have been questioned. The conventional method, with the rear limbs pulled caudal, is not a position normally adopted by the dog. In this position the joint capsule is tightened, and the muscles have an unnatural strain placed on them. Therefore, certain young dogs who have some palpable joint laxity may have hips that appear radiographically normal. Those dogs who do reveal minimal subluxation on the conventional radiographic view obviously have excess joint laxity.

The wedge or fulcrum technique was developed to improve the radiographic evaluation of hip joints in young dogs by revealing coxofemoral joint laxity in hip joints that otherwise appeared radiographically normal.[6,58] The principle of this technique is extremely valuable in determining an early diagnosis of hip dysplasia. It is most useful when used in conjunction with palpation of the hips when attempting to detect joint laxity during a physical examination. However, the technique has not met with wide acceptance because of a lack of standardization for the procedure and the material used to create the wedge.

A new stress radiographic positioning technique provides a method for quantitative measurement of hip joint laxity in the dog.[163] For this procedure the dogs must be anesthetized or heavily sedated. They are positioned on the radiographic table in dorsal recumbency. The hocks are grasped and the stifles maintained in a neutral flexion/extension and adduction/abduction position. Stress radiography is done with the hips in compressed and distracted positions. In the compressed position the femoral head is seated into the acetabulum in the most congruent position. In the distracted position the femoral head can be distracted laterally from the acetabulum. The distance the femoral head can be distracted is directly related to the degree of joint laxity present. This stress radiographic technique may be more sensitive for measuring hip joint laxity than the standard hip-extended position. Further studies need to be done using this new procedure in many dogs of various breeds and ages to determine the difference between normal and abnormal hip joint laxity. Although this new technique shows promise, further studies must be completed to correlate laxity with potential development of degenerative joint disease later in life.[163]

The dog's age when radiographs are taken varies depending on the purpose of the films. For example, if a dog is to be OFA certified, it must be 2 years of age. At one time, dogs could be OFA certified at 1 year. However, as more investigations on the disease were published, it was shown a significant number of dogs did not have the radiographic changes of hip dysplasia at age 1 year but did at 2 years. It has been reported that 95% of dysplastic dogs will have radiographic evidence of hip dysplasia by the time they are 2 years old. However, it is not necessary to wait until 2 years to take films of the hips of dogs with clinical signs. Radiographic views to diagnose lameness or to determine in a screening procedure if a clinically asymptomatic dog has early evidence of hip dysplasia may be taken as early as age 2 months.[56,136,137] Early diagnosis of hip dysplasia is also important if some type of reconstructive surgery on the hip joint is to be done.

Hip palpation. The diagnosis of hip dysplasia in humans can be made in the newborn infant by palpating the hip joint and detecting a positive Ortolani sign.[118,119] The Ortolani sign signifies the presence of excess joint laxity and confirms coxofemoral subluxation in the newborn. When the technique is done properly, a positive Ortolani sign is detected by feeling and sometimes hearing the resounding "click" as the subluxed femoral head is reduced back into the acetabulum. The presence of an Ortolani sign in pups has been reported.[56,137] However, all newborn pups have a normal hip joint with no laxity. In most cases, laxity in the hip joint severe enough to result in a positive Ortolani sign will not be detected until the pup is at least 4 to 8 weeks of age.

A technique for palpating the hip joints of 4-week-old pups to detect joint laxity in predicting which ones would become dysplastic was first published by Bardens and Hardwick in 1968.[8] Bardens later determined that the best age to palpate pups for hip joint laxity was 8 to 9 weeks of age.[7] This technique estimates the distance of lateral displacement of the femoral head out of the acetabulum. Based on the amount of joint laxity present, a prediction was made as to whether the pup would be normal or dysplastic as an adult and was verified on follow-up radiographic studies. This study initiated a new interest in hip palpation of pups to obtain an early diagnosis of hip dysplasia. Additional studies were done to evaluate the Bardens technique and the reliability of detecting hip joint laxity and predicting which pups would become dysplastic. In general, most of these studies were done on 8- to 12-week-old pups while they were anesthetized.[26,43,92,145] A correlation may exist between the degree of hip joint laxity in 8-week-old pups and the radiographic signs of hip dysplasia when the dog is 1 year old. Dogs with a greater degree of joint laxity tend to show the radiographic signs of hip dysplasia as they mature.

The technique of determining joint laxity by estimating the distance the femoral head can be displaced from the acetabulum is a subjective test. Therefore the palpation score obtained by one person can be quite different from that of another on the same pup. Using this technique, erroneous data can be obtained from an inadequate depth of anesthesia, improper positioning of the pup on the table, and improper manipulation of the limb of the hip to be examined. Accuracy in palpating the hips of pups should improve with training and experience. Some who have used this palpation procedure for several years report an accuracy of 83% or greater in detecting the predysplastic pup when it is 4 to 8 weeks of age.[7,8,43] In most cases, once a pup has reached age 11 to 12 weeks, the technique's accuracy decreases because of the increased size of the hind limb. A slight amount of normal joint laxity may be present as the hip joint grows and develops. Not all pups with a tight (no laxity) hip joint at age 8 weeks are going to be normal, and conversely, not all pups with a slight amount of joint laxity are going to become dysplastic. Palpation of the hip joints in 8-week-old puppies is a screening procedure for detecting those pups with extreme joint laxity who *may* become dysplastic.

In older dogs a closer correlation exists between palpable joint laxity and the radiographic signs of hip dysplasia.[145] During the orthopedic examination of dogs 3 months of age and older, the technique described[28] to detect an Ortolani sign in dogs should be used for evaluation of hip joint stability. An Ortolani sign is diagnostic of hip joint subluxation, which will be confirmed radiographically in most cases. However, some dogs at age 12 to 18 months may not reveal much, if any, degree of subluxation on radiographs but have a positive Ortolani sign on palpation of the hips. If followed over a longer time, most but not all dogs will develop radiographic signs consistent with hip dysplasia. In such cases a radiographic procedure using the new stress radiographic technique[65] may be of value in documenting the subluxation. Some dogs with a positive Ortolani sign as a juvenile have been found to have normal hip joint laxity at age 2 years.

Control

Hip dysplasia is an inherited disease with a polygenetic mode of inheritance. Although disease progression is influenced by various factors, such as body size, body type, rapid growth, and weight gain, the genetic transmission of the disease is controlled by not breeding affected animals. Numerous studies have been done showing how the incidence of canine hip dysplasia can be decreased using selective breeding programs.[55,63,70,135]

Medical Treatment

A medical (nonsurgical) approach is indicated in dogs with mild signs or a first episode of lameness. Each patient's physical status and response to activity and environmental conditions must be evaluated to determine the best treatment modalities. The patient should be kept in a warm, dry environment if cold, damp weather incites clinical signs. Obesity must be avoided. All overweight patients should be placed on a weight reduction program. Excessive weight adds more stress to the arthritic joint, causing more pain and the need for analgesic or antiinflammatory medication. After losing weight, many dogs no longer need daily analgesic medication.

Nonsteroidal antiinflammatory drugs (NSAIDs). One of the NSAIDs approved for use in dogs is generally used to provide relief of pain from the osteoarthritis in the affected joint(s). The NSAIDs work by inhibiting cyclooxygenase, which is responsible for the production of prostaglandins from arachidonic acid.[47] Prostaglandins play a very specific role as mediators in the inflammatory process and may augment pain perception.[30] The cell types that secrete prostaglandins in an arthritic joint include polymorphonuclear leukocytes, lymphocytes, macrophages, and synovial membrane cells.[156]

Data are available to show that NSAIDs may influence chemotaxis of polymorphonuclear leukocytes and, by increasing cyclic adenosine monophosphate (cAMP), stabilize lysosomal membranes and prevent the release of enzymes involved in inflammation.[33,47,157] Inhibitors of prostaglandin synthesis have been found to reduce greatly the emigration of monocytes in an acute inflammatory reaction.[156] Therefore, by inhibiting prostaglandin synthesis, the inflammatory process can be decreased and pain relief achieved. Although the NSAIDs are quite effective in providing pain relief for the patient, they do not reverse or completely stop the progression of osteoarthritis.[69] However, aspirin has been shown to have some protective effect against the degeneration of articular cartilage, probably through the inhibition of prostaglandin synthesis.[77] In general, these drugs simply allow the patient to be more comfortable for an unpredictable period. The most frequently used NSAIDs approved for clinical use in the dog are aspirin, phenylbutazone, and meclofenamic acid.

Aspirin. Aspirin products are often used for treating osteoarthritis because they are readily available, reasonably effective, and inexpensive. If aspirin is used, it should be in the form of one of the buffered products, such as Ascriptin (William H. Rorer, Inc., Fort Washinginton, Pa) or Bufferin (Bristol-Meyers Co., NY). Aspirin in the non-buffered form is much more irritating to the gastric mucosa of dogs and therefore should be avoided. Based on serum salicylate concentrations, the recommended dose for either of these buffered aspirin products is 25 mg/kg of body weight every 8 hours.[79] Some patients show an effective clinical response to Ascriptin or Bufferin at a dose of 25 mg/kg every 12 hours. It has also been reported that some dogs attain pain relief from aspirin therapy at a lower dose of 10 to 20 mg/kg every 12 hours.[32] Unlike the opiates, aspirin acts as an analgesic peripherally rather than centrally.[4] The patient is started on a dose of 25 mg/kg every 8 hours for 5 days, then every 12 hours, based on the patient's response, for as long as necessary.

When used with care at its recommended therapeutic dose, aspirin is relatively free of serious side effects.[4] At the previous therapeutic dose, vomiting may be caused by the irritation of the gastric mucosa. The gastric intolerance seen in these patients can sometimes be eliminated by administering the drug after giving the patient some food or preceding administration with one of the oral antacid drugs, such as Maalox (aluminum hydroxide gel and magnesium hydroxide) (Rorer). Maalox is available in both tablet and liquid preparations.

Phenylbutazone. This NSAID has been used for many years in the treatment of osteoarthritis in dogs and other animals and has a mechanism of action similar to aspirin. Phenylbutazone may be effective in canine patients that cannot tolerate a buffered aspirin product. The dosage varies widely from 1 mg/kg total dose divided every 8 hours,[20] 1 mg/kg every 8 hours,[4] or 10 to 15 mg/kg every 8 hours, with a maximum of 800 mg daily.[15,30] The higher dose should only be used for 48 hours and then decreased to the lowest effective dose for the patient. Regardless of which dosage regimen is used, the patient should be treated every 8 hours and should not receive any more than 800 mg in a 24-hour period. One of the major adverse effects of phenylbutazone when used over a long period is bone marrow depression. Therefore, patients should not be treated for more than 2 weeks at a time.

Meclofenamic acid. Meclofenamic acid (Arquel) is NSAID approved for use in the dog. Arquel will soon be available for specific use in the canine in 10 and 20 mg scored tablets (Fort Dodge Laboratories, Fort Dodge, Iowa). Currently, it is only available in the equine (Arquel) and human (Meclomen) (Parke-Davis & Co., Ann Arbor, Mich) preparations. Arquel is prepared in the granular form with a concentration of 500 mg meclofenamic acid in each 10 g package. It has been found to be very effective in the treatment of osteoarthritis in the dog.

In patients that require long-term NSAID therapy for their osteoarthritis, meclofenamic acid is recommended by some over all other approved drugs for treating osteoarthritis in the canine patient with hip dysplasia. The most effective dose is 1.1 mg/kg administered once daily, at the same time each day, after a full meal. For ease of administration, the granules are placed in a small meatball and given to the patient after the regular meal has been eaten. The previous dosage and schedule are continued for 14 days. If the patient obtains relief on this dose and schedule, the same dose is continued but is given every other day for another 2 weeks. If the patient is still responding, 1.1 mg/kg is administered in the same way every third day for five treatments. If during the alternating interval of drug administration (every other day or every third day) the patient shows discomfort, administration should be returned to the regimen in which symptomatic relief of pain was evident.

In author Wallace's experience, approximately 5% of the dogs treated with Arquel develop diarrhea, which, if related to the drug, is evident by the third to fifth day of treatment. Owners must be warned of this side effect, since the diarrhea develops acutely and generally is of a watery consistency. If this occurs, the owner must discontinue administering the drug, give the patient a gastrointestinal (GI) protectant such as Kaopectate, and seek veterinary advice. The intestinal protectant is continued until the diarrhea stops. The regular diet is stopped for the first 24 hours, then patients are fed a diet of cooked rice until they have a normal stool. Diarrhea generally stops within 48 hours.

In about 3% of the 5% of dogs that develop diarrhea, Arquel therapy can be resumed at a dose of 0.5 mg/kg every other day for 14 days, administered at the same time each day after a full meal and an antacid such as Maalox. If the patient's GI tract tolerates this treatment regimen but the patient fails to show symptomatic relief of arthritic pain, the dose can be increased up to 1.1 mg/kg on an every-other-day schedule for another 10 to 14 days. If the patient responds to this dose, one should attempt to administer the drug every third day. If the discomfort returns, the previous schedule of every other day is resumed. For patients unresponsive to the previous treatment, a different drug should be selected. Approximately 2% of the 5% of patients that have an adverse effect from Arquel will never be able to tolerate the drug. Although vomiting can be an adverse reaction to Arquel, it has been a rare occurrence. When the tablet form of this drug

becomes available, its administration will be easier and the dosage more accurate.

Adverse effects. All the NSAIDs just mentioned have the potential for causing certain adverse effects, which include, but are not limited to, GI irritation, renal toxicity, platelet aggregation, and in the case of meclofenamic acid and phenylbutazone, hepatotoxicity. Therefore, one must be familiar with the patient's medical history and avoid using any of these drugs when they are contraindicated. In patients that require long-term therapy, certain laboratory tests, such as a hemogram, chemistry profile (especially liver and kidney studies), and urinalysis, should be done periodically. Owners must be advised of the potential adverse effects of any of these drugs and what to look for, such as melena, diarrhea, vomiting, or lethargy. If any adverse reaction is observed, the drug must be discontinued and the veterinarian contacted immediately. A reference describing the adverse effects, contraindications, drug interactions, and pharmacology of these drugs has been published.[125]

Several other NSAIDs are available for the treatment of osteoarthritis in humans but have not been approved for use in the dog. The disposition of NSAIDs in dogs, other than the ones previously mentioned, may differ greatly from that in humans; therefore, in the absence of evidence to the contrary, human dosages of NSAIDs should not be modified for use in dogs based on weight considerations.[79] Until further information regarding the pharmacology of the newer NSAIDs in dogs is available, the clinical use of these drugs should be avoided.[69]

Corticosteroids. Corticosteroids such as prednisone and prednisolone have been used frequently over the years for treating osteoarthritis in dogs. They are potent and effective antiinflammatory drugs that often provide quick relief from the discomfort caused by the pathologic changes of an arthritic joint. They are most useful in the treatment of inflammatory joint disease associated with immune-mediated polyarthritis (see Chapter 21). Corticosteroids should not be used simultaneously with any of the ulcerogenic drugs (e.g., NSAIDs) because this may increase the risk of GI ulceration.[125]

The overall adverse effects of long-term parenteral and oral administration of corticosteroids are well known.[125] The intraarticular administration of corticosteroids has been used for the treatment of degenerative joint disease in both animals and humans.[20] Only those corticosteroids specifically manufactured for intraarticular administration, such as Depo-Medrol (Upjohn Co., Kalamazoo, Mich), should be used for this purpose. Abundant evidence in the literature describes the various deleterious effects of corticosteroids on articular cartilage after single or multiple intraarticular administrations.* Experimental studies in the

---

*References 2, 97, 98, 101, 106, 107.

rabbit have shown that articular cartilage ultrastructure was minimally affected by a single dose of corticosteroids; however, biochemical changes in the cartilage were obvious.[10] In articular cartilage that does not already have apparent morphologic changes, the biochemical alteration precedes histological and ultrastructural changes. Therefore, one intraarticular injection of a corticosteroid will temporarily alter the cartilage biochemistry; however, without repeated intraarticular corticosteroid injections, the cartilage biochemistry will return to normal in several weeks.

A study in rabbits showed that repeated administration of an intraarticular corticosteroid caused a decreased synthesis of proteoglycans, hastening cartilage destruction that resembles chondromalacia.[97] The term *Charcot arthropathy* has been applied to the steroid-induced degeneration of articular cartilage in weight-bearing joints.[156] Although corticosteroids may induce a Charcot arthropathy in otherwise healthy articular cartilage, the arthropathy is enhanced if the articular cartilage is already damaged from preexisting osteoarthritis. Not only chronic intraarticular administration of corticosteroids, but also chronic parenteral administration of these drugs, have been proved to cause cartilage matrix degeneration and progression of osteoarthritis.[10,98,101,106,107]

A major precaution when considering the use of intraarticular steroids is to make sure the joint in question is not already infected. If infection is present, it would be greatly potentiated by the injection of corticosteroids. Although joint sepsis is a rare complication resulting from intraarticular corticosteroid administration, it does occur. Septic arthritis can be life-threatening to the patient or can have disastrous effects on the joint. It usually results from the deposition of skin bacteria into the joint space via the needle. The skin over the joint must be aseptically prepared, and aseptic injection technique is essential. It must not be done if the skin over the joint is not normal.

Because of the chronic nature of the degenerative osteoarthritis, such as that occurring in dogs with hip dysplasia, posttraumatic injury to the hip joint, or primary degenerative osteoarthritis, corticosteroids are not the long-term drugs of choice. It may be necessary to use them as a last resort when NSAIDs or other drugs have been ineffective and the quality of the dog's life is worsening. Although the continuous use of corticosteroids is not usually recommended in the treatment of degenerative osteoarthritis of the hip joint, it may be necessary when the owner does not consent to surgery or the patient's general health prevents surgery. When corticosteroids are used, the drug's lowest effective dose should be administered. Repeated intraarticular injection of the hip joint with corticosteroids should be limited to only those patients with severe osteoarthritis, when surgery is not possible, and when other antiarthritic drugs are not

effective in providing the patient a reasonably pain-free hip joint.

Polysulfated glycosaminoglycans. A polysulfated glycosaminoglycan, Adequan (Lutipold Pharmaceuticals, Inc., Animal Health Division, Shirley, NY), is being advocated by some veterinarians for use in treating osteoarthritis in dogs with hip dysplasia. Its experimental use in a dog stifle arthritis model has shown that it does have a chondroprotective effect on articular cartilage.[2,3,50] Other studies in both rabbits and dogs have also shown that intramuscular (IM) injection of Adequan has a chondroprotective effect on articular cartilage subjected to various types of trauma.[27,45,46,50,62] Adequan is known to retard the catabolic process in articular cartilage, decrease joint inflammation, and increase synovial fluid viscosity. It is a potent enzyme inhibitor. It is essential that viable articular cartilage is present in the joint for this drug to be effective.

The results from all experimental work using osteoarthritis animal models have shown that the glycosaminoglycan polysulfuric acid ester reduces cartilage breakdown. The exact mechanism for the beneficial effect is still being studied, but chondrocyte regulation or inhibition of degradative mechanisms may be involved.[3] The beneficial effect probably is achieved from multiple actions on or within the articular cartilage. The dose of Adequan has varied from 1 to 4 mg/kg, the frequency of IM administration has been either once or twice weekly, and the reported duration of administration also has varied. In one study, beagle dogs were treated for 6 months.[15] No adverse or toxic reactions to Adequan have been reported.

In another study, two groups of pups susceptible to hip dysplasia received IM Adequan from 6 weeks to 8 months of age. One group received 2.5 mg/kg twice weekly, and the other received 5 mg/kg twice weekly. A third untreated control group of 6-week-old pups also susceptible to hip dysplasia received saline injections for the same period.[95]

Radiographic evaluation of coxofemoral joint congruity, with the dogs positioned in the standard hip-extended position and using the Norberg angle of measurement, revealed significant improvement in the treated groups. Hip joint laxity was also measured using a distraction method during the radiographic evaluation.[163] The distraction technique revealed no significant difference in hip joint laxity between the treated and control groups. The fibronectin content of femoral head articular cartilage was less in the treated groups compared with the untreated group. At necropsy, the joint pathology scores indicated a trend toward improvement in the treated versus the untreated groups, but the overall scores were not statistically significant. The proteoglycan content in the femoral head articular cartilage was not different in treated and untreated dogs. The exact mechanism of action of the polysulfated glycosaminoglycan in this study remains unknown.[95]

Further studies using Adequan in pups genetically prone to develop hip dysplasia appear to be warranted. In addition, further well-documented studies on the clinical use of Adequan in the treatment of young and adult dogs with hip joint osteoarthritis associated with hip dysplasia are needed.

Other medical regimens. Vitamin C has been recommended as a preventive treatment for canine hip dysplasia. One report stated that vitamin C administered to pregnant females and their offspring until they were 18 to 24 months of age was effective in preventing hip dysplasia.[12] Data on blood and tissue levels of vitamin C and follow-up radiographic studies were not included in the report. At this time, no controlled scientific data are available to show a definite cause-and-effect relationship between vitamin C and the prevention of hip dysplasia.[12,13] Over the years, numerous other vitamin, mineral, and chemotherapeutic agents (e.g., selenium, vitamin E, orgotein) have been used in the treatment of osteoarthritis in the dog with hip dysplasia. Although the clinical signs may improve in some patients after use of these drugs, the improvement is at best temporary. The clinical signs recur as the regenerative process in the joints continues.

Another medical treatment for canine hip dysplasia is a form of physical therapy done daily on pups with excess hip joint laxity from 6 to 16 weeks of age.[3] The manipulation, applied to each hip 100 times a day, consisted of properly placing the pup on its back, properly positioning the femurs, and manipulating them in a way that forced the femoral heads deep into the acetabulum. Reportedly, most pups would have clinical relief from pain in 1 month. Although this type of therapy was reported to be successful, no data correlated clinical findings with the degree of joint laxity through radiographic evidence of normal or dysplastic hips at the end of the therapy or when the patients reached adulthood. The effect on promoting normal development of the hip joint was not documented.

A dysplasia-prone hip joint can develop into a normal joint, but this requires full congruity between the femoral head and acetabulum for several weeks. In the human infant, this has been done by placing the legs in an abduction-flexion position using diapers or a brace. This would not be applicable in the canine patient. It has been shown that by confining the young dog to a small cage (1 m³), where the dog spends most of its time sitting on its haunches (abduction-flexion position), the development of hip dysplasia may be prevented in the young canine genetically predisposed.[149] This is not a recommended method for treating hip dysplasia.

The medical treatment programs previously described have played and will continue to play a very important role in managing patients with hip dysplasia. Medical treatment is frequently selected because the owner will not allow or cannot afford the surgical procedure that is best indicated for the patient at the time. The owner must be informed about the progression of degenerative joint disease associated with conservative management of the dysplastic patient.

Because the initial joint laxity and associated abnormal biomechanical forces in hip joints lead to articular cartilage degeneration and osteoarthritis, medical management of these patients with various drugs may become ineffective at some point in the patient's life. When this occurs, surgical management may provide the patient with a good quality of life free of hip pain and with functional hip joint(s).

Surgical Treatment

The main reasons for performing surgery on dysplastic patients are (1) to relieve pain, (2) to return the patient to as near-normal functional use of the limb as possible, and (3) to prevent or significantly reduce the progressive degenerative osteoarthritic changes that begin in the unstable hip joints of young dogs.

The most frequently used surgical procedures for treating patients with hip dysplasia include excision of the femoral head and neck, pectineus tenonectomy or myectomy (partial or complete), triple pelvic osteotomy, intertrochanteric osteotomy, and total hip replacement. Another surgical procedure advocated by some surgeons is the biocompatible osteoconductive polymer (BOP) shelf arthroplasty. Clinical and research studies are being done at various universities and surgical practices to evaluate the efficacy of this technique. To select the proper surgical procedure for treating the dysplastic patient the surgeon must (1) understand the advantages, disadvantages, indications, and contraindications of the various surgical procedures; (2) know regional hip anatomy; (3) understand the biomechanics of normal and dysplastic hips; and (4) know abnormal hip joint pathology. With this information the surgeon can select the surgical procedure that is most suited for a given patient.

Excision of the femoral head and neck. This procedure, also referred to as *excision arthroplasty,* was first reported as a treatment for dogs with hip dysplasia in 1961.[117,165] It was described for treating unilateral osteoarthritis of the hip joint in humans by Girdlestone in 1945.[44] Since 1961, studies on its use and on modifications for treating painful disorders of the hip joint in both the dog and the cat have been reported.* Excision of the

---

*References 14, 19, 21, 34, 38-40, 42, 44, 51, 73, 77, 80-83, 96, 99, 117, 124, 142, 153, 165, 168, 171, 180.

femoral head and neck is a salvage procedure that relies on the formation of a scar tissue joint. The abnormal ball-and-socket joint is sacrificed to eliminate pain and preserve or improve limb function.

Indications. Indications for excision arthroplasty include (1) hip dysplasia, (2) LCPD, (3) nonreparable fractures of the acetabulum or femoral head, (4) degenerative joint disease (osteoarthritis) that is unresponsive to medical treatment, (5) chronic recurring hip luxations, (6) osteomyelitis and septic arthritis of the hip,[153] and (7) villinodular synovitis of the hip joints.[73]

The expected result of surgery is a functional pseudoarthrosis. Therefore the hip weight-bearing load in a patient with an excision arthroplasty is eventually supported by a thick, fibrous, false joint and surrounding muscles. Patients also shift weight to the opposite hip and to the front limbs, placing more stress on the thoracolumbar spine. When considering this procedure, one must carefully evaluate the patient for evidence of facet joint osteoarthritis, especially in the thoracolumbar and lumbosacral regions. Patients with facet joint osteoarthritis, especially if they are older and overweight, can be expected to have more difficulty in the early convalescent period.

Several general factors must be considered when selecting a patient for this surgical procedure. They include, but are not limited to, the following:

1. *Body size.* Excellent results are usually achieved in cats and toy and miniature breeds of dogs. Good to excellent results are normally found in dogs weighing up to 22 kg (48½ pounds). Dogs weighting more than 22 kg should not be ruled out for this procedure, but the results are less predictable. Excision arthroplasty has been successfully done in both the equine and the bovine species.[51,171] Although data have indicated no difference in the success rate of excision arthroplasty between large and small breeds,[80,168] larger dogs can be expected to be less active and have weaker rear limbs when functioning with a pseudoarthrosis than with a normal hip joint.
2. *Patient temperament.* Active patients that adapt to the surgery and therapy generally recover more quickly than those who are sedentary, obese, and unable to adapt.
3. *Patient age.* Younger patients in good physical condition respond faster and function better than middle-age and older patients.
4. *Obesity.* In general, overweight patients have a more difficult rehabilitation period. Many obese patients are sedentary, and extensive therapy by the owner is frequently required to get them to use the operated limb. All obese patients should be put on a postoperative weight reduction program.
5. *Chronicity of the disease.* A patient with longstanding painful osteoarthritis of the hip joint has disuse muscle atrophy in the affected limb(s). These patients require extensive physical therapy to get them to use the limb and rebuild muscle strength.
6. *Concurrent musculoskeletal problems.* Patients who have other muscle, tendon, or ligament problems or osteoarthritis in other major weight-bearing joints have more difficulty during recovery.
7. *Owner considerations.* It is important to inform the owner how a patient may function after surgery. The owner should be aware the patient may not perform the same or have the same endurance as with a normal hip joint. The owner must be willing to perform any necessary physical therapy.
8. *Need for unilateral or bilateral excision arthroplasty.* In the best of circumstances, patients will have a functional false joint if the opposite hip joint is normal. Some hunting dogs with an excision arthroplasty have returned to satisfactory hunting activities when the opposite hip was normal. Larger patients have a more difficult time with bilateral excision arthroplasties. Rear limbs fatigue with exercise faster after bilateral procedures.

Procedure. The surgical approaches to the hip joint include craniolateral, dorsal, caudal, and ventral.[153] The approach used will vary depending on the reason for the excision arthroplasty and the surgeon's preference. For LCPD and hip dysplasia, the craniolateral approach to the hip joint is typically used. A partial tenotomy of the deep gluteal muscle's tendon of insertion may be necessary for proper exposure. Extreme caution must be used in placing retractors on or around the biceps femoris muscle caudally and dorsally to the hip joint to avoid injury to the sciatic nerve. The joint capsule incision runs from the acetabular rim parallel to the femoral neck and continues around the neck at the capsule's insertion. A periosteal elevator removes muscle fibers, thus exposing of the neck's base and the lesser trochanter. The ligament of the femoral head is severed if it is intact. The limb is rotated outward 90 degrees, exposing the femoral head and neck for an accurate osteotomy and using either a sharp osteotome and mallet or an oscillating bone saw. The line of the cut for the osteotomy should extend ventrally from where the neck joins the femur's medial wall and should continue to the medial portion of the greater trochanter (Fig. 17-6). When using an osteotome, the cut for the excision should never be started dorsally on the femoral neck and directed ventrally, since this may split the femoral shaft.

If the cut is started too far proximal on the neck, a sharp bony protrusion of the femoral neck will remain and impinge on the dorsal rim of the acetabulum, causing pain and loss of limb function in the postoperative period. The entire excision site is inspected after the cut to make sure the cut is smooth and no portion of the neck is left. Irregularities must be removed. Leaving a portion of the

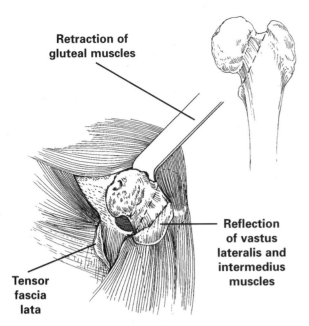

Fig. 17-6   Osteotomy line for an excision arthroplasty (*dashed line*) should extend from the trochanter's medial edge to the most ventral point where the femoral neck joins the medial femoral shaft. When the craniolateral approach is used, the femur is rotated 90 degrees and the vastus lateralis muscle is elevated from its origin to expose the site of osteotomy.

femoral neck is the most common reason for failure to achieve good postoperative function.[19] Large osteophytes on the acetabulum should also be removed.

After the excision procedure has been completed, the limb is placed in a normal position and the proximal femur moved through complete ROM. If evidence of bone-on-bone contact is felt, the excision site must be reinspected. With the limb in normal position, the hip is pushed dorsally, causing the excision site to pass over the acetabulum. If there is interference from a bony protuberance, it must be removed. Suturing the joint capsule over the acetabulum is up to the surgeon's preference.

Some surgeons interpose various soft tissue structures between the proximal femur and the acetabulum. This is done as a final step in the procedure. Some authors have reported obtaining better postoperative results if soft tissue is interposed between the acetabulum and the excision site on the femur.[14,83] However, experimental studies have reported no objective difference in postoperative results with interposition of soft tissues compared with no interposition.[77] Other authors have observed a more rapid return to active use of the limb but generally no difference in long-term results when the deep gluteal muscle pedicle is used.[19] Author Wallace prefers the use of the biceps femoris muscle sling procedure.[83] Care must be taken to identify the sciatic nerve so that it will not be injured when cutting the muscle or entrapped when applying the sling around the proximal femur.

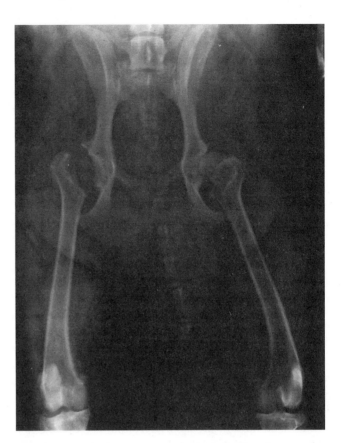

Fig. 17-7   Immediate postoperative radiographs after excision arthroplasty of the dog in Fig. 17-5.

Postoperative radiographs should always be taken to document the position of the osteotomy (Fig. 17-7). If too much femoral neck is left or irregularities are present, the patient should be immediately returned to surgery for removal of the unwanted bone.

Postoperative care. The patient is encouraged to use the limb as soon as possible after surgery. Physical therapy is started the day after surgery and may be essential for return of functional limb use. Physical therapy consists of 35 to 50 slow flexion-extension-abduction exercises two or three times a day until limb use is satisfactory. During the first 10 to 14 postoperative days, an aspirin product (e.g., Ascriptin, 10 to 25 mg/kg) may be given 1 hour before the physical therapy. Owners must be advised that initial discomfort may be associated with the physical therapy, which should lessen over 2 weeks. Swimming is an excellent exercise for rehabilitation after suture removal.

Patients must not be allowed to become overweight. Those who are overweight at surgery should be put on a weight reduction program, then a weight control program once they have attained the proper weight.

The more disuse muscle atrophy present in the affected limb at surgery, the longer it will take to regain functional use of the limb. Patients who have had this surgery done for hip dysplasia or LCPD may bear some weight when standing or walking very slowly within a few days after surgery. Gradual improvement should be observed over 3 to 4 months, when the patient may have regained use of the limb without a limp. Some patients may not regain functional use of the limb for 6 or 8 months or more after surgery. Regaining functional use of the limb depends on a properly done surgical procedure, diligent physical therapy, and the amount of disuse muscle atrophy in the affected limb. Patients failing to make progressive improvement after this surgery must be carefully examined. If infection is suspected, a deep aspirate for culture should be taken from the surgical site. Radiographs should always be taken to determine if any bony spurs have developed or if other abnormalities are present.

The surgical limb will be functionally shorter than the nonsurgical limb. The operated proximal femur will be displaced higher relative to the pelvis than the unoperated limb. As a result, some patients will extend the stifle and hock of the operated limb more than normal. A pain response should not be obtained during physical examination once the scar tissue joint has completely developed. Smaller breeds usually have less gait changes than larger breeds.

When this surgery is needed on both hip joints, the one causing the patient the most pain should be operated on first. Once the patient is bearing weight on that limb, the second hip can be done. Generally, it is not recommended to do this surgery on both hips at the same time.

Pectineus tendon surgery. The pectineus muscle originates from the pubic bone's iliopectineal eminence and extends distally just beyond where a muscular branch of the femoral artery and vein crosses its medial surface. Approximately 0.5 to 1.0 cm distal to this vascular bundle, the tenomuscular junction is found in most dogs, where the tendon of insertion continues to its attachment on the distal femur. The pectineus muscle and its tendon of insertion lie between the adductor magnus et brevis muscle caudally and the vastus medialis muscle cranially.

Procedure. The patient is positioned in dorsal recumbency. The femurs are secured perpendicular to the midline, making the pectineus muscles easily palpated and/or seen. Improper positioning makes the pectineus muscles more difficult to identify and increases the risk of surgical iatrogenic injury to the femoral artery or vein. The patient is aseptically draped, isolating both pectineal muscles.

The skin incision is started about 3.0 cm above where the vessels cross the muscle belly and continues about 4.0 cm distal to the vascular bundle. The distal belly of the pectineus muscle, vascular bundle, and tenomuscular junction are exposed. A curved Kelly forceps is passed cranially between the pectineus tendon of insertion and the vastus medialis muscle, under the tendon and between the adductor muscle and pectineus tendon caudally. The sur-

geon avoids incorporating the femoral artery and vein with the forceps. The Kelly forceps brings the muscle belly and proximal end of the tendon into view. The tendon is clamped with two Kelly forceps about 1.0 cm apart. The tendon is cut between the two forceps. The small part of tendon of insertion left on the muscle belly is sutured to the muscle (Fig. 17-8). The remaining tissues are closed in layers, and the procedure is repeated on the opposite limb.

If only a tenotomy was performed, a fibrotic reattachment of the severed ends is possible. If this reattachment occurs, relief of pain is only temporary, with a return of the original clinical signs in 3 to 12 weeks. Using the technique of suturing the tendon of insertion to the pectineus muscle belly has eliminated any reattachment of the tendon's severed ends.

Postoperative care. Owners are advised to keep their dog's activity restricted on a short hand-held leash when outside for the first 14 days after surgery. After that time, regular activity can resume. During the first 10 to 12 days

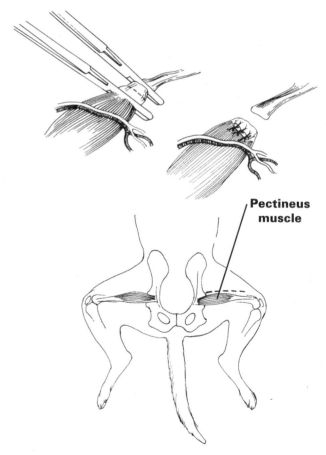

Fig. 17-8 With the dog placed in ventral recumbency in the frog-leg position, both pectineus muscles can be operated on at the same time. A section of the tendon is isolated between two forceps and severed. The portion of the tendon of insertion left with the muscle belly is folded back on the muscle and sutured in place.

after surgery, the owner should check the incision sites daily for any evidence of seroma formation or infection. If a seroma develops but is not too large, activity restriction alone allows the seroma to reabsorb within 14 to 21 days. If a seroma becomes extremely large, aseptic aspiration may be necessary.

Results. This procedure is not a cure for hip dysplasia; its objective is to relieve pain. Tendon surgery has been highly successful in meeting this objective. It is believed relief of pain results from a combination of releasing the tension on the joint capsule and an increased range of abduction. The tension on the joint capsule is created by the upward force on the joint from the tense pectineus muscle. The increased abduction of the femur allows the femoral head to articulate better within the acetabulum. Thus, there is improved weight loading of femoral head articular cartilage within the acetabulum. Some pain relief may also result from the release of tension on the pectineus muscle itself.

With the techniques just described, there is less risk of fibrotic reattachment of the tendon's severed ends, and the incidence of seroma formation is decreased. Several different surgical techniques have been developed, including tenotomy of the tendons of origin or insertion, tenectomy of the tendon of insertion, tenomyectomy, and myotomy or total myectomy of the pectineus muscle. Either a partial or a complete pectineus myectomy or tenomyectomy can be performed with good results when the proper technique is used. Muscle hemorrhage must be controlled, and

seroma formation may occur more frequently than with a tenectomy at the tendon of insertion. A myotomy of the pectineus muscle by itself is not recommended because fibrotic reattachment of the muscle's severed ends is likely and muscle hemorrhage is prevalent.

Pectineus surgery usually will not restore normal gait. In many affected dogs, sufficient pathological and remodeling changes are present in the femoral head and acetabulum, and thus abnormal gait persists even when hip pain is alleviated. Young dogs (5 to 6 months of age) have developed a normal or near-normal gait after surgery; however, this cannot be predicted or expected.

After pectineus tendon surgery, many dogs clinically affected with dysplasia have shown one or more of the following improvements: increased activity, increased abduction of the rear limbs, relief of hip pain, improved ability in rising to a standing position from sternal or lateral recumbency, increased ease in getting in or out of a motor vehicle and in going up and down stairs, improved disposition, and ability to hunt for longer intervals.

None of the surgical procedures on the pectineus tendon or muscle stabilize the hip joint. Therefore the degenerative changes of osteoarthritis will continue even though the patient is clinically improved (Fig. 17-9). Since the degenerative changes in the hip will progress, lameness and hip pain may recur. The time of recurrence of the hip pain and lameness is unpredictable and may take months or years. Many patients have gone 5 to 6 years before recurrence of lameness from the hip pain.

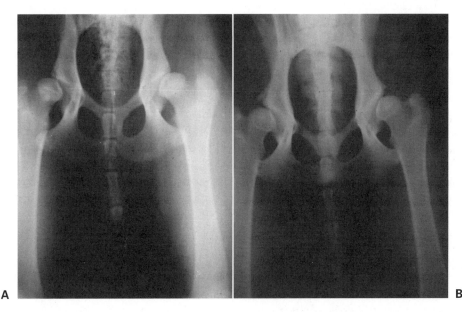

Fig. 17-9 **A,** Ventrodorsal radiographs of a 6-month-old Labrador retriever at the time bilateral pectineus tendonectomy was performed for pain associated with hip dysplasia. **B,** Even though the osteoarthritis has progressed in this dog, as shown by these radiographs taken 14 months after surgery, the dog's activity levels are normal and no pain was detected on manipulation of the hip joints.

BOP shelf arthroplasty

Clinical reports. This procedure has been described as a surgical treatment for canine hip dysplasia.[65,66,155] The procedure uses a co-polymer referred to as *biocompatible osteoconductive polymer* (BOP). It is composed of two monomers, homopolymers *N*-vinyl-pyrrolidine and methylmethacrylate, in combination with calcium gluconate and polysemide-6 fibers to form BOP-F, the fiber form. Under heat and pressure, the fibers are formed into BOP-B, the block or solid form.[158] It has been reported to be biocompatible and osteoconductive, with a molecular weight of 80,000 daltons, and acts as a scaffold for bone ingrowth or osteoconduction. The BOP-B and BOP-F are reported to be partially degradable by hydrolysis, allowing for ingrowth of bony tissue or osteoconduction.[66] The procedure requires creation of a hole in the caudal ilium and dorsal aspect of the acetabulum for placement of the BOP block and BOP fibers, with the intent of creating a shelf over the cranial and dorsal acetabulum. Autogenous cancellous bone harvested from the ilium is packed between the BOP fibers.

The principal objective of the BOP graft in the treatment of hip dysplasia is to form an extension or shelf over the shallow acetabulum. The new bony complex is supposed to improve the lever arm effect of the abductor muscles, thus increasing medial vector loads on the femoral head and decreasing cranial dorsal loads. Supporters of the procedure report that the improved seating of the femoral head decreases subluxation and luxation of the femoral head, reduces stretching of the joint capsule, and subsequently eliminates or reduces pain in the joint. Those animals with significant degenerative osteoarthritis but without instability are not considered candidates for the BOP shelf arthroplasty because the procedure's purpose is to improve stability.[66]

One report provides data on 105 patients with 200 surgically treated hips.[66] Patients ranged from age 6 months to 11 years, with an average age of 18 months. This study's authors recommend that, because of decreased osteogenic ability in older dogs, patients older than 5 years should not be considered for this procedure. The report provides data on follow-up evaluations on 67 dogs from 3 to 48 months postoperatively, with a reported high success rate. Minor complications were reported in 4.5% of the patients (sciatic neuropraxia, broken screws, seromas). Serious complications attributable to infection with chronic draining tracts, which did not respond to antibiotic therapy, were reported in 2.5% of the hips.[66]

Experimental studies. The use of the BOP material in the shelf arthroplasty procedure has created much controversy and has been the subject of controlled research studies.[29,86,109,170] One study was designed to evaluate the biocompatibility and osteoconductive properties of the synthetic BOP implant over 6 months.[170] Based on the results of this study, it was concluded that BOP was not osteoconductive within 6 months when implanted without the addition of cancellous bone in femoral subtrochanteric defects or when placed extraperiosteally on the proximal portion of the humerus of clinically normal dogs.[29] Although the BOP fibers were infiltrated by fibrovascular connective tissue, bone did not incorporate the BOP material. The physical presence of BOP fibers appeared to impede healing of the bone defects. No evidence exists to suggest the BOP fiber is biocompatible. It was concluded that although the BOP block was not osteoconductive, it may be considered biocompatible, unlike the BOP fiber.[170]

A 3-month study in dogs evaluated the formation of new bone in a standardized fracture gap model, which involved the installation of no material, autogenous cancellous bone alone, BOP plus autogenous cancellous bone, and BOP alone.[29] Untreated and autogenous cancellous bone–grafted defects had a cortical union at 3 months. Defects treated with BOP alone or with the combination of BOP plus autogenous cancellous bone did not heal in the same period. Histomorphometric analysis showed that less new bone was produced in ostectomies treated with BOP plus autogenous cancellous bone or with BOP alone. Data analysis indicated a possible inhibitory effect of BOP on new bone formation.[170]

One investigation evaluated the osteointegration of BOP at the site of the BOP shelf arthroplasty in normal dogs over a 39-month period.[158] Minimal mineralization of the shelf was noted by radiography at 26 and 39 weeks postoperatively. A moderate to large amount of mature fibrous connective tissue was observed around the BOP fibers. Bone growth occurred around the BOP fibers but was minimal between them. The results of this study suggest that either the BOP has no osteoconductive properties or the purported osteoconductive properties are overwhelmed by a simultaneous foreign body reaction. The investigators did not observe sufficient osteoconduction of BOP in the location of the shelf arthroplasty to encourage its use in the treatment of canine hip dysplasia.[158]

Another experimental study evaluated the BOP shelf arthroplasty procedure on dysplastic dogs.[109] Ten young dogs with bilateral hip joint laxity were evaluated before surgery based on lameness assessment, hip joint palpation, manual goniometry, thigh circumference measurements, standard ventrodorsal radiographs, and coxofemoral distraction pelvic radiographic studies. A BOP shelf arthroplasty was done on the right hip, and a "sham" procedure was done on the left hip. The same evaluations just listed were repeated on these dogs at specific periods from 1 to 52 weeks postoperatively. The only parameter that differed between the right and left hips was periarticular bone, which was significantly greater in the right hip. However, no dog developed a large, bony shelf. At necropsy, all BOP implants were in their original position, encapsulated by fibrous tissue. Radiographs showed complete healing of the periarticular slot on the left side but no evidence of healing on the right side. No evidence indicated that the BOP shelf arthroplasty alters the progression of hip dysplasia in young dogs.[109]

Based on the data reported from all these studies, the BOP material does not appear to be osteoconductive and may impede bone formation in the defect where it is placed. Evidence from one study indicates that the BOP fiber is not biocompatible.[61] Although the BOP shelf arthroplasty is intended to enhance joint stability, the loading forces on the articular cartilage of the femoral head and acetabulum remain abnormal (Fig. 17-10). Therefore, progression of the hip joint osteoarthritis can be expected and was reported to occur in the clinical and research studies.

Triple pelvic osteotomy. The first published report describing pelvic osteotomy as a treatment for canine hip dysplasia appeared in 1969.[61] Since then, other studies have used similar or significantly modified techniques to perform canine pelvic osteotomies.[59,152,154,159-162,169] In children an innominate osteotomy was reported in 1961 and 1966 for the treatment of congenital subluxation of the hip.[143,144] Triple osteotomy on the pelvis for correction of dislocated or subluxated femoral heads in older people was reported in 1973 and 1977.[166,167]

The triple pelvic osteotomy procedure consists of separate osteotomies on the pubis, ischium, and ilium. This creates a free acetabular segment that can be rotated over the femoral head with the objective of increasing hip joint stability (Fig. 17-11). The acetabular rotation is maintained using a specifically designed bone plate to fix the ilial osteotomy. The two more frequently used bone plates are the triple pelvic osteotomy plate (Synthes, Paoli, Pa) (Fig. 17-12) and the Slocum canine pelvic osteotomy plate (Slocum Enterprises, Eugene, Ore). Another technique for triple pelvic osteotomy without bone plates requires a step cut of the ilium. After the acetabulum has been rotated, the ilium is fixed in position using a screw and wire.[152,154]

The triple pelvic osteotomy is suited for treating the young, growing dog with clinical and radiographic signs of hip dysplasia and no radiographic evidence of osteoarthritis. By reestablishing normal function of the hip joint in these patients, the prognosis is excellent for full activity. Age, however, is not a limiting factor for selecting the patient for this surgery. This procedure can be done on dogs as early as 4 months of age and on into adulthood. The main limiting factor in performing a triple pelvic osteotomy is the degree of degenerative osteoarthritis and remodeling changes present in the hip joint. Patients with severe osteoarthritis are not candidates for the surgery.

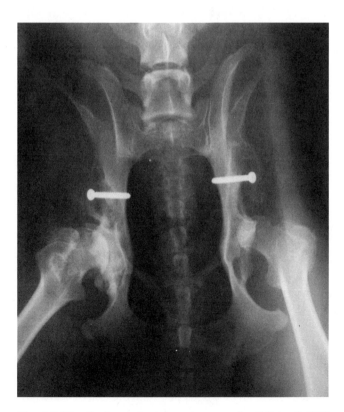

Fig. 17-10 Radiographs taken 4 years after bilateral BOP shelf arthroplasty was performed on a Labrador retriever. In addition to severe osteoarthritis in both hip joints, both ilial shafts exhibit a significant periosteal reaction.

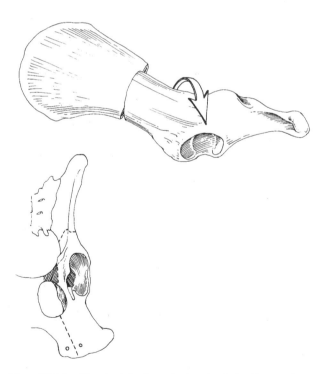

Fig. 17-11 Hemipelvis is osteotomized in three places (ilium, pubis, ischium) to create a free pelvic segment containing the acetabulum. This segment is rotated to increase coverage of the femoral head. The segment will be stabilized in the rotated position with a special bone plate. Two holes have been drilled in the ischial segment on either side of the osteotomy for the wire used to stabilize this bone.

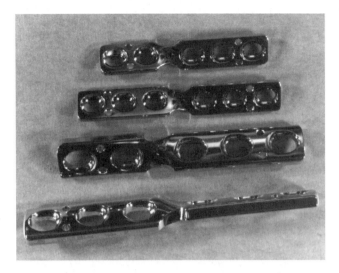

Fig. 17-12 Triple pelvic osteotomy plate shown here comes as either a 2.7 mm or 3.5 mm plate with either five or six Dynamic Compression Holes. The plate is twisted in the center at a 45-degree angle. Two small holes are present near the ends of the plates, through which orthopedic wire can be passed to help secure the plate to the bone.

However, patients with mild osteoarthritis in their hips have a reasonable prognosis, as long as there is good contour of the femoral head, adequate depth of the acetabulum, and no osteophyte formation around the femoral head or acetabulum. Patients with mild osteoarthritis must be carefully evaluated. In addition to standard hip radiographic views, the frog-leg view and dorsal acetabular rim view[162] may be helpful in determining the full extent of their osteoarthritis. The combination of hip palpation and radiographic correlation is essential when evaluating patients for this surgery.

Besides the presence of preexisting osteoarthritis, other contraindications to a triple pelvic osteotomy include a neurological deficit involving hip muscles and significant coxa valga; however, a patient with the latter condition may be a candidate for intertrochanteric osteotomy.

Once the diagnosis of hip dysplasia has been made, it is important to do the surgery as soon as possible to prevent further deterioration of the hip joint. This is especially true in immature dogs, in whom abnormal forces acting in or on the joint may induce rapid remodeling and degenerative changes. The second hip should be operated on as soon as possible after the first surgery, since it is subject to increased loading forces after the first hip has been treated.

Procedure. The entire rear limb is clipped on all sides from the hock joint proximally to include the entire inguinal region medially and over the dorsal midline laterally from the base of the tail cranial to the ilial wing. The patient is placed in lateral recumbency and draped to allow surgical approaches ventrally to the pubis, caudally

to the ischium, and laterally to the ilium via a gluteal roll-up approach.

To osteotomize the pubic bone, the rear limb is abducted 90 degrees. A skin incision about 6 cm in length is made parallel to the ventral midline and centered over the iliopectineal eminence. The tendon of origin of the pectineus muscle is transected, allowing a clear view of the pubic bone. The obturator nerve is identified at the caudolateral aspect of the pubic bone to protect it. A 5 to 7 mm section of pubic bone medial to the acetabulum is removed using either a sharp osteotome or an oscillating saw. No extension of the pubic bone should be left attached to the medial side of the acetabulum. Any part of the pubic bone left attached on the acetabulum would be rotated into the pelvic canal and could impinge on the pelvic viscera. The pectineus muscle is left in its retracted position. The subcutaneous tissue and skin are closed in a routine manner. The limb then is returned to its normal position.

The osteotomy on the ischium is done from a caudal approach. A skin incision is made midway between the tuber ischii and the lateral border of the ischial arch. Another incision is made at the origin of the hamstring muscles, and the ventral ischium is exposed. The internal obturator muscle is elevated from the dorsal ischium to the obturator foramen. Using a small drill or intramedullary pin, two holes are made 1 cm cranial to the end of the ischium. One hole is made just lateral to the ischial arch, and the second is made 1.5 cm lateral to the first one. An orthopedic wire is preplaced through both holes. A loop of wire on the dorsal side of the ischium is left large enough to allow insertion of an index finger under the loop.

A sharp osteotome is placed on the caudal surface of the ischium and driven cranially with a mallet into the lateral edge of the obturator foramen. The osteotomy passes an equal distance between the holes containing the wire. The osteotomy is palpated with an index finger to make sure the entire ischium has been cut.

The lateral approach (gluteal roll-up approach) is used to for doing the osteotomy on the ilium.[153] The cranial gluteal nerve is protected. The ilium is exposed by elevation and dorsal retraction of the middle and deep gluteal muscles. The iliacus muscle on the ventral surface of the ilium immediately below the caudodorsal iliac spine is subperiosteally elevated for a distance of 1 to 1.5 cm. A sciatic nerve guard (Eickemeyer Co., Tuttlingen, Germany), used by author Wallace, is inserted from where the iliacus muscle was elevated, with its tip against the bone to the caudoventral aspect of the sacrum. The nerve guard is moved off the sacrum and advanced dorsally to a point caudal to the caudal iliac spine. The osteotomy will be perpendicular to an imaginary line from the tuber ischii to the ventral one half of the ilial wing and just caudal to the sacrum. An oscillating bone saw is used to make the ilial osteotomy.

A Kern bone-holding forceps is clamped on the dorsal and ventral ilial surfaces, and a second Kern forceps is applied to the ischium lateral to the wire. The bone-holding forceps is used to maintain axial rotation of the acetabulum over the femoral head at the position where a positive Ortolani sign is eliminated. If the acetabulum is rotated too far, it will interfere with hip abduction by impingement of the femoral neck on the dorsal acetabular rim. If the acetabulum is not rotated far enough, the hip joint will remain unstable and progressive osteoarthritis may occur. A pelvic osteotomy bone plate (Synthes) is contoured and applied to cranial and caudal ilial segments. These plates are manufactured with a 45-degree torque in their center. If a greater or lesser angle is required, it can be achieved with plate benders.

The small tip of bone on the dorsal surface of the ilium caudal to the osteotomy is removed so that it will not protrude into the middle gluteal muscle and be a source of postoperative discomfort. In younger dogs with softer bone, additional fixation of the plate to the ilial wing can be achieved by using orthopedic wire passed through a small hole in the plate. A hole is drilled through the ilium using the small hole in the plate as a guide. The wire is grasped with a forceps and pulled around the ventral side of the ilial wing. The wire is twisted tight, cut, and bent in against the bone. An autogenous cancellous bone graft may be harvested from the ilial wing and placed around the dorsolateral and ventrolateral aspects of the ilial osteotomy. All tissues and skin are closed in a routine manner.

The ischial osteotomy is fixed by drawing the preplaced wire tightly over the dorsal side of the ischium and twisting the wire ventrally. The wire will cut through soft bone if it is twisted too tightly. The deep tissues and the skin over the ischium are closed in a routine manner.

Postoperative care. The patient is to be kept on restricted activity until radiographic evidence shows the osteotomies are healed, usually in 6 to 8 weeks. The patient can go for short walks three or four times daily when restrained with a short hand-held leash. Stairs are to be avoided if possible. The second hip is generally operated on within 1 to 4 weeks after the first hip. Some surgeons perform surgery on both hips the same day. Almost all patients are bearing a slight amount of weight at a slow walk after recovery from anesthesia. Weight bearing on the limb should improve progressively. Full weight bearing without any limp is expected 8 to 12 weeks after surgery. Follow-up radiographs of the pelvis are taken immediately after surgery and at the sixth postoperative week or sooner depending on when the second hip is surgically treated (Fig. 17-13). Additional postoperative radiographs may be needed depending on what is seen on the 6-week radiographs. Radiographs at week 6 after surgery should reveal a femoral head well seated in the acetabulum and evidence of good healing at the osteotomy sites. On physical examination, the hip joint should be stable on palpation and nonpainful in all ranges of motion. Pain-free hip motion and increased activity levels, potentially for the animal's lifetime, are the expected results from this surgery. Some dogs exhibit a narrow-based gait because of the alterations in pelvic anatomy.

One study on triple pelvic osteotomies used force plate analysis.[102] The study included 15 dogs 6 to 13 months old with bilateral hip dysplasia. Force plate analysis was performed preoperatively and at 5, 10, 15, and 28 weeks postoperatively. Ten normal dogs served as controls. Young dysplastic dogs transmitted significantly less vertical force through the hip joints than normal dogs. The force transmitted through treated hips reached or approached that of the control animals by postoperative week 28, at which time clinical lameness was completely gone in 92% of the treated dogs.

Potential complications. Complications associated with the triple pelvic osteotomy occur infrequently provided soft tissues are handled carefully and the surgery is technically correct. Injury to the obturator, sciatic, and cranial gluteal nerves should be avoided. The sciatic nerve can potentially be injured by inappropriate placement of retractors or sawing or drilling through the ilium. All linear bone plates must be contoured to conform to the concave lateral surface of the ilium to prevent excessive narrowing of the pelvic canal. Constipation could result if the canal is narrowed. Dysuria is avoided if the pubic ramus is ostectomized correctly.

If plates are properly applied to the ilium, implant failure is infrequent. On occasion a screw(s) may loosen, but loss of axial rotation occurs infrequently. Screws loosen more often when wire fixation of the ischial osteotomy is not used. Failure of the owner to restrict the patient's activity during healing can lead to implant loosening.

Intertrochanteric osteotomy. Intertrochanteric osteotomy of the femur for treating canine hip dysplasia using the specially designed double hook plate (Synthes) was first described in 1980.[130] Several papers have reported on the use of this procedure for treating dogs with hip dysplasia.[17,18,128,129,173] The best long-term results can be expected when the procedure is used in patients without radiographic evidence of osteoarthritis. Patients who have advanced osteoarthritis of the hip joint with severe remodeling of the femoral head and acetabulum are better candidates for a total hip replacement or excision arthroplasty.

The surgical objective of intertrochanteric osteotomy is to reduce the angle of inclination of the femur from a coxa valga position to normal and to decrease the femoral anteversion angle to near a neutral position (Fig. 17-14). The femoral head will be seated deeper in the acetabulum, thus providing a more stable hip joint. The loading forces will be more evenly distributed over the

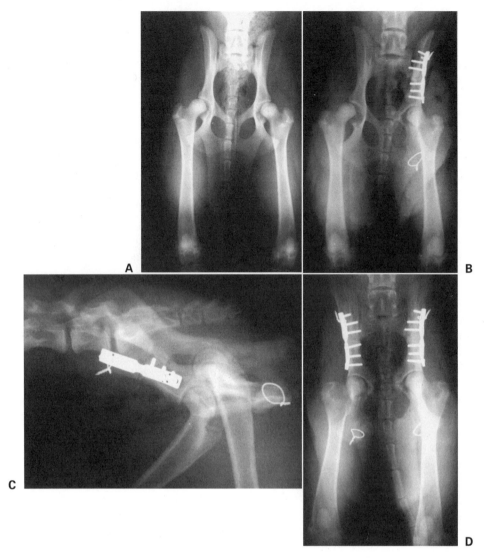

Fig. 17-13 **A,** Preoperative radiographs of a 6-month-old golden retriever with bilateral subluxation of both hips and no arthritic or structural changes in the joints. The dog was lame and had pain on palpation of each hip. **B,** Immediate postoperative ventrodorsal radiographs showing a triple pelvic osteotomy of the left hemipelvis. **C,** Immediate postoperative lateral radiographs of the same hip. **D,** Triple pelvic osteotomy was performed on the right side 3 weeks after the left side was done. These radiographs were taken 9 weeks after the first surgery.

articular cartilage of the acetabulum and femoral head than in the subluxated hip. This may stop or retard the progression of osteoarthritis. The desired angle of inclination with the intertrochanteric osteotomy is 135 degrees.[17] The anteversion angle of the femoral head and neck should be reduced to between 0 and 5 degrees. The femoral head and neck should not be placed in a position of retroversion.

Preoperative planning. When preparing to perform this procedure, some surgeons plan the osteotomy cuts to reduce the angle of inclination on paper before surgery. From ventrodorsal radiographic views of the pelvis that include extended femurs with the patellas centered in the trochlear groove, an outline of the proximal half of the femur is drawn on transparent paper. The angle of inclination is drawn on the paper and measured. From this, the size of bone wedge needed to be removed to reduce the angle of inclination to 135 degrees is determined. The paper tracing of the femur is cut out, and an appropriately sized paper wedge is removed at the intertrochanteric osteotomy site. The proximal and distal paper femoral segments are reduced, and the hook plate to be used in the surgery is contoured to fit the femur. These paper drawings can be used to serve as a guide during the surgery.

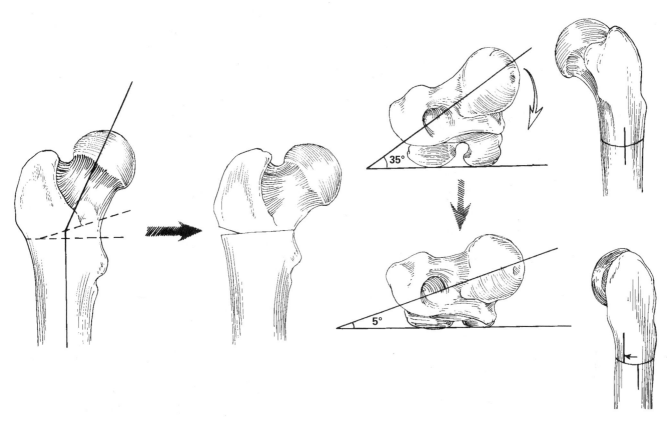

Fig. 17-14 The objective for the intertrochanteric osteotomy procedure is to decrease the femoral neck's angle of inclination and anteversion. This positions the femoral head deeper into the acetabulum. A wedge of bone is removed from the subtrochanteric area, and the proximal fragment is rotated caudally to accomplish this objective. The proximal femoral fragment is secured in its new position with a bone plate.

Procedure. A routine lateral approach to the proximal two thirds of the femur is made. The superficial gluteal muscle is incised at its insertion and reflected dorsally. The vastus lateralis muscle is incised at its origin and retracted cranially. The vastus lateralis and biceps femoris muscles are retracted away from the surgical site. The sciatic nerve is identified and protected.

To evaluate the degree of anteversion present, a small intramedullary pin is passed parallel to the cranial femoral neck and seated into the femoral head. The pin should move when the femur is rotated. The pin is cut at the level of the greater trochanter.

A drill guide specifically designed for this procedure is placed on the lateral aspect of the greater trochanter. A mark on the drill guide is aligned over the planned intertrochanteric osteotomy line. Two holes are drilled in the proximal trochanter through the two proximal drill sleeves in the drill guide. These holes will accommodate the plate's hooked portion. The guide is removed, and an osteotomy guide, which is anchored in the two previously drilled holes, is aligned over the osteotomy site. The osteotomy guide has an adjustable wing, and an angle scale on this wing is used to ensure that a bone wedge with the predetermined angles can be removed. With an oscillating saw guided by the wing, an intertrochanteric osteotomy is made perpendicular to the femoral long axis at the level of the lesser trochanter. The wing is adjusted to the predetermined angle, and the bone wedge is cut from the proximal fragment.

The osteotomy surfaces are held in reduction while the hook plate is applied to the femur's lateral side. The two hooks in the plate are inserted into the holes in the proximal trochanter. The proximal femoral segment is rotated using the pin placed in the femoral head as a marker until the anteversion angle is near 0 degrees. The plate is fixed laterally to the proximal and distal femoral segments with bone screws. Ideally, one of the screws in the distal segment should be placed across the fracture line into the femoral neck as a lag screw. The pin in the femoral head is removed after the plate is secured in place. The soft tissues and skin are closed in layers. Immediate postoperative radiographs are taken (Fig. 17-15).

Postoperative care. The owner is instructed to restrict the patient's activity for 8 weeks. During this period, the patient must always be outside on a short hand-held leash. During the first 2 weeks after surgery, the owner observes the surgical site daily for any evidence of swelling, drainage, or sutures being chewed out. Follow-up radiographs to

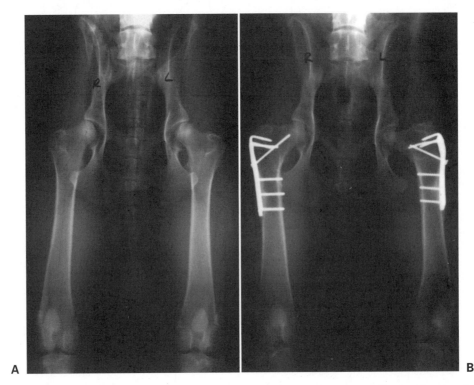

Fig. 17-15 **A,** Preoperative radiographs of a 15-month-old male German shepherd with subluxation of both femoral heads. The dog was lame and had pain on palpation of each hip. An intertrochanteric osteotomy was performed in each hip 2 months apart. **B,** Follow-up radiographs 29 months after the first surgery on the right femur.

evaluate osteotomy healing should be done at 8 weeks. When the opposite hip requires this surgery, the usual recommendation is that it be done 3 to 4 weeks after the first surgery.

Results. The ultimate goal of intertrochanteric osteotomy is to allow the patient to have pain-free function of the hip joints and to stop or slow the progression of osteoarthritis. This is accomplished by improving the biomechanical loading between the femoral head and acetabulum and decreasing the abnormal tension on the periarticular muscles.

Two retrospective studies have evaluated intertrochanteric osteotomies.[18,173] In one study of 183 dogs with follow-ups of 1 to 7 years, 89.6% were rated as having an excellent or good return to function. "Excellent" was defined as walking and running normally without pain for long distances. "Good" was defined as walking and running normally without pain but with a slight limp after exercise. Better results were obtained in dogs treated before radiographic evidence of osteoarthritis was present. Excellent results were found in 12.1% of the dogs with severe osteoarthritis, 45.8% with moderate osteoarthritis, and 51.4% with no osteoarthritis at surgery.[173]

The second retrospective study reported on 37 dogs with early-stage hip dysplasia that had 43 hip surgeries over 7 years. The dogs were evaluated on the basis of a questionnaire sent to the owners, an orthopedic examination of the patient, and/or a telephone conversation with the owner. For this study, "excellent" was defined as normal function and "good" as normal weight bearing with joint stiffness after strenuous exercise or a long rest. From the orthopedic examination, 82% (27 of 33 hips) were rated as good or excellent at 15 months after surgery.[18]

This study indicated patients benefited from the surgery for up to 3 years. Of the owners contacted, 91.6% (33 of 36) reported they would have the same surgery done again given the same circumstances. Although radiographic evidence of osteoarthritis continues to progress in the hip joints, patients may continue to function normally, and clinical signs of pain may be alleviated for many years.

Canine total hip replacement. In veterinary medicine a widely accepted prosthesis is available only for the canine hip joint. The hip joint is a simple ball-and-socket joint and has the easiest joint motion to duplicate with a prosthesis. It is also a joint often affected by disabling conditions, and thus a significant segment of the dog population needs treatment for a hip problem.

Since the mid 1970s, prosthetic canine hip joints have been very successfully used.* Since 1976, an ongoing

---

*References 35, 60, 76, 78, 100, 104, 111-115, 120.

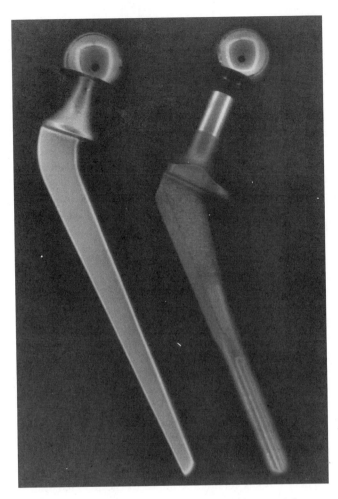

Fig. 17-16 Fixed-head femoral component and modular-system femoral stem and head of a prosthetic canine hip joint.

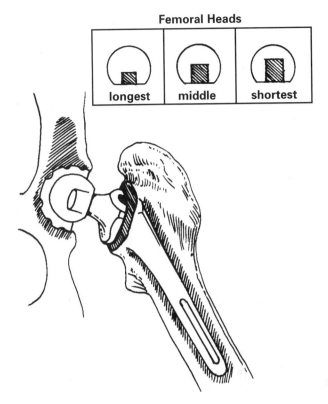

Fig. 17-17 Components of a modular hip replacement cemented into place in the acetabulum and femur. The femoral head, which is a separate piece from the femoral stem, is available with different depths of holes. The hole depth in the femoral head dictates the length of the femoral neck. The deepest hole gives the shortest neck, and the most shallow hole gives the longest neck.

Courtesy of BioMedtrix, Ltd.

prospective study has been performed at Ohio State University to evaluate the effectiveness of canine hip prosthesis.[111-115] In this study, more than 1800 prostheses have been implanted, establishing indications, contraindications, the most effective surgical technique, a complication rate, and long-term functional evaluation for canine total hip replacement. Until 1990 the prosthesis used in this study was a fixed-head system (Richards Medical Company, Memphis) comprised of a cobalt-chrome femoral component with a combined head, neck, and stem and a high-density polyethylene plastic cup for the acetabulum.

More recently, a newly designed modular system (BioMedtrix, Ltd., Allendate, NJ), which is made up of a stem, a separate cobalt-chrome femoral head, and a high-density polyethylene cup, is being used (Fig. 17-16). The first stems of the modular prosthesis were made of titanium (six aluminum, four vitallim) alloy, but since spring 1995 the stems are cobalt-chrome. These two systems were both secured in the patient's femur and acetabulum with polymethylmethacrylate (PMMA), or "bone cement."

Other surgeons have done work on various cementless prostheses, which have had short-term clinical results similar to results with cemented prostheses but are not yet commercially available.[35,104] Cementless prostheses are technically more demanding to implant than cemented prostheses.

The modular system has several advantages over the fixed-head system. In the modular system the femoral component is made of two separate pieces: a stem that is inserted in the femoral shaft and a head that is impacted onto the stem's neck portion. The hole in the head that the stem's neck inserts into is cut to three different depths. This allows three different neck lengths to be achieved with each prosthesis (Fig. 17-17). The proper neck length is determined by using plastic trial heads on the stem before the implantable cobalt-chrome head is impacted.

The head and neck have a locking taper design. When the head is properly impacted on the neck, the head locks in place and is capable of resisting physiological rotation and distraction loads. Five different stem sizes are available, allowing prosthesis implantation in dogs as small as 14 kg (30 pounds), with no upper weight limit. Four sizes of acetabular cups are available, ranging from 23 to 29 mm in outside diameter (OD), which accept the femoral head with a 17 mm OD. For dogs with a small acetabulum, a 20 mm OD cup is also available, which accepts a femoral head with a 14 mm OD. The variation in acetabular cup size and femoral neck length achieved with the modular system allows greater flexibility in the size of patients treated and allows the surgeon to adjust to the patient's needs at surgery.

Preoperative evaluation. Preoperative evaluation is very important in selecting the proper patient to receive a total hip prosthesis. Dogs must be in good general health except for their disabling hip condition. Although hip dysplasia is the most common disabling condition of the canine hip, other conditions have been treated with a prosthesis, such as osteoarthritis not associated with hip dysplasia, malunions of the femoral head and neck or acetabulum, chronically dislocated hips, failed excision arthroplasty, severely comminuted femoral heads, and avascular necrosis of the femoral head. The dogs must be at least 9 months of age and more than 14 kg to be potential candidates for total hip replacement. There is no upper age or weight limit if the dog is in good overall health.

Contraindications for total hip replacement include infection anywhere in or on the body, neoplastic disease, neurological dysfunction affecting the hind limbs, and pathology in the joints other than the hip. Thus a dog with hip dysplasia and a ruptured cranial cruciate ligament or degenerative myelopathy would not be considered a good candidate for a hip prosthesis. Also, any dog with normal hind limb function, no matter how extensive the coxofemoral joint osteoarthritis appears on radiographs, is not a candidate for hip replacement.

A complete general physical and orthopedic examination is performed on every animal being considered for joint replacement. All causes of lameness other than those related to the hip should be ruled out. Pain and other abnormalities in the hip should be confirmed. The hip should be evaluated for the angle of greatest flexion and extension as well as inward and outward rotation. Any pain response elicited while evaluating these angles should be noted. The joint should be checked for laxity. Neurological evaluation is conducted to eliminate spinal disorders as a cause of the lameness.

A ventrodorsal radiograph that includes the stifles and pelvis and a lateral radiograph of the pelvis must be taken. This helps evaluate the extent of hip joint disease and provides information on bone size so that a properly sized prosthesis can be implanted. These radiographs may also reveal other causes of lameness that will alter the treatment plan, such as panosteitis, low lumbar diskospondylitis, or bone tumors.

Procedure. The dog's hind limb is clipped the day before surgery, and if necessary, the dog is bathed. Intra-

venous antibiotics (sodium cephalexin, 25 mg/kg) are administered immediately before surgery. Special draping of the patient with sterile paper and plastic drapes provides a barrier impermeable to bacteria. Strict aseptic technique is followed.

The hip joint is exposed via a modified craniolateral approach. The skin incision starts dorsal and caudal to the greater trochanter and curves distally along the front edge of the femur. The tensor fascia lata is reflected cranially. The deep gluteal muscle, which is exposed by reflecting the middle and superficial muscles dorsally, is incised at its origin. The joint capsule is incised. With the femur externally rotated, an osteotomy template is aligned with the long axis of the femoral shaft and the axis of the femoral neck. An osteotomy of the femoral neck is performed and the diseased femoral head removed.

Instrumentation developed specifically for the modular system allows power reaming of the femur and acetabulum. The acetabular bed is prepared first using the acetabular reamer. Three to five holes are drilled around the rim of the acetabulum using a drill bit and special tissue guard to protect soft tissues.

The femoral shaft is drilled with a bit to a size corresponding to the femoral stem to be implanted. A fluted reamer widens the hole in the femoral shaft to accommodate the stem taper. Final preparation of the femoral shaft is done by hand with a finishing file and sometimes a broach. The femoral implant fits easily into the femoral canal with proper preparation.

The PMMA is mixed according to the manufacturer's specifications. Sodium cephalexin can be added sterilely during mixing of the cement at a rate of 1 antibiotic to 20 PMMA. PMMA is injected through a catheter tip syringe into the acetabular bed first. Only PMMA with a liquid phase of 3 to 7 minutes can be injected. The acetabular cup positioner, aligned with specific anatomical landmarks, is used for proper cup positioning. The femoral shaft is cleared of any blood and debris, and the shaft is injected with PMMA using a 60 ml catheter-tip syringe or a cement gun. The femoral stem is inserted and the PMMA allowed to harden.

A trial plastic head is placed on the femoral stem so that neck length can be assessed. Once the proper neck length has been determined, the cobalt-chrome head is impacted on the neck. The head is reduced into the acetabular cup. Cultures are taken, and the joint capsule is tightly closed. The surgical site is then closed in layers.

Postoperative care. Lateral and ventrodorsal pelvic radiographs are taken for assessment of the position of the acetabular and femoral components and the fill of the PMMA. Antibiotic therapy is continued until the culture results are known to be negative. The dogs are maintained on limited activity for 2 months after surgery. No activity more strenuous than a walk is allowed, and the dog is to be outside only on a leash. After that period the dog can gradually return to normal activity.

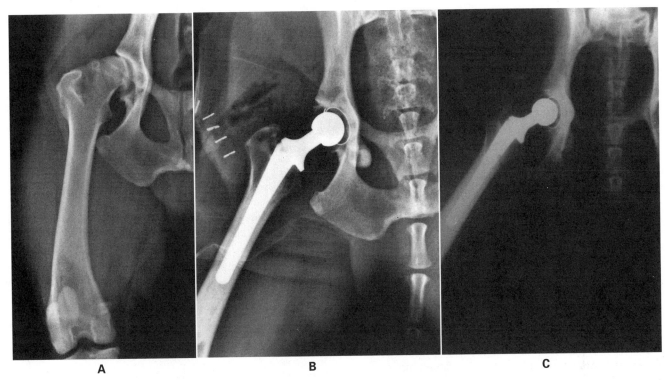

Fig. 17-18   Preoperative (**A**), immediate (**B**), and 1-year postoperative (**C**) radiographs of the hips of a working dog that received a modular hip prosthesis. The dog had significant lameness associated with hip dysplasia. After surgery the dog returned to successful field trail work. The owner observes pain-free movement, a marked increase in exercise tolerance, and an increased muscle mass in the limb with the total hip replacement.

Potential complications. Complications associated with fixed-head total hip replacements have been evaluated through a prospective study done at Ohio State University.[112,115] The number of dogs with complications decreased from 20% to 6% as the surgeons gained more skill and understanding.[112] The complications encountered with the fixed-head prosthesis include dislocations, infections, femoral fractures, aseptic loosening of the implants, and sciatic neuropraxia. The most common complication is dislocation, while the most serious is infection.

Proper positioning of the implants and controlled convalescent activity greatly reduce the risk of dislocation. Surgical reduction of the prosthesis, sometimes combined with realignment of the acetabular cup, is the usual method of treating dislocations. Breaks in sterile technique during surgery greatly increase the risk of infection. Animals that have had previous surgery in the area of the hip joint are five times more likely to develop an infection.[111] Infections can spread to the hip via hematogenous routes months or years after surgery. Infected implants are removed. Complete femoral fractures are fixed with internal fixation (AO* techniques) when encountered. Loose implants that are not infected are reimplanted or removed, depending on the quality of the bone around

them. Sciatic neuroparaxia is caused by the heat released during hardening of the PMMA, if the PMMA is next to the nerve. This occurs when the medial cortical wall is inadvertently penetrated during preparation of the acetabular bed. The nerve will regain its function in weeks to months without treatment.

Results. With the fixed-head prosthesis, the dog achieves normal or near-normal hind limb function 95% of the time.[112] This rate of success is being equalled or bettered by the modular prosthesis. A pain-free hip joint, full-range hip motion, increased exercise tolerance, increased muscle mass, and improved quality of life are standard findings. Working dogs return to field or police work, and pets exercise more without pain (Fig. 17-18). It has been found that 80% of the dogs will not need surgery on the untreated hip. The total hip replacement provides enough relief that surgery on the other side is not necessary. Often, neither hip is painful on reevaluation, even when both are painful before surgery. The thigh circumference of the side with the total hip replacement is routinely 1 to 3 cm larger than the other side. The prosthesis usually functions well for the dog's lifetime. Author Olmstead's longest case follow-up is 16 years, and he has reported on 50 cases with 5- to 10-year follow-ups.[112] Because the prosthesis provides the normal ball-and-socket arrangement of the hip joint, the femur maintains its normal position

---

*Arbeitsgmeinschaft für Osteosynthesefragen.

relative to the pelvis, and the hind limb is able to generate maximum propulsion forces during locomotion. This is not the case if the ball-and-socket joint configuration is not present.

As part of an ongoing prospective study, owners have been asked to fill out questionnaires on their dog's function after total hip replacement with the modular system.[113] Owners evaluated the dog's various activities, such as walking, standing, sitting, running, getting in and out of motor vehicles, climbing stairs, and play or exercise. Owners rated these activities with one of five levels, ranging from normal to severely abnormal. Comparing the preoperative activity levels with postoperative levels, owners reported marked improvement in their pets' ability to perform various activities. Greatly improved quality of life for the pet was reported by 85% of the owners and somewhat improved quality by 12%. When asked if they would have the procedure done again in the same circumstances, 90% indicated they would and 10% were undecided. Although the results of the evaluation of the modular system are preliminary, it is clear that canine total hip replacement continues to be a very effective method of treating disabling conditions of the canine hip.

REFERENCES AND SUGGESTED READINGS

1. Aegerter E, Kirkpatrick JA Jr: *Orthopedic diseases*, ed 3, Philadelphia, 1968, Saunders.
2. Altman RD, and others: Prophylactic treatment of canine osteoarthritis with glycosaminoglycan polysulfuric acid ester, *Arthritis Rheum* 39:759-766, 1989.
3. Altman RD and others: Therapeutic treatment of canine osteoarthritis with glycosaminoglycan polysulfuric acid ester, *Arthritis Rheum* 32:1300-1307, 1989.
4. Arnoczky SP, Lipowitz AJ: Degenerative joint disease. In Slatter DH, editor: *Textbook of small animal surgery*, Philadelphia, 1985, Saunders.
5. Arnoczky SP, Torzilli PA: Biomechanical analysis of forces acting about the canine hip, *Am J Vet Res* 42:1581-1585, 1981.
6. Bardens JW: Palpation for the detection of dysplasia and wedge technique for pelvic radiography. In *Proceedings of the 39th Annual Meeting of the American Animal Hospital Association*, Denver, 1972.
7. Bardens JW: Palpation for the detection of joint laxity. In *Proceedings of the Hip Dysplasia Symposium and Workshop*, St Louis, 1972, Orthopedic Foundation for Animals.
8. Bardens JW, Hardwick H: New observations on the diagnosis and cause of hip dysplasia, *Vet Med Small Anim Clin* 63:238-245, 1968.
9. Bardet JF, Rudy RL, Hohn RB: Measurement of femoral torsion in dogs using a biplanar method, *Vet Surg* 12:1-6, 1983.
10. Barker WD, Martinek J: An ultrastructural evaluation of the effect of hydrocortisone on rabbit cartilage, *Clin Orthop* 115:286, 1976.
11. Bassett FH, Wilson JW, Allen BL Jr.: Normal vascular anatomy of the head of the femur in puppies with emphasis on the inferior retinacular vessels, *J Bone Joint Surg* 51A:1139, 1967.
12. Belfield WO: Chronic subclinical scurvy and canine hip dysplasia, *Vet Med Small Anim Clin* 71:576-577, 1961.
13. Bennett D: Hip dysplasia and ascorbate therapy: fact or fancy? *Semin Vet Med Surg Small Anim* 2:152, 1987.
14. Berzon JL, and others: A retrospective study of the efficacy of femoral head and neck excisions in 94 dogs and cats, *Vet Surg* 9:88-92, 1980.
15. Booth NH: Nonnarcotic analgesics. In Booth NH, McDonald LE, editors: *Veterinary pharmacology and therapeutics*, Ames, 1988, Iowa State University Press.
16. Bowen JM: Electromyographic analysis of reflex and spastic activities of canine pectineus muscles in the presence and absence of hip dysplasia, *Am J Vet Res* 35:661-668, 1974.
17. Braden TD, Prieur WD: Three-plane intertrochanteric osteotomy for treatment of early stage hip dysplasia, *Vet Clin North Am Small Anim Pract* 22:623-643, 1992.
18. Braden TD, Prieur WD, Kaneene JB: Clinical evaluation of intertrochanteric osteotomy for treatment of dogs with early stage hip dysplasia: 37 cases (1980-1987), *J Am Vet Med Assoc* 196:337-341, 1990.
19. Brinker WO, Piermattei DL, Flo GL: Diagnosis and treatment of orthopedic conditions of the hindlimb. In *Handbook of small animal orthopedics and fracture treatment*, ed 2, Philadelphia, 1990, Saunders.
20. Brinker WO, Piermattei DL, Flo GL: *Handbook of small animal orthopedics and fracture treatment*, Philadelphia, 1990, Saunders.
21. Brown SG, Rosen H: Craniolateral approach to the canine hip: a modified Watson-Jones approach, *J Am Vet Med Assoc* 159:1117, 1971.
22. Calvé J: Sure one forme particuliere de pseudocoxalgie freffee sur des deformations characteristiques de L-extremite superieure du femur, *Rev Chir* 42:54, 1910.
23. Candlin FT: The diagnosis and treatment of hip dysplasia: one point of view, *J Am Hosp Assoc* 8:323-325, 1972.
24. Cardinet GH, Fedde MR, Tunell GL: Correlates of histochemical and physiologic properties in normal and hypotrophic pectineus muscles of the dog, *Lab Invest* 27:32-38, 1972.
25. Cardinet GH, Guffy MM, Wallace LJ: Canine hip dysplasia: effects of pectineal tenotomy on the coxofemoral joints of German shepherd dogs, *J Am Vet Med Assoc* 164:591-598, 1974.
26. Cardinet GH and others: Developmental myopathy in the canine, *Arch Neurol* 21:620-630, 1969.
27. Carreno MR, Muniz OE, Howell DS: The effect of glycosaminoglycan polysurfic acid ester on articular cartilage in experimental osteoarthritis: effects on morphologic variables of disease severity, *J Rheumatol* 13:490-497, 1984.
28. Chalman JA, Butler HC: Coxofemoral joint laxity and the Ortolani sign, *J Am Anim Hosp Assoc* 21:671-676, 1985.
29. Clark DM, Fry TR: A comparison of the bone forming properties of compatible osteoconductive polymer (BOP) versus autogenous cancellous bone in a canine fracture gap model. In *Scientific Presentation Abstracts of the American College of Veterinary Surgery 28th Annual Meeting*, San Francisco, 1993.
30. Colon PD: Nonsteroidal drugs used in the treatment of inflammation, *Vet Clin North Am* 18:1115, 1988.
31. Corley EA, Hogan PM: Trends in hip dysplasia control: analysis or radiographs submitted to the Orthopedic Foundation for Animals, 1974-1984, *J Am Vet Med Assoc* 187:805-809, 1985.
32. Davis LE: Clinical pharmacology of salicylates, *J Am Vet Med Assoc* 176:65, 1980.
33. Dawson J, Lees P, Segwick AD: Actions of nonsteroidal anti-inflammatory drugs on equine leucocyte movement in vitro, *J Vet Pharmacol Ther* 10:150, 1987.
34. DeAngelis M, Hohn RB: The ventral approach to excision arthroplasty of the femoral head, *J Am Vet Med Assoc* 152:135, 1968.
35. DeYoung DJ and others: Implantation of an uncemented total hip prosthesis technique and initial results of 100 arthroplasties, *Vet Surg* 21:168-177, 1992.
36. Douglas SW, Williamson HD: *Veterinary radiological interpretation*, Philadelphia, 1970, Lea & Febiger.
37. Dueland DJ: Femoral torsion and its possible relationship to canine hip dysplasia, *Vet Surg* 9:48, 1980 (abstract).

38. Dueland R, Bartel DL, Antonson E: Force plate technique for gait analysis of the total hip and excision arthroplasty, *J Am Anim Hosp Assoc* 13:544-552, 1977.

39. Duff R, Campbell JR: Long term results of excision arthroplasty of the canine hip, *Vet Rec* 101:181-184, 1977.

40. Duff R, Campbell JR: Effects of experimental excision arthroplasty of the hip joint, *Res Vet Sci* 24:174, 1978.

41. Gambardella P: Legg-Calvé-Perthes disease in dogs. In Bojrab MJ, editor: *Pathophysiology in small animal surgery*, Philadelphia, 1981, Lea & Febiger.

42. Gendreau C, Cawley AJ: Excision of the femoral head and neck: the long term results of 35 operations, *J Am Anim Hosp Assoc* 13:605-608, 1977.

43. Giardina JF, MacCarthy AW Jr: Hip palpation: evaluation of a technic for early determination of predysplastic dogs, *Vet Med Small Anim Clin* 63:878-882, 1971.

44. Girdlestone GR: Pseudoarthrosis: discussion on the treatment of unilateral osteoarthritis of the hip joint, *Proc R Soc Med* 38:363, 1945.

45. Golding J, Gosh P: Drugs for osteoarthrosis. I. The effects of pentosan polysulphate (SP54) on the degradation and loss of proteoglycans from articular cartilage in a model of osteoarthrosis induced in the rabbit knee joint by immobilization, *Curr Ther Res* 33:173-184, 1983.

46. Golding J, Gosh P: Drugs for osteoarthrosis. II. The effects of a glycosaminoglycan polysulphate ester (ArTe paron) on proteoglycan aggregation and loss from articular cartilage of immobilized rabbit knee joints, *Curr Ther Res* 34:67-80, 1983.

47. Goodwin JS: Mechanism of action of nonsteroidal anti-inflammatory agents, *Am J Med* 77(1A):57, 1984.

48. Gustafsson PO, Beling CG: Estradiol induced changes in beagle pups: effects of prenatal and postnatal administration, *Endocrinology* 85:481-491, 1969.

49. Haas J: *Congenital dislocation of the hip*, Springfield, Ill, 1951, Thomas.

50. Hannan N and others: Systemic administration of glycosaminoglycan polysulfate (ArTe paron) provided partial protection of articular cartilage from damage produced by meniscectomy in the canine, *J Orthop Res* 5:47-59, 1987.

51. Hauptman JH: Orthopedics of the hind limb. The hip joint, In Slatter DH, editor: *Textbook of small animal surgery*, Philadelphia, 1985, Saunders.

52. Hauptman JH and others: The angle of inclincation of the canine femoral head and neck, *Vet Surg* 8:74-77, 1979.

53. Hauptman JH and others: Angles of inclination and anteversion in hip dysplasia in the dog, *Am J Vet Res* 46:2033-2036, 1985.

54. Hedhammar A, and others: Overnutrition and skeletal disease: an experimental study in growing Great Dane dogs, *Cornell Vet* 64:1-160, 1974.

55. Hedhammar A and others: Canine hip dysplasia: study of heritability in 401 litters of German shepherd dogs, *J Am Vet Med Assoc* 9:1012-1016, 1979.

56. Henricson B, Norberg I, Olson SE: On the etiology and pathogenesis of hip dysplasia: a comparative review, *J Small Anim Pract* 7:673-688, 1966.

57. Henry JD: A modified technique for pectineal tendonectomy in the dog, *J Am Vet Med Assoc* 163:465-468, 1973.

58. Henry JD Jr, Park RD: Wedge technique for demonstration of coxofemoral joint laxity in the canine. In *Proceedings of the Canine Hip Dysplasia Symposium and Workshop*, St Louis, 1972, Orthopedic Foundation for Animals.

59. Henry WB, Wadsworth PL: Pelvic osteotomy in treatment of subluxation associated with hip dysplasia, *J Am Anim Hosp Assoc* 11:636, 1975.

60. Hoefle WD: A surgical procedure for prosthetic total hip replacement in the dog, *J Am Anim Hosp Assoc* 10:269-276, 1974.

61. Hohn RB, Janes JM: Pelvic osteotomy in the treatment of canine hip dysplasia, *Clin Orthop* 62:70-78, 1969.

62. Howell DS, Muniz O, Carreno MR: Effect of glycosaminoglycan polysulphate ester on proteoglycan degrading enzyme activity in an animal model of osteoarthritis, *Adv Inflamm Res* 11:197-205, 1986.

63. Hutt FB: Genetic selection to reduce the incidence of hip dysplasia in dogs, *J Am Vet Med Assoc* 151:1041-1048, 1967.

64. Ihemelandu EC, and others: Canine hip dysplasia: differences in pectineal muscles of healthy and dysplastic German shepherd dogs when two months old, *Am J Vet Res* 44:411-416, 1983.

65. Jenson DJ, Sertl GO: BOP shelf arthroplasty: a new correction to canine hip dysplasia, *Vet Form*, June 24, 1989.

66. Jenson DJ, Sertl GO: Sertl shelf arthroplasty (BOP procedure) in the treatment of canine hip dysplasia, *Vet Clin North Am Small Anim Pract* 22:683-701, 1992.

67. Jessen CR, Spurrell FA: Heritability of canine hip dysplasia. In *Proceedings of the Canine Hip Dysplasia Symposium and Workshop*, St Louis, 1972, Orthopedic Foundation for Animals.

68. Jessen CR, Spurrell FA: Radiographic detection of canine hip dysplasia in known age groups. In *Proceedings of the Canine Hip Dysplasia Symposium and Workshop*, St Louis, 1972, Orthopedic Foundation for Animals.

69. Johnston SA: Conservative and medical management of hip dysplasia, *Vet Clin North Am* 22:595-606, 1992.

70. Kaman CH, Gossling HP: A breeding program to reduce hip dysplasia in German shepherd dogs, *J Am Vet Med Assoc* 151:562-571, 1967.

71. Kasstrom H: Nutrition, weight gain, and development of hip dysplasia: an experimental investigation in growing dogs with special reference to the effect of feeding intensity, *Acta Radiol* 344:135-179, 1975.

72. Kolde DL: Pectineus tenectomy for treatment of hip dysplasia in a domestic cat: a case report, *J Am Anim Hosp Assoc* 10:564-565, 1974.

73. Kusba JK, and others: Suspected villinodular synovitis in a dog, *J Am Vet Med Assoc* 182:390, 1983.

74. Lee R, Fry PD: Some observations on the occurrence of Legg-Calvé-Perthes disease (coxa plana) in the dog and an evaluation of excision arthroplasty as a method of treatment, *J Small Anim Pract* 19:309, 1969.

75. Legg AT: An obscure affection of the hip joint, *Boston Med Surg J* 162:202, 1910.

76. Leighton RL: The Richard's II canine hip prosthesis, *J Am Anim Hosp Assoc* 15:73-76, 1979.

77. Lewis DL and others: Postoperative examination of the biceps femoris muscle sling used in excision of the femoral head and neck in dogs, *Vet Surg* 17:269-277, 1988.

78. Lewis RG, Jones JP: A clinical study of canine total hip arthroplasty, *Vet Surg* 9:20-23, 1980.

79. Lipowitz AJ, Boulay JP, Klausner JS: Serum salicylate concentrations and endoscopic evaluation of the gastric mucosa in dogs after oral administration of aspirin-containing products, *Am J Vet Res* 47:1586, 1986.

80. Lippincott CL: Improvement of excision arthroplasty of the femoral head and neck utilizing a biceps femoris muscle sling, *J Am Anim Hosp Assoc* 17:668-673, 1981.

81. Lippincott CL: Excision arthroplasty of the femoral head and neck utilizing a biceps femoris muscle sling. Part two. The caudal pass, *J Am Anim Hosp Assoc* 20:377-384, 1984.

82. Lippincott CL: Excision arthroplasty of the femoral head and neck, *Vet Clin North Am Small Anim Pract* 17:857-871, 1987.

83. Lippincott CL: Femoral head and neck excision in the management of canine hip dysplasia, *Vet Clin North Am Small Anim Pract* 22:721-737, 1992.

84. Ljunggren GL: Conservative vs. surgical treatment of Legg-Perthes disease, *Anim Hosp* 2:6, 1966.

85. Ljunggren GL: Legg-Perthes disease in the dog, *Acta Orthop Scand* (suppl):95, 1967.

86. Lussier B, Lanthier T, Martinear-Doize B: Evaluation of compatible osteoconductive polymer (BOP) shelf arthroplasty in normal dogs. In *Scientific Presentation Abstracts of the American College of Veterinary Surgery 28th Annual Meeting*, San Francisco, 1993.

87. Lust G, Kindlon CC: Biochemical studies on hip dysplasia in dogs. In *Proceedings of the 19th Gaines Vet Symposium*, Lafayette, Ind, 1969, Purdue University Press.

88. Lust G, Summers BA: Early, asymptomatic stage of degenerative joint disease in canine hip joints, *Am J Vet Res* 42:1849-1855, 1981.

89. Lust G, Beilman WT, Rendano VT: A relationship between degree of laxity and synovial fluid volume in coxofemoral joints of dogs predisposed for hip dysplasia, *Am J Vet Res* 41:55-60, 1980.

90. Lust G, Geary JC, Sheffy BE: Development of hip dysplasia in dogs, *Am J Vet Res* 34:87-91, 1973.

91. Lust G, Rendano VT, Summers BA: Canine hip dysplasia: concepts and diagnosis, *J Am Vet Med Assoc* 187:638-640, 1985.

92. Lust G and others: Changes in pelvic muscle tissues associated with hip dysplasia, *Am J Vet Res* 33:1097-1108, 1972.

93. Lust G and others: Studies on pectineus muscles in canine hip dysplasia, *Cornell Vet* 62:628-645, 1972.

94. Lust G and others: Intra-articular volume and hip joint instability in dogs with hip dysplasia, *J Bone Joint Surg* 62A:576-582, 1980.

95. Lust G and others: Effects of intramuscular administration of glycosaminoglycan polysulfates on signs of incipient hip dysplasia in growing pups, *Am J Vet Res* 53:1836-1840, 1992.

96. Mackay-Smith MP: Management of fracture and luxation of the femoral head in two ponies, *J Am Vet Med Assoc* 145:248, 1964.

97. Mankin HJ: The reaction of articular cartilage to injury and osteoarthritis, *N Engl J Med* 291:1285-1292, 1974.

98. Mankin HJ, Conger KA: The acute effects of intra-articular hydrocortisone on articular cartilage in rabbits, *J Bone Joint Surg* 48A:1383, 1966.

99. Mann FA and others: A comparison of two methods of femoral head and neck and excision in the dog, *Vet Surg* 16:223-230, 1987.

100. Massat BJ, Vasseur PB: Clinical and radiographic results of total hip arthroplasty in dogs: 96 cases (1986-1992), *J Am Vet Med Assoc* 205:3, 448-454, 1994.

101. McIlwraith CW: Current concepts in equine degenerative joint disease, *J Am Vet Med Assoc* 180:239, 1982.

102. McLoughlin RM Jr and others: GI: Force plate analysis of triple pelvic osteotomy for the treatment of canine hip dysplasia, *Vet Surg* 20:291-297, 1991.

103. Moltzen-Nielsen H: Calvé-Perthes Krankheit, Malum Deformans Juvenilis Coxas bei Hunden, *Arch Wiss Prakt Tierheillk* 72:91, 1938.

104. Montgomery RD and others: Total hip arthroplasty for treatment of canine hip dysplasia, *Vet Clin North Am Small Anim Pract* 22:703-719, 1992.

105. Morgan JP: Radiographic diagnosis of hip dysplasia in skeletally mature dogs. In *Proceedings of the Canine Hip Dysplasia Symposium and Workshop*, St Louis, 1972, Orthopedic Foundation for Animals.

106. Moskowitz RL: Treatment of osteoarthritis. In McCarty DJ, editor: *Arthritis and allied conditions: a textbook of rheumatology*, ed 11, Philadelphia, 1989, Lea & Febiger.

107. Moskowitz RW and others: Experimentally induced corticosteroid arthropathy, *Arthritis Rheum* 13:236, 1970.

108. Nunamaker DM: Legg-Calvé-Perthes disease. In Newton CD, Nunamaker DM, editors: *Textbook of small animal orthopedics*, Philadelphia, 1985, Lippincott.

109. Oakes MG, and others: An experimental investigation of the BOP Sertl Shelf Arthroplasty in the treatment of canine hip dysplasia.

In *Scientific Presentation Abstracts of the American College of Veterinary Surgery 28th Annual Meeting*, San Francisco, 1993.

110. Olmstead ML: Fractures of the femoral head and neck. In Brinker WO, Hohn RB, Prier WD, editors: *Manual of internal fixation in small animals*, New York, 1984, Springer-Verlag.

111. Olmstead ML: Total hip replacement, *Vet Clin North Am* 17:943-955, 1987.

112. Olmstead ML: Total hip replacement, *Semin Vet Med Surg Small Anim* 2:131-140, 1987.

113. Olmstead ML: The canine cemented modular total hip prosthesis, *J Am Hosp Assoc* 31:2, 109-124, 1995.

114. Olmstead ML, Hohn RB: Ergbisse mit der hufltoltal-prostheses bei 103 klinischen fallen an der Ohio State University, *Klin Prox* 25:407-415, 1980.

115. Olmstead ML, Hohn RB, Turner TM: A five year study of 221 total hip replacements in the dog, *J Am Vet Med Assoc* 183:191-194, 1983.

116. Olsson SE: Canine hip dysplasia. In Kirk RW, editor: *Current veterinary therapy VII*, Philadelphia, 1980, Saunders.

117. Ormond AN: Treatment of hip lameness in the dog by excision of the femoral head, *Vet Rec* 73:576-577, 1961.

118. Ortolani M: Un segno poco noto e sua importanza per la diagnosis procece de prelussazione congenita dellanea, *Pediatria (Napoli)* 45:129, 1937.

119. Ortolani M: The classic: congenital hip dysplasia in the light of early and very early diagnosis, *Clin Orthop* 119:6-10, 1976.

120. Parker RB and others: Canine total hip arthroplasty: a clinical review of 20 cases, *J Am Anim Hosp Assoc* 20:97-104, 1984.

121. Peiffer RL Jr, Blevins WE: Hip dysplasia and pectineus resection in the cat, *Feline Pract* 4:40-43, 1974.

122. Perthes G: Uber arthritis deformans juvenilis, *Deutsche Ztschr Chir* 107:111, 1910.

123. Pierce KR, Bridges CH: The role of estrogens in the pathogenesis of canine hip dysplasia: metabolism of exogenous estrogens, *J Small Anim* 8:383-389, 1967.

124. Piermattie DL: Femoral head ostectomy in the dog: indication, techniques, and results in 10 cases, *J Am Anim Hosp Assoc* 1:180-188, 1965.

125. Plumb DC: *Veterinary drug handbook*, White Bear Lake, Minn, 1991, Pharma. Vet.

126. Priester WA, Mulvihill JJ: Canine hip dysplasia: relative risk by sex, size, and breed, and comparative aspects, *J Am Vet Med Assoc* 160:735-739, 1972.

127. Prieur WD: Coxarthrosis in the dog. Part I. Normal and abnormal biomechanics of the hip joint, *Vet Surg* 9:145-149, 1980.

128. Prieur WD: Intertrochanteric osteotomy in the dog: theoretical consideration and operative technique, *J Small Anim Pract* 28:3-20, 1987.

129. Prieur WD: Intertrochanteric osteotomy. In Bojrab MJ, editor: *Current techniques in small animal surgery*, ed 3, Philadelphia, 1990, Lea & Febiger.

130. Prieur WD, Scartazzini R: Grundlagen und Ergenbnisse der InTerTrocanTaren Variation sostoeotomie bei Huftdysplasie, *Kleintierpraxia* 24:393, 1980.

131. Rhodes WH, Jenny J: A canine acetabular index, *J Am Vet Med Assoc* 137:97-100, 1960.

132. Richards DA, Hinko PJ, Morse EM Jr: Pectinecotmy vs. pectinotomy in the treatment of hip dysplasia, *Vet Med Small Anim Clin* 67:976-977, 1972.

133. Riser WH: Producing diagnostic pelvic radiographs for canine hip dysplasia, *J Am Vet Med Assoc* 141:600-603, 1962.

134. Riser WH: A new look at developmental subluxation and dislocation: hip dysplasia in the dog, *J Small Anim Pract* 4:421-434, 1963.

135. Riser WH: Progress in canine hip dysplasia control, *J Am Vet Med Assoc* 155:2047-2052, 1969.

136. Riser WH: The dog as a model for the study of hip dysplasia, *Vet Pathol* 12:229-234, 1975.

137. Riser WH, Shirer JF: Hip dysplasia: coxofemoral abnormalities in neonatal German shepherd dogs, *J Small Anim Pract* 7:7-12, 1966.

138. Riser WH, Shirer JF: Correlation between canine hip dysplasia and pelvic muscle mass: a study of 95 dogs, *Am J Vet Res* 124:769-777, 1967.

139. Riser WH, Rhodes WH, Newton CD: Hip dysplasia. In Newton CD, Nunamaker DM, editors: *Textbook of small animal orthopedics*, Philadelphia, 1985, Lippincott.

140. Riser WH, and others: Influence of early rapid growth and weight gain on hip dysplasia in the German shepherd dog, *J Am Vet Med Assoc* 145:661-668, 1964.

141. Rosenthal JJ, Poqust HN: Pectineus myotomy: a photographic synopsis of a procedure to surgically rehabilitate the lame dysplastic dog, *Vet Med Small Anim Clin* 67:781-784, 1972.

142. Sahu S, Saxena OP: Excision arthroplasty of the hip in bovines: a report of two cases, *Indian Vet J* 53:294, 1976.

143. Salter RB: Innominate osteotomy in the treatment of congenital dislocation and subluxation of the hip, *J Bone Joint Surg* 43B:518, 1961.

144. Salter RB: Role of innominate osteotomy in the treatment of congenital dislocation and subluxation of the hip in the older child, *J Bone Joint Surg* 48A:1413, 1966.

145. Samuelson ML: Correlation of palpation with radiography in diagnosis and prognosis of canine hip dysplasia. In *Proceedings of the Canine Hip Dysplasia Symposium and Workshop*, St Louis, 1972, Orthopedic Foundation for Animals.

146. Schales O: Genetic aspects of dysplasia of the hip joint, *North Am Vet* 37:476-478, 1956.

147. Schales O: Hereditary patterns in dysplasia of the hip, *North Am Vet* 38:152-155, 1957.

148. Schnelle GB: Some new diseases in dogs, *Am Kennel Gaz* 52:25-26, 1935.

149. Schnelle GB: Congenital subluxation of the coxofemoral joint in a dog, *Univ Pa Bull* XXXVII(65), Jan 15, 1937.

150. Schnelle GB: Regional radiography—the pelvic region. Part I, *North Am Vet*. 18:53-57, 1937.

151. Schnelle GB: The veterinary radiologist: coxa plana, *North Am Vet* 18:46, 1937.

152. Schrader SC: Triple osteotomy of the pelvis as a treatment for canine hip dysplasia, *J Am Vet Med Assoc* 178:39-44, 1981.

153. Schrader SC: Septic arthritis and osteomyelitis of the hip in six mature dogs, *J Am Vet Med Assoc* 181:894-898, 1982.

154. Schrader SC: Triple osteotomy of the pelvis and trochanteric osteotomy as a treatment for hip dysplasia in the immature dog: the surgical technique and results of 77 consecutive operations, *J Am Vet Med Assoc* 189:659-665, 1986.

155. Sertl GO, Jensen DJ: The pelvis and osteoconductive polymer (BOP) shelf arthroplasty for the surgical treatment of hip dysplasia. In Whittic WG, editor: *Canine orthopedics,* ed 2, Philadelphia, 1990, Lea & Febiger.

156. Short CR, Beadle RE: Pharmacology of antiarthritic drugs, *Vet Clin North Am* 8:401-417, 1978.

157. Simon LS, Mills JA: Nonsteroidal anti-inflammatory drugs. Part I, *N Engl J Med* 302:1179, 1980.

158. Skondia V and others: Chemical and physicomechanical aspects of compatible orthopedic polymer (BOP) in bone surgery, *J Int Med Res* 15:293-302, 1987.

159. Slocum B, Devine T: Pelvic osteotomy technique for axial rotation of the acetabular segment in dogs, *J Am Anim Hosp Assoc* 22:331-338, 1986.

160. Slocum B, Devine T: Pelvic osteotomy in the dog as treatment for hip dysplasia, *Semin Vet Med Surg* 2:107, 1987.

161. Slocum B, Devine T: Pelvic osteotomy. In Whittick WG, editor: *Canine orthopedics,* ed 2, Philadelphia, 1990, Lea & Febiger.

162. Slocum B, Slocum TD: Pelvic osteotomy for axial rotation of the acetabular segment in dogs with hip dysplasia, *Vet Clin North Am Small Anim Pract* 22:645-682, 1992.

163. Smith GK, Biery DN, Gregor TP: New concepts of coxofemoral joint stability and the development of a clinical stress-radiographic method for quantitating hip joint laxity in the dog, *J Am Vet Med Assoc* 196:59-70, 1990.

164. Snavely JG: The genetic aspects of hip dysplasia in dogs, *J Am Vet Med Assoc* 135:201-207, 1959.

165. Spruell JSA: Excision arthroplasty as a method of treatment of hip joint diseases in the dog, *Vet Rec* 73:573-576, 1961.

166. Steel HH: Triple osteotomy of the innominate bone, *J Bone Joint Surg* 55A:343, 1973.

167. Steel HH: Triple osteotomy of the innominate bone: a procedure to accomplish coverage of the dislocated or subluxated femoral head in the older patient, *Clin Orthop Rel Res* 122:116, 1977.

168. Stoyak JS: Legg-Perthes disease in the dog. In Bojrab MJ, editor: *Current techniques in small animal surgery*, Philadelphia, 1975, Lea & Febiger.

169. Tarvin GB, Lenehan TM: Pelvic osteotomy. In Bojrab MJ, editor: *Current techniques in small animal surgery*, ed 3, Philadelphia, 1990, Lea & Febiger.

170. Trevor PB and others: Evaluation of compatible osteoconductive polymer as an orthopedic implant in dogs, *J Am Vet Med Assoc* 200:1651-1660, 1992.

171. Vasseur PB: Femoral head and neck osteotomy. In Bojrab MJ, editor: *Current techniques in small animal surgery,* ed 3, Philadelphia, 1990, Lea & Febiger.

172. Vaughan LC, Jones DGC, Lane JG: Pectineus muscle resection as a treatment for hip dysplasia in dogs, *Vet Rec* 96:145, 1975.

173. Walker T, Prieur D: Intertrochanteric femoral osteotomy, *Semin Vet Med Surg Small Anim* 2:117-130, 1987.

174. Wallace LJ: Clinical investigations and surgery on the pectineus muscle and its relationship to canine hip dysplasia. In *Scientific Proceedings of the AAHA 38th Annual Meeting*, Las Vegas, 1971.

175. Wallace LJ: Pectineus tendonectomy or tenotomy for treating clinical canine hip dysplasia, *Vet Clin North Am* 1:455-465, 1971.

176. Wallace LJ: Canine hip dysplasia: past and present, *Semin Vet Med Surg Small Anim* 2:92, 1987.

177. Wallace LJ: Pectineus tendon surgery for the management of canine hip dysplasia, *Vet Clin North Am Small Anim Pract* 22:607-621, 1992.

178. Wallace LJ, Guffy MM, Cardinet GH: Pectineus tendon surgery for treating canine hip dysplasia. In *Scientific Proceedings of the AAHA 39th Annual Meeting*, 1972.

179. Wallace LJ, Guffy MM, Cardinet GH: Pectineus tendon or muscle surgery for treatment of clinical hip dysplasia in the dog. In Bojrab MJ, editor: *Current techniques in small animal surgery,* Philadelphia, 1975, Lea & Febiger.

180. Wallace LJ and others: Surgical rehabilitation of the dysplastic dog. In *Proceedings of the Conference on Research to Expand the Usefulness of the Military Working Dog*, San Antonio, Texas, 1970.

181. Whittington K and others: Report of the Panel on Canine Hip Dysplasia, *J Am Vet Med Assoc* 139:791-806, 1961.

18

The Stifle Joint

DONALD A. HULSE

PATELLA LUXATION

Limb dysfunction caused by medial or lateral patella luxation is one of the most common problems seen in veterinary practice. To choose the most appropriate treatment method, the surgeon must know the normal anatomy, function, and interrelationships of the hip joint, femur, and tibia (Fig. 18-1).

In the normal canine the angle of the femoral neck–femoral shaft axis in the frontal projection is approximately 135 to 145 degrees. *Coxa valga* is an increase in the angle of the femoral neck–femoral shaft axis, whereas *coxa vara* is a decrease in that angle. *Anteversion* of the femoral head and neck is an external rotation of the proximal femur in relation to the distal femur. *Retroversion* is the opposite: an internal rotation of the femoral head relative to the distal femur. The normal anteversion angle in puppies is near 0 degrees and increases to approximately 27 degrees in the adult.

Distally, the angle of the transcondylar–femoral shaft axis in the frontal projection is approximately 93 degrees. The femoral trochlear sulcus is the wide articular groove

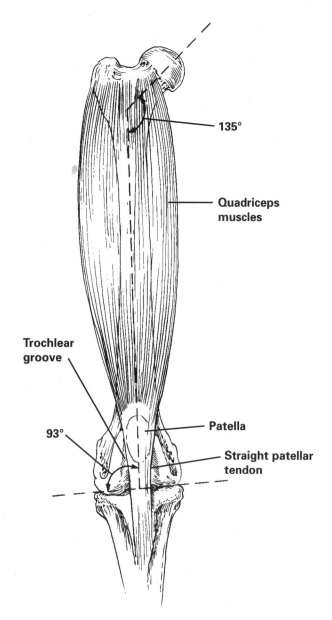

Fig. 18-1 The normal relationship between the hip joint and stifle joint. The quadriceps muscle group, patella, trochlear groove patellar tendon, and its insertion onto the tibial tuberosity are in alignment with the stifle in a neutral position.

femoris, vastus lateralis, vastus intermedius, and vastus medialis. The vastus medialis and vastus lateralis are fixed to the patella by the medial and lateral parapatellar fibrocartilages. The fibrocartilages ride on the ridges of the femoral trochlea and, along with the medial and lateral retinacula, aid in patella stability. The medial and lateral retinacula are groups of collagen fibers that course from the fabella to blend with the medial and lateral parapatellar fibrocartilages, respectively. The function of the quadriceps muscle group is extension of the stifle joint. In addition, the quadriceps, along with the entire extensor mechanism, aids in the stability of the stifle joint. The quadriceps muscle group converges on the patella and continues distally as the straight patellar tendon.

The patella is a sesamoid bone embedded in the tendon of the quadriceps muscle. The inner articular surface is smooth and curved so as to articulate fully with the trochlea. The normal gliding articulation of the patella and trochlea is necessary for maintaining the nutritional requirements of the trochlear and patellar articular surfaces. Lack of normal articulation, as shown experimentally through patellectomy, results in degeneration of the trochlear articular cartilage. The patella is also an essential component of the functional mechanism of the extensor apparatus. The patella maintains even tension when the stifle is extended and also acts as a lever arm, increasing the mechanical advantage of the quadriceps muscle group. A 15% to 30% increase in contractile force is necessary in humans when patellectomy has removed the mechanical advantage of the patella.

The tibial tuberosity is located cranial and distal to the tibial condyles. Its location and prominence are important for the mechanical advantage of the extensor mechanism. The alignment of the quadriceps, patella, trochlea, patellar tendon, and tibial tuberosity must be normal for proper function. Malalignment of one or more of these structures may lead to luxation of the patella.

Etiology and Pathophysiology

Because medial patella luxation is the more common abnormality seen in veterinary practice, this discussion regarding pathophysiology relates to the development of abnormalities when the patella luxates medially. Since abnormalities associated with lateral patella luxation are mirror images of those seen with medial luxations, one simply needs to transpose the images discussed next to understand the pathophysiology of lateral patella luxation.

The following musculoskeletal abnormalities are associated with medial patella luxation in the dog (Fig. 18-2):

1. Medial displacement of the quadriceps muscle group
2. Lateral torsion of the distal femur

on the cranial surface of the femur that articulates with the patella. The groove is bounded medially and laterally by prominent trochlear ridges that aid in maintaining stability of the patella. The trochlear groove is normally in alignment with the quadriceps mechanism, patellar ligament, and tibial tuberosity. This anatomical alignment is necessary for stability of the stifle joint and efficiency of the extensor mechanism.

The extensor mechanism of the stifle joint is composed of the quadriceps muscle group, patella, trochlear groove, straight patellar ligament, and tibial tuberosity. The quadriceps muscle group is formed by the rectus

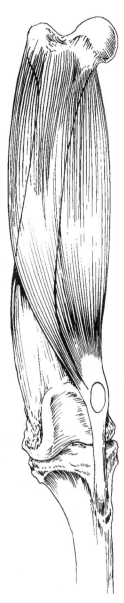

Fig. 18-2 The abnormal relationship between the hip joint and stifle joint in a dog having a medial displacement of the patella. The quadriceps muscle group, patella, patellar tendon and its insertion onto the tibial tuberosity are no longer in alignment with the trochlear groove. A bowing of the distal femur tilting of the joint line are evident.

3. Lateral bowing of the distal one third of the femur
4. Dysplasia of the femoral epiphysis
5. Rotational instability of the stifle joint
6. Tibial deformity

The degree of anatomic derangement depends on the severity of patella luxation and the degree of growth plate activity. Although the changes vary, most patients with patella luxation show some type of structural abnormality just listed. The skeletal deformities noted result from changes within the metaphyseal growth plates. In young animals, a great potential for axial and torsional growth exists in the cartilage columns of the metaphyseal growth plates. Since the growth plate is very active, the cells within the growth plates yield to physiological forces very rapidly by either increasing or decreasing rate of growth. The torsional and angular deformities of the skeleton associated with patella luxations are caused by abnormal pressures exerted on the growth plate by displacement of the quadriceps muscle group. In contrast, existing bone responds to increased force through bone deposition or resorption; therefore, remodeling of existing bone occurs more slowly.

It may be concluded that the growth plates are the primary reason for the rapid formation of skeletal deformities in the immature animal. An abnormal torsional force leads to a deflection of the cartilage columns of the growth plate in a spiral pattern. Therefore a lateral or medial torsion of the femur may result, depending on the direction of the deforming force. With medial luxation, lateral torsion of the distal femur occurs; therefore the torsional force must be in a lateral direction. Abnormal compression or tension forces (axial forces) also affect the growth of the cartilage columns. Disparity between medial and lateral axial forces can lead to bowing of the distal one third of the femur in dogs with medial patella luxation. This abnormal bowing results from shortening of the longitudinal length of the medial cortex relative to the lateral cortex.

The pathogenesis of this mechanism may be explained by increased pressure parallel to the growth plate retarding growth and decreased pressure parallel to the growth plate accelerating growth. The pressure need not be extreme. On the contrary, mild forces originating from postural abnormalities, gravitational forces, or muscle forces are sufficient to affect the growth plate. A medial malalignment of the quadriceps muscles occurs in dogs with medial patella luxation, which produces sufficient pressure on the medial aspect of the growth plate to retard growth. At the same time, less pressure is placed on the plate's lateral aspect, which accelerates growth. The result is retarded growth of the femur's medial cortex and accelerated growth of its lateral cortex. Decreased length of the medial cortex relative to the increased length of the lateral cortex results in the lateral bowing of the distal femur.

Abnormal growth continues as long as the quadriceps is displaced medially and the growth plates are active. Therefore the degree of lateral bowing depends on the severity of patella luxation and age of the patient at the onset of luxation. With mild luxations, the quadriceps is rarely displaced medially and has minimal abnormal effect on the growth plate. However, with severe luxations, the quadriceps is medially displaced at all times, and maximal effect on the growth plate results in severe lateral bowing of the distal femur in the young patient.

The tibial deformities seen with patella luxations are the result of abnormal forces acting on the proximal and distal growth plates. The tibial deformities described with medial patella luxation are (1) medial displacement of the tibial tuberosity, (2) medial bowing (varus deformity) of the proximal tibia, and (3) lateral torsion of the distal tibia.

The articular cartilage is the "growth plate" for the epiphysis and responds to increased or decreased pressure in the same manner as the metaphyseal growth plate. That is, increased pressure retards growth, whereas decreased pressure accelerates growth. Abnormal development of the trochlear groove is present in dogs with medial patella luxation. The degree of abnormality varies from a near-normal trochlea to an absent trochlear groove. The articulation of the patella within the trochlear groove exerts physiological pressure on the articular cartilage, which retards cartilage growth. Continued pressure by the patella is responsible for the development of normal depth of the trochlear groove. If the physiological pressure exerted by the patella is not present on the trochlear articular cartilage, the trochlear groove fails to gain proper depth. An immature patient with a mild luxation shows minimal loss of depth to the trochlear groove, since the patella is in normal position during development. However, an immature patient with a severe luxation has an absent trochlear groove, since the normal pressure responsible for groove development is not present.

The pathological changes are multiple and may vary from mild soft tissue changes to marked skeletal abnormalities. Currently, insufficient experimental evidence exists to establish definitively the cause and sequence of events leading to the anatomical derangements just described. However, an explanation of the pathophysiological events is given based on the present experimental and clinical evidence.

Classification

Patella luxation is classified as acquired traumatic luxation or developmental luxation. Developmental luxation is more common, and the patella can be displaced medially or laterally. Medial luxation occurs more often and is seen most frequently in small and toy breeds of dogs. Lateral luxation is less common and is most often diagnosed in larger breeds of dogs. Acquired traumatic medial patella luxation is not common but can be seen in any breed of dog subjected to a trauma that tears the lateral retinacular structures.

The degree of skeletal pathology associated with patella luxation varies considerably between the mildest and severest forms (Figs. 18-3 and 18-4). Because of the variable degree of clinical and pathological changes, a system for classifying canine patella luxation has been developed.

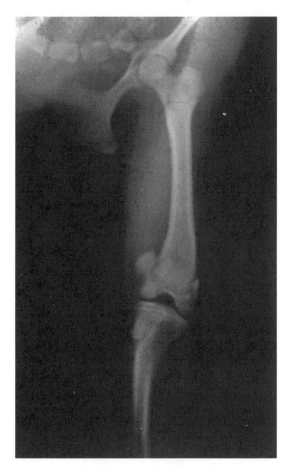

Fig. 18-3 Craniocaudal radiograph showing skeletal abnormalities associated with a Grade III medial patella luxation.

Grade I. The patella can be luxated, but spontaneous luxation of the patella during normal joint motion rarely occurs. Manual luxation of the patella may be accomplished during physical examination, but the patella reduces when pressure is released. Flexion and extension of the joint are essentially normal.

Grade II. Angular and torsional deformities of the femur may be present to a mild degree. The patella may be manually displaced with lateral pressure or may luxate with flexion of the stifle joint. The patella remains luxated until it is reduced by the examiner or by extension and derotation of the tibia by the patient.

Grade III. The patella usually remains luxated medially but may be manually reduced with the stifle in extension. However, after manual reduction, flexion and extension of the stifle result in reluxation of the patella. The quadriceps muscle group is medially displaced. Abnormalities of the supporting soft tissues of the stifle joint and deformities of the femur and tibia may be demonstrated.

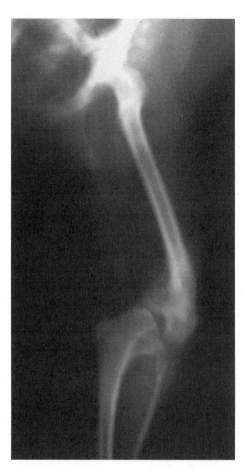

Fig. 18-4 Craniocaudal radiograph showing skeletal abnormalities associated with a Grade IV medial patella luxation.

Grade IV. The proximal tibial plateau may be medially rotated 80 to 90 degrees. The patella is permanently luxated and cannot be manually repositioned. The femoral trochlear groove is shallow or absent, and the quadriceps muscle group is medially displaced. Abnormalities of the supporting soft tissues of the stifle joint and deformities of the femur and tibia are severe.

History and Physical Findings

Clinical signs and physical findings vary and depend on the severity of luxation. Patients with grade I luxations generally exhibit no lameness, and the diagnosis is made as an incidental finding on physical examination. Patients with grade II luxations occasionally "skip" when walking or running. These patients may stretch the lateral retinacular structures and have a non-weight-bearing lameness. Lameness in patients with a grade III patella luxation varies from an occasional skip to a weight-bearing lameness. Patients with grade IV luxations walk with the rear quarters in a crouched position because of the inability to extend the stifle joints fully. The patella is hypoplastic and

may be found displaced medially alongside the medial femoral condyle.

Differential diagnoses include avascular necrosis of the femoral head, coxofemoral luxation, ligamentous sprain, and muscle strain. Diagnosis is based on the finding of medial patella luxation during physical examination and the absence of other causes of lameness. Careful examination of the hip joint is essential, since a significant percentage of patients with avascular necrosis of the femoral head also have patella luxation. Craniocaudal and mediolateral radiographs should be taken to assess skeletal deformity.

Methods of Treatment

Treatment of medial patella luxation may be nonsurgical or surgical. Deciding which method is applicable for a patient depends on the clinical history, physical findings, and age. An older patient in whom patella luxation is noted as an incidental finding on physical examination and in whom the client reports no clinical lameness does not warrant surgical intervention. Rather, the client should be informed as to the clinical signs associated with patella luxation. Surgery is advised in the young adult patient even though no clinical problem is apparent, since intermittent luxation may prematurely wear the articular cartilage. Surgery is indicated in any aged patient exhibiting lameness and is strongly advised in one with active growth plates because skeletal deformity may worsen rapidly. However, the surgical techniques used in actively growing animals should not adversely affect skeletal growth.

Numerous surgical techniques are aimed at restraining the patella within the trochlear groove. Tibial tuberosity transposition, collateral restraint release, collateral restraint reinforcement, trochlear groove deepening, femoral osteotomy, and tibial osteotomy have all been advocated for correction of patella luxation. Generally, a combination of techniques is required. The techniques used depend on the severity of luxation, the skeletal deformity, and the surgeon's preference. The techniques are described in detail here for medial patella luxation because it is more frequently encountered than lateral luxation. However, the same basic techniques are employed for both types of luxation; most techniques for medial luxation are simply reversed for lateral luxation in relation to the anatomical alteration that occurs.

The techniques also depend on the pathology present. Not every patient with a luxating patella needs all the techniques listed next for surgery to be successful. The surgeon must recognize which abnormalities are present in a given stifle and then use the technique(s) that addresses each problem.

Tibial tuberosity transposition. Tibial tuberosity transposition is an effective treatment for grades II, III, and IV patella luxations (Fig. 18-5). A craniolateral skin

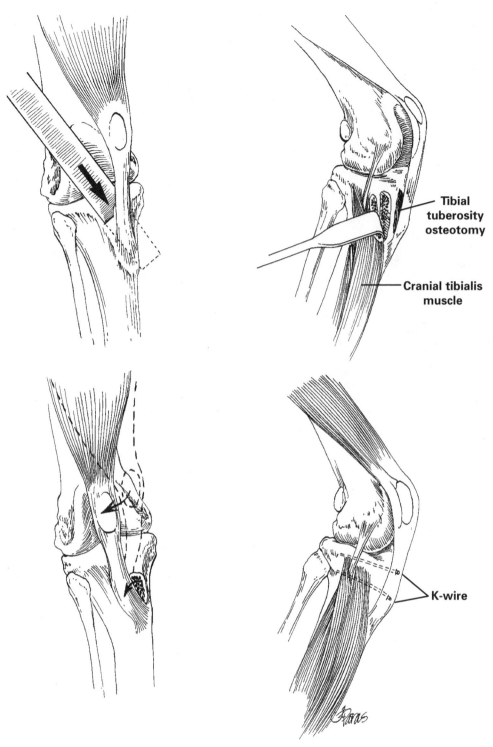

Fig. 18-5 Steps taken to perform a transposition of the tibial tuberosity. An osteotome is slipped beneath the insertion of the patellar tendon 5 to 6 mm caudal to its insertion. The tuberosity is released and moved laterally to align the tibial tuberosity with the trochlear groove and the quadriceps muscle group. The tuberosity is secured in position with 1 or 2 small pins (K-wires).

incision extends from proximal to the patella to the tibial tuberosity. The subcutaneous tissue is incised along the same line. A lateral parapatella incision is made through the fascia lata and is carried distally onto the tibial tuberosity below the joint line. The cranialis tibialis mus-

cle is reflected from the lateral tibial tuberosity and tibial plateau caudally to the level of the long digital extensor tendon. Careful sharp dissection is used to gain access to the deep surface of the patella tendon for placement of the osteotome. Beginning at the level of the patella, a

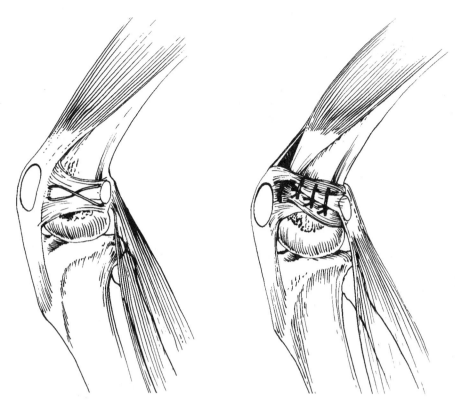

Fig. 18-6   Two methods by which the surgeon may reinforce the lateral retinaculum to help restrain the patella within the trochlear groove. A nonabsorbable suture is placed from the fabella to the parapatella fibrocartilage, or restraint is provided with a fascial graft passed beneath the femoral-fabellar ligament and sutured to the parapatella fibrocartilage.

medial parapatella incision is made through the fascia and through the periosteum of the tibial tuberosity to allow lateral movement of the tibial tuberosity. An osteotome is positioned beneath the patella tendon 3 to 5 mm caudal to the cranial point of the tibial tuberosity. A mallet is used to complete the osteotomy in a proximal-to-distal direction.

The distal periosteal attachment should not be transected to lever the tuberosity laterally. The degree of lateral movement of the tibial tuberosity is subjective but is based on its longitudinal realignment relative to the trochlear groove. Once the site of relocation is chosen, the thin layer of cortical bone is removed with a rasp or the osteotome. The tibial tuberosity is levered into position and stabilized with one or two small Kirschner wires directed caudally and slightly proximally. It is important to gauge the depth and direction of pin placement. The pin should not exit the tibia caudally but should only engage the caudal cortex. If the pin protrudes too far from the caudal cortex of the tibia, persistent lameness results.

Lateral reinforcement. Reinforcement of the lateral retinaculum is accomplished with suture placement and imbrication of the fibrous joint capsule, by placement of a

fascia lata graft from the fabella to the parapatella fibrocartilage, or excision of redundant retinaculum (Fig. 18-6). For suture reinforcement, polyester suture is passed through the femoral-fabellar ligament and lateral parapatella fibrocartilage. A series of imbrication sutures are preplaced through the fibrous joint capsule and lateral edge of the patella tendon. With the leg in slight flexion, the femoral-fabellar suture and imbrication sutures are tied. The lateral retinaculum may also be reinforced through transposition of fascia lata. A section of fascia lata equal in width to the patella and in length to twice the distance from the patella to the fabella is isolated. The graft is freed proximally and left attached to the proximal pole of the patella distally. The free end of the graft is passed deep to the femoral-fabellar ligament and back to the lateral parapatella fibrocartilage. The graft is sutured to itself and the femoral-fabellar ligament with the leg in slight flexion.

If the patella is out of position most of the time, the retinaculum opposite the side of the luxation is stretched; with medial luxations, there is redundant lateral retinaculum. Once the patella is reduced, the excess retinaculum and joint capsule can be excised, allowing tight closure of the arthrotomy. None of the reinforcement techniques alone is adequate to permanently prevent reluxations. If the mechanical forces pulling the patella out of the trochlear groove are not neutralized, the reinforced retinaculum stretches again with time.

Medial release. The medial joint capsule is thicker than normal and contracted in patients with a grade III or IV patella luxation (Fig. 18-7). In these patients the medial joint capsule and retinaculum must be released to allow lateral placement of the patella. A medial parapatella incision is made through the medial fascia and joint capsule with a scalpel. The incision is begun at the level of the proximal pole of the patella and extends distally to the tibial crest. The wound is allowed to separate, and the cut edges are not sutured when surgery is completed. Rather, medial subcutaneous tissue is sutured to the cranial cut edge of the incision. If dynamic contraction of the cranial sartorius muscle and vastus medialis muscle directs the patella medially, the insertions of these muscles at the proximal patella are released. The insertions are redirected and sutured to the vastus intermedius.

Deepening of the trochlear groove. If the medial and lateral trochlear ridges do not constrain the patella, the trochlear groove must be deepened (Figs. 18-8 and 18-9). This technique is most commonly used in patients with a grade III or IV luxation. This may be achieved with a

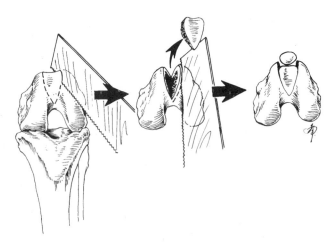

Fig. 18-8 Steps taken to deepen the trochlear groove with a trochlear wedge recession. An osteochondral wedge is removed, and the recess deepened by removing more bone from the recess's lateral edge. The osteochondral wedge is replaced into the deepened recess.

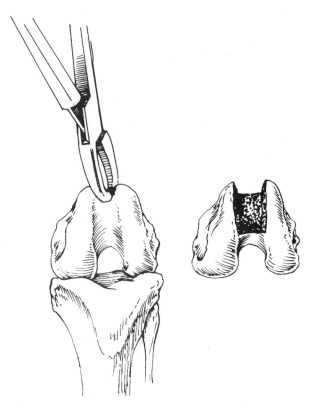

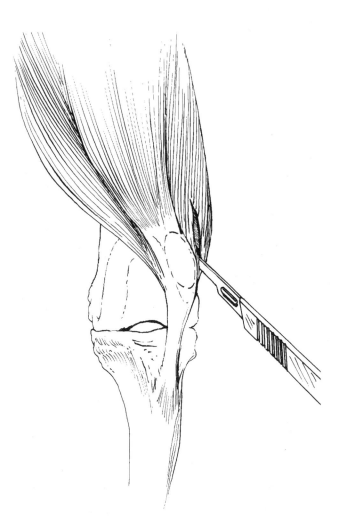

Fig. 18-7 Release of the medial restraints to allow lateral displacement of the patella.

Fig. 18-9 The method of deepening the trochlear groove by removing bone and articular cartilage. The width of the deepened groove must be such that it accommodates the patella.

trochlear wedge recession or a trochlear resection. A trochlear wedge recession is technically more demanding but preserves the articular cartilage, whereas a simple trochlear resection is less demanding but destroys the articular cartilage.

Trochlear wedge recession deepens the trochlear groove to restrain the patella and maintains the integrity of the patellofemoral articulation. A diamond-shaped outline is cut into the articular cartilage of the trochlea with a scalpel. The width of the cut must be sufficient at its midpoint to accommodate the patella's width. An osteochondral wedge of bone and cartilage is removed by following the outline previously made. The osteotomy is made so that the two oblique planes that form the free wedge intersect distally at the intercondylar notch and proximally at the dorsal edge of the trochlear articular cartilage. In larger patients an oscillating saw is used, but in smaller and toy breeds of dogs a fine-tooth hand-held saw or the cutting edge of a no. 20 scalpel blade and mallet are used. The osteochondral wedge is removed, and the recession in the trochlea is deepened by removing additional bone from one or both sides of the newly created femoral groove. With medial luxations, it is often best to take more bone from the lateral side of the groove, thus preserving as much of the medial ridge as possible. Remodeling the free osteochondral wedge with rongeurs may also be necessary to allow the wedge to seat deeply into the new femoral groove. The wedge can also be rotated 180 degrees when it is returned to the femoral groove if doing so aids in heightening the medial ridge. When the depth is sufficient to house 50% of the patella's height, as determined through periodic replacement of the free osteochondral wedge, it is replaced into the trochlea. The free osteochondral wedge remains in place because of the net compressive force of the patella and the friction between the cancellous surfaces of the two cut edges.

Trochlear resection is a method of deepening the trochlear groove through removal of articular cartilage and subchondral cancellous bone. The measured width of the patella's articular surface is used to determine the proper width of the trochlear resection. Articular cartilage and bone are removed with a bone rasp, power burr, or rongeurs. The length of the trochlear resection should extend to the proximal margin of articular cartilage and distally to the cartilage margin just above the intercondylar notch. The groove's depth should accommodate 50% of the patella's height and allow the parapatella fibrocartilage to articulate with the newly formed medial and lateral trochlear ridges. The medial and lateral trochlear ridges are made parallel to each other and the groove's base perpendicular to each trochlear ridge. The advantage of this technique is its simplicity. The disadvantages are that it removes the trochlear articular cartilage, and patella articulation on the rough cancellous surface

results in wearing of patella articular cartilage. Nevertheless, the trochlear groove eventually fills with a combination of fibrous tissue and fibrocartilage, and patients appear to have acceptable limb function.

Osteotomy of the femur. This procedure is used only in patients with severe skeletal deformity in whom it is determined that maintaining patella reduction is not possible with the techniques described previously. The deformities usually seen are a varus bowing of the distal femur and medial torsional deformity of the proximal tibia. The goal of surgery is to realign the stifle joint in the frontal plane where the transverse axis of the femoral condyles is perpendicular to the longitudinal axis of the femoral diaphysis. This requires accurate preoperative measurement and wedge osteotomy of the femur. Transposition of the tibial crest, lateral retinacular reinforcement, medial restraint release, and deepening of the trochlear groove are also required for success. These techniques require special equipment and a trained specialist.

Lateral Patella Luxation

Lateral patella luxation is seen most frequently in large breeds of dogs but does occur in small and toy breeds. The cause is unknown but thought to be related to abnormal anteversion or coxa valga of the hip joint. Either condition shifts the line of force produced by the pull of the quadriceps lateral to the longitudinal axis of the trochlear groove. Clinical signs and physical findings are similar to those seen with medial patella luxations. One difference is that the lameness associated with lateral luxation is usually more pronounced. As with medial luxations, there are four grades of lateral luxation; grade I is the least severe and grade IV the most severe.

Differential diagnoses include hip dysplasia, osteochondritis dissecans (OCD) of the stifle or tarsal joints, panosteitis, HOD, capital physeal injury, cranial cruciate ligament rupture, and muscle strain. Diagnosis is determined by the finding of lateral patella luxation on physical examination and by eliminating other causes of rear limb lameness. Many patients with lateral patella luxation concurrently have evidence of hip dysplasia. Both conditions may be contributing to clinical lameness and need appropriate treatment.

Goals and methods of treatment for lateral patella luxation are similar to those described for medial patella luxation. The surgical exposure is identical, as is the technique for osteotomy of the tibial tuberosity. However, with lateral luxations, the tuberosity is repositioned and stabilized medially. The medial retinaculum is reinforced with suture reconstruction, fascia lata transposition, and/or excision of redundant joint capsule. The lateral restraints are released, which helps neutralize lateral forces acting on the patella. Methods for deepening the trochlear groove are the same as described for medial patella luxation. Osteotomies of the femur and tibia may be required to correct severe angular and torsional deformities. Corrective osteotomies are best performed by a specialist with the necessary equipment and training to perform these complex procedures.

Prognosis

The clinical results of surgical correction of medial patella luxation in dogs have been reviewed. The results were based on clinical assessment of the dog's gait and physical and radiographic examination of the stifle joints. The dogs were grouped according to age at presentation and examined after a minimum of 1 year after surgery. Group 1 included dogs 3 to 6 months of age, group 2 included dogs 8 to 20 months, and group 3 included dogs 2.2 to 12 years. One year after surgery, six of seven joints in group 1 had moderate to severe degenerative changes of the patellofemoral joint radiographically. Groups 2 and 3 exhibited mild radiographic changes of the patellofemoral joint. Twenty-five of 52 (48%) of the joints evaluated showed recurrent luxation. However, the majority were grade I luxations, which did not affect clinical function. Forty-eight of 52 stifle joints functioned well enough that lameness was not apparent during examination, and the client did not report clinical dysfunction. Most patients with recurrent luxations exhibited reluxation only on physical examination when manual force was used to displace the patella. Reluxation was not correlated to the method(s) of surgical correction, so it is not possible to determine if a particular corrective measure was more or less successful in this group of patients.

Overall, the prognosis for patients undergoing surgical correction of a patella luxation is excellent for return to normal limb function.

LIGAMENT INJURIES OF THE STIFLE JOINT
Cranial Cruciate Ligament Injury

Anatomy and function of the cranial cruciate ligament. The cranial cruciate ligament (CCL) originates from the inside (medial) surface of the lateral femoral condyle (Fig. 18-10). The CCL is a complex arrangement of longitudinally oriented collagen fiber bundles that functions to prevent excessive cranial translation of the tibia relative to the femur. The ligament fibers course distal and medial, spiral 90 degrees, and insert onto the craniomedial surface of the tibial plateau. The CCL is divided into two major fiber groups according to their insertional position on the tibial plateau: the craniomedial band and the caudolateral band. The craniomedial band is taut during all phases of flexion and extension; the caudolateral band is taut in extension but becomes lax with flexion. The CCL also functions to limit internal rotation of the tibia; as the stifle is flexed, the cranial and caudal cruciate ligaments twist

on each other and limit the degree of internal rotation of the tibia relative to the femur. The interaction of the cranial and caudal cruciate ligaments during flexion also provides limited varus-valgus support to the flexed stifle joint.

Mechanoreceptors and afferent nerve endings have been identified within the interfiber layers of the CCL. The CCL's innervation serves as a proprioceptive feedback mechanism to prevent excessive flexion or extension of the stifle joint. This protective action is through stimulation or relaxation of muscle groups that lend support to the joint. The major blood supply to the CCL enters the ligament through the synovial sheath. The synovial vessels give rise to smaller intraligamentous arteries that course through the ligament as endoligamentous vessels; others leave the synovial sheath to enter the ligament transverse to the longitudinal axis of the ligament.

Mechanism of injury. The mechanism of injury to the CCL directly reflects its function as a constraint to joint motion. Injury can be purely traumatic; however, other factors may be involved in the pathogenesis of cruciate disease. One factor is age-related change in the CCL's structural and histological properties. Histologically, there is a loss of fiber bundle organization and metaplastic

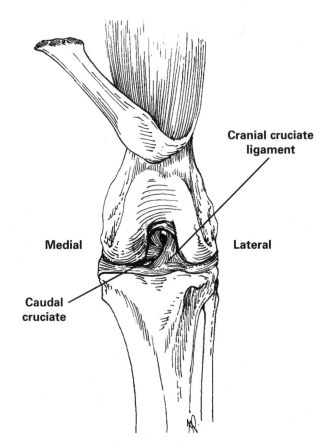

Fig. 18-10 The normal appearance and intraarticular position of the cranial cruciate and caudal cruciate ligament.

changes of the cellular elements. Biomechanically, loss of structural and material strength and stiffness occurs. Abnormal conformation also may contribute to CCL rupture. Certain breeds, such as the Rottweiler and chow chow, appear to have a greater standing angle of the stifle joint. This may predispose them to complete or partial tearing of the CCL's craniomedial band by the roof of the intercondylar notch. Partial tearing of the CCL may lead to the formation of anticollagen antibodies that can destroy the CCL's structure. Anticollagen antibodies and immune complexes have been detected in the synovial fluid and sera of dogs with CCL rupture.

Traumatic CCL rupture is most often seen in small breeds of dogs and young, athletic, sporting breeds of dogs. Complete traumatic CCL rupture diagnosed in the young sporting breeds may reflect a change in the owner's activity level in recent years. The history often shows that these patients are "weekend" athletes; that is, they are sedentary during the week when the owners are busy but very active on weekends. The strenuous weekend activity (e.g., hunting, jogging, playing frisbee) without proper physical conditioning may predispose to ligament injury. Smaller dogs tend to rupture their CCL later in life; this reflects on an age-related change in the strength of cruciate ligaments.

The most common mechanism of CCL injury is associated with a violent internal rotation. When this occurs, the cruciate ligaments begin to twist and become wound tightly on themselves. As internal rotation progresses, the CCL is subject to injury from the caudomedial edge of the lateral femoral condyle as the condyle rotates against the ligament. Another mechanism of CCL injury is hyperextension of the stifle. When the stifle joint is hyperextended, the roof of the intercondylar notch may act as a knife in transecting the CCL.

Sporting breeds of dogs have an increased incidence of partial CCL tearing. The anatomical components of the CCL provide specific stability in flexion and extension, and each component may be injured independent of the other, giving rise to partial CCL tearing. The activities that cause partial tearing are most likely the same as those already described for complete rupture, but the force is not great enough to tear the ligament completely. Also, conformational characteristics of the breed can predispose the dog to partial CCL tearing. It appears that partial tears subsequently progress to total rupture within 1 year.

Clinical presentation. Three clinical presentations are associated with injury: (1) acute injury, (2) chronic injury, and (3) partial tears.

Acute injury. Patients with acute tears have an acute non-weight-bearing or partial weight-bearing lameness. The patient is apprehensive during examination of the stifle joint, but pain, if present, is usually mild. Joint effusion may be palpable alongside the patella tendon. Instability can be difficult to elicit because of patient apprehension and resulting muscle contraction.

Chronic injury. Patients with more chronic injury have a history as previously described, but lameness has improved with time. In most dogs the lameness appears to be resolving without treatment 3 to 4 weeks after injury. This is particularly true in patients weighing less than 10 kg (22 pounds). Retrospective studies of this population of patients (smaller dogs) seem to indicate they may have adequate clinical function with nonsurgical treatment. In patients weighing greater than 10 kg, the lameness improves but the patient never returns to preinjury activity without evidence of recurring periodic lameness. Physical examination shows a decrease in thigh muscle mass compared with the normal limb, and crepitus may be evident through flexion and extension. When the joint is extended from a flexed position, a clicking or popping may be heard and felt; this is usually associated with a meniscal tear. However, the presence or absence of joint noise neither confirms nor denies the presence of meniscal injury. Osteophytes are present along the medial and lateral trochlear ridges, and a palpable enlargement of the joint's medial surface is evident. Craniocaudal instability can be difficult to elicit in this group of patients because of the proliferative response of the fibrous joint capsule. This is particularly true in larger, apprehensive patients.

Partial tears. Patients with partial CCL tears are difficult to diagnose in the early stages of injury. In the beginning, they have a mild weight-bearing lameness associated with exercise. However, before the development of degenerative changes, the lameness resolves when the dog is rested. As the CCL continues to tear and the stifle becomes more unstable, the degenerative changes worsen and the lameness is more evident. At this point, the lameness does not resolve with rest. Instability of the stifle joint is difficult to detect early because a section of the CCL is still intact.

Tearing of the caudolateral band alone does not produce instability if the craniomedial band is preserved, since the latter is taut in both flexion and extension. If an isolated injury to the craniomedial band occurs (caudolateral band remains intact), the joint is stable in extension because the caudolateral band remains taut; however, instability is present in flexion because the caudolateral band normally becomes lax during flexion. Initially, there is no pain, detectable synovial effusion, or crepitus, but as time progresses, signs of instability and degenerative joint disease (DJD) become evident.

Differential diagnoses. Differential diagnoses include mild joint sprains or muscle strains, patella luxation, caudal cruciate ligament injury, long digital extensor tendon avulsion, and primary or secondary arthritis. Cranial drawer (excessive craniocaudal movement) is diagnostic of cruciate ligament injury. With partial tears the cranial drawer sign may reveal only 2 to 3 mm of instability, and then only when the test is done in flexion. Since almost all isolated cruciate ligament tears involve the CCL, craniocaudal instability is usually associated with CCL injury.

The *cranial drawer test* is performed with the patient in lateral recumbency. Lack of adequate patient relaxation is the most common cause of failure to elicit cranial drawer movement. Therefore, if the examiner suspects that the lameness originates with a stifle joint problem, general anesthesia or heavy sedation is necessary to negate the influence of muscle tension. Once the dog is in lateral position, the examiner stands to the patient's rear and positions the thumb and forefinger of one hand on the femur. The thumb is placed directly behind the fabella and the forefinger over the patella. The remaining fingers are wrapped around the thigh. The other hand is placed on the tibia with the thumb directly behind the fibular head and the forefinger over the tibial crest. The three remaining fingers are wrapped around the tibial shaft. The femur is stabilized with the one hand while the tibia is moved forward and back with the second hand parallel to the transverse plane of the tibial plateau. The pressure to move the tibia forward should be applied through the thumb behind the fibular head. The tibia must be held in neutral position, as determined by the position of the fingers on the patella and tibial tuberosity, and must not be allowed to rotate internally. If this occurs, internal joint rotation may appear as cranial drawer movement. The examiner must test for signs of instability with the stifle joint in extension, normal standing angle, and 90 degrees of flexion. If the degree of movement is questionable, comparison with the opposite limb is helpful. A positive test is craniocaudal movement beyond the normal 0 to 2 mm found in normal stifle joints.

After the cranial drawer test, the stifle should be flexed and extended though a range of normal movement. With the leg in extension, collateral stability should be assessed. After assessment of the joint's ligamentous integrity, craniocaudal and mediolateral radiographs should be taken. With acute tears, radiographs are helpful to rule out other causes of stifle joint lameness. Radiographic findings in patients with chronic ligament tears include osteophyte formation along the trochlear ridge, caudal surface of the tibial plateau, and inferior pole of the patella. Also, thickening of the medial fibrous joint capsule and subchondral sclerosis are evident. If joint palpation and radiographs are inconclusive, joint centesis and synovial fluid examination are helpful. This is particularly true with partial ligament tears to help identify stifle joint involvement as the cause of the lameness. Increased joint fluid and a twofold to threefold increase in the number of cells (6000 to 9000) indicate secondary DJD.

Methods of treatment. Patients with CCL tears should have surgical reconstruction of the injured stifle joint.

Although patients weighing less than 7 to 10 kg (15½ to 22 pounds) appear to function adequately after conservative treatment, they may have future problems. After nonsurgical treatment in smaller patients, the lameness may resolve within 6 weeks, and they appear to function normally on the injured leg. However, instability persists and secondary DJD develops. These patients may injure the cruciate ligament of the opposite limb 12 to 18 months later. With both limbs having ruptured cruciate ligaments, the patient may be nonambulatory and appear to have an acute neurological problem. With accurate historical information and physical examination, it becomes evident that the patient's problem is bilateral cruciate ligament injury. Although the patient appeared to function adequately after injury to the first limb, body weight was merely shifted to the uninjured leg. Abnormal stress coupled with the increasing mechanical weakness of the cruciate ligament associated with aging lead to cruciate ligament rupture in the opposite stifle joint. Treatment of patients with bilateral cruciate ruptures is not as successful as in patients with only one injured stifle joint. For this reason, surgical reconstruction is recommended in small patients with CCL injury.

Surgical therapy is divided into reconstruction techniques and primary repair with augmentation. Primary repairs are not used often and are always supplemented with a reconstructive technique.

Reconstruction. The reconstruction method chosen for an individual patient is usually the surgeon's preference. Retrospective studies of reconstructive techniques show the success rate to be near 90% regardless of the technique chosen. Intracapsular and extracapsular reconstructions of the CCL share equal popularity among veterinary surgeons. Intracapsular reconstructions consist of passing autogenous tissue through the joint using the "over-the-top" method or passing the tissue through predrilled holes in the femur and tibia. Extracapsular reconstructions involve the placement of sutures outside the joint or redirection of the lateral collateral ligament. It is often useful to combine intracapsular and extracapsular reconstructions in the large and giant breeds of dogs.

Intracapsular reconstruction. The most frequently used intracapsular reconstruction is the over-the-top placement of autogenous tissue. Three autogenous tissues have been described for use in veterinary orthopedics: (1) medial one-third of the patella tendon and proximal fascia, (2) central third of the patella tendon and proximal fascia, and (3) lateral fibers of the patella tendon and distal fascia lata. Of these, the central and lateral grafts are stronger and stiffer. Because the lateral graft is easier to harvest, I prefer this graft when choosing an intracapsular reconstruction.

To perform an intracapsular reconstruction with fascia lata, the limb is surgically prepared to allow manipulation during surgery, and the patient is placed in lateral recumbency with the affected limb uppermost. The skin incision is begin from a point proximally midway between the greater trochanter and superior pole of the patella. From this point, the incision courses along the craniolateral surface of the thigh and extends distally to the level of the tibial plateau. The subcutaneous tissue and loose connective tissues are reflected from the fascia lata medially to the border of the cranial sartorius muscle and laterally to the biceps femoris muscle. The superficial surface of the patella tendon is freed of loose connective tissue. The limb is flexed to tighten the patella tendon and lateral retinacular tissue. An incision is made beginning at the lateral edge of the distal pole of the patella and extending through the lateral third of the patella tendon and retinaculum to the tibial crest distally. The limb is then extended to relax the retinacular tissues lateral to the patella. With the scalpel and periosteal elevator, the retinacular tissue overlying the lateral patella surface is reflected. Scissors are placed deep into the incision and forced proximally along the medial edge of the cranial sartorius muscle. The incision through the fascia lata is carried proximally the full length of the skin incision. When the proximal extent of the incision is reached, the fascia lata is incised caudally to the reflection of the biceps femoris muscle. The incision is continued distally along the cranial edge of the biceps muscle to the tibial plateau. When bringing the fascial incision distally, it is extremely important to maintain equal width of the fascial graft along its entire length (Fig. 18-11). The graft needs to be undermined from proximal to distal and freed from the loose connective tissue attachments. This process is stopped midway between the patella and tibial crest to ensure vascularity of the graft.

The joint capsule is incised from the distal pole of the patella to the tibial crest. At the patella level, the capsule incision is directed proximally and caudally along the vastus lateralis border to the lateral fabella region. The patella is luxated, medially exposing the cranial view of the stifle. Remnants of the torn CCL are excised and the joint's internal structures examined. To visualize the caudomedial joint compartment, a Hohmann retractor is used. The tip is placed on the caudal tibial spine and the body set against the distal trochlea. Caudal pressure on the retractor handle forces the tibia forward and down, exposing the medial meniscus. Damage in the form of tears or folding of the caudal body of the medial meniscus is seen in 50% to 75% of patients with a torn CCL. In patients with a damaged medial meniscus, the damaged section of meniscus is excised.

The fascial graft is passed beneath the intermeniscal ligament with a right-angle forceps. The over-the-top maneuver is completed by passing an Adson curved hemostatic forceps over the top of the fabella and by gliding next to the lateral condyle, penetrating the caudal joint capsule. The graft's free end is grasped and pulled through the joint (Fig. 18-12). An incision is made through the femoral-fabellar ligament and the graft passed through the ligament. The fascial graft is secured to the lateral femoral condyle with a spiked polyacetyl washer and bone screw or sutured to the femoral-fabellar ligament, fibrous joint capsule, and patella tendon.

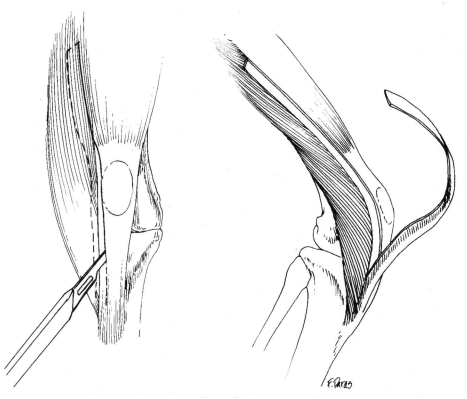

Fig. 18-11   Isolation of a patella tendon-fascia lata graft.

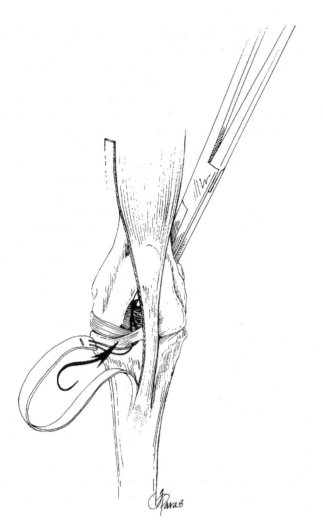

Fig. 18-12 Passage of an intracapsular graft through the joint using the under and over method. The graft is first passed beneath the intermeniscal ligament and then through the joint adjacent to the lateral condyle.

Lameness and occasional draining tracts have been associated with the use of the screw and washer. If a screw and washer are used, removal 2 to 3 months postoperatively is recommended. When the graft is being secured to the femoral condyle, no attempt should be made to eliminate all the cranial drawer, since this places excessive tension within the graft. As a rule, all but 2 to 3 mm of cranial drawer should be eliminated while the leg is positioned in normal standing angle. The fibrous joint capsule, cut edge of fascia lata, and subcutaneous tissues are sutured with absorbable suture using a simple interrupted pattern. The skin is sutured with nonabsorbable suture with a simple interrupted pattern.

Extracapsular reconstruction. Various surgical techniques have been described for extracapsular suture placement as a method to treat the CCL-deficient stifle joint. All the techniques involve placement of nonabsorbable sutures or orthopedic wire to eliminate or

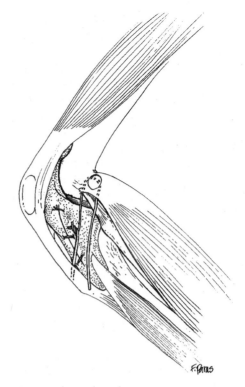

Fig. 18-13 Correct placement of a suture from the fabellar to tibial crest for extracapsular stabilization of the cranial cruciate deficient stifle joint. Note the placement around the fabella and through predrilled holes in the tibial crest.

reduce cranial drawer. Surgical exposure and inspection of the joint's internal structures are identical to those described for intracapsular reconstruction. The arthrotomy is then closed with absorbable suture using a simple interrupted pattern. The biceps femoris muscle is elevated from the joint capsule surface laterally and caudally to expose the muscle fibers of the gastrocnemius muscle. Polyester suture or monofilament wire is passed deeply through the femoral-fabellar ligament, passing around the fabella. The suture size depends on the patient's weight, but as a general rule, no. 2 to 5 polyester suture or 20-to-18 gauge wire is used. The femoral-fabellar ligament is located just proximal to the fabella and is the dense fibrous tissue that incorporates the insertion of the fabella and gastrocnemius muscle onto the femur's caudolateral metaphysis. The suture or wire is then passed through a predrilled hole through the tibial crest. The stifle is flexed to 90 degrees and the suture tied (or wire twisted) until it engages the joint capsule (Fig. 18-13). In addition to the stabilizing suture, a series of imbricating sutures can be placed through the fibrous joint capsule with nonabsorbable suture (Fig. 18-14). Each suture passes through the fibrous capsule caudal to the arthrotomy line, crosses superficial to the arthrotomy, and penetrates the fibrous capsule cranial to the arthrotomy. Individual sutures are preplaced and not tied until the series of sutures is in

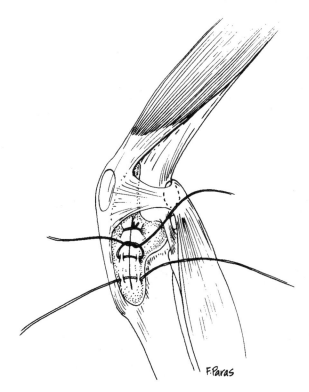

Fig. 18-14   Preplacement and tying of sutures used for imbricating the joint capsule for gaining additional extracapsular support for the cruciate deficient stifle joint. Note the sutures are placed to cross the arthrotomy line to prevent separation of the arthrotomy.

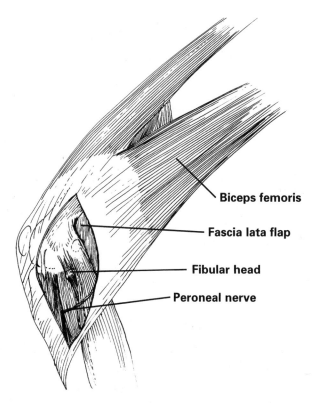

Biceps femoris

Fascia lata flap

Fibular head

Peroneal nerve

Fig. 18-15   Lateral and caudal reflection of the fascia lata parallel to the joint line to expose the fibular head. Note the position of the peroneal nerve.

place. The extracapsular sutures can be augmented with tissue advancements. Typically, advancement of the biceps femoris muscle by suturing the cranial edge of the biceps fascia incision to the patella tendon aids in restricting cranial drawer. The subcutaneous tissue is sutured with continuous pattern using absorbable suture and the skin sutured with nonabsorbable suture using a simple interrupted pattern.

Postoperatively, patient activity is limited to exercise on a leash only for 8 weeks. If wire is used, it ultimately breaks; generally this does not occur until periarticular fibrous tissue is formed to stabilize the joint. Occasionally a dog becomes lame when the wire breaks, but this often resolves with 2 weeks of rest and administration of nonsteroidal antiinflammatory drugs. If polyester suture material is used, the suture loosens with increasing postoperative time. Again, this may not occur until after the stifle has been stabilized by fibrosis. Polyester suture causes a draining tract in 15% to 20% of patients, whereas orthopedic wire rarely causes a problem of draining tracts. Removal of the suture resolves the problem.

Static advancement of the lateral collateral ligament. Static advancement of the lateral collateral ligament (LCL) is another useful technique for elimination of instability in the CCL-deficient stifle joint. This is accomplished by advancing the fibular head, which is the LCL's

point of insertion. Surgical exposure and inspection of the joint are the same as described before. The arthrotomy is sutured with absorbable suture using a simple interrupted pattern. The fascia lata is reflected caudally. This is facilitated by a craniocaudal transverse incision of the fascia lata 2 to 3 cm distal to the joint line (Fig. 18-15). Care must be taken to identify and protect the peroneal nerve at this time and throughout the remainder of the procedure. The fibular head is freed cranially and caudally from the tibial epiphysis with sharp dissection and elevation (Fig. 18-16). An incision is made along the LCL's cranial and caudal edges. Being careful not to injure the popliteal tendon or lateral meniscus, the surgeon frees the LCL's deep surface from its origin to insertion onto the fibular head. This is most easily accomplished with a small periosteal elevator. The fibularis longus muscle and lateral digital extensor muscle are incised from caudal to cranial at the joint line and reflected craniodistal to allow redirection of the LCL. The tibia is externally rotated and the fibular head with the attached ligament advanced cranially using bone-holding forceps.

The fibular head is stabilized with a small Steinmann pin and tension-band wire (Fig. 18-17). The wire is placed through predrilled holes in the tibial crest, deep to the extensor muscles and around the pin's protruding end. As the wire is tightened, further advancement of the LCL is

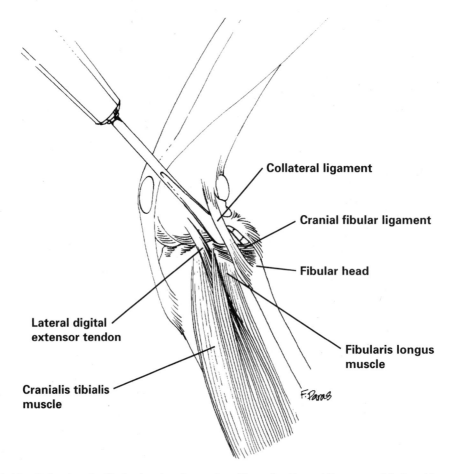

Fig. 18-16 Releasing the fibular head and associated lateral collateral ligament with the aid of a periosteal elevator. Sharp dissection and elevation are combined to separate the fibular head from the tibia.

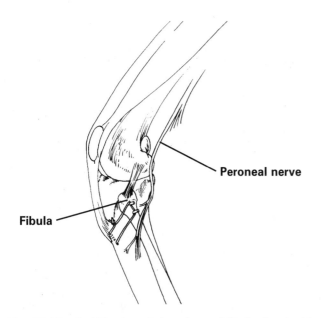

Fig. 18-17 Stabilization of the advanced fibular head with wire and pins. Note the wire is passed through predrilled holes in the tibial crest and around the ends of two small pins used to stabilize the position of the fibular head.

obtained. The incised extensor muscles and fascia lata are sutured with absorbable suture using a simple interrupted pattern. The subcutaneous tissue and skin incisions are sutured as described before. Postoperatively, the limb is placed in a soft, padded bandage for 10 to 14 days. After this, exercise is limited to leash activity for an additional 3 weeks. Prognosis for return of function is good with all breeds of dogs.

Primary repair. Primary repair with augmentation is reserved for a small percentage of patients that have experienced failure of the CCL at the point of insertion on the tibial plateau or failure from the CCL's origin on the femur. This mode of ligament failure may occur following trauma to the stifle joint in patients less than 1 year of age. The most frequently seen site of failure is the point of insertion onto the tibial plateau. Surgical exposure is the same as described for intracapsular or extracapsular reconstruction. A reconstructive procedure is always used in addition to primary repair. When the arthrotomy is made, the CCL is identified. Often a small piece of cancellous bone remains attached at the site of failure. Nonabsorbable suture is passed through the ligament using a locking loop

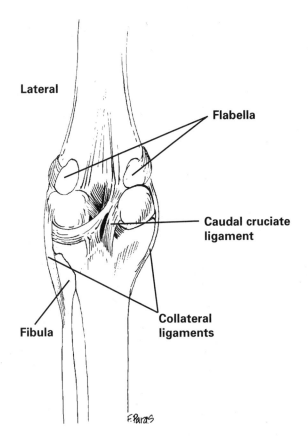

Lateral

Flabella

Caudal cruciate ligament

Fibula

Collateral ligaments

F.Paras

Fig. 18-18 A caudal view of the stifle joint. The insertion of the caudal cruciate ligament into the popliteal notch and its position relative to other joint structures is shown.

pattern. Two small parallel drill holes are made from the medial tibial metaphysis to exit within the joint at the CCL's insertion point. Wire loops are used to pass the suture's free ends through the predrilled holes. The previously isolated fascial graft is passed through the joint and secured to the femoral condyle as described earlier to eliminate cranial drawer and augment the primary repair. Once the joint is stable, the sutures in the ligament are tied outside the joint. The surgical wound is closed using the technique previously described.

Postoperatively, the limb is placed in a padded, soft bandage to prevent overextension and flexion of the stifle joint. Enforced rest and the bandage are necessary for 3 to 4 weeks postoperatively. Supervised activity on a leash only is encouraged for an additional 8 weeks. After this, the patient must gradually return to normal activity. Prognosis for return of function is good for all breeds of dogs.

Caudal Cruciate Ligament Injury

Anatomy and function of caudal cruciate ligament. The caudal cruciate ligament (CaCL) originates from the intercondyloid fossa of the distal femur; specifically, from the craniolateral (inside) surface of the medial condyle

(Fig. 18-18). From the point of origin, the CaCL courses distally to insert into the tibia's popliteal notch. The CaCL has functionally been separated into two components; the larger cranial portion is taut in flexion and lax in extension, whereas the smaller caudal section is taut in extension and lax in flexion. The cranial and caudal bands function to prevent caudal translation (sliding) of the tibia during flexion. The CaCL also functions in concert with the CCL to provide rotational stability in flexion and varus-valgus stability in extension.

Mechanism of injury. Isolated CaCL tears are rare in small animals for several reasons. First, the CaCL is positioned in the joint such that the loads that typically cause ligament injury are directed more toward the CCL. Second, the CaCL is stronger than the CCL. Third, the types of accidents that can cause CaCL rupture are not usually encountered. Nevertheless, isolated CaCL ruptures do occur and are generally caused by a cranial-to-caudal blow directed against the proximal tibia. This type of injury is most frequently associated with an automobile accident or falling on the limb with the stifle joint flexed.

CaCL injuries are more often associated with severe derangement of the stifle joint. In these patients, a combination of primary and secondary joint restraints are ruptured; the cause is a severe traumatic episode, usually an automobile accident. Primary restraints usually injured are the CCL, CaCL, and medial collateral ligament (MCL). Secondary restraints injured are the joint capsule, muscle tendon units, and meniscocapsular ligaments.

Clinical presentation. Patients with an isolated CaCL rupture initially have a non-weight-bearing lameness in association with the traumatic episode. The lameness progressively improves, but the patient does not regain athletic status. The patient may have a normal gait at a walk but is lame when running. This is because the CaCL functions to stabilize the joint primarily when the joint is in flexion and the patient does not need to flex the stifle joint beyond 90 degrees when walking. However, with running the stifle is flexed beyond 90 degrees, allowing caudal instability to occur.

Diagnosis of isolated CaCL tears is based on the presence of craniocaudal instability. It can be difficult to determine if the craniocaudal movement is caused by CCL or CaCL injury. Perceived cranial drawer movement may actually be a forward reduction of the tibia to a normal position. The following points may help in the differentiation between CCL and CaCL injury:

1. When the joint is held in extension, the degree of palpable instability is less with CaCL tears compared with that present with CCL tears.
2. With a normal joint, the tibial tuberosity forms a distinct prominence cranial to the patella; when a

CaCL injury is present, there is a loss of the tuberosity prominence.

3. If the CaCL is ruptured, when the tibia is moved forward, there is a distance end point to the cranial movement.

4. With the tibia in the forward position, there is a distinct caudal subluxation of the tibia when the stifle joint is flexed and internally rotated.

Radiographs are often helpful in the diagnosis of CaCL injuries. Small bone densities may be apparent on the lateral projection just behind and distal to the femoral condyles. Also, the tibial plateau is displaced caudal relative to the femoral condyles in the lateral projection. CaCL tears that are part of a multiple ligament injury are diagnosed because of the presence of severe instability.

Methods of treatment. Long-term evaluation of dogs having reconstruction of isolated CaCL tears shows the prognosis to be good and independent of treatment methods. Experimental studies question the need for CaCL reconstruction, but clinical experience dictates that reconstruction is warranted in larger breeds of dogs and athletic dogs. As with CCL injury, treatment may be done by extracapsular reconstruction or intracapsular reconstruction.

Extracapsular reconstruction is performed by suture stabilization, redirection of the MCL, or popliteal tendon tenodesis. Suture stabilization has been described by Brinker and consists of imbrication of the caudomedial joint capsule and placement of a stabilizing suture from the proximal patella tendon through a predrilled hole in the caudomedial corner of the tibial epiphysis. On the lateral side, the caudal joint capsule is imbricated and a stabilizing suture placed from the proximal patella tendon through a predrilled hole in the fibular head. Extracapsular reconstruction can also be accomplished through redirection of existing autogenous tissue. A technique described by Egger is to redirect the MCL caudally and entrap the ligament with a bone screw and washer. A medial approach allows incision through the insertion of the caudal sartorius muscle and medial fascia along the tibial metaphysis. The muscle and fascia are reflected caudally to expose the MCL. The ligament body is freed with a periosteal elevator and directed caudally to course in the same sagittal plane as the CaCL. The ligament is then secured in this position with a bone screw and spiked washer. Another method of CaCL reconstruction is entrapment of the popliteal tendon. A lateral approach and reflection of the fascia lata allow isolation of the popliteal tendon as it passes beneath the LCL. Tenodesis of the popliteal tendon is done by entrapping the popliteal tendon with a suture as it passes caudal and proximal to the fibular head.

Intracapsular reconstruction of the CaCL may be performed by transposition of the origin of the popliteal tendon. The origin of the popliteal tendon is found just cranial and deep to the origin of the long digital extensor tendon on the lateral condyle's cranial surface. A small osteotome is used to free the origin of the popliteal tendon along with a small section of bone. The tendon/bone complex is passed deep to the LCL, through the caudal joint capsule, and into the joint. A bone tunnel is drilled through the medial condyle from outside the joint to emerge at the CaCL's origin. The tendon/bone complex is passed into the drill hole and secured with suture or an interference screw.

Collateral Ligament Injury

Anatomy and function of the medial and lateral collateral ligaments. The MCL originates from the medial femoral epicondyle and courses distally to insert onto the proximal tibial metaphysis. As the MCL crosses the medial joint line, it forms a strong attachment to the joint capsule and medial meniscus. This is important in stabilizing the medial meniscus but predisposes the caudal body of the meniscus to injury from the medial femoral condyle when CCL rupture is present. The LCL originates from an oval area on the lateral femoral epicondyle; it then courses distally to insert onto the fibular head.

The MCL and LCL function in concert to limit varus-valgus motion of the stifle joint. This is most important when the stifle joint is in extension, the point at which both the MCL and the LCL are taut. As the stifle joint flexes, the MCL remains tight, but the LCL becomes more relaxed to allow internal rotation of the tibia. This motion permits the foot to turn inward beneath the body during ambulation. As the stifle joint extends, the LCL becomes taut once again to assist in external rotation of the tibia. This motion aligns the foot into proper position for the weight-bearing phase of the gait.

Mechanism of injury. Isolated MCL or LCL tears are rare in small animals. Most injuries that involve the MCL or LCL occur in conjunction with injury to other primary and secondary restraints of the stifle joint. These multiple ligament injuries are often the result of severe trauma directed to the stifle joint and involve injury to a myriad of stifle joint ligaments.

Clinical presentation. Diagnosis of collateral ligament injury, whether an isolated ligament tear or as part of a complex injury, is based on palpation. It is important to remember that the stifle joint must be positioned in extension when examining for collateral restraint injury. The valgus stress test is used to evaluate the integrity of the MCL. With the patient in lateral recumbency, one hand is used to stabilize the femur while the other hand grasps the distal tibia and applies an upward force (abduction). If the medial joint restraints (MCL, joint capsule, peripheral meniscal ligaments) are torn, opening of the medial joint line is apparent. The varus stress test is used to evaluate the integrity of the LCL. One hand stabilizes the femur while the other hand grasps the distal tibia and applies an inward force (adduction). If the lateral joint restraints (LCL, joint capsule, peripheral meniscal ligaments) are torn, opening of the lateral joint is apparent. Radiographs should be taken to assess the presence or absence of bone chips associated with ligament damage. Additional stress radiographs can be taken to help assess the severity of collateral restraint injury.

Methods of treatment. The decision to use conservative or surgical treatment for isolated collateral ligament injury is based on the degree of injury to the ligament and secondary joint restraints (joint capsule, peripheral meniscal ligaments). This assessment is made based on palpation and radiographs. Minimal swelling and only slight opening of the joint space when the joint is placed under stress indicate conservative treatment. This method of treatment is supported by in vivo experiments, which have shown that selected transection of a collateral ligament heals well when treated only with immobilization. Patients in this category should have a fiberglass cast applied for 2 weeks followed by controlled activity for 6 weeks.

Patients with moderate to severe swelling and significant opening of the joint space when the joint is placed under stress have significant injury to the collateral restraints (Fig. 18-19). In this group of patients, operative treatment is recommended. Surgery includes reconstruction of the collateral ligament, meniscocapsular ligaments, and joint capsule. A medial or lateral parapatella incision is made, depending on which ligament is injured. The MCL is exposed by incising the insertion of the caudal head of the sartorius muscle and deep fascia along the craniomedial border of the proximal tibia. The muscle and fascia are retracted caudally to expose the MCL and medial joint capsule. The LCL is exposed by making a parapatella incision through the fascia lata from proximal to distal. The incision is carried distally 4 cm below the tibial crest and courses caudally parallel to the joint line. Care is exercised not to injure the peroneal nerve. The fascia lata is reflected caudally to expose the LCL and lateral joint capsule.

Primary repair of the collateral ligament is undertaken if the point of failure is the origin or insertion of the ligament. Occasionally, a small fragment of bone may be present on the end of the ligament, which can be incorporated into the repair. The ligament is replaced in its anatomical site and secured with a screw and polyacetyl spiked washer (Fig. 18-20). If the ligament injury is an intrasubstance tear, primary repair is accomplished by

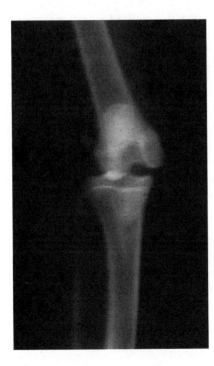

Fig. 18-19 Craniocaudal radiograph showing joint widening assoicated with medial collateral ligament injury.

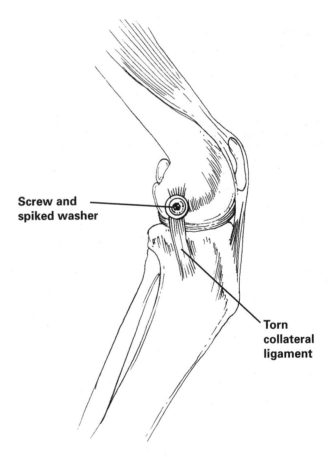

Screw and spiked washer

Torn collateral ligament

Fig. 18-20 Primary repair of a collateral ligament that failed at the site of origin onto the femoral condyle. A screw is tightened to compress a spiked washer to hold ligament in position.

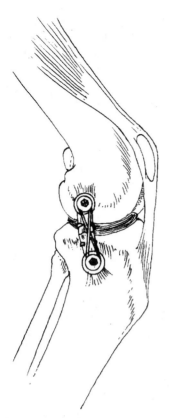

Fig. 18-21 Primary repair of an interstitial tear of the collateral ligament. Following apposition of the torn ends, the repair is supported with screws placed at the anatomical origin and insertion of the ligament. Nonabsorbable suture is placed around the screw heads.

suturing the ligament ends; a locking loop suture pattern using small, nonabsorbable suture is recommended. The primary repair must be supplemented with screws and figure-eight support (Fig. 18-21). Following repair of the collateral ligament, careful reconstruction of the meniscocapsular ligaments and joint capsule must be performed. Interrupted sutures of small, nonabsorbable suture material (prolene or nylon) are preferred.

MENISCAL INJURY
Anatomy and Function

The lateral and medial menisci are two semilunar fibrocartilage disks interposed between the femur and tibia (Fig. 18-22). They are positioned in the joint with the open side of the C facing the midline and are held in place by cranial meniscotibial ligaments, caudal meniscotibial ligaments, and meniscocapsular ligaments. The lateral meniscus has an additional ligament, which inserts into the caudal intercondyloid fossa of the femoral condyles. This ligament, along with its loose meniscocapsular ligaments, renders the lateral meniscus more mobile than the medial meniscus. Clinically, the lack of mobility of the medial meniscus predisposes it to injury. The menisci are

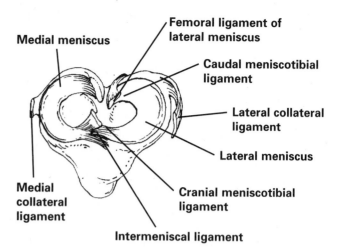

Fig. 18-22 Dorsal view of the normal anatomy of the lateral and medial meniscus.

important intraarticular structures; functions attributed to the menisci include (1) load transmission and energy absorption, (2) rotational and varus-valgus stability, (3) lubrication, and (4) rendering joint surfaces congruent.

Mechanism of Injury

Isolated meniscal injuries are not common in the dog. Occasionally, I have seen isolated meniscal tears involving the midbody of the lateral meniscus; these have been associated with a fall and twisting motion. Almost all meniscal tears causing clinical lameness in dogs are associated with CCL ruptures. The incidence of meniscal tears in conjunction with CCL ruptures may be as high as 75% and almost always involve the caudal body of the medial meniscus. This is because the craniocaudal instability associated with CCL rupture displaces the medial femoral condyle caudally during flexion of the stifle joint. The caudal body of the medial meniscus becomes wedged between the femur and tibia and is crushed on weight bearing and joint extension. The most common type of tear is a "bucket handle" tear of the medial meniscus. This is a transverse tear in the caudal body of the medial meniscus that extends from medial to lateral in a transverse direction (Fig. 18-23). The free portion of the meniscus is frequently folded forward with these tears. The second most frequently seen meniscal injury is a peripheral meniscal tear. These injuries are associated with a severe traumatic episode that results in multiple ligament injures. Ruptures of the medial meniscocapsular ligaments are frequently seen.

Methods of Treatment

The treatment of meniscal tears continues to be a controversial subject and one of ongoing research. The methods of treatment include partial meniscectomy, total

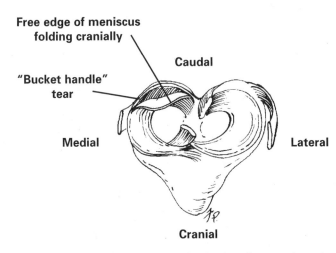

Fig. 18-23 Diagram showing a "bucket handle" tear through the caudal body of the medial meniscus. Note the cranial advancement of the "free" section of the meniscus.

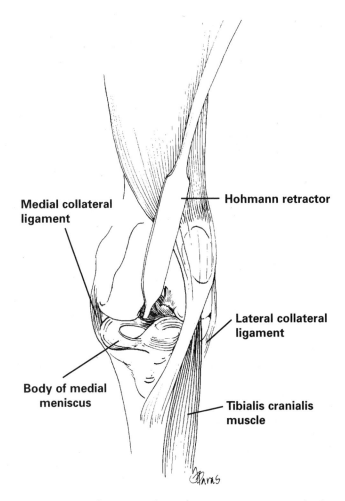

Fig. 18-24 Placement of a Hohmann retractor to assist in visualizing the medial compartment of the stifle joint. Note the tip of the retractor is placed directly behind the tibial plateau and the body of the retractor levered against the distal femur.

meniscectomy, and primary repair of peripheral meniscal injuries. A partial meniscectomy involves removal of the torn section of meniscus. Experimentally, partial meniscectomy carries less morbidity than does a total meniscectomy and is the treatment of choice for "bucket handle" tears of the medial meniscus. When performing a partial meniscectomy, adequate exposure of the torn meniscus is necessary. Exposure is facilitated with suction and by levering the tibial plateau down and forward. Levering is accomplished by placing the tip of a small Hohmann retractor behind the caudal edge of the tibial plateau and forcing the retractor's body against the nonarticular portion of the trochlear groove (Fig. 18-24). Once the damaged section of meniscus is visualized, it is removed with a no. 11 scalpel blade. The most medial attachment of the "bucket handle" is incised first, followed by the most lateral attachment. After removal of the torn section of meniscus, the remaining meniscus must be inspected for additional tears.

Primary repair of a torn meniscal body is advocated by some physicians in human orthopedics. However, because of the low morbidity associated with partial meniscectomy in the dog and the difficulty in suturing meniscal body tears in the dog, primary repair is reserved for peripheral tears on the meniscocapsular ligaments. Tearing of the peripheral meniscocapsular ligaments generally occurs following significant trauma and subsequent injury to both primary and secondary restraints of the stifle joint. The medial meniscus is more often involved in conjunction with injury of the medial collateral restraints. Meticulous repair with interrupted sutures using an absorbable suture allows for healing of the meniscocapsular tissue.

Total meniscectomy should only be considered when the peripheral rim of the meniscus is damaged to a point where primary suturing of the meniscocapsular tissue is not possible.

MULTIPLE LIGAMENT INJURIES

Most often, multiple ligament injuries occur following automobile accidents or, more rarely, gunshot wounds. CCL and CaCL tears, failure of the primary and secondary medial restraints, and peripheral medial meniscal tears are a common triad of injuries seen at our hospital. Diagnosis is determined by palpation and radiographs. Combined CCL and CaCL tears are characterized by marked craniocaudal translation of the tibia relative to the femur. Medial or lateral restraint injury is determined by palpation. Medial or lateral restraint injury denotes tears involving both the collateral ligament complex and joint capsule complex. With the leg in extension, a varus (inward) stress applied to the distal tibia causes opening of the lateral joint line if the lateral restraints are injured. A valgus (outward) stress causes opening of the medial joint line if the medial restraints are injured. Radiographs show subluxation of the stifle joint. Careful assessment of both craniocaudal and mediolateral radiographs may show small bone chips at the origin or insertion of ligaments.

Surgical treatment involves careful reconstruction of the CCL and CaCL, collateral restraints, and menisci. Repair of the collateral ligament complex is performed first, followed by reconstruction of the cruciate ligaments. Specific repair and reconstruction techniques depend on the surgeon's preference and are described in the discussion of each individual ligament repair. Postoperative care includes a support bandage and controlled activity. The support bandage is placed before the patient recovers from anesthesia. This allows accurate placement of the bandage with the leg in extension. The purpose of the bandage is to provide comfort in the early postoperative period by immobilizing the soft tissues and to prevent overextension and flexion of the stifle joint. The bandage should be changed as necessary but no less than once each week. The patient should be sedated with a narcotic/tranquilizer combination for bandage change. Sedation provides patient comfort and allows accurate replacement of the bandage. A bandage should be maintained for 3 to 4 weeks following surgery. Exercise is limited to that on a leash only for 8 weeks postoperatively. During this period, passive flexion and extension of the stifle are recommended to maintain a good range of motion.

SUGGESTED READINGS

1. Arkin AM: The effects of pressure on epiphyseal growth: a mechanism of plasticity of growing bone, *J Bone Joint Surg* 5:38, 1956.
2. Aron DN: Traumatic dislocation of the stifle joint: treatment of 12 dogs and 1 cat, *J Am Anim Hosp Assoc* 24:333-340, 1988.
3. Boone E, Hohn B, Weisbrode S: Trochlear recession wedge technique for patella luxation: an experimental study, *J Am Anim Hosp Assoc* 19:735-742, 1983.
4. Dulish ML: Suture reaction following extra-articular stifle stabilization in the dog: a retrospective study of 161 stifles, *J Am Anim Hosp Assoc* 17:569-571, 1981.
5. Egger E: Caudal cruciate ligament repair. In Bojrab MJ, editor: *Current techniques in small animal surgery*, Philadelphia, 1990, Lea & Febiger.
6. Evans HE, Christensen GC: *Miller's anatomy of the dog*, Philadelphia, 1979, Saunders.
7. Gambardela PC and others: Lateral suture technique for management of anterior cruciate ligament rupture in dogs: a retrospective study, *J Am Anim Hosp Assoc* 17:33-38, 1981.
8. Hulse DA, Shires PK: The meniscus: anatomy, function and treatment, *Comp Cont Educ* 5:765, 1983.
9. Hulse DA, Shires PK: The stifle joint. In Slatter DH, editor: *Textbook of small animal surgery*, Philadelphia, 1985, Saunders.
10. Hulse DA, Shires PK: Multiple ligament injury of the stifle joint in the dog, *J Am Anim Hosp Assoc* 22:105, 1986.
11. Johnson AL, Olmstead ML: Caudal cruciate ligament rupture: a retrospective analysis of 14 dogs, *Vet Surg* 16:202-206, 1987.
12. Moore J, Banks W: Repair of full-thickness defects in the femoral trochlea of dogs after trochlear arthroplasty, *Am J Vet Res* 50(8):1406-1413, 1989.
13. Niebauer GW and others: Antibodies to canine collagen types 1 and 11 in dogs with spontaneous cruciate ligament rupture and osteoarthritis, *Arthritis Rheum* 30:319-327, 1987.
14. Olmstead, ML: The use of orthopedic wire as a lateral suture for stifle stabilization, *Vet Clin N Am: Sm Anim Prac* 23:735-753, 1993.
15. Smith GK, Torg JS: Fibular head transposition for repair of cruciate deficient stifle in the dog, *J Am Vet Med Assoc* 187:375-383, 1985.
16. Vasseur PB: Clinical results following non-operative management for rupture of the cranial cruciate ligament in dogs, *Vet Surg* 13:243-246, 1984.
17. Vasseur PB and others: Correlative biomechanical and histological study of the cranial cruciate ligament in dogs, *Am J Vet Res* 9:1842-1854, 1985.
18. Willauer C, Vassuer P: Clinical results of surgical correction of medial luxation of the patella in dogs, *Vet Surg* 16:31-36, 1987.

19

Musculoskeletal Neoplasia: Biology and Clinical Management

RODNEY L. PAGE

Evaluation and treatment of musculoskeletal neoplasia (primary or metastatic bone tumors and peripheral soft tissue sarcomas [STSs]) represent a significant time and energy commitment in small animal medicine and surgery. It is estimated that 15% and 8% to 10% of all canine and feline neoplasms, respectively, are of primary mesenchymal origin.[33] Mammary gland tumors and lymphoproliferative disorders are the only malignant tumors more prevalent. Moreover, the dramatic onset of clinical signs associated with bone neoplasia and the aggressive behavior of many STSs seem to amplify the perception that these tumors are particularly numerous. Since pets with musculoskeletal neoplasia often die as a result of the tumor, improved tumor control would be a major achievement in pet health and longevity. To achieve this goal, clinicians must first accept the problem's magnitude, understand the tumor's natural history and biology, and clearly communicate the treatment options, benefits, and risks to clients.

Successful management of cancer in veterinary medicine can be defined in many ways. A satisfactory out-come can be achieved even when dealing with a pet that has a grave prognosis if the process of arriving at the conclusion is thoughtful and thorough. Essential factors to the success of such a process include patient status, tumor extent and biological behavior, the client's emotional and financial ability to cope with cancer, resources available for therapy, and current information regarding success or failure of specific therapeutic options. This review focuses primarily on the initial management of musculoskeletal neoplasia, including tumor biology, biopsy, and treatment options (Fig. 19-1).

BIOPSY CONSIDERATIONS

The importance of biopsy planning is generally overlooked compared with the urgency of tumor treatment, but proper biopsy methodology is essential to the optimum management of cancer. The goal of any biopsy procedure is to obtain tissue that is representative of the entire mass, provide prognostic information, and not deleteriously affect treatment outcome. Considerations include (1) type of biopsy procedure (incisional versus excisional) and (2) appropriate biopsy site selection to avoid unnecessary compartmental contamination and not deleteriously affect treatment.

It is important to realize that a *comprehensive* treatment plan must be based on accurate information of tumor type, tumor grade, and extent of host invasion. An excisional biopsy of any mass should never be considered a therapeutic procedure except for small, superficial, cutaneous lesions or mammary gland neoplasia. Even when wide surgical margins can be easily obtained, consideration of additional treatment or more extensive reexcision of the tumor site is necessary if the biopsy indicates a high grade of malignancy. Incisional or punch-style biopsy procedures can often be performed without general anesthesia, provide information regarding tumor

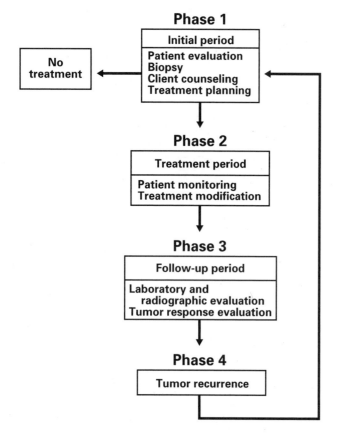

Fig. 19-1 Management scheme for musculoskeletal neoplasia.

grade, and if obtained from the tumor/normal tissue interface, can help estimate the extent of resection necessary in a subsequent, definitive procedure. Such information obtained from a presurgical biopsy improves tumor control by identifying when close, marginal resection may be sufficient (low-grade, well-differentiated tumor) from those instances where more aggressive resections or multimodality therapy should be considered (intermediate-grade and high-grade malignancies). An individualized, definitive treatment plan that is developed after review of the biopsy and staging information *and* is compatible with client expectations should be the goal of the initial management period.

BONE TUMORS
Primary Bone Neoplasia

From 3% to 7% of all canine neoplasms are primary bone tumors.[33] This represents more than 8000 dogs with bone neoplasia each year in the U.S. canine population. For comparison, approximately 1200 humans are diagnosed annually with bone neoplasia.[12] The similarities between canine and human osteosarcoma are striking; similar size, stage, metaphyseal site on long bones, and predilection for metastasis exist for both species. This similarity has resulted in attempts to investigate novel

therapeutic strategies in dogs with osteosarcoma as a relevant model of human osteosarcoma.[19,21,42] These studies have obvious benefits for canine tumor management as well.

The pathological classification of many primary bone tumors in dogs is confounded by uncertainty of the primary cell type. In general, about 90% of primary tumors of bone are osteosarcoma; 75% of osteosarcomas occur on appendicular, or "long," bones and 25% arise on the skull or axial skeleton.[5] The most common sites of occurrence for osteosarcoma are, in order, distal radius, proximal humerus, and either proximal or distal sites of the femur and tibia. Large and giant breeds are predisposed to osteosarcoma, with more than 90% of the tumors occurring in dogs weighing over 20kg (44 pounds). Males tend to have a slight predisposition for development of osteosarcoma. The median age of tumor occurrence is 7 years. Bone neoplasia is usually advanced at the time of diagnosis, and therefore staging of bone tumors is of little clinical use.

Diagnosis. The diagnosis of canine bone neoplasia is often straightforward. A history of lameness or poorly defined bone pain often precedes clinical detection of the tumor. Any such complaint in a middle-aged, large dog should alert the clinician to the possibility of an underlying bone neoplasm, and prompt radiographic evaluation of the suspected region should be done.

The radiographic appearance of long bone osteosarcoma is characterized by osteolysis, osteoproliferation, or a mixture, with an extremely variable degree of periosteal reaction. Pathological fracture may occur at the tumor site. Although definitive diagnosis requires tissue biopsy, a strong case for a tentative diagnosis of a primary bone tumor can be made after survey radiographic examination that demonstrates a characteristic lesion located in a preferred site in a large dog. The differential diagnoses include other primary bone tumors, lymphoproliferative disorders that arise from or involve the bone marrow (lymphoma, multiple myeloma), and osteomyelitis of bacterial or systemic mycotic origin. Benign bone lesions occur much less frequently.

Radiographic survey of the entire skeleton and nuclear imaging techniques have recently been evaluated as methods to identify polyostotic (multicentric) osteosarcoma involvement. Skeletal survey studies identified 4 of 42 dogs with multicentric osteosarcoma in one report.[18] Nuclear imaging studies report considerable variation in the incidence of multicentric osteosarcoma in dogs (less than 1% and up to 30%).[9,14,17,30] The reason for such variation is not clear at this time. Although skeletal surveys or nuclear imaging techniques may have significant impact on treatment recommendations in particular circumstances, such as when limb-sparing procedures are being considered, a uniform recommendation for the pretreatment evaluation of all dogs with osteosarcoma for multicentric bone involvement using nuclear techniques seems unwarranted at this time. Continued characterization of the biological properties of bone tumors through the use of imaging technologies, however, should be encouraged.

Radiographic evaluation of the thoracic cavity with two lateral views and one ventrodorsal view should be conducted on each dog or cat with suspected osteosarcoma. The incidence of pulmonary metastasis detected at the time of original diagnosis is approximately 10%.[5] However, metastasis has likely occurred by the time the tumor is observed, since the principal reason for failure

after amputation of the tumor-bearing limb is pulmonary metastasis.

As previously mentioned, the definitive diagnosis of bone neoplasia requires a tissue diagnosis. The tumor may occupy a relatively small percentage of the total area involved radiographically, making accurate biopsy site selection difficult and the frequency of nondiagnostic samples frustratingly high. A recent technique has been described for bone biopsy that represents an attempt to reduce the time and trauma associated with the procedure and has been shown to result in a high rate of success.[32] Fig. 19-2 illustrates the recommended

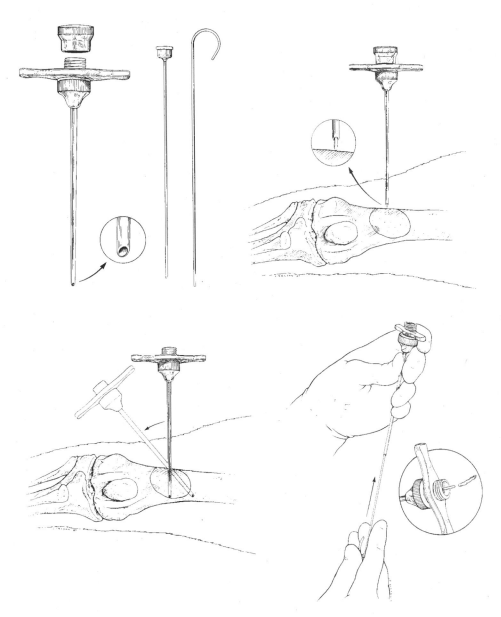

Fig. 19-2 Jamshidi bone biopsy intrument and biopsy technique. Cannula and stylet are advanced until bone is contacted. Stylet is removed and the cannula is advanced through the cortex into the lesion. Instrument is withdrawn, stylet inserted into tip of cannula and biopsy specimen expelled retrograde through the base. Redrawn from Powers BE, and others: Jamshidi needle biopsy for diagnosis of bone lesions in small animals, J Am Vet Med Assoc 193: 205-210, 1988.

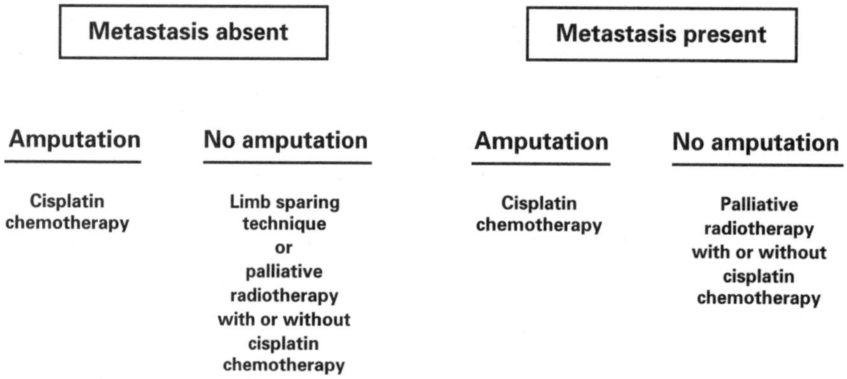

Metastasis absent		Metastasis present	
Amputation	**No amputation**	**Amputation**	**No amputation**
Cisplatin chemotherapy	Limb sparing technique or palliative radiotherapy with or without cisplatin chemotherapy	Cisplatin chemotherapy	Palliative radiotherapy with or without cisplatin chemotherapy

Fig. 19-3 Treatment options for dogs with appendicular osteosarcoma.

technique using a Jamshidi bone marrow biopsy needle.* Several biopsy specimens can be obtained through the same small skin incision by redirecting the biopsy needle. The biopsy tract can be easily excised if limb sparing is planned. After either amputation or limb sparing, the tumor should be evaluated histologically.

Treatment. Numerous options are available for dogs with appendicular osteosarcoma (Fig. 19-3). The classical treatment for osteosarcoma of any appendicular bone has been amputation. This procedure is palliative only, since occult metastasis occurs in 90% of the dogs with osteosarcoma by the time of amputation. However, significant improvement in lifestyle can be realized after an amputation in dogs that are otherwise able to ambulate on three legs. Owners are generally pleased with the decision despite initial reluctance. The 1-year survival rate was originally determined to be about 10% after amputation.[4] This was recently confirmed in a large, multi-institutional descriptive study.[36] The median survival time is approximately 4 months.

Adjuvant or planned postoperative treatment with cisplatin[†] may prolong survival in dogs.[22,35,38] The 1-year survival of dogs treated with a minimum of two courses of cisplatin (60 to 70 mg/m^2 every 3 weeks) is approximately 40%, and the median survival time is approximately 9 to 10 months. Although no prospective, randomized trial exists to prove the benefit of adjuvant cisplatin in dogs, improved survival of this magnitude (10% versus 40% 1-year survival rate) indicates adjuvant chemotherapy should be the standard treatment recommendation. Adequate pretreatment evaluation of renal function and the routine evaluation of both hematological parameters and renal function before each course of therapy must be emphasized if cisplatin is to be considered. Safe handling and administration of chemotherapeutic agents in veterinary medicine require considerable commitment from the physician as well as the client, and such commitment is essential for successful adjuvant treatment.[40]

Adjuvant immunotherapy has also been evaluated for dogs with osteosarcoma. Liposome-encapsulated muramyl tripeptide (MTP) has significantly prolonged survival in dogs after amputation.[21] This agent stimulates macrophage function, which results in direct tumor cell destruction. Liposomal encapsulation increases the intracellular concentration of MTP. Combination of MTP with cisplatin is a logical strategy that may delay metastatic development to a greater extent than either agent alone after amputation. Evaluation of such a combination is currently underway.[20]

Several techniques for limb sparing have been developed and refined recently.[19,37,42] Currently, this approach involves some form of definitive surgical procedure to remove the tumor and stabilize the bone defect with the use of cortical or cancellous bone allografts. Cisplatin and radiation have been used before surgery to consolidate the tumor, thus making removal less difficult. Cisplatin should be continued after surgery for control of metastatic disease.

Limb sparing is indicated when amputation is not possible because of expected orthopedic or biomechanical problems or owner dissatisfaction with the concept of amputation. Survival rates are not significantly prolonged after limb sparing compared with amputation plus cisplatin (approximately 300 days), but dogs are able to ambulate on four legs without pain for the remainder of their lives.[37] It is suggested that clients who want to consider limb-sparing alternatives for their dogs with osteosarcoma discuss specific available protocols with a variety of individuals, including their general practitioner and a surgical or oncological specialist, since the outcome depends on the total commitment of the entire team.

Adjuvant chemotherapy and techniques to preserve limb function have improved the survival and quality of

---

*American Pharmaseal Co., Valencia, Calif.
†Platinol, Bristol Laboratories, Evansville Ind.

life for many dogs with long bone osteosarcoma in recent years. This is a result of a multimodality therapeutic approach. Further improvement may be realized if refinements in techniques, improved antineoplastic agents, and new modalities can be incorporated into a comprehensive approach to tumor management. Furthermore, improvements observed in dogs with osteosarcoma should serve as an example for the potential of multimodality treatment in the management of other tumor types.

Radiation therapy can be administered in a palliative strategy to relieve pain temporarily and possibly improve limb function. A three-fraction course of cobalt-60 radiotherapy (10 Gy administered on days 0, 7, 21) has recently been evaluated for this purpose in twelve dogs with osteosarcoma.[25] Ten of twelve dogs showed improvement in limb function within 7 to 22 days of treatment. The median duration of this response was 149 days. No serious side effects as a result of this therapy were observed. When amputation of limb sparing cannot be considered, palliative radiation therapy may improve limb function temporarily.

Osteosarcoma that occurs on axial, or "flat," bones is also extremely difficult to manage and may require aggressive surgical resection or multimodality therapy, such as combination radiation and surgery, to achieve local control.

Feline osteosarcoma is histologically and clinically similar to osteosarcoma in the dog. However, metastasis occurs less frequently and long-term survival may be possible after amputation in cats with an appendicular osteosarcoma.[1]

Bone cancer, other than osteosarcoma, in dogs accounts for only 10% of all primary bone tumors. Fibrosarcoma and chondrosarcoma are the principal tumor types that have been reported. The management of these neoplasms is similar to osteosarcoma in that primary tumor control should be aggressive. Amputation or aggressive resection may be necessary to manage the neoplasm adequately. Combined-modality treatment is equally logical as a treatment plan, and limb-sparing techniques may provide adequate limb function for dogs affected with fibrosarcoma/chondrosarcoma of appendicular sites. The response of these tumor types to cisplatin has not been fully investigated because of the decreased frequency of these tumors relative to osteosarcoma. Adjuvant therapy, therefore, should only be initiated with the owner's consent after discussing the *potential* benefits.

Metastatic Bone Neoplasia

Many tumor types have been reported with metastasis to the skeletal system; however, bone is a much less frequent site for metastasis than reported in humans. The diagnosis of bony metastasis is generally determined by the onset of lameness or pain. Nuclear scintigraphy is helpful in defining the extent of bone involvement.

Therapy for metastatic neoplasia to a bony site should be considered palliative at this time. The pain associated with bony metastasis may be temporarily alleviated with the palliative radiation therapy schedule previously outlined.

SOFT TISSUE SARCOMAS

The term *soft tissue sarcome* (STS) refers to a group of tumors of mesenchymal origin that have similar biological characteristics and are more easily evaluated by histological grade than by histological type. This is not to imply that they are not a diverse group of tumors. Clinical presentations may vary considerably. However, the response of STSs, as a group, to treatment can be compared collectively, and therefore management recommendations can be made collectively. STSs can be further subdivided into the classical sarcomas occurring on the trunk or extremities and the visceral or thoracic sarcomas. Box 19-1 lists the histological types of peripheral tumors that are classified as STSs for this review. Mast cell tumors and hemangiosarcomas, although of mesenchymal origin, have been specifically excluded from this discussion, since these tumor types differ significantly from other STSs in their biological behavior. Recent reviews are available on the management of these neoplasms.[15,28]

Diagnosis

The radiographic imaging of tumor volume and invasion is essential to accurate treatment planning for STS. Survey radiographs may define tumor boundaries, but improved imaging is possible with computed tomography (CT) or nuclear magnetic resonance spectroscopy (MRS). This is particularly helpful when tumors appear clinically invasive and potentially difficult to resect completely. Fig. 19-4 illustrates several images through an undifferentiated sarcoma on the medial thigh of a dog. Complete excision, short of amputation, is essentially impossible in this patient. The use of CT is essential for accurate radiation therapy treatment planning. Improved tumor response can be expected when the optimum treatment strategy increases the radiation dose to the tumor and minimizes exposure to normal tissue. Ultrasonographic evaluation can also be useful to determine proximity of the tumor to large vessels, cavitation, or intraabdominal lymph node enlargement.

The importance of a *thorough* diagnostic evaluation, including accurate histological diagnosis and staging, is mentioned earlier but must be reemphasized in particular for STS. The initial attempt at tumor management

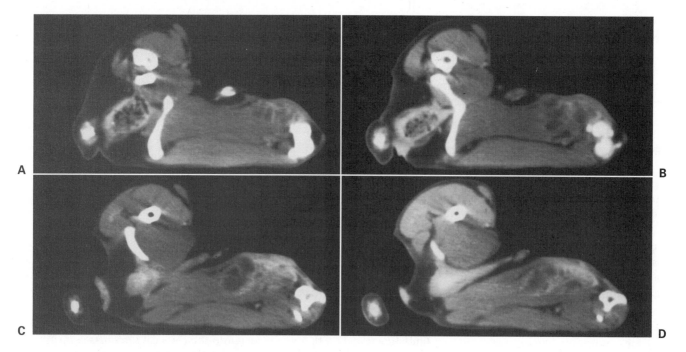

Fig. 19-4   A to **D,** Computed axial tomographic evaluations of canine soft tissue sarcoma. Four consecutive images demonstrate the infiltrative nature and tissue heterogeneity of this neoplasm.

represents the best chance for successful control. The failure of surgery to control many STSs is usually related to incomplete excision of the mass or a tumor classified as intermediate or high grade that may have occult extension or metastasis at the time of surgery. Therefore, knowing the extent of surgery required for long-term control before resection is essential.

BOX 19-1

HISTOLOGICAL CLASSIFICATION OF PERIPHERAL SOFT TISSUE SARCOMAS

Hemangiopericytoma
Neurofibrosarcoma
Myxosarcoma
Liposarcoma
Undifferentiated sarcoma
Fibrosarcoma
Malignant fibrous histiocytoma
Sarcoma—not otherwise specified

Ideally, tumor staging should be based on prognostic information that helps guide the treatment decision. Unfortunately, this is often not the case for clinical staging schemes in veterinary oncology. The current staging system for STS in companion animals is based on tumor size as well as the presence or absence of lymph node involvement and metastasis. The size groupings used to determine the staging system in dogs and cats were

assigned empirically without adequate clinical trial assessment. In addition, lymph node involvement at the time of diagnosis is rare (less than 7%).[33] Histological grade, percent tissue necrosis observed on histological examination, and normal tissue margins (i.e., quality of resection) have been identified as prognostic factors in humans with STS and have been incorporated into the staging system.[6] Mitotic index was found to be of prognostic significance in one report in dogs with STS treated with surgery alone.[2] A systematic review of the staging criteria for STS in dogs and cats and characterization of prognostic factors are long overdue. Until clinical staging schemes that accurately reflect the treatment outcome can be produced, determination of histological grade should be used to suggest treatment direction. Pathologists should include such information in all reports.

Treatment

Surgery. Accurate data regarding recurrence of STS in companion animals after simple resection are difficult to obtain. Evaluation of the existing reports indicates a recurrence rate of 20% to 50%.[2,13,31] STSs are usually located in the deeper planes of the musculoaponeurotic structures and are therefore difficult to dissect without substantial soft tissue disruption. Compartmental disruption has been associated with increased recurrence in humans after STS resection because of contamination or extension of tumor beyond the gross tumor boundary.[10] STSs often have the appearance of being encapsu-

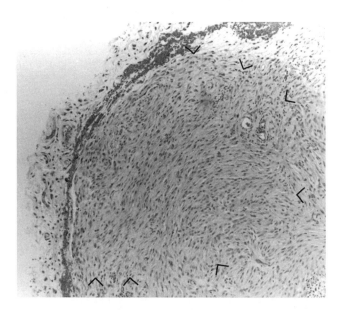

Fig. 19-5 Photomicrographs of a 'pseudocapsule' around the border of a fibrosarcoma in a cat. Arrows indicate tumor cells extending beyond the pseudocapsule into adjacent skeletal muscle.

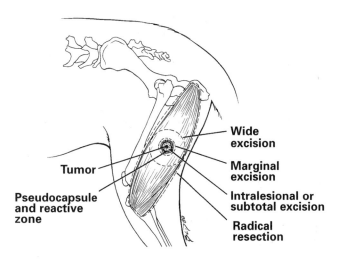

Fig. 19-6 Various surgical options for removal of a neoplasm. From Gilson SD, Stone EA: Principles of oncologic surgery, *Comp Cont Educ* 12:1047-1058, 1990.

Table 19-1 Recurrence and Survival of Dogs With Soft Tissue Sarcomas after Marginal Resection as a Function of Mitotic Index (Tumor Grade)

Mitotic index*	Recurrence at 3 years (%)	Median Survival (weeks)	Dogs with metastasis (%)
0-8	25	118	1.6
≥9	63[†]	49[‡]	15[‡]

*Number of mitotic figures/10 fields at 400×.
[†]$p<0.01$.
[‡]$p<0.05$.

From: Bostock DE, Dye MT: Prognosis after surgical excision of canine fibrous connective tissue sarcomas, *Vet Pathol* 17:581-588, 1980.

lated and thus easy to resect. In fact, this "capsule" is compressed tumor tissue and surrounding fibrous tissue that affords no barrier to tumor extension. Careful histological evaluation of these regions usually reveals microscopic extension beyond the confines of the pseudocapsule (Fig. 19-5).

Local extension of STS is usually by longitudinal growth along intermuscular fascial planes. However, these tumors rarely cross major muscular septa (compartments). Current recommendations for resection of STS in humans involve resection of the compartment enclosing the tumor, being careful not to disrupt or excessively manipulate the tumor. For instance, if a STS is located within the quadriceps group, all components of the quadriceps and sartorius muscles, including origin and insertion, are removed. If underlying bone involvement is also detected, a limb-sparing technique or amputation is recommended. Such procedures have reduced local recurrence of STS in humans from more than 50% for excisional resection and 30% to 40% for wide marginal resection to less than 20%.[10] Fig. 19-6 graphically defines resections just discussed.

Bostock and Dye[2] evaluated control of canine STS in 187 dogs after marginal resection.[2] Recurrence and metastasis were found to be related to mitotic index (i.e., tumor grade) but not to tumor volume (Table 19-1). Hemangiopericytomas appeared to have a favorable prognosis compared with other STSs. However, histological type of tumor was not significant when tumors were compared by mitotic index. This merely implies that more hemangiopericytomas are generally low grade relative to other STS.

Aggressive surgical procedures have been shown to prolong tumor control considerably in dogs and cats.[3,34,43,44] Mandibulectomy and maxillectomy for oral neoplasia are currently considered recommended procedures if tumor-free margins can be achieved (usually 2 to 3 cm). One-year and 2-year survival rates for 81 dogs with oral tumors treated with mandibulectomy/maxillectomy were approximately 45% and 30%, respectively.[34] Cosmetic appearance and function have been generally acceptable to pet owners after such procedures. Less information is available regarding aggressive therapy for extremity or truncal STS. Postorino and others[31] reported improved tumor control rates for hemangiopericytomas after a staging excision followed by a planned definitive resection or adjuvant therapy (radiotherapy) based on biopsy results and assessment of margins. The mean disease-free interval was 16 months, and median survival was 26 months in dogs treated with this approach.

Surgical recommendations for management of STS can be developed from the previous information. A presurgical biopsy is a prerequisite for optimum results. It is important to consider the most aggressive yet appropriate procedure as early in the treatment course as possible. Multimodality therapy should be considered if (1) the histological appearance of the tumor is of intermediate-grade or high-grade malignancy, (2) tumor volume is large (more than 3 cm in diameter), or (3) normal tissue margins are contaminated and reresection is not feasible. Referral of the patient with an advanced STS to a comprehensive cancer treatment center or consultation with a surgical specialist is warranted.

Radiation therapy. The role of radiation therapy in the management of STS in dogs and cats is undergoing considerable reevaluation. Several early reports suggested that the response of STS to radiotherapy was moderate at best.[11,41] However, the current use of more accurate treatment plans based on CT images of the tumor volume, increased total radiation doses delivered in a more biologically relevant schedule, and continued critical evaluation of indications for radiotherapy administration have demonstrated improved tumor control.

McChesney and others[23] reported that 50% of dogs with STS treated with 45.3 Gy (4530 rads, megavoltage radiotherapy administered in 10 fractions) experience tumor control for 1 year. This dose is well tolerated by surrounding normal tissue. The tumor control rates for 1 and 2 years after orthovoltage radiotherapy (approximately 45 Gy divided into 10 fractions) and surgical resection for dogs with hemangiopericytomas were 60% and 41%, respectively.[8] Small tumor volume was a positive prognostic factor in both these studies. These data support the use of radiation therapy for long-term control of STS. Further improvements in treatment schedules have been implemented that may result in continued improvement in tumor control with radiation therapy. However, it is unlikely that even optimum radiation therapy will sufficiently control all STSs. Therefore, consideration of combined-modality treatment is necessary when planning the management of a large, infiltrative, or high-grade STS.

Chemotherapy. Chemotherapy has generally not been effective as a single modality of treatment in solid tumors. However, doxorubicin* is the most active single agent for STS. A recent evaluation of doxorubicin administered at 30 mg/m² as a slow intravenous bolus (10 to 15 minutes) every 3 weeks for six treatment courses revealed a 20% objective response rate (more than 50% reduction in tumor volume) in dogs with STS.[27] Fifty percent of dogs with STS treated in such a manner had stabilization of tumor growth or reduction in tumor size. A combination chemotherapy protocol has recently been evaluated in dogs with STS.[16] This protocol involves com-

Table 19-2 Chemotherapeutic Protocol for Soft Tissue Sarcomas

Treatment day	Drug	Dose
1	Doxorubicin	30 mg/m² IV
	Cyclophosphamide	100 mg/m² IV
8	Vincristine	0.7 mg/m² IV
15	Vincristine	0.7 mg/m² IV
21	Restart 3-week cycle	

bination of vincristin,† cyclophosphamide,‡ and doxorubicin ("VAC" protocol; Table 19-2). This drug cycle can be continued for six treatment courses as long as bone marrow suppression and cardiac function remain adequate. Concurrent use of antibiotics with this protocol may be helpful in reducing potential complications from excessive myelosuppression. Careful attention to the safe handling of all cytotoxic chemotherapeutic agents should be standard procedure for any physician engaged in chemotherapy.[40] In dogs with STS (excluding those with hemangiosarcoma) a 60% objective response rate was noted using the VAC protocol. This suggests that combination chemotherapy may be associated with improved tumor response compared with doxorubicin alone. The added expense, time commitment, and potential for toxicity must be considered when designing each treatment plan.

Multimodality therapy. Multimodality therapy may be broadly defined as the use of agents that may enhance the tumor's response relative to single-modality therapy. Some combinations may influence tumor response in an additive, superadditive, or synergistic fashion. The principles that should govern appropriate combination of treatment include substantial demonstrated activity of the single agent on the specific tumor class and nonoverlapping toxicity. This implies that a greater therapeutic index or therapeutic gain may be achieved. Little information is currently available in dogs or cats that confirms improved response after combined treatment. However, surgery, radiation, and chemotherapy all appear to produce acceptable responses as single modalities, and logical strategies for combining treatments have been evaluated in preliminary studies.

Radiation combined with surgery has resulted in a significant improvement in the control of STS in humans.[39] Improved tumor control can be accomplished when postoperative or preoperative radiation therapy is administered. With preoperative irradiation of STS, a closer, marginal resection can be considered because microscopic tumor in the peritumoral zone can be sterilized. Less frequent compartmental resection or ampu-

---

*Adriamycin, Adria Laboratories, Columbus, Ohio.

†Oncovin, Eli Lilly and Co., Indianapolis.
‡Cytoxan, Merck Sharp & Dohme, West Point, Pa.

tation means improved function and cosmesis. A summary of the clinical strategies of combined radiation and surgery for control of tumors in companion animals has been published.[26]

Hyperthermia (heat) is undergoing extensive investigation as a means to improve tumor control rates when combined with radiation or chemotherapy.[29] Considerable evidence in human and veterinary oncology supports the addition of hyperthermia to radiation treatment for control of solid tumors. A recent prospective, randomized study revealed that the median time to tumor recurrence was 360 days and 700 days for dogs with STS treated with radiation or radiation plus hyperthermia, respectively.[24] Further study is obviously required to confirm and refine the combination of radiation/hyperthermia. Unfortunately, at this time, availability of hyperthermia is limited.

The combined use of chemotherapy and surgery may also provide improved tumor control. Chemotherapy can be used in a neoadjuvant (preoperative) or adjuvant (postoperative) setting. The same principles that apply to combined surgery/radiotherapy likely make evaluation of surgery/chemotherapy an attractive alternative to single-modality therapy. Neoadjuvant chemotherapy may be used to reduce tumor volume and thus make surgical resection more likely.

SUMMARY

A concerted effort has been made over the past 5 to 10 years to improve cancer management in veterinary medicine. No options existed for dogs with osteosarcoma other than amputation. We now can discuss adjuvant chemotherapy, limb sparing, or palliative radiotherapy with clients as options for control. In addition, sophisticated multimodality treatment plans have substantially increased tumor control for dogs and cats with STS. These accomplishments are encouraging and provide hope for further improvements. However, the greatest single improvement that could be made in veterinary oncology is to improve initial tumor management by recommending early, aggressive surgical resection or multimodality therapy.

REFERENCES

1. Bitetto WV, and others: Osteosarcoma in cats: 22 cases (1974-1984), *J Am Vet Med Assoc* 148:2943, 1987.
2. Bostock DE, Dye MT: Prognosis after surgical excision of canine fibrous connective tissue sarcomas, *Vet Pathol* 17:581-588, 1980.
3. Bradley RL, and others: Mandibular resection for removal of oral tumors in 30 dogs and 6 cats, *J Am Vet Med Assoc* 184:460-463, 1984.
4. Brodey RS, Abt DA: Results of surgical treatment of 65 dogs with osteosarcoma, *J Am Vet Med Assoc* 168:1032-1035, 1976.
5. Brodey RS, Riser WH: Canine osteosarcoma: a clinicopathologic study of 194 cases, *Clin Orthop* 62:54-64, 1969.
6. Costa J, and others: The grading of soft tissue sarcomas: results of a clinicohistopathologic correlation in a series of 163 cases, *Cancer* 53:530-541, 1984.
7. Dorn CR, and others: Survey of animal neoplasms in Alameda and Contra Costa counties, California. II. Cancer morbidity in dogs and cats from Alameda County, *J Natl Cancer Inst* 40:307-318, 1968.
8. Evans SM: Canine hemangiopericytoma: a retrospective analysis of response to surgery and orthovoltage radiation: *Vet Radiol* 28:13-16, 1987.
9. Forrest LJ, and others: Bone scintigraphy in limb sparing for osteosarcoma: prediction of tumor response, allograft incorporation and assessment of metastasis, *Proceedings of the American College of Veterinary Radiology Meeting*, Chicago, 1990 (abstract).
10. Gerner RE, and others: Soft tissue sarcomas, *Ann Surg* 181:803-808, 1975.
11. Gillette EL: Radiation therapy of canine and feline tumors, *J Am Anim Hosp Assoc* 12:359-362, 1976.
12. Goorin AM, and others: Osteosarcoma: fifteen years later, *N Engl J Med* 313:1637-1643, 1985.
13. Graves GM, and others: Canine hemangiopericytoma: 23 cases (1967-1984), *J Am Vet Med Assoc* 192:99-102, 1988.
14. Hahn KA, and others: Single-phase methylene diphosphate bone scintigraphy in the diagnostic evaluation of dogs with osteosarcoma, *J Am Vet Med Assoc* 196:1483-1486, 1990.
15. Hammer AS, Couto CG: Adjuvant chemotherapy for sarcomas and carcinomas, *Vet Clin North Am* 20:1015-1036, 1990.
16. Helfand SC: Chemotherapy for non-resectable and metastatic soft tissue tumors, *Kal Kan Symposium*, Columbus, Ohio, 1986.
17. Lamb CR, and others: Preoperative measurement of canine primary bone tumors, using radiography and bone scintigraphy, *J Am Vet Med Assoc* 196:1474-1478, 1990
18. LaRue SM, and others: Radiographic bone surveys in the evaluation of primary bone tumors in dogs, *J Am Vet Med Assoc* 5:514-516, 1986.
19. LaRue SM, and others: Limb-sparing treatment of osteosarcoma in dogs, *J Am Vet Med Assoc* 195:1734-1743, 1989.
20. MacEwen EG: Adjuvant chemotherapy and immunotherapy for canine osteosarcoma *Proceedings of the 8th Annual ACVIM Forum*, 1990.
21. MacEwen EG, and others: Therapy for osteosarcoma in dogs with intravenous injection of liposome-encapsulated muramyl tripeptide, *J Natl Cancer Inst* 81:935-938, 1989.
22. Mauldin GN, and others: Canine osteosarcoma treatment by amputation versus amputation and adjuvant chemotherapy using doxorubicin and cisplatin, *J Vet Intern Med* 2:177-180, 1988.
23. McChesney SL, and others: Radiotherapy of soft-tissue sarcomas in dogs, *J Am Vet Med Assoc* 194:60-63, 1989.
24. McChesney-Gillette SL, and others: Response of canine soft tissue sarcomas to radiation or radiation plus hyperthermia: a randomized phase II study, *Int J Hyperthermia* 8:309-320, 1992.
25. McEntee MC, and others: Palliative radiotherapy for canine appendicular osteosarcoma, *Vet Radiol* 34:367-371, 1993.
26. McLeod DA, Thrall DE: The combination of surgery and radiation in the treatment of cancer: a review, *Vet Surg* 18:1-6, 1989.
27. Ogilvie GK, and others: Phase II evaluation of doxorubicin for treatment of various canine neoplasms, *J Vet Med Assoc* 195:1580-1583, 1989.
28. O'Keefe DA: Canine mast cell tumors, *Vet Clin North Am* 20:1105-1117, 1990.
29. Page RL, Thrall DE: Clinical indications and applications of radiotherapy and hyperthermia in veterinary oncology, *Vet Clin North Am* 20:1075-1092, 1990.
30. Parchman MB, and others: Nuclear medical bone imaging and targeted radiography for evaluation of skeletal neoplasms in 23 dogs, *Vet Surg* 18:454-458, 1989.
31. Postorino NC, and others: Prognostic variables for canine hemangiopericytoma: 50 cases, *J Am Anim Hosp* 24:501-509, 1988.
32. Powers BE, and others: Jamshidi needle biopsy for diagnosis of bone lesions in small animals, *J Am Vet Med Assoc* 193:205-210, 1988.

33. Preister WA, McKay FW: The occurrence of tumors in domestic animal, *Natl Cancer Inst Monogr* 54, 1980.

34. Schwarz PD, Withrow SJ: Mandibular and maxillary resection as a treatment of oral cancer: long term follow-up and survival, *Proceedings of the Veterinary Cancer Society 8th Annual Conference*, Estes Park, Col, 1988.

35. Shapiro W, and others: Use of cisplatin for the treatment of appendicular osteosarcoma in dogs, *J Am Vet Med Assoc* 4:507-511, 1988.

36. Spodnick GJ, and others: Prognosis for dogs with appendicular osteosarcoma treated by amputation alone: 162 cases (1978-1988), *J Am Vet Med Assoc* (in press).

37. Straw RC, and others: Management of canine appendicular osteosarcoma, *Vet Clin North Am* 20:1141-1161, 1990.

38. Straw RC, and others: Amputation and cisplatin for treatment of canine osteosarcoma, *J Vet Int Med* 5:205-210, 1991.

39. Suit HD, and others: Treatment of the patient with stage M_0 soft tissue sarcoma, *J Clin Oncol* 6:854-862, 1988.

40. Swanson LV: Potential hazards associated with low-dose exposure to antineoplastic agents. *Comp Cont Educ* 10:293-300, 1988.

41. Thrall DE: Orthovoltage radiotherapy of oral fibrosarcomas in dogs, *J Am Vet Med Assoc* 179:159-162, 1981.

42. Thrall DE, and others: Radiotherapy prior to cortical allograft limb sparing in dogs with osteosarcoma: a dose-response assay, *Int J Radiol Oncol Biol Phys* 18:1351-1357, 1990.

43. Withrow SJ, Holmberg DL: Manidbulectomy in the treatment of oral cancer, *J Am Anim Hosp Assoc* 19:273-386, 1983.

44. Withrow SJ, and others: Premaxillectomy in the dog, *J Am Anim Hosp Assoc* 21:49-55, 1985.

20

Diseases Affecting Bone

PAUL MANLEY

HYPERTROPHIC OSTEODYSTROPHY

Hypertrophic osteodystrophy (HOD) is an uncommon developmental disease that affects immature large and giant breeds of dogs. The metaphyseal areas of long bones are primarily affected and become swollen and painful.

HOD results from a disturbance in endochondral ossification in the metaphyseal growth plates. A compromise of metaphyseal blood supply may cause a delay or failure of ossification of the hypertrophic zone.[28] Secondary hemorrhage, inflammation, necrosis, and fracture may occur in the metaphyseal bone adjacent to the growth plate. A periosteal response may occur in response to this activity.[28]

Although several theories have been proposed, the etiology of HOD is unknown. Vitamin C deficiency is one of the more popular theories; however, low serum and urine vitamin C levels are not consistent findings associated with this disease.[28,44] Oversupplementation with vitamins and minerals has been linked with this disease, but again not as a consistent finding.[21] An infectious agent has been sought as a predisposing factor, since the changes in the metaphyses are largely caused by inflammation. However, attempts to isolate a bacteria or virus have been unsuccessful.[18,48] Finally, as in many developmental diseases, a heritable cause has been sought but has not been conclusively demonstrated.[18,48]

Diagnosis

HOD occurs most often in large and giant breeds of dogs 3 to 6 months of age (range, 2 to 8 months); no sex predilection exists. Animals often have an acute history of lameness. The lameness may vary from a mild limp to an animal that is recumbent and reluctant to stand. The lameness is caused by the pain associated with swelling in the metaphyseal areas of the long bones. In mild cases the clinical signs may be episodic and involve only the distal radius and ulna. In severe cases the pain is unrelenting, and all metaphyseal areas are affected. The lesions are bilateral and usually symmetrical. In the most severe cases the animal may be systemically ill and may have a history of anorexia, depression, pyrexia, and weight loss.

The earliest and most consistent radiographic sign is soft tissue swelling in the metaphyseal region. Also, an irregular radiolucent line is apparent as a second line, or *double physeal line* (Fig. 20-1).[28] Periosteal new bone is less frequently observed in the metaphysis and rarely may extend into the diaphyseal region.

Other diseases causing lameness in young growing animals must be ruled out as differential diagnoses for HOD. Panosteitis, hypertrophic osteopathy (HO), and craniomandibular osteopathy can be ruled out based on signalment, history, and radiographic distribution of lesions.

Treatment

No specific treatment exists for HOD other than supportive care. Analgesics are prescribed for pain (Ascriptin or buffered aspirin, 10 to 25 mg/kg orally three times daily), and any dietary imbalances are corrected. If the animal is moribund, forced nutrition and parenteral therapy may be necessary. No conclusive evidence exists to recommend the use of vitamin or mineral supplementation in the treatment of HOD.

The prognosis is good to excellent in patients with mild HOD. Complications associated with growth disturbances occur infrequently unless the animal is

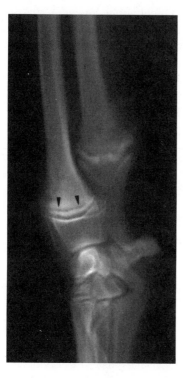

Fig. 20-1 Lateral radiographic view of the distal antebrachium. The arrows demonstrate the *double physeal line* at the metaphyseal growth plate of the distal radius. A similar change is evident in the metaphyseal growth plate of the distal ulna.

severely affected with HOD. In severe cases, however, the prognosis is guarded because of the problems encountered in treatment of a moribund patient. Complications may include decubital ulcers and secondary bacterial infections associated with the recumbent animal.

CRANIOMANDIBULAR OSTEOPATHY

Craniomandibular osteopathy (CMO) is a nonneoplastic, proliferative bone disease of growing animals primarily involving the flat bones of the skull. The mandible, temporal, and occipital bones are most often involved, and the lesions are bilaterally symmetrical. This condition is predominantly seen in terrier breeds, including the Scottish, West Highland white, and Cairn terriers, but has also been reported in the Labrador retriever, Great Dane, English bulldog, Doberman pinscher, and boxer.*

In CMO the normal lamellar bone is resorbed, and woven (immature) bone is laid down in its place.[35,38] The woven bone is deposited on the periosteal and endosteal surfaces of the flat bones of the skull in a random, disorganized fashion. This process may occur in cycles until the entire medullary cavity is occupied by immature bone. Once the animal reaches skeletal maturity, the woven bone may be replaced by mature bone; however, the bone rarely returns to its normal architecture.[1,35,40]

The etiology of CMO is not known, although the occurrence of this disease in select breeds suggests a genetic relationship.[1] The histological picture of CMO bears some resemblance to Paget disease in humans.[24]

Diagnosis

CMO is most often encountered in terrier breeds 4 to 10 months of age; no sex predilection exists. Animals have a history that reflects discomfort when the mouth is opened. Excess salivation, dehydration, weight loss, and lethargy are variable clinical signs, depending on the severity of this discomfort. Physical examination reveals bilateral swelling of the mandibles with temporomandibular muscle atrophy. Difficulty may be encountered when attempting to open the mouth, even with the patient under general anesthesia.[38]

Radiographic examination reveals bilateral, symmetrical, proliferative bony lesions involving the mandible and temporal bones (Fig. 20-2).[38] In severe cases the angular processes of the mandibles and bullae may appear to fuse together. At skeletal maturity the proliferative lesions become less aggressive and the edges of the bone smoother.

Rarely, radiographic changes in the metaphyses of long bones may demonstrate a diffuse periosteal reaction. It

*References 4, 8, 20, 37, 42, 47.

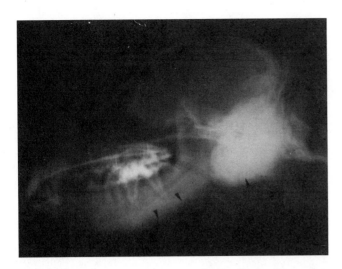

Fig. 20-2 Lateral radiographic view of the skull. The arrows demonstrate the periosteal new bone along the mandible and the tympanic bulla.

is important to differentiate these lesions from those seen in HOD and HO. CMO rarely affects the long bones, and HOD and HO rarely affect the flat bones. CMO may also be confused radiographically with neoplastic disease and bacterial or fungal osteomyelitis. Signalment, history, radiographic appearance, and sometimes biopsy are necessary to distinguish these conditions.[38]

Treatment

Treatment is largely supportive because this disease is self-limiting once skeletal maturity is reached. Therapy may include the use of analgesics, parenteral supplementation, and a gastrostomy or enterostomy tube for nutritional maintenance. Surgical attempts to decrease the bone mass and increase jaw mobility have not been successful.[35]

The prognosis depends on the extent of bony involvement. If bony lesions are severe enough to compromise jaw function, the prognosis is guarded. Complications are usually associated with the animal's impaired nutritional status.

PANOSTEITIS

Panosteitis is a self-limiting developmental disease of young, large, and giant breeds of dogs resulting in pain and lameness in one or more limbs.[29] Although it is most often seen in the German shepherd breed, it has been reported in most other large and giant breeds.

Panosteitis is a primary disease of fatty bone marrow with secondary effects on the long bones.[29] The condition is usually cyclical, with one or more bones affected at any one time. Degeneration of the medullary adipocytes often begins in the region of the nutrient

foramen and is followed by stromal cell proliferation and the production of osteoid, which becomes calcified. The fatty marrow is gradually replaced by osteoid, beginning in the area of the nutrient foramen and spreading proximally and distally within the medullary cavity. As the vascular sinusoids within the medullary cavity become congested, a secondary endosteal and periosteal response may occur. Eventually, this new bone is resorbed, and the fatty and hematopoietic marrow are restored. The entire cycle from degeneration of the fatty marrow to its restoration may take 60 to 90 days.[29,45]

The etiology is unknown, although several possibilities have been proposed and include viral and bacterial osteomyelitis, stress, transient vascular abnormalities, metabolic disorders, parasite migration, autoimmune reactions, allergic reactions, and hyperestrinism.[6,29,45]

Diagnosis

Panosteitis is most frequently seen in large or giant breeds of dogs with a history of acute lameness. It is usually diagnosed in dogs 5 to 12 months of age but has been reported in German shepherd dogs as young as 2 months and as old as 5 years.[6] The condition occurs most often in males, and if it occurs in females, it is often associated with the first estrus.[45] The disease is episodic, and the cycles often occur at 2- to 3-week intervals. Physical examination reveals pain on deep palpation of the affected long bone with varying degrees of lameness. The clinical signs often resolve in one long bone, only to occur in another long bone of a different limb. Generally the entire cycle resolves by the time the animal reaches 18 to 20 months of age.[6]

The earliest radiographic sign is an increased radiolucency in the region of the nutrient foramen. This is rarely observed; solitary or multifocal increases in intramedullary density are seen more often (Fig. 20-3). The lesion may appear small with indistinct margins or may be spread along the entire length of the medullary cavity.[45] Secondary periosteal reaction is an inconsistent finding and is usually mild. In later stages the medullary opacity regresses but may remain for several months after the lameness has resolved.[2] No correlation exists between the radiographic lesion and the severity of the clinical disease.

Other cases of lameness must be differentiated from panosteitis by physical examination and the presence of supporting radiographic lesions.

Treatment

The treatment is supportive and includes the use of analgesics as necessary for discomfort. Client education is important so that the owner is aware of the likelihood of recurrence of the disease process in different limbs.

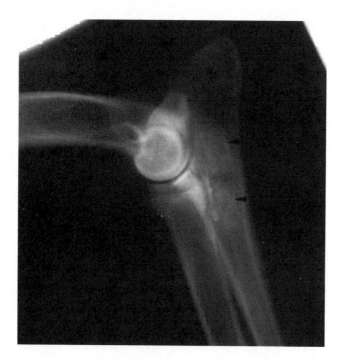

Fig. 20-3 Lateral radiographic view of the distal humerus and proximal antebrachium. The arrows demonstrate an area of increased medullary density.

The prognosis is excellent because the disease is self-limiting. Complications are rarely observed and are usually associated with chronic lameness and disease recurrence.

MULTIPLE CARTILAGINOUS EXOSTOSIS

Multiple cartilaginous exostosis (MCE) is a proliferative disease of cartilage and bone that has been reported in dogs, cats, horses, and humans. The disease is characterized by the presence of multiple ossified protuberances that arise from the cortical surfaces in the metaphyseal region of long bones, in the vertebrae, or in the ribs.[7,14,30]

MCE results from a displacement of chondrocytes from the growth plate and differentiation of these cells into cartilage and bone in a juxtacortical position.[34] The nodules are often located adjacent to the growth plate but may also be seen in the diaphyseal region of long bones. The masses grow in size as the animal develops but usually cease their growth once the growth plate closes.

The etiology of MCE is unknown, although MCE is a heritable disease in humans, and a familial tendency has been reported in dogs.[11,15,34]

Diagnosis

MCE occurs in young, growing animals with open growth plates. The animals may have multiple firm swel-

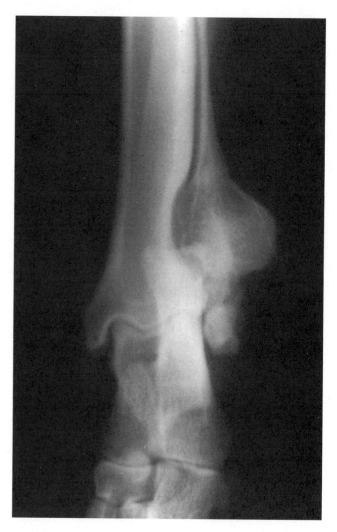

Fig. 20-4 Craniocaudal view of the distal tibia and the tarsal joint. On the lateral side of the distal tibia, a large bony nodule is evident.

Courtesy Dr. Wendy Myer.

lings in several locations of long bones, vertebrae, and ribs. The swellings may cause few clinical signs unless they encroach on surrounding soft tissue structures. A biopsy of the mass reveals hyaline cartilage and bone in various stages of differentiation.[14]

Radiographic examination confirms the presence of multiple bony nodules arising from various bones (Fig. 20-4).

Differentiation of these masses from multiple tumors is based on age at presentation, radiographic appearance, and biopsy.

Treatment

Treatment is not necessary unless the nodules cause a mechanical interference with the overlying soft tissue.

Local excision of the offending nodules is usually adequate. Occasionally the nodules become malignant, and more aggressive therapy is warranted.

The prognosis is good to excellent unless the masses mechanically interfere with soft tissue structures. Transformations of the growths to chondrosarcoma or osteosarcoma have been reported.[13,34,36] Periodic radiographic evaluation is indicated, which may reveal an early tendency toward malignant transformation.

HYPERTROPHIC OSTEOPATHY

Hypertrophic osteopathy (HO) is a condition that affects long bones but is secondary to a primary thoracic or abdominal mass. The bony lesions are characterized by bilateral, symmetrical swellings affecting the distal extremities of all four limbs.[28] Hypertrophic pulmonary osteoarthropathy, pulmonary osteoarthropathy, and hypertrophic pulmonary osteopathy are other names that have been assigned to this condition. However, since this condition seldom involves the joints and is not restricted to masses in the thorax, hypertrophic osteopathy is the more descriptive term.

The pathogenesis is poorly understood but is believed to be associated with an increase in peripheral blood flow secondary to stimulation of afferent neural pathways by the primary thoracic or abdominal mass. The increased peripheral blood flow causes congestion of periosteal tissue and a secondary periosteal reaction.[16]

Diagnosis

HO is most often associated with metastatic pulmonary lesions, although the condition has been reported with primary pulmonary neoplasia, chronic bronchopneumonia, pulmonary tuberculosis, pulmonary abscesses, spirocercosis, dirofilariasis, blastomycosis, foreign bodies, rib tumors, bacterial endocarditis, liver adenocarcinoma, and various bladder neoplasias.[19,43,46]

The animal usually has a history of gradual swelling of all four limbs with associated lameness. Palpation reveals firm swelling and may elicit pain. The condition is most often observed in older animals. The swelling may be seen early in the course of the primary disease, which may offer a signal for the early detection and treatment of the thoracic or abdominal mass. Later in the disease, the systemic signs associated with the primary lesion may predominate.

Radiographic examination reveals bilaterally symmetrical, periosteal reactions involving the long bones. The metacarpal and metatarsal bones are often affected first, but as the condition progresses, all the long bones and some of the flat bones (pelvis, mandible) become involved. The condition does not primarily involve the joints, but if the periosteal reaction is aggressive, new

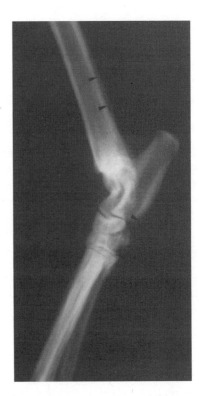

Fig. 20-5 Lateral radiographic view of the distal tibia, tarsal joint, and metatarsal bones. The arrows demonstrate periosteal proliferation on the caudal aspect of the tibia, the calcaneus, and the distal tarsal bones.

bone formation may inhibit normal articulation (Fig. 20-5). Early in this condition, soft tissue swelling may be the only radiographic sign.

Treatment

Treatment is directed toward the recognition and elimination of the primary lesion. Radiographic survey of the thorax and abdomen and the use of alternate imaging techniques are important to identify the cause of the HO. Elimination of the primary disease should result in resolution of the bony lesions, although the response is not immediate.[22,26]

The prognosis depends on the nature of the primary lesion and is favorable only if the primary disease can be eliminated. Complications are usually related to the primary disease.

BONE CYSTS

Bone cysts are benign, fluid-filled cavities that are found rarely in the long bones of young, large breeds of dogs. Monostotic, polyostotic, and aneurysmal bone cysts have been described in dogs and cats. Aneurysmal bone cysts are very rare and are large multicompartment cysts filled with blood.[5,17]

Bone cysts are found in the metaphysis, the epiphysis, or the diaphysis of long bones and may form after an initial vascular insult results in local venous obstruction.

The etiology is unknown, although a hereditary predisposition has been reported in Doberman pinschers.[10,41]

Diagnosis

Monostotic and polyostotic bone cysts occur in young animals. The lesions may be clinically inapparent and go unnoticed for years. If lameness is associated with the lesions, it often results from a pathological fracture.[17]

Monostotic and polyostotic bone cysts appear as large radiolucent defects in the metaphysis or diaphysis of long bones. Pathological fractures are secondary to cortical thinning. Aneurysmal bone cysts also appear as radiolucent defects that are compartmentalized by trabecular bone and connective tissue, giving a "soap bubble" appearance (Fig. 20-6).[5]

Treatment

Drainage, curettage, and autogenous cancellous grafting constitute the recommended treatment if the cyst causes clinical lameness.[41] Good results have been reported with a technique that uses multiple drill holes into the cyst as the definitive treatment.[12] A biopsy may be necessary to distinguish bone cysts from bone neoplasia or infection. If a pathological fracture occurs, a period of immobilization is necessary for the fracture to unite.

The prognosis is good unless the cyst or fracture occurs close to the joint or to the growth plate in a

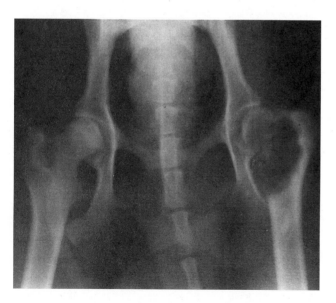

Fig. 20-6   Ventrodorsal view of the pelvis and proximal femora of a dog. Note the radiolucent defect in the proximal femur ("soap bubble" appearance).

Courtesy Dr. David Biller.

growing animal. The prognosis is guarded for aneurysmal bone cysts because complete removal is difficult.[5]

HYPERPARATHYROIDISM

Parathroid hormone (PTH) is produced and released from the parathroid glands in response to low serum calcium to maintain the normal serum calcium/phosphorus ratio. PTH exerts its effects on bone, kidney, and intestine. In bone, PTH causes calcium mobilization and release from skeletal reserves by stimulating osteoclastic and osteocytic bone resorption.[9] In kidney, PTH inhibits renal tubular phosphate resorption and increases urinary phosphate excretion. PTH also stimulates the hydroxylation of 25-hydroxycholecalciferol to 1,25-dihydroxycholecalciferol in the renal mitochondria. 1,25-dihydroxycholecalciferol is the active form of vitamin D responsible for stimulating calcium absorption from the intestine. Primary and secondary hyperparathyroidism results in an increase in PTH production and release with subsequent increased resorption of bone.

Diagnosis

Primary hyperparathyroidism is associated with hyperplastic parathyroid glands that produce excess PTH. Neoplasia and hyperplasia of the glandular tissue often result in increased PTH release. The condition occurs infrequently in the dog but should be suspected when the glandular tissue becomes enlarged and clinical signs reflect hyperparathyroidism.

Renal secondary hyperparathyroidism may result from the kidney's inability to excrete phosphorus or to hydroxylate 25-hydroxycholecalciferol to its active form. Hyperphosphatemia indirectly lowers blood calcium, whereas a decrease in 1,25-dihydroxycholecalciferol decreases intestinal absorption of calcium.[9] In young animals, renal secondary hyperparathyroidism may be linked to congenital renal insufficiency. In older animals, it is most often associated with chronic renal failure.

Nutritional secondary hyperparathyroidism results from a decrease of calcium in the diet, an increase in phosphorus in the diet with normal or decreased calcium intake, or a decrease in vitamin D. Agents that bind calcium in the intestine (mineral oil) and prevent calcium absorption have also been implicated in this condition.

The clinical signs of renal secondary hyperparathyroidism reflect the severity of the renal disease. Polydipsia, polyuria, vomition, dehydration, and azotemia are signs attributed to renal failure. Acute lameness and masticatory problems may reflect pathological fractures of affected bones.

The history and clinical signs for nutritional secondary hyperparathyroidism often reflect a diet with high phosphorus and low calcium. An all-meat diet or a diet supplemented with phosphorus and calcium in abnormal ratios are typical examples.[9] Immature animals may develop clinical signs of the disease within a week, whereas it may take several months of an abnormal diet in a mature animal before clinical signs become evident. Lamenesses associated with pathological fractures and growth abnormalities are often the reasons for presentation.

Radiographically, skeletal involvement is first recognized in the bones of the mandible and maxilla. Resorption of the alveolar bone and loss of lamina dura dentes occur early in the disease process. Subsequent loosening of the teeth and mastication problems may be associated with loss of alveolar support to the teeth or with pathological fractures of the bones.[9] Diffuse demineralization of the entire skeleton may be evident on survey skeletal films. Thin cortices and generalized loss of bone density are often noted in the long bones. In renal-based disease, abdominal radiographs and ultrasound may reveal small, misshapen kidneys.

Treatment

In renal secondary hyperparathyroidism, treatment is directed toward the restoration of normal renal function. Dietary protein restriction (high quality, low quantity) and the use of phosphate-binding gels are basic therapeutic principles aimed at the renal disease. Supplementation with calcium lactate or calcium gluconate and vitamin D may decrease the severity of the skeletal lesions.[9]

In nutritional secondary hyperparathyroidism, treatment is directed toward correction of the dietary imbalance of calcium and phosphorus. The calcium/phosphorus ratio should be maintained at 2:1 during the healing of pathological fractures. It may take 8 to 10 weeks for the cortical fractures to heal and for bone density to return to normal.[9,27] Pathological fractures should be treated as any other fracture, with consideration of the best technique to achieve rigid fixation and fracture union.

The prognosis is guarded for renal secondary hyperparathyroidism and is based on the stage of renal disease. Complications are related to renal failure and secondary effects on the skeletal system. Delayed union of pathological fractures should be anticipated.

The prognosis for nutritional secondary hyperparathyroidism is favorable unless significant skeletal deformities have occurred. Complications are usually associated with delayed unions and malunions of pathological fractures.

VITAMIN D DEFICIENCY (RICKETS, OSTEOMALACIA)

Vitamin D is necessary for the normal absorption of calcium from the intestine. Rickets occurs in the immature animal with open growth plates; osteomalacia occurs in the adult animal after growth plate closure. The diseases occur infrequently because of the natural availability of vitamin D. Vitamin D is present in small amounts in pet foods and can be synthesized by activation of sunlight on 7-dehydrocholesterol, which is present in the epidermis of the skin.[25] The liver and kidney hydroxylate 7-dehydrocholesterol to its active form, which is responsible for calcium absorption from the intestine.[3,9]

In young animals, calcium is necessary for bone growth and maturation of the growth plates. If vitamin D is deficient, calcium is unavailable for mineralization of the hypertrophic zone of the growth plate. Normal growth of long bones becomes affected. In the mature animal, vitamin D deficiency prevents the osteoclasts and osteocytes from responding to PTH. Bone resorption is inhibited, and serum calcium levels cannot be maintained.

The etiology of vitamin D deficiency relates to a dietary deficiency or an environmental situation that does not allow the animal to be exposed to natural sunlight.

Diagnosis

Lameness, a stiff gait, deformity of long bones, and pathological fractures are the predominant clinical signs.

Radiographic signs are similar to hyperparathyroidism. A generalized decrease in cortical density, pathological fractures, and loss of lamina dura dentes are the most common radiographic lesions in vitamin D deficiency. In the immature animal the growth plates may appear wider than normal, with extension of cartilage cores into the metaphysis (Fig. 20-7). Shortened bones and abnormal curvature of bones may result from interference with normal growth.

Treatment

Treatment is directed toward correction of the dietary or environmental abnormalities. Pathological fractures are managed according to general principles of fracture treatment. Initially, vitamin D supplementation may be used to correct obvious deficiencies. The vitamin D levels should not exceed 10 to 20 IU/kg/day.[32]

The prognosis is favorable unless the pathological fractures are severe or growth plate abnormalities are permanent. Complications are related to malunions and premature growth plate arrests.

RETAINED CARTILAGE CORE

Retained cartilage core, retained endochondral core, and retained enchondral core are terms used to describe a maturation defect of the hyaline cartilage in the metaphyseal growth plate. This condition is rare but has been reported in the distal ulnar growth plate of large and giant breeds of dogs. It may be observed as an incidental

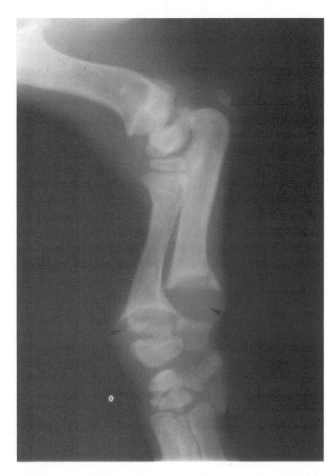

Fig. 20-7 Lateral radiographic view of the antebrachium. The arrows point to areas of widened growth plates (unmineralized cartilage).

Courtesy Dr. Kenneth Johnson.

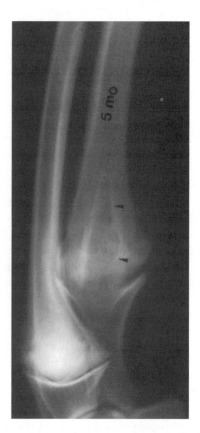

Fig. 20-8 Lateral radiographic view of the antebrachium of a 5-month-old Great Dane. The arrows demonstrate the extension of uncalcified cartilage from the metaphyseal growth plate of the ulna.

Courtesy Dr. Paul Howard.

finding on radiographic examination of the antebrachium or may be associated with premature retardation of ulnar growth.[23,31]

Retained cartilage core results from a defect in endochondral ossification of the metaphyseal growth plate's hypertrophic zone. The hypertrophic zone becomes thicker than normal, and a central zone of uncalcified cartilage extends into the long bone's metaphysis. Histologically, the hypertrophic chondrocytes located in the center of the growth plate do not follow the normal sequence of enlargement, vacuolation, and degeneration. Also, provisional mineralization of the longitudinal septae between these hypertrophic chondrocytes is absent. This maturation defect of the growth plate cartilage may be a separate disease or a manifestation of osteochondrosis.[23,33,39]

Diagnosis

Retained cartilage core has been reported in large and giant breeds of dogs 4 to 8 months of age. Clinical signs may vary from swelling of the metaphyseal area to cranial bowing of the radius with external deviation of the forepaw.[23] The condition is usually bilateral, and pain may be apparent with deep palpation of the metaphyseal area of the distal antebrachium. In some cases, no clinical abnormalities are noted, and only radiographic evidence of the condition is apparent.

The most consistent radiographic sign is a radiolucent defect extending proximally from the distal ulnar metaphyseal growth plate (Fig. 20-8). Cranial bowing of the radius and external deviation of the foot may be apparent, depending on the degree of growth plate retardation.

Other diseases causing swelling of the metaphyseal region (e.g., HOD, HO) can be ruled out by radiographic examination.

Treatment

In the mildest forms of retained cartilage core, treatment is unnecessary. Clinical and radiographic reexamination ensures that premature growth retardation is not of clinical significance. If curvature of the radius is a problem, a partial ulnar ostectomy with interpositional fat graft is recommended to prevent further deviation of the antebrachium. A definitive osteotomy of the radius may be necessary, depending on the severity of the deformity.

The prognosis is excellent if premature retardation of the distal ulnar growth plate has not occurred. The prognosis is guarded if premature closure of the distal ulna is present. Bowing of the antebrachium, external deviation of the foot, and subluxation of the antebrachiocarpal joints are complications seen with this condition.

REFERENCES

1. Alexander JW: Selected skeletal dysplasias: craniomandibular osteopathy, multiple cartilaginous exostoses, and hypertrophic osteodystrophy, *Vet Clin North Am Small Anim Pract* 13:55-70, 1983.
2. Alexander JW: Orthopedic diseases. In Slatter DH, editor: *Textbook of small animal surgery*, Philadelphia, 1985, WB Saunders.
3. Allen LH: The role of nutrition in the onset and treatment of metabolic bone disease, *Nutr Update* 1:263-281, 1983.
4. Battershell D: Craniomandibular osteopathy, *J Am Vet Med Assoc* 155:1735-1736, 1969.
5. Biller DS, and others: Aneurysmal bone cyst in a rib of a cat, *J Am Vet Med Assoc* 190:1193-1195, 1987.
6. Bohning R and others: Clinical and radiologic survey of canine panosteitis, *J Am Vet Med Assoc* 156:870-883, 1970.
7. Brown RJ, Trevethan WP, Henry VL: Multiple osteochondroma in a Siamese cat, *J Am Vet Med Assoc* 160:433-435, 1972.
8. Burk RL, Broadhurst JJ: Craniomandibular osteopathy in a Great Dane, *J Am Vet Med Assoc* 169:635-636, 1976.
9. Capen CC: Calcium-regulating hormones and metabolic bone disease. In Newton CD, Nunamaker DM, editors: *Textbook of small animal orthopaedics*, Philadelphia, 1985, JB Lippincott.
10. Carrig CB, Seawright AA: A familial canine polyostotic fibrous dyspasia with subperiosteal cortical defects, *J Small Anim Pract* 10:397-405, 1969.
11. Chester DK: Multiple cartilaginous exostoses in two generations of dogs, *J Am Vet Med Assoc* 159:895-897, 1971.
12. Chigira M, and others: The aetiology and treatment of simple bone cysts, *J Bone Joint Surg* 65B:633-637, 1983.
13. Doige CE, Pharr JW, Withrow SJ: Chondrosarcoma arising in multiple cartilaginous exostoses in a dog, *J Am Anim Hosp Assoc* 14:605-611, 1978.
14. Gambardella PC, Osborne CA, Stevens JB: Multiple cartilaginous exostoses in the dog, *J Am Vet Med Assoc* 166:761-768, 1975.
15. Gee BR, Doige CE: Multiple cartilaginous exostoses in a litter of dogs, *J Am Vet Med Assoc* 156:53-59, 1970.
16. Gerbode F, Birnstingl M, Braimbridge M: Experimental hypertrophic osteoarthropathy, *Surgery* 60:1030-1035, 1966.
17. Goldschmidt MH, Biery DN: Bone cysts in the dog. In Newton CD, Nunamaker DM, editors: *Textbook of small animal orthopaedics*, Philadelphia, 1985, JB Lippincott.
18. Grondalen J: Metaphyseal osteopathy (hypertrophic osteodystrophy) in growing dogs: a clinical study, *J Small Anim Pract* 17:721-735, 1976.
19. Halliwell WH, Ackerman N: Botryoid rhabdomyosarcoma of the urinary bladder and hypertrophic osteoarthropathy in a young dog, *J Am Vet Med Assoc* 165:911-913, 1974.
20. Hathcock JT: Craniomandibular osteopathy in an English bulldog, *J Am Vet Med Assoc* 81:389, 1982.
21. Hedhammar A, and others: Overnutrition and skeletal disease: an experimental study in growing Great Dane dogs, *Cornell Vet* 64 (suppl 5):1-160, 1974.
22. Jaffe HL: Pulmonary hypertrophic osteoarthropathy. In Jaffe HL, editor: *Metabolic, degenerative, and inflammatory diseases of bones and joints*, Philadelphia, 1972, Lea & Febiger.
23. Johnson KA: Retardation of endochondral ossification at the distal ulnar growth plate in dogs, *Aust Vet J* 57:474-478, 1981.
24. Jubb KVF, Kennedy PC: Craniomandibular osteopathy of dogs. In *Pathology of domestic animals*, New York, 1970, Academic Press.
25. Kallfelz F: Skeletal and neuromuscular diseases. In Lewis L, Morris M, Haud MS, editors: *Small animal clinical nutrition*, ed 3, Topeka, Kan, 1982, Mark Morris.
26. Kelly MJ: Long-term survival of a case of hypertrophic osteopathy with regression of bony changes, *J Am Anim Hosp Assoc* 20:439-444, 1984.
27. Krook L: Reversibility of nutritional osteoporosis: physiochemical data on bone from an experimental study in dogs, *J Nutr* 101:233-246, 1971.
28. Lenehan TM, Fetter AW: Hypertrophic osteopathy. In Newton CD, Nunamaker DM, editors: *Textbook of small animal orthopaedics*, Philadelphia, 1985, JB Lippincott.
29. Lenehan TM, Van Sickle DC, Biery DM: Canine panosteitis. In Newton CD, Nunamaker DM, editors: *Textbook of small animal orthopaedics*, Philadelphia, 1985, JB Lippincott.
30. Morgan JP, Carlson WD, Adams OR: Hereditary multiple exostoses in the horse, *J Am Vet Med Assoc* 140:1320-1322, 1962.
31. Newton CD: Radial and ulnar osteotomy. In *Textbook of small animal orthopaedics*, Philadelphia, 1985, JB Lippincott.
32. Nutrient requirements of dogs, pub no. 0-309-03496-5, National Academy of Sciences, Washington, DC, 1985, National Academic Press.
33. Olsson SE: Osteochondrosis: a growing problem to dog breeders, *Gaines Progress*, 1976.
34. Owen LN, Bostock DE: Multiple cartilaginous exostoses with development of a metastasizing osteosarcoma in a Shetland sheepdog, *J Small Anim Pract* 12:507-512, 1971.
35. Pool RR, Leighton RL: Craniomandibular osteopathy in a dog, *J Am Vet Med Assoc* 154:657-660, 1969.
36. Resnich D, Kyriakos M, Greenway GD: Tumors and tumor-like lesions of bone: imaging and pathology of specific lesions. In Resnich D, Niwayama G, editors: *Diagnosis of bone and joint disorders*, Philadelphia, 1988, WB Saunders.
37. Riser WH: What is your diagnosis? Craniomandibular osteopathy in a Labrador puppy, *J Am Vet Med Assoc* 148:1543-1547, 1966.
38. Riser WH, Newton CD: Craniomandibular osteopathy. In Newton CD, Nunamaker DM, editors: *Textbook of small animal orthopaedics*, Philadelphia, 1985, JB Lippincott.
39. Riser WH, Shirer JF: Normal and abnormal growth of the distal foreleg in large and giant dogs, *J Am Vet Radiol Soc* 6:50-64, 1965.
40. Riser WH, Parkes LJ, Shirer JF: Canine craniomandibular osteopathy, *J Am Vet Radiol Soc* 8:23-30, 1967.
41. Schrader AC, Burk RL: Bone cysts in two dogs and a review of similar cystic bone lesions in the dog, *J Am Vet Med Assoc* 182:490-495, 1983.
42. Schulz S: A case of craniomandibular osteopathy in a boxer, *J Small Anim Pract* 19:749-757, 1978.
43. Susanek SJ: Hypertrophic osteopathy, *Comp Cont Educ* 4:689-693, 1982.
44. Tear JA, and others: Ascorbic acid deficiency and hypertrophic osteodystrophy in the dog: a rebuttal, *Cornell Vet* 69:384-401, 1979.
45. Van Sickle DC, Hohn RB: Selected orthopedic problems in the growing dog, *Am Anim Hosp Assoc Monogr*, 1975, p 20.
46. Vulgamott JC, Clark RG: Arterial hypertension and hypertrophic pulmonary osteopathy associated with aortic valvular endocarditis in a dog, *J Am Vet Med Assoc* 177:243-246, 1980.
47. Watson ADJ, Huxtable CRR, Farrow BRH: Craniomandibular osteopathy in Doberman pinschers, *J Small Anim Pract* 16:11-19, 1975.
48. Woodard JC: Canine hypertrophic osteodystrophy: a study of the spontaneous disease in littermates, *Vet Pathol* 19:337-354, 1982.

21

Joint Diseases of the Dog and Cat

STEVEN C. SCHRADER

PRINCIPLES OF DIAGNOSIS

Historical and physical examinations provide the basis for diagnosis of joint disease. Radiographic examination and joint fluid analysis are subsequently used to confirm, deny, or otherwise modify the clinical assumptions. The diagnosis of joint disease is rarely based only on laboratory findings or on a specific laboratory test; radiographic and laboratory results should always be interpreted with the clinical situation in mind. It is much more important for the student (clinician) to learn to examine peripheral joints and to be able to locate the site of swelling or pain than to be able to launch into a learned discourse on the basic science of anti-deoxyribonucleic acid (anti-DNA) antibodies or immune complexes.[51] The principles of historical and physical examinations and the ancillary methods of diagnosis are described in Chapter 1.

PRINCIPLES OF TREATMENT

Most treatments for joint disease in dogs and cats are symptomatic and palliative. Nonsurgical methods include rest, massage, physical therapy, weight loss, and treatment with analgesic or antiinflammatory drugs. Acupuncture appears to be effective in the treatment of certain joint disorders;[63] however, additional investigation is needed to define further its indications and limitations. Surgical procedures have been used to reduce or eliminate pain by improving range of motion, stabilization, or by correcting deformity or structural abnormality. Specific surgical procedures are described elsewhere in this chapter and in the chapters that detail traumatic joint disease, cruciate ligament and meniscal injuries, and hip dysplasia.

Rest, physical therapy, weight control, or administration of analgesic or antiinflammatory drugs may be used alone, in combination with each other, or in combination with surgical therapy. These methods are frequently the first to be employed in animals with lameness caused by joint disease. Knowledge of the animal's response to rest, weight loss, and drug therapy provides the clinician with valuable insight regarding prognosis and the need for surgery or other forms of therapy. Although customary, it is somewhat misleading to refer to these methods of therapy as conservative treatments; use of nonsurgical methods in situations that call for surgical intervention is not reasonable, moderate, or restrained.

The owner is an essential element in determining suitability and success of both surgical and nonsurgical treatments. Therapeutic failure can be the result of poor compliance. The veterinarian must ascertain which methods or protocols are reasonable for the client to follow. As such, the veterinarian must have knowledge of the client's lifestyle and understand the role that the animal plays in the household. Instructions must be clear and their significance understood. Clients must be able and willing to apply the treatment and accurately assess the animal's response.

Rest

Confinement to a small area or employing other means of restricting physical activity may relieve pain and facilitate recovery in animals with acute joint and soft tissue injuries. In addition, restricting physical activity may ensure the success of stabilization or reconstructive procedures. In chronic situations, only those activities that seem to exacerbate clinical signs might need to be curtailed. The owner must be aware of the types of activity that tend to aggravate the condition; the owner is responsible for imposing the necessary restrictions.

Rest is generally easiest to enforce when the animal is placed in a secluded area away from encounters with other pets and children; this is easier to accomplish indoors than outdoors. Although rest would appear to be a natural protective mechanism, many dogs and cats remain physically active even though they have serious joint injury or disease. Certain animals remain active despite attempts to keep them quiet. These animals may require sedation or confinement to a small cage in a very isolated area of the home.

The level of physical activity should be gradually increased as healing occurs or when clinical signs abate. The level of physical activity that can be ultimately achieved depends on the nature and degree of the problem.

Exercise and Physical Therapy

Exercise and certain physical therapies are as important as rest in the management of animals with joint disease. Lack of activity causes joint stiffness, muscle atrophy, and a decline in overall conditioning. Weight gain may occur in sedentary animals or in animals receiving corticosteroids. Efforts must be made to maintain a certain level of activity to avoid these problems. Many pets seem to enjoy walking, running, and playing; that is, they seem to derive mental as well as physical benefits from exercise.

Activities that maximize the benefits and minimize the adverse effects of physical exercise should be encouraged in animals with joint disease. In this regard, swimming, jogging, and long walks on a regular basis seem to be better than intermittent field work, hard play, or spurts of activity. Intermittent drug therapy may be necessary to ensure that a certain level of activity can be maintained. Surgical intervention may be indicated to help maintain an adequate degree of physical function when drug therapy is ineffective or results in adverse side effects.

Active exercise is of greater benefit in maintaining joint mobility and muscle mass than passive movement; however, in humans, gentle manipulation or massage plays an important role in the management of joint, bursal, and soft tissue pain. Although the animal's temperament or pain may limit the use of passive therapy, many pets seem to enjoy gentle massage of the affected part and continue to seek it from their owner. Clients are often able to determine what the animal will tolerate, what manipulations the pet seems to enjoy and what manipulations they resist. Owners should be encouraged to experiment and try different techniques; however, manipulations that the animal will resist or that might result in injury to the owner or veterinary assistant should not be prescribed. To be of value, passive manipulations should be performed several times each day with duration and intensity gradually increased until rehabilitation is complete.

Weight Control

Weight control or weight reduction is essential in the treatment of dogs and cats with joint disease. Many older dogs with degenerative joint disease (DJD) are obese; a vicious cycle is established as they continue to gain weight with declining levels of physical activity. Dogs with severe arthritis, especially those receiving corticosteroids, are particularly difficult to manage, since weight control or weight loss is almost impossible to achieve. Sympathetic owners often cannot resist the urge to give food to their pet; they may perceive food as the animal's only source of enjoyment. Pets do not (or should not) feed themselves, so an obese pet indicates that the owner has a problem with food.[17]

Successful obesity therapy, whether through exercise, pharmacological treatment, or starvation, requires that the clinician recognize current behavior and provide training to permit new "nonfattening" patterns of interaction.[17] Specific dietary strategies should be formulated and followed; the goals that are established should be reasonable. Compliance can be achieved only if the owner understands and accepts the recommendations. Weight management strategies and their execution have been described.[17] Optimum "normal" weights (Box 21-1) provide the basis for weight loss plans (Fig. 21-1).

Drug Therapy

Drug therapy is, for the most part, intended to reduce inflammation/pain, thereby lessening the physical disability that accompanies joint disease. Few drugs are used specifically for one type of joint disease or another; instead, a single drug or class of drugs may be effective in treatment of disorders that have varied etiologies. Since many noninfectious inflammatory joint disorders seem to be associated with autoimmune mechanisms, treatment of such disorders usually includes administration of corticosteroids and other immunomodulating drugs. The use of corticosteroids is not limited to treatment of immune-mediated joint disease; they are used in certain cases of noninflammatory joint disease as well. Similarly, aspirin has been used in the treatment of DJD, regardless of its cause.

Few drugs are capable of effecting a cure; signs may be controlled, but complete resolution is rarely achieved. There are exceptions: antibiotics are used specifically in cases of bacterial arthritis, and the infection may be resolved; permanent remission is sometimes achieved with corticosteroid therapy of idiopathic inflammatory joint disease.

One drug may produce different results in different animals with the same type of joint disorder. The veterinarian must have the knowledge and experience necessary to modify dosages, select alternative drugs, or concoct drug combinations that meet the needs of the patient and the owner. However, it is unrealistic to expect the student or clinician to become familiar with the indications and limitations of all drugs used in the treatment of joint disease. It is better to have a good understanding of the benefits and limitations of a few frequently used drugs than an incomplete understanding of many.

BOX 21-1
OPTIMUM WEIGHTS FOR VARIOUS BREEDS (lb)

TOY BREEDS

Chihuahua	2-6
Lhasa apso	10-15
Miniature dachshund	5-10
Pekinese	10-14
Toy poodle	8-12
Yorkshire terrier	4-7
Miniature schnauzer	12-15

SMALL BREEDS male (female)

Beagle	25-35 (-5)
Boston terrier	15-25 (-5)
Cocker spaniel	25-30 (-5)
Dachshund	20-25 (-5)
Miniature poodle	15-25 (-5)

MEDIUM BREEDS

Bassett hound	45-55 (-5)
Brittany spaniel	30-40 (-5)
Collie	45-65 (-5 to 10)
Siberian husky	45-60 (-10)
Pointer	55-70 (-10)
Samoyed	55-70 (-5)
Standard poodle	40-50 (-5)

LARGE BREEDS

Boxer	55-70 (-5)
German shepherd	70-85 (-10)
Irish setter	55-70 (-10)
Labrador retriever	60-75 (-5)

GIANT BREEDS

Great Dane	120-150 (-20)
St. Bernard	140-200 (-40 to 60)

Modified with permission from Buffington T: Obesity better prevented than treated: involve owner in treatment, DVM Mag 21(6):27-31, 1990.

A. Daily Energy Needs for Weight Loss

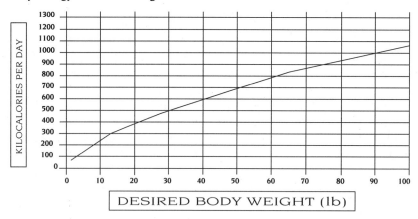

B. **Current weight – desired weight = pounds to lose**

C. **Pounds to lose ÷ weight loss expected per week = weeks required for weight loss**

Weight loss expected per week:
Cats/toy breeds	¼ - ½ lb
Small breeds	½ - 1 lb
Medium breeds	1 - 1½ lb
Large breeds	1½ - 2½ lb
Giant breeds	2-3 lb

D. **Example Diet Foods (Kcal/unit)**

Dog	Dry Cup	Can	Cat	Dry Cup	Can
Hill's r/d	200	260	Hill's r/d	180	300
w/d	220	420	w/d	220	400
Science Diet Light	250		Science Diet Light	260	
Cycle 3	240	310	Tender	110/	
Fit 'n Trim	280		Vittles Light	pouch	
Iams Lite	320				
Alpo Lite	310				

Fig. 21-1   Weight loss planning for dogs and cats.

Modified with permission from Buffington T: Obesity better prevented than treated: involve owner in treatment, *DVM Mag* 21(6):27-31, 1990.

As with other methods of nonsurgical management, the owner must be able and willing to comply with instructions. The owner must administer the drug as prescribed and be able to provide an accurate assessment of the response, or lack thereof. With long-term drug therapy, it is helpful for the client to purchase a calendar that has enough space to allow daily notations concerning amount of drug administered and the animal's physical status. The calendar provides the clinician with valuable information and is often more accurate and concise than owner recall.

Finally, veterinarians and clients must avoid extrapolating dosages and other information that have been obtained from studies in other species. For example, serious gastrointestinal (GI) side effects have been associated with naproxen administration in dogs.[25,37,87] In these reports the dosage of naproxen was similar to or exceeded the daily recommended adult (human) dose. Pharmacological studies suggest that, in dogs, the half-life of naproxen is exceedingly long and that therapeutic levels are maintained at a fraction of the human dose.[34] Based on these studies, the dose of naproxen in dogs is only 7% to 14% of the daily adult dose used in humans. At this dosage, naproxen appears to be relatively safe and effective. Aspirin-like drugs are relatively more toxic to cats than dogs,[53] and acetaminophen is toxic in cats and should not be used.[73] Adverse reactions have been reported in dogs and cats that have received any one of a number of analgesic drugs that are used in humans.*

---

*References 25, 30, 37, 47, 87, 101, 104.

Unfortunately, little information is available on the use and effectiveness of many analgesic and antiinflammatory drugs that are used in dogs and cats; most such drugs are still used empirically.

Medications used in the management of joint disease in man have been grouped into several broad categories: nonsteroidal antiinflammatory drugs (NSAIDs) or aspirin-like drugs, corticosteroids (prednisone, others), slow-acting remittive agents (gold salts, penicillamine), antimalarial agents (hydroxychloroquine), cytotoxic agents (azathioprine, cyclophosphamide), and hypouricemics (allopurinol, probenecid).[89] NSAIDs and corticosteroids are typically used in the treatment of joint disorders in dogs and cats. They are available, effective, and relatively safe. The use of hypouricemic drugs does not appear to have indications in dogs and cats because true gout has not been reported to occur. In addition, little information is available that supports the use of gold salts, penicillamine, or hydroxychloroquine in the treatment of canine and feline joint disease; a number of toxic effects have been associated with their administration in humans.[89] Azathioprine and cyclophosphamide are used with some frequency in dogs with noninfectious inflammatory or immune-mediated arthritis. Although little clinical information suggests one drug or drug combination is more effective than another, these drugs do appear to produce beneficial results. Recommendations on the use of cyclophosphamide and azathioprine can be found at the end of this chapter.

Aspirin and NSAIDs. Aspirin is the most well known and widely used NSAID; it serves as the prototype for this group (Table 21-1). Aspirin (acetylsalicylic acid) is a potent analgesic, antiinflammatory, and antipyretic agent; properties related to aspirin's ability to interfere with prostaglandin synthesis via irreversible inactivation of cyclooxygenase.[32] The drug is relatively inexpensive and readily available (Table 21-2); more than 60 aspirin-containing preparations are listed in the 44th (1990) edition of the *Physicians' Desk Reference*.[5] As such, the veterinarian must be specific when prescribing aspirin products.

Aspirin is generally well tolerated by dogs and is effective in the management of various types of joint disease. In the dog the antiinflammatory dosage of aspirin is 25 to 35 mg/kg every 8 to 12 hours (10 to 15 mg/lb every 8 to 12 hours); antipyresis and analgesia can be achieved at about one-half this dosage.[19,112] The half-life of aspirin in cats is considerably longer than in dogs.[26] In the cat, analgesic and antipyretic effects can be maintained by a dosage of 10 to 12 mg/kg every 48 hours (4 to 5 mg/lb every 48 hours).[26,107]

The severe toxic effects of aspirin generally do not occur until the amount ingested greatly exceeds the amount needed for antipyresis or analgesia.[19] When aspirin is administered at therapeutic dosages, most of its adverse effects can be associated with gastric irritation. Vomiting (with or without blood), melena, abdominal pain, anorexia, and anemia are clinical signs of aspirin-induced GI disease.

Gastroduodenal ulceration is common with aspirin therapy; it has been associated with administration of other NSAIDs as well. Contrary to popular belief, buffering aspirin probably does not offer significant protection against ulcer formation.[60,97] Time-release preparations of aspirin are of limited value, and absorption of enteric-coated products is sometimes incomplete.[32] H_2-receptor antagonists have been used in an attempt to reduce gastric acid secretion and subsequent ulcer formation in patients receiving aspirin. Such drugs are probably more useful in treatment than prevention. It has been shown that cimetidine, an H_2-receptor antagonist, does not prevent gastric hemorrhage caused by the administration of aspirin in dogs[13] or accelerate healing of ulcers in people who continue to take aspirin.[33,106]

In suspected cases of NSAID-induced gastroduodenal ulceration and blood loss, anemia should be evaluated by means of red blood cell (RBC) indexes and by the degree of regeneration.[106] Most affected dogs have a normocytic normochromic anemia, consistent with short-term blood loss, and have some evidence of regeneration. Evaluation of serum proteins is helpful to confirm that the anemia is caused by blood loss; fecal analysis helps to rule out parasitism as a cause of anemia and melena.[106]

Aspirin therapy should be discontinued when vomiting occurs or when blood loss is evident. Antacid, H_2-receptor antagonist, or sucralfate therapy appears to be beneficial. The use of a single agent is less expensive, less inconvenient, and probably as effective as the use of combination therapy.[106] If the animal does not appear to improve clinically, a different drug or drug combination is indicated; other causes of ulceration (renal failure) or of bleeding should be ruled out by serum biochemical analysis and evaluation of coagulation.[106]

Finally, the ubiquitous use of aspirin and advertising campaigns of companies promoting a plethora of aspirin alternatives have contributed to the erroneous notion that aspirin is less effective than these products. Aspirin is such a potent drug that if it had to meet current requirements of the U.S. Food and Drug Administration (FDA), it might not be licensed for over-the-counter use.[19] Clients should be informed of the potency of aspirin and warned against the indiscriminate use of it or any NSAIDs that have been touted as being safer or more effective. Efficacy, availability, low cost, and availability of pharmacological data on the use of aspirin in dogs and cats favor its use over other NSAIDs whenever such drugs are indicated for use. Another NSAID may prove effective when aspirin therapy has failed.

Table 21-1 Nonsteroidal Antiinflammatory Drugs (NSAIDs)

Drug category	Specific drug	Treatment of joint disease*		Comments
		Dosage: canine	Dosage: feline	
Salicylates	Acetylsalicylic acid (aspirin, many trade names)	25-35 mg/kg q8-12h	10-12 mg/kg q48h	Various dosages reported
	Salicylsalicylic acid (Salfex, Monogesic, Disalcid)	ND	ND	
	Choline magnesium trisalicylate (Trilisate)	ND	ND	
Pyrazolon derivatives	Phenylbutazone (Butazolidin)	10-12 mg/kg q12h	NR	Dosage should not exceed 800 mg/day
	Oxyphenbutazone (Oxalid, Tandearil)	ND	NR	
Paraaminophenol derivatives	Acetaminophen (Tylenol, many trade names)	NR	NR (Toxic)	Not clinically effective in treatment of joint disorders
Fenamates	Meclofenamate (Meclomen, Arquel)	1 mg/kg/day	ND	
Propionic acid derivatives	Ibuprofen (Motrin, many trade names)	5 mg/kg q8-12h†	ND	Narrow therapeutic index
	Naproxen (Naprosyn, Anaprox, others)	2.2 mg/kg once daily†	ND	
	Fenoprofen (Nalfon, others)	ND	ND	
	Flurbiprofen (Ansaid, Froben)	ND	ND	
	Ketoprofen (Alrheumat, Orudis)	ND	ND	
Oxicams	Piroxicam (Feldene)	ND	ND	
Phenylacetic acid derivative	Diclofenac sodium (Voltaren)	ND	ND	
Others	Tolmetin (Tolectin)	ND	ND	
	Indomethacin (Indocin)	NR	NR	
	Sulindac (Clinoril, others)	ND	NR	

*Adverse effects have been associated with the use of various NSAIDs in these species. All NSAIDs should be used with caution in cats. Recommended dosages should be adjusted downward until the minimum effective dose is reached. Dosages should not be extrapolated from those recommended for humans.
†Not approved for use in dogs.
ND, Not determined; NR, not recommended.

Table 21-2 Various Nonprescription Aspirin-Containing Preparations

Name (manufacturer)	Aspirin content grains (mg)	Comments
Aspirin USP (various)	5 (325)	Not buffered
Bayer: Genuine Tablet/Caplet (Glenbrook)	5 (325)	Not buffered
Bayer: Children's Chewable	1.25 (81)	Not buffered
Bayer: Maximum Tablets/Caplets	7.7 (500)	Not buffered
Bayer: 8 Hour Timed-Release Caplet	10 (650)	Microencapsulated
Bufferin: Tri-Buffered (Bristol Myers)	5 (325)	Buffered
Bufferin: Extra Strength Tri-Buffered	7.7 (500)	Buffered
Bufferin: Arthritis Strength Tri-Buffered	7.7 (500)	Buffered
Ecotrin: Regular Strength Tablet/Caplet (Smith Kline)	5 (325)	Enteric coated
Ecotrin: Maximum Strength Tablet/Caplet	7.7 (500)	Enteric coated
Anacin: Tablet/Caplet (Whitehall)	6.1 (400)	Contains caffeine (32 mg)
Anacin: Maximum Strength Tablet	7.7 (500)	Contains caffeine (32 mg)
Excedrin: Extra Strength Tablet/Caplet (Bristol Myers)	3.8 (250)	Contains acetaminophen (250 mg) and caffeine (65 mg)
Vanquish: Caplets (Glenbrook)	3.5 (227)	Contains acetaminophen (194 mg) and caffeine (33 mg)
Ascriptin: Regular Strength (Rhone-Poulenc Rorer)	5 (325)	Buffered
Ascriptin: Extra Strength	7.7 (500)	Buffered
Ascriptin: A/D	5 (325)	More buffer than regular strength

Table 21-3 Relative Potencies, Equivalent Doses, and Uses of Corticosteroids

Compound	Relative antiinflammatory potency	Relative sodium-retaining potency	Duration of action*	Adapted for alternate-day use	Approximate equivalent dose (mg)†
Cortisone	0.8	0.8	S	No	25
Hydrocortisone	1.0	1.0	S	No	20
Prednisone	4.0	0.8	I	Yes	5
Prednisolone	4.0	0.8	I	Yes	5
Methylprednisolone	5.0	0.5	I	Yes	4
Triamcinolone	5.0	0.0	I	No	4
Paramethasone	10.0	0.0	L	No	2
Dexamethasone	25.0	0.0	L	No	0.75
Betamethasone	25.0	0.0	L	No	0.75

* S, short or 8- to 12-hour biological half-life; I, intermediate or 12- to 36-hour biological half-life; L, long or 36- to 72-hour biological half-life.
† Dose relationships apply only to oral or intravenous administration; relative potencies may differ greatly when injected intramuscularly or into joint spaces.

Modified with permission from Haynes RC, Murad F: Adrenocorticotropic hormone; adrenocortical steroids and their synthetic analogs; inhibitors of adrenocortical steroid biosynthesis. In Gilman AG, Goodman L, Goodman A, editors: *The pharmacological basis of therapeutics*, ed 6, New York, 1980, Macmillan.

Corticosteroids. The medical use of corticosteroids began in 1949 when humans with rheumatoid arthritis were treated with cortisone and were reported to experience marked improvement.[20,45] Exogenous glucocorticoids are the corticosteroids used by clinicians to treat a number of inflammatory and immunological diseases, including those that affect the musculoskeletal system. As a result, "corticosteroids" is generally assumed to mean glucocorticoids.[20] Chastain[20] has composed an excellent discussion and review of the use of corticosteroids in the dog.

In the United States a number of corticosteroids are commercially available in numerous single-item prepara-tions or in combination with antibiotic or various other drugs.[20] Of these, prednisone and prednisolone are probably best suited for treatment of musculoskeletal injuries and joint disease. They are inexpensive, have an intermediate duration of action, and can be given on an alternate-day program to minimize hypothalamic-pituitary-adrenal (HPA) axis suppression.[20] They have minimum mineralocorticoid effect.[20,44] Prednisone does not have antiinflammatory activity until hepatic metabolism converts the drug to prednisolone. Severe liver disease can impair this conversion.[20] Basic information concerning potency, duration of action, and use of various corticosteroids is found in Table 21-3.

Table 21-4 Indications for Corticosteroid Use and Required Dosages

Indication	Initial required dosage of prednisone or prednisolone
Glucocorticoid replacement therapy	0.1 mg/lb (0.25 mg/kg) per day
Antiinflammatory therapy	0.2-0.5 mg/lb (0.5-1 mg/kg) per day
Immunosuppressive therapy	1-2 mg/lb (2-4 mg/kg) per day

Although corticosteroid therapy is largely empirical, certain principles of use should be followed.[20,44] Whenever corticosteroids are to be administered over long periods, the dose must be the smallest one that will achieve the desired effect. This dose is found by trial and error.[44] Corticosteroids having an intermediate duration of action, such as prednisone, prednisolone, and methylprednisolone, are suitable for long-term therapy and for alternate-day administration. The initial dosages of prednisone or prednisolone that have been suggested in various situations are listed in Table 21-4.

Administering prednisone/prednisolone for up to 3 days at a dosage of 1.0 mg/kg/day (0.5 mg/lb/day), so-called burst or pulse therapy,[20] can be useful in the treatment of acute musculoskeletal injuries such as severe strain or sprain injuries. This method of treatment may be useful in dogs that have DJD and are experiencing an acute onset of swelling or pain after overactivity or trauma to the affected joint. No lasting suppression of the HPA axis is expected with pulse therapy; however, certain adverse effects such as GI ulceration or pancreatitis are possible.[20,67]

Long-term (greater than 2 weeks) corticosteroid therapy is rarely indicated for treatment of DJD and other so-called noninflammatory joint disorders. Long-term therapy is indicated in the treatment of the various immune-mediated joint disorders. At antiinflammatory dosages, the extraadrenal adverse effects of corticosteroids become evident with 2 weeks of continuous therapy.[20,21] Administering the recommended daily dosage of prednisone in divided doses throughout the day causes more adverse effects than a single daily dose.[3] Divided daily doses of prednisone are appropriate when an attempt is made to put such corticosteroid-responsive diseases as idiopathic immune-mediated joint disease into remission. Divided doses are not appropriate to maintain remission. Once-a-day therapy should be instituted as soon as possible.[20] With immune-mediated (inflammatory) joint disease, once-a-day therapy is generally possible by the second to fourth week of treatment. Whenever the duration of daily oral therapy exceeds 2 weeks, it is prudent to slowly taper the dosage of corticosteroid before discontinuing the drug. Abrupt cessa-

tion of prolonged corticosteroid therapy is associated with a significant risk of adrenal insufficiency.[44] The rate at which the dosage is decreased depends on the type of disorder being treated and the clinical response that occurs during the course of dose reduction.

Using prednisone or prednisolone at antiinflammatory doses once every 48 hours produces little HPA axis suppression.[3,20] Alternate-day oral prednisone or prednisolone therapy should be considered in every animal that requires systemic corticosteroid therapy for longer than 2 weeks.[21] This is the case with such immune-mediated joint disorders as systemic lupus erythematosus and idiopathic immune-mediated polyarthritis. Conversion of once-a-day to alternate-day therapy should be gradual. This can be achieved by tapering the daily dose to the effective minimum, then doubling that dose and administering it every other day while discontinuing or gradually tapering the dose on the "off" day.[93] Alternate-day dosages that meet or exceed 1.1 mg/kg (0.5 mg/lb) every other day saturate the dog's ability to metabolize fully the last dose before the next dose is given, therefore negating the primary advantage of alternate-day therapy.[21,56] The dosage of prednisone/prednisolone given on alternate days should be tapered to the effective minimum and then, if possible, discontinued.

Finally, the use of fixed-dose corticosteroid combination preparations (corticosteroid-aspirin, corticosteroid-antibiotic) should be questioned. The use of such combinations may result in adverse side effects and imposes certain therapeutic limitations, which often preclude their use in the treatment of joint disease. Likewise, slowly absorbed forms of corticosteroid should be used with caution. Methylprednisolone acetate (2.5 mg/kg) suppresses the adrenal cortex for at least 5 weeks;[14,54] triamcinolone acetonide (0.22 mg/kg) suppresses the adrenal cortex for about 4 weeks.[55] These drugs should not be used for their systemic effects. They are occasionally used in the treatment of monoarticular noninfectious joint disease and bursitis. They are ideal for intraarticular administration because the required dose is small, the local concentration of steroid is high, and systemic effects are probably minimal.[20]

PROGNOSIS ASSOCIATED WITH JOINT DISEASE

Complete resolution of pain or dysfunction is rarely achieved in animals having joint disease. Even with correct diagnosis and appropriate therapy, control is more likely than cure. Clinical benefits are associated with surgical treatment of cruciate ligament injuries in large breeds of dogs; however, DJD is inevitable in dogs that have undergone a stabilization procedure. Remodeling changes continue to progress even when good stability seems to have been achieved with surgery. Likewise, infection may be eliminated in animals with septic arthritis, but the aftermath of infection can cause significant long-term disability.

Although many dogs and cats with noninflammatory joint disease continue to experience some pain or clinical disability, most will be able to lead reasonably active lives or be functional companions to their owners. Animals with inflammatory joint disease, especially those with associated systemic manifestations, do not fare as well; the long-term prognosis with feline progressive arthritis, rheumatoid or rheumatoid-like arthritis, and systemic lupus erythematosus is poor.

The goals and expectations associated with therapy should be reasonable and be understood by all. It is not unusual for an owner of a pet with joint disease to become frustrated and disenchanted with treatment. Clear explanations, sound advice, and a sympathetic attitude help overcome frustration, prevent misunderstanding, and foster confidence and loyalty. The veterinarian and owner must work together for treatment to be successful.

CLASSIFICATION OF JOINT DISORDERS OF THE DOG AND CAT

Numerous disorders affect the joints of dogs and cats.[85,92] Joint disease is encountered more frequently in dogs, probably because the small size, light weight, and agile but somewhat sedentary nature of cats preclude the development or detection of certain joint problems.

The joint disorders that occur in dogs and cats are listed in Box 21-2. The most clinically prevalent of these disorders are described here or elsewhere in this textbook. Joint disorders that are rarely encountered in clinical practice or that are incompletely documented are not discussed; selected references are cited to assist readers who are interested in learning more about these disorders.

Different methods have been used to classify disorders that affect joints; certain flaws and inconsistencies are associated with each. Inflammation is present in almost all joint disorders that affect dogs and cats; however, an inflammatory-noninflammatory scheme of classifying joint disease has clinical merit (Box 21-2).[85] With this classification scheme, joint disorders are differentiated on the basis of the degree to which the inflammatory process is involved in the pathogenesis of the disorder. DJD is considered a noninflammatory disorder; that is, although a certain degree of inflammation is usually present in affected joints, inflammation does not appear to play a significant role in its onset or pathogenesis. The inflammatory process associated with infection or immune-mediated joint disease is considered central to

the onset or pathogenesis of the disorder; thus, these are considered inflammatory disorders. The clinician must be able to distinguish inflammatory from noninflammatory disease because it provides an insight to treatment and prognosis (see Chapter 1).

NONINFLAMMATORY JOINT DISORDERS

Numerous noninflammatory joint disorders are encountered by the practicing veterinarian (Box 21-2); DJD is especially common. The noninflammatory joint disorders are rarely associated with systemic signs; affected animals tend to exhibit clinical signs in only one or two joints even though multiple joints may be affected. These historical and physical findings help to differentiate this group of joint disorders from inflammatory disease.

Degenerative Joint Disease

DJD is a progressive disease characterized by degeneration and destruction of articular cartilage; this occurs with (secondary) or without (primary) known predisposing cause or injury. The consequences of cartilage degeneration, and the instability or incongruency that may cause it, are collapse of the joint space (cartilage space), remodeling of subchondral bone, synovitis, and periarticular fibrosis and osteophyte formation. Each of these contributes to the historical, physical, radiographic, and clinical pathological features of this disorder.

The unifying theme in DJD is degeneration and destruction of articular cartilage. The cause of primary DJD has not been identified. Secondary DJD is often associated with abnormal joint mechanics (instability or incongruency) or caused by direct trauma to the cartilage itself. Both primary (idiopathic) and secondary forms of DJD are clinically prevalent in dogs and cats.

Softening of the articular cartilage occurs early in the course of the disease. Chondromalacia involves loss of matrix, that is, the supporting substance for collagen fibers. As matrix is lost, enzymes and other substances are released that may lead to further destruction and weakening of the cartilage and a chemical synovitis (Fig. 21-2).[22] Collagen is exposed (fibrillation), and fissures develop and propagate.

Continued interval loading of affected cartilage causes mechanical destruction and physiological alterations within the cartilage that remains. Normal articular cartilage can be likened to a sponge. Waste products move from the cartilage and into the synovial fluid as the cartilage is loaded (squeezed); fluid containing nutrients is taken in as load is removed. Thus, intermittent loading and unloading of the joint are essential to the survival of

BOX 21-2

CLASSIFICATION OF JOINT DISORDERS OF THE DOG AND CAT*

I. Noninflammatory joint disease
  A. Degenerative joint disease
    1. Primary
    2. Secondary
  B. Traumatic joint disease
    1. Supporting soft tissue damage
    2. Cartilage damage
    3. Disruption of bone
  C. Luxation and subluxation
    1. Traumatic
    2. Developmental/congenital
      a. Hip dysplasia
      b. Patellar luxation
      c. Shoulder dysplasia/instability
      d. Temporomandibular luxation/instability
      e. Axial-atlanto-occipital malformation
      f. Caudal cervical spinal instability
      g. Ruptured cruciate ligament
  D. Other developmental disorders
    1. Conformational abnormalities
      a. Varus/valgus deformities (coxa valga, genu valgum)
      b. Joint malformation/malalignment secondary to physeal growth disturbance
    2. Osteochondritis dissecans
    3. Fragmented medial coronoid process
    4. Ununited anconeal process—nonchondrodystrophoid dog
    5. Avascular necrosis—femoral head
    6. Elbow incongruity (may be associated with fragmented coronoid or ununited anconeal process)
  E. Other intervertebral joint disorders
    1. Spondylosis
    2. Lumbosacral instability/subluxation
    3. Intervertebral disc protrusion/herniation
  F. Meniscal disorders
    1. Primary
    2. Secondary (ruptured cruciate ligament)
  G. Constitutional disorders
    1. Chondrodystrophy
      a. Intervertebral joint (disc) disease
      b. "Ununited" anconeal process—chondrodystrophoid dog
      c. Hip joint instability
    2. Mucopolysaccharidosis[42,43,52]†
    3. Congenital hypothyroidism
    4. Hemophilia A
  H. Dietary disorders
    1. Hypervitaminosis A[‡23,95]†
  I. Neoplastic/neoplasia-like disorders
    1. Synovial cell sarcoma
    2. Osteosarcoma‡
    3. Osteocartilaginous exostosis‡
    4. Villonodular synovitis[59,100]
    5. Lymphosarcoma†
  J. Other
    1. Multicentric periarticular calcinosis[29]
    2. Synovial chondrometaplasia[31]
    3. Hypertrophic osteopathy[‡15]
    4. Carpal weakness/laxity syndromes[1,96]

II. Inflammatory joint disease
  A. Infectious arthritis
    1. Bacterial arthritis
      a. Synovial joint
      b. Intervertebral joint (discospondylitis)
    2. Bacterial L forms
    3. Mycoplasmal arthritis[48,71]†
    4. Rickettsial arthritis[7,102]
    5. Spirochetal arthritis
    6. Viral arthritis[84] (includes postvaccinal reactions)
    7. Fungal arthritis[38,64,79]
    8. Protozoal arthritis
  B. Noninfectious arthritis
    1. Immune-mediated arthritis
      a. Deforming or erosive arthritis
        (1) Rheumatoid/rheumatoid-like arthritis of dogs[18,49,11]
        (2) Polyarthritis syndrome of greyhounds[18,49,11]†
        (3) Feline chronic progressive arthritis (rheumatoid form)†
      b. Periosteal proliferative arthritis: feline chronic progressive arthritis†
      c. Nondeforming or nonerosive arthritis
        (1) Idiopathic nondeforming arthritis—no associated abnormalities (type I)§
        (2) Arthritis associated with chronic infection (type II)
        (3) Arthritis associated with enteric disorder (type III)
        (4) Arthritis associated with neoplasia (type IV)
        (5) Systemic lupus erythematosus
        (6) Plasmacytic-lymphocytic synovitis
        (7) Drug-induced arthritis
        (8) Periarteritis nodosa[2]
        (9) Juvenile polyarthritis syndrome of Akitas[27]
    2. Crystal-induced arthropathy
      a. Gout[68]
      b. Pseudogout[35]

*References cited for rare, poorly understood, or incompletely documented disorders. Most disorders are of equal or greater prevalence or are better documented in dogs versus cats. Exceptions are denoted with a dagger (†).
‡Lesions are primarily extracapsular, but clinical signs mimic those of joint disease.
§See later text discussion.

Modified with permission from Pederson NC and others: Joint diseases of dogs and cats. In Ettinger SJ, editor: *Textbook of veterinary internal medicine,* ed 3, Philadelphia, 1989, Saunders.

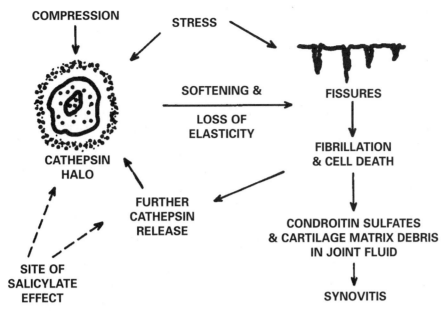

Fig. 21-2   Vicious cycle of degenerative joint disease.

From Chrisman OD: Biochemical aspects of degenerative joint disease, *Clin Orthop Rel Res* 64:77-86, 1969.

the articular cartilage. Biomechanical alterations that affect the degree of loading adversely affect cartilage homeostasis; instability and incongruency are important in this regard (Fig. 21-3).

As destruction of articular cartilage continues, substances are released that may contribute to synovitis and result in pain. Excessive production of joint fluid or failure to absorb it causes distention of the capsule and contributes to pain. The capsule is well endowed with sensory nerve endings.[4]

Loss of cartilage exposes subchondral bone to forces that normally would be dampened by overlying cartilage. There is sclerosis of the subchondral bone, and the denuded apposing articular surfaces take on a polished appearance (eburnation).

Microfractures and fissures in the subchondral bone may allow subsequent leakage of synovial fluid into the bone, resulting in subchondral cyst formation. Healing processes are initiated as the fissure propagates; these processes result in alternate resorption and deposition of bone. Continued interval loading and filling of the crack with joint fluid may prevent bridging of the gap. Continued resorption leads to cavitation; deposition of bone at the periphery of the cyst isolates it from surrounding bone and potential blood supply. This process is analogous to that associated with fracture nonunion. Subchondral cyst formation is a more prominent feature of DJD in humans and horses than in dogs or cats.

Periarticular osteophyte production is an especially prominent feature of DJD whenever instability is present.

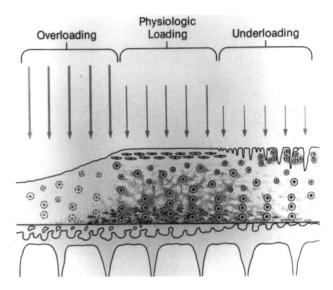

Fig. 21-3   Continued optimum functional integrity of connective tissue depends on balanced rates of matrix production and breakdown by the cells. Healthy tissue (*center*) results from a physiological range of stress that maintains optimum cell activity. If this range of stress is exceeded (*left*), the result is cell injury and, eventually, necrosis (chondrolysis). If the stress is inadequate (*right*), disuse atrophy, that is, lack of adequate matrix production by the cells, may occur. In cartilage, this is associated with increased water content and fibrillation of the collagen.

From Bullough PG, Vigorita VJ: *Atlas of orthopaedic pathology with clinical and radiologic correlations*, New York, 1984, Gower Medical.

Osteophytes are invariably located where the synovial membrane and fibrous capsule insert on the bone. The presence of abnormal mechanical factors and a blood supply appear to be necessary for the development of osteophytes at these sites. The pathogenesis of osteophyte formation has been described by Marshall.[65]

Diagnosis. Generally speaking, there are no breed or sex predispositions for DJD in dogs and cats; however, the ubiquitous nature of hip dysplasia in large breeds of dogs and the prevalence of specific disorders such as osteochondritis dissecans in some breeds increase the rate at which DJD is diagnosed in specific breeds and in certain joints. The prevalence of hip dysplasia and cruciate ligament rupture helps make the hip and stifle common sites for DJD in the dog.

Primary DJD and DJD that is secondary to developmental disorders such as hip dysplasia are usually characterized as having an insidious onset and slowly progressive course. In animals having subclinical or mildly symptomatic DJD, the onset of signs may occur suddenly after strenuous activity or trauma. Joint trauma may cause an acute onset of lameness in normal animals; resolution of lameness may be total or incomplete. Subsequent development of DJD may result in recurrent or intermittent lameness.

DJD is usually characterized as having a slowly progressive, waxing-waning course. Whenever the onset or course of lameness seems somewhat unusual or atypical for DJD, the clinician must consider the possibility that it is caused by some other or concurrent problem. A change in the character of lameness in an animal with confirmed DJD should cause some concern and prompt a careful review of the historical and physical findings.

Many animals with DJD have only one or two affected joints; however, polyarticular DJD has been documented in laboratory colonies of dogs and occurs with some frequency in aged dogs and cats.[77] Many dogs and cats with polyarticular DJD are asymptomatic or exhibit clinical signs referable to one or two joints only. Few systemic manifestations are associated with DJD. These features help the veterinarian distinguish DJD from many of the inflammatory joint disorders in which polyarticular involvement is often apparent and systemic manifestations are commonplace.

The physical abnormalities associated with DJD include muscle atrophy, joint stiffness, and thickening of the periarticular soft tissues. The degree of abnormality is largely determined by the duration of disease. Crepitus may be detected as cartilage destruction advances and osteophytes develop. Crepitus is not a consistent finding; little or no crepitus may be detected in dogs having DJD secondary to hip dysplasia even when remodeling and osteophyte production are severe. Certain maneuvers are more likely to produce crepitus than others; it is easier to produce crepitus in the hip by abduction and rotation than by flexion or extension of the joint. There may be joint effusion in animals with DJD; effusion is usually not a prominent feature of DJD unless recent trauma or injury has occurred to the affected joint.

Animals with DJD resist palpation or manipulation of the affected joint, especially if the examiner attempts to exceed the limit of normal range of motion (see Chapter 1). Hyperextension and hyperflexion of the affected joint are good methods of eliciting a response from animals with DJD. Abduction is a good method of eliciting a response from an animal with hip disease. The response to these maneuvers and to digital pressure is usually mild to moderate; the clinician should consider other causes when the animal is very sensitive to manipulation or is unwilling to bear weight on the limb. Animals with DJD usually stand or walk on the affected limb.

The radiographic findings associated with DJD have been previously alluded to and include collapse of the joint space, sclerosis or remodeling of subchondral bone, subchondral cyst formation, and periarticular osteophyte formation. The value and limitations of radiographic examination in the diagnosis of joint disease are discussed in Chapter 1. The width of the joint (cartilage) space is often difficult to define accurately; width is distorted by the practice of making radiographs while traction is being applied to the limb. In addition, cyst formation is generally not a prominent feature of DJD in dogs and cats. Subchondral remodeling changes, cyst formation, and periarticular osteophytes are slow to develop. Three or 4 weeks must elapse before osteophyte formation becomes evident with rupture of the cranial cruciate ligament. Even in chronic DJD, it is rare to appreciate fully the extent of osteophyte production by radiographic examination alone.

Great care should be exercised whenever the physical, historical, or radiographic findings suggest that something other than DJD exists. Other disorders may occur concurrently with DJD; the radiographic abnormalities associated with DJD may predominate and preclude the proper diagnosis (see Chapter 1, Fig. 1-24).

Treatment. Nonsurgical treatment is beneficial to most patients with lameness caused by DJD. Rest and NSAIDs are used initially; an exercise program is outlined and instituted to help maintain range of motion and muscle mass. Weight reduction is recommended in patients that are obese; dietary management is an important consideration in all patients with DJD. Drug therapy is monitored and adjusted to fit the patient's individual needs. When a favorable response occurs, drug dosages can usually be progressively decreased and sometimes discontinued. Administering NSAIDs on an intermittent or as-needed basis is probably better than everyday administration.

Surgical options should be considered when symptomatic therapy has failed to produce an acceptable response or maintain adequate function. Surgical treatment might be employed when drug therapy has or is likely to produce undesired effects. The veterinarian must be certain that the owner has complied with instructions and that the diagnosis is correct before surgery is performed. The use of an alternative analgesic/antiinflammatory drug might be warranted before surgical treatment is attempted; however, using more than one NSAID at a time or the concurrent use of corticosteroids and NSAIDs is not recommended.

Early surgical treatment is warranted whenever the underlying cause of DJD can be successfully dealt with by surgical means. Weight control, rest, exercise, and drug therapy are used in conjunction with surgical treatment. The indication for one procedure over another depends on the underlying cause, severity, and location of disease. The outcome of surgery should be anticipated; for example, arthrodesis of the carpus tends to allow good function, whereas arthrodesis of the elbow does not.

A short-term clinical benefit seems to be associated with lavage of an affected joint. A possible explanation is that irritants such as cartilage debris and enzymes are removed. In addition, scarification of synovial membrane may alter the inflammatory response and result in some clinical improvement; synovectomy may be beneficial as well. Lavage, scarification, and synovectomy might be used alone or in combination whenever surgical findings suggest the presence of DJD; they might be of value when used in conjunction with stabilization or reconstructive techniques. Removal of periarticular osteophytes is of questionable value unless they are large enough or positioned in such a way that they mechanically interfere with joint motion. They are easily removed with a sharp osteotome or rongeur. The value of such procedures as lavage, synovial scarification, synovectomy, and resection of osteophytes in the surgical management of DJD needs to be investigated by controlled studies in dogs and cats.

The joint should be thoroughly explored any time an arthrotomy is performed, especially if the underlying cause of DJD has not been established. Loose bodies, cartilage flaps, and remnants of disrupted ligaments are generally removed. With rupture of the cranial cruciate ligament, the medial meniscus should be carefully evaluated. All abnormalities should be recorded in the surgical record.

The surgical treatment of joint injuries, growth deformities, and the hip and stifle problems that lead to development of DJD are described elsewhere in this textbook. Early surgical intervention may help diminish the significance of the degenerative changes that are likely to occur in affected animals. So-called salvage procedures, such as excisional arthroplasty, total hip replacement, and arthrodesis, are described in other chapters as well. They are performed when other treatments have been tried and have failed, that is, when pain and clinical dysfunction persist. Salvage procedures are indicated when surgical methods that spare the joint are not possible or not expected to produce an acceptable result. The surgical treatments of a few of the more important clinical conditions that result in DJD are described later.

Osteochondritis Dissecans

Osteochondritis dissecans (OCD) is a relatively common condition that affects young, large breeds of dogs. It is characterized by the development of a cartilaginous flap on the articular surface of various bones. In dogs the most frequently diagnosed site of involvement is the caudomedial aspect of the humeral head. OCD lesions are often found to be bilateral.

The etiology of OCD is unknown. OCD is considered to be one of various manifestations of disturbance in enchondral ossification known as osteochondrosis.[78] At affected sites, the articular cartilage seems thicker than normal; enchondral ossification apparently lags behind cartilage growth. Necrosis occurs in the deepest layers of the articular cartilage, perhaps because of inadequate diffusion of nutrients from the synovial fluid or subchondral vessels. Clefts develop and propagate to form the flap. OCD lesions may develop secondary to overnutrition, that is, excessive caloric intake. Also, trauma and genetic predisposition have been described as possible etiological factors.

Diagnosis. The clinical signs of OCD are first noticed at 5 to 10 months of age. The disorder usually occurs in large breeds of dogs but may develop in medium-sized animals as well (cocker spaniel, Brittany spaniel, etc.). Males are affected more than females.[61] OCD has been reported in a cat.[24]

The onset of clinical signs is usually insidious; however, the owner may be able to associate onset with an episode of trauma or strenuous activity. The lameness associated with OCD tends to be mild to moderate in intensity; lameness is generally persistent, although its intensity may wax and wane. Clinical signs may remain subtle or inapparent, particularly with lesions of the humeral head. Bilateral lesions may be overlooked when one of the lesions is clinically predominate.

OCD lesions are most often found on the humeral head but may also be found on the medial portion of the humeral condyle, the medial or lateral trochlear ridge of the talus, and the lateral condyle of the femur. OCD lesions are occasionally found at other sites as well.[61]

Pain can generally be elicited by full extension and sometimes flexion of the affected joint(s). Atrophy of the supraspinatus and infraspinatus muscles is often detectable in dogs having OCD of the humeral head. Joint swelling or effusion may be detected with lesions within the elbow, stifle, or tarsus. Joint swelling also may be present with lesions of the humeral head but may be more difficult to detect because of surrounding soft tissues. Joint effusion is not usually a prominent or consistent clinical feature of OCD.

Radiographs are useful in diagnosis of OCD. Routine craniocaudal and mediolateral projections are usually sufficient; flexed dorsoplantar and oblique projections of the talocrural joint may facilitate identification of OCD of the talus.[70,110] Radiographs should be made of the opposite joint whenever a diagnosis of OCD has been made or is suspected. This protocol allows detection of bilateral lesions and, when the opposite side is unaffected, provides a comparison that might substantiate the presence of an abnormality on the affected side.

Joint capsular distention or soft tissue swelling may be apparent on radiographic examination of an affected elbow or tarsus; joint distention and soft tissue swelling are more difficult to detect with lesions of the shoulder or stifle. Defect, flattening, irregularity, and sclerosis of subchondral bone are important and consistent radiographic findings (Fig. 21-4). Loss or remodeling of subchondral bone simulates widening of the joint space at the site of the lesion (Fig. 21-4, B). Irregular or sclerotic subchondral bone may occasionally be noted on the opposing bone, so-called kissing lesions. The flap of cartilage can be seen if it becomes mineralized. Mineralized flaps may be seen lying over the subchondral defect; mineralization is more often present in flaps that have broken away from the parent bone and subsequently become attached to the synovial membrane (Fig. 21-4, A). Radiographic signs of DJD are noted in chronic cases.

Treatment. OCD lesions are not always clinically apparent. In addition, clinical signs may spontaneously regress without treatment. The development of clinical signs may be influenced by the depth and size of the lesion. Paradoxically, both rest and exercise have been advocated for dogs with OCD of the humeral head. Rest and NSAID therapy may provide symptomatic relief; however, resting the dog with the hope that the flap will reattach seems, at best, wishful thinking. With OCD of the humeral head, Olsson[78] believes that encouraging exercise might hasten detachment of the flap, thus allowing the flap to move into the caudal cul-de-sac of the joint, in effect, a nonsurgical flap removal.

It would seem prudent to attempt nonsurgical management for 3 to 6 weeks after the onset of clinical signs. Surgical intervention is probably not indicated for treatment of clinically quiescent lesions. Little clinical evidence suggests that leaving a flap in an asymptomatic dog will have serious untoward effects; in fact, few operated dogs having an asymptomatic contralateral lesion ever become symptomatic on the unoperated side.

A bias exists toward surgical intervention as treatment for OCD because many reports concerning treatment are written by veterinary surgeons. The results obtained with surgical treatment of humeral head lesions are good to excellent; with lesions at other sites, they seem to be less favorable or, at least, less predictable.

Surgical exploration with removal of the flap or loose bodies combined with curettage of exposed subchondral bone is the most widely accepted treatment for OCD. Several surgical approaches have been described that facilitate treatment of lesions of the humeral head. Exposure of the lesion is accomplished via infraspinatus tenotomy or one of a number of modifications of the caudolateral approach to the shoulder.[86] Exposure gained by infraspinatus tenotomy is illustrated in Fig. 21-5.

When the chondral flap is found to be partially attached and is complete, the attachment site is incised and the flap removed. The cartilage that remains at the periphery of the defect is carefully inspected; any cartilage that appears separated from or is only loosely attached to subchondral bone is removed using a sharp curette. Experimental work suggests that the cartilaginous rim of the defect should be cut perpendicular to the articular surface, not beveled.[88] The exposed subchondral bone is curetted. Reestablishing blood flow apparently ensures that the defect will fill with fibrocartilage.

A thorough search for fragments of cartilage should be performed whenever the cartilaginous flap is detached or is attached but incomplete. The detached flap or loose fragments may remain hidden from view when they settle in the caudal cul-de-sac of the shoulder joint or become lodged in the intertubercular groove. All loose bodies should be removed.

Activity is restricted for 7 to 10 days after surgery; thereafter, normal activities are allowed. Most dogs that have been treated for humeral head lesions are able to function at a presurgical level within a month and continue to improve. The prognosis for clinical recovery is excellent; DJD is inevitable but rarely becomes symptomatic.

Compared with OCD of the humeral head, the results of surgical treatment of OCD at other sites are apparently not as good or predictable. Joint biomechanics undoubtedly play a role in the outcome. Surgical treatment did not alleviate clinical signs or slow the progression of secondary degenerative change in dogs with OCD of the medial trochlear ridge of the talus.[99] Nevertheless, surgery is probably warranted in the treatment of OCD of the talus or of the humeral or femoral condyle if nonsurgical methods have proved ineffective.

A standard lateral parapatellar approach[86] allows visualization of lesions of the femoral condyle. Exposure of

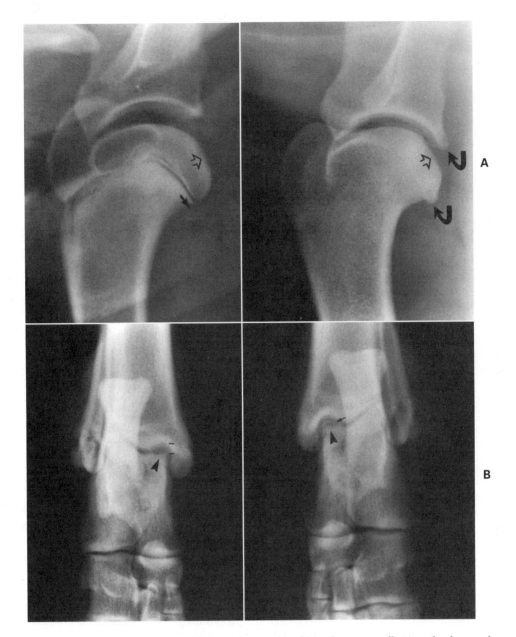

Fig. 21-4   A, Radiographic examples of osteochondritis dissecans affecting the humeral head. There is flattening and irregularity of the subchondral bone of the caudal aspect of both humeral heads (*open arrows*). The bony abnormalities are more pronounced on the right than on the left. On the left, a portion of the cartilage flap is located in the caudal cul-de-sac of the shoulder joint where it has become mineralized (*closed straight arrow*). Periarticular osteophytes are present in the shoulder joint on the right (*curved arrows*). **B**, Radiographic example of bilateral osteochondritis dissecans affecting the medial trochlear ridge of the talus. Soft tissue swelling is evident in both joints, and there is irregularity of the affected subchondral bone (*arrow heads*). On one side (*left*) the medial trochlear ridge appears flattened and the joint space widened (*solid lines*). On the opposite side (*right*) the trochlear ridge is present, but a subchondral fissure is seen at its base (*small arrow*).

lesions within the elbow and tarsal joints may be somewhat more difficult to accomplish. Transection of the medial collateral ligament or osteotomy of the medial epicondyle of the humerus allows entry to the medial portion of the elbow joint.[86] Osteotomy of the medial

malleolus of the tibia[86] or medial or lateral arthrotomy[6,39] has been used to allow inspection of the talus.

Osteotomy of the medial epicondyle of the humerus may be used for exposure of OCD lesions of the medial portion of the condyle and fragmented medial coronoid

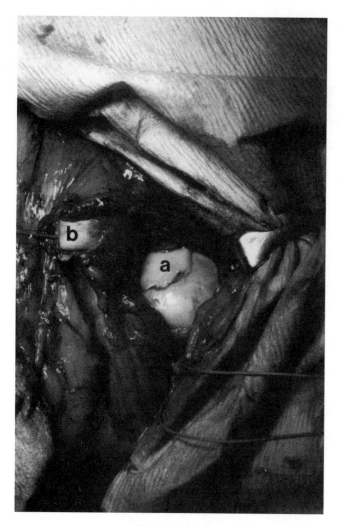

Fig. 21-5 Osteochondritis dissecans of the humeral head. The cartilage flap is located on the caudomedial aspect of the humeral head (*a*). Exposure has been gained by a craniolateral approach via tenotomy of the infraspinatus muscle. The muscle has been retracted caudodorsally while the shoulder has been flexed and internally rotated (*b*).

process of the ulna.[86] Lag screw fixation of the detached bone allows stable closure of the joint. Osteotomy of the medial malleolus of the tibia is usually not necessary for exposure of lesions of the talus. Lesions on the medial trochlear ridge of the talus can usually be visualized by incision of the soft tissues caudal or cranial to the medial malleolus. Likewise, incisions caudal or cranial to the lateral malleolus are used to expose lesions of the lateral trochlear ridge.[6,39] Flexion or extension of the joint may be needed to bring the lesion into view. Osteotomy of the medial malleolus does allow good visualization of the talus; however, it is more laborious and has a relatively high rate of complication when compared with the previously mentioned methods.

With or without surgery, the radiographic signs of DJD usually become quite evident in dogs having OCD of the elbow, stifle, or tarsus. As such, clients should be forewarned of the limitations of surgical treatment and consoled by the fact that the intensity of the lameness is not always in agreement with the severity of radiographic change. Symptomatic therapy, as described earlier, is helpful in the long-term management of these animals.

Ununited Anconeal Process

Ununited anconeal process (UAP) is a relatively uncommon condition that affects young growing dogs. It is characterized by separation of the anconeal process from the remainder of the ulna (chondrodystrophoid dogs) or by failure of the anconeal center of ossification to unite with the parent bone (nonchondrodystrophoid dogs).[62,85] Secondary remodeling changes are progressive and severe. The associated lameness is usually mild to moderate; it may be severe following injury or strenuous activity.

The etiology of UAP is not completely understood. It may be one of the many manifestations of a disturbance of enchondral ossification known as osteochondrosis.[78] OCD or fragmented coronoid process may be found in affected elbows. UAP has been diagnosed in German shepherd and certain other large breeds of dogs in whom the anconeal process may develop from a separate center of ossification.[62,85] Elbow incongruity may play a role in the development of UAP. UAP is practically unheard of in greyhounds, even though they tend to have a separate center of ossification;[109] elbow incongruity is not usually seen in this breed.[85] Excessive forces may be generated, which might disrupt an abnormal or incomplete union between the anconeal process and the remainder of the ulna. Asynchronous growth of the radius and ulna, that is, slowed ulnar growth, may produce an upward force on the anconeal process and cause a fracture. This has been reported to occur in large chondrodystrophoid dogs such as the basset hound and English bulldog.[85] The use of the term *ununited* can be disputed in such cases.

Diagnosis. UAP is usually diagnosed between 5 and 18 months of age; occasionally, clinical signs do not become evident until the dog is older, when degenerative joint changes are more severe. Large breeds of dogs are most often affected, especially the German shepherd. UAP occurs in chondrodystrophic breeds such as basset hounds and bulldogs as well (see previous discussion). Males may be affected more often than females.[98]

The onset of lameness is usually insidious. The intensity of the lameness is mild to moderate; it tends to wax and wane. On close observation, affected dogs rarely have full function of the affected limb, although most dogs function remarkably well despite evidence of substantial DJD. Bilateral involvement has been reported.

Chronically affected dogs may experience an acute onset of lameness after strenuous activity or trauma. The owner may not have noted any previous lameness; however, it is obvious from physical and radiographic examinations that the anconeal process has been detached for a long time.

Diagnosis of UAP is straightforward; soft tissue swelling, bony crepitus, and stiffness are found on examination of the affected elbow. Early remodeling changes are generally more pronounced with UAP than with other elbow problems, such as OCD of the humeral condyle or fragmented medial coronoid process. The abnormal anconeal process is readily identified when the joint is radiographed.

Radiographs reveal a cleavage line between the anconeal process and the remainder of the ulna (Fig. 21-6). The mediolateral projection is most useful, particularly if the elbow has been held in a flexed position as the film is exposed. The abnormal anconeal process may be located near its normal position or displaced cranially or dorsally; dorsal displacement may occur after a traumatic event.[69]

The diagnosis can be relatively certain if the anconeal process is unattached and in an abnormal position. The radiographic findings need to be carefully considered in animals having a separate center of ossification. Fusion may not occur until 20 weeks of age in the German shepherd dog.[62,85] In this breed, if the anconeal process appears nondisplaced, it is probably best to wait until the dog is 5 months old before making a diagnosis of UAP.

Treatment. Symptomatic therapy, as outlined earlier in this chapter, is useful in most dogs with UAP. In addition, positive effects are associated with arthrotomy and removal of the abnormal process; partial resolution of lameness is common, even in dogs with associated DJD.

A lateral approach to the elbow allows sufficient visualization of the anconeal process.[86] Flexing the elbow facilitates visualization. The anconeal process is usually found to be attached to the ulna or, in some cases, to the olecranon fossa of the humerus by fibrous connective tissue. An Adson periosteal elevator or ¼-inch osteotome is wedged between the anconeal process and adjacent bone and used as a lever to pry the process loose and lift it from the joint cavity. The surgery is not difficult; there is minimal aftercare or exercise restriction.

Surgical removal of UAP is not always indicated. Clinical disability is probably related to the presence of a loose body and the joint instability/DJD that accompany it. Although removal of the abnormal anconeal process is said to slow the progression of DJD,[98] the radiographic changes of DJD become quite severe whether surgery is performed or not. In the symptomatic patient,

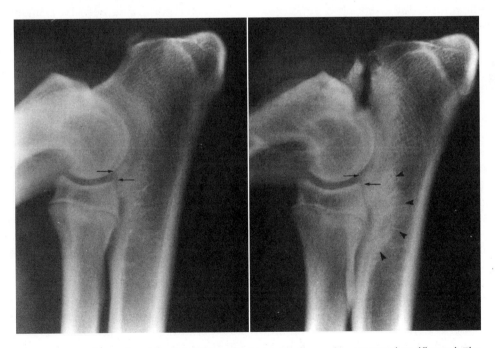

Fig. 21-6   Radiographs of the left (*left*) and right (*right*) elbow of a young Irish wolfhound. The right anconeal process is deformed, and a cleavage plane is present between the process and the remaining ulna. Also, bony sclerosis is located caudal and distal to the trochlear notch of the right ulna, and apparent narrowing of the adjacent medullary cavity (*arrowheads*) is present; these changes suggest a fragmented coronoid process. There appears to be an incongruency at the radioulnar articulation (*arrows*) in both joints.

removal of the anconeal process eliminates one of the factors that might be causing pain. In the asymptomatic or mildly affected patient, the significance of the loose body should be carefully considered. Surgical removal of the anconeal process should be reserved for use in dogs that have obvious disability or those that fail to respond to nonsurgical treatment.

Open reduction and internal fixation of the abnormal anconeal process have been successful in a few cases.[46,62] This method of treatment has been recommended in early cases when the process appears to be well formed and is minimally displaced and when minimal remodeling changes are evident. A successful fixation leads to union of the anconeal process and apparently reestablishes joint stability, thereby minimizing or preventing secondary DJD. Unfortunately, in many dogs the process is deformed and has undergone fibrous replacement by the time the diagnosis is made. Fibrous replacement, changes in shape, and the small size of the process interfere with reduction and fixation. Repair under these circumstances can be likened to inadequate fixation of a fibrous nonunion in a dynamic environment (joint); failure of the repair is likely in this situation.

Fragmented Coronoid Process

Fragmented medial coronoid process (FCP) affects large breeds of dogs. The clinical and radiographic findings associated with the disorder are often subtle or nonspecific; neither the fissure nor the detached medial coronoid process is usually seen on radiographs of the affected joint. Clinical signs may develop as early as 5 to 6 months of age; some dogs remain asymptomatic or become lame later in life as DJD progresses. Bilateral involvement is common.

As with OCD and UAP, FCP may be a clinical manifestation of osteochondrosis.[78] FCP may develop as the result of excessive loading of the medial coronoid process. Many dogs with FCP have elbow incongruity; an association with elbow dysplasia has been identified in Bernese mountain dogs.[108] FCP may result from trauma. A genetic predisposition has been implied.[85]

Diagnosis. Lameness usually begins between 5 and 9 months of age. The disorder occurs most frequently in large dogs such as the Rottweiler, Labrador retriever, Bernese mountain dog, and Newfoundland.

The onset of clinical signs is usually insidious. Most affected dogs experience lameness that is subtle or mild and waxes and wanes in intensity. As a result, lameness is not always observed at the time of physical examination; the owner or veterinarian may not be able to localize the lameness, especially if both elbows are affected.

Careful physical examination is especially important in the diagnosis of FCP, not because physical findings are obvious or diagnostic, but because historical and physi-

cal findings are often nonspecific and subtle. Physical abnormalities are especially difficult to detect in early cases. Early diagnosis of FCP is often made by the process of exclusion; careful physical examination is necessary to rule out other causes of lameness as well as to detect abnormalities associated with FCP.

Many dogs have no apparent abnormality except subtle resistance to palpation of the elbow. Direct pressure applied over the medial coronoid process and pronation and supination with the elbow in flexion are useful in eliciting a response (see Chapter 1). Comparing the response to that obtained from the opposite elbow may be helpful. Joint effusion and crepitus may be detected; effusion and crepitus are inconsistently present in affected elbows.

Definitive radiographic diagnosis of FCP is rare. The fragmented portion of the coronoid process is rarely displaced and cannot usually be seen; the fissure is almost impossible to detect even when multiple radiographic projections are made. Ossicles and mineralization located in the joint capsule or of periarticular soft tissues should not be confused with FCP (Fig. 21-7). Likewise, a small sesamoid bone may be located just cranial to the radial head in some large breeds of dogs. Incongruency of the radioulnar joint may be seen, and as time goes by, sclerosis of the subchondral bone of the trochlear notch of the ulna becomes evident. Subchondral sclerosis may be subtle; the opposite elbow should be radiographed for comparison and, because bilateral involvement is common, to assess the status of the opposite elbow (Fig. 21-8).

In chronic cases, there is periarticular osteophyte formation proximal to the anconeal process on the cranial surface of the olecranon and along the medial portion of the humeral condyle. As time passes, remodeling changes associated with DJD become more pronounced; they may obscure the underlying cause.

FCP is probably the most frequent developmental disease of the canine elbow.[108] One author[12] found most dogs with FCP also had OCD of the medial portion of the humeral condyle; this has not been substantiated by others.[41,66] Few dogs with FCP have cartilaginous flaps or full-thickness defects typical of OCD; however, cartilage erosions on the medial humeral condyle and trochlear notch of the ulna are common. Perhaps these represent so-called kissing lesions.

Treatment. Surgical exploration of the elbow is warranted in dogs thought to have FCP if other causes of lameness have been ruled out and symptomatic therapy has failed, that is, if clinical signs are persistent or recurrent. The surgical approaches are similar to those described for visualization of lesions of the medial portion of the humeral condyle (see Osteochondritis Dissecans). The cleavage plane between the fragment and parent bone is not always complete or readily identifiable; only a

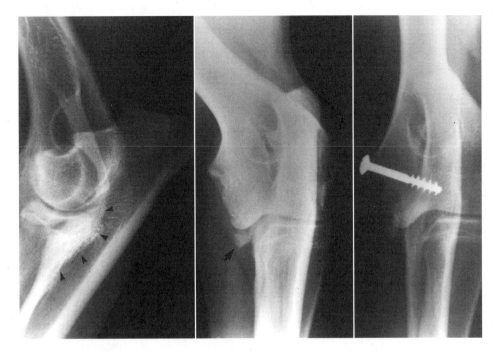

Fig. 21-7   Mediolateral (*left*) and craniocaudal (*center*) radiographs of the elbow of a dog having fragmented medial coronoid process of the ulna. Sclerosis of the bone is located caudal and distal to the trochlear notch of the ulna (*left, arrowheads*), and a radiopaque mass is located on the medial aspect of the joint (*center, arrow*). Craniocaudal radiograph of the same joint (*right*) immediately after humeral epicondylar osteotomy and removal of the detached portion of the coronoid process. The osteotomized portion of bone has been reattached using a screw. Notice that the radiopaque mass is still present. Ossicles and mineralization located in the periarticular soft tissues should not be confused with the fragmented coronoid process. The detached portion of the coronoid process is usually minimally displaced and is only rarely identified on radiographic examination of the affected joint.

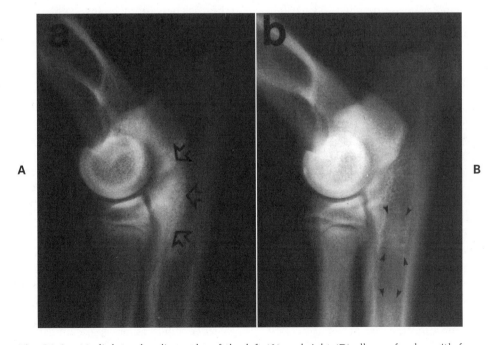

Fig. 21-8   Mediolateral radiographs of the left (**A**) and right (**B**) elbow of a dog with fragmented medial coronoid process of the left ulna. Notice the sclerosis located in the bone caudal and distal to the trochlear notch of the left ulna (*open arrows*). In addition, changes within the medullary canal of the right ulna suggest panosteitis (*arrowheads*).

slight alteration in the articular surface may be apparent. Alternate pronation and supination of the antebrachium help one to appreciate the radioulnar relationship and may help identify the fissure. An Adson periosteal elevator or ¼-inch osteotome can be wedged between the process and parent bone to dislodge the fragment and lift it from the joint cavity. The joint should be inspected before the capsule is closed; any cartilaginous flaps or loose bodies are removed. Rest is enforced for 3 to 5 weeks depending on the surgical approach and security of closure.

Unfortunately, the response to surgical treatment is not consistently good or predictable. Lameness subsides, at least temporarily, in some dogs, whereas in others it is unabated. Even when performed early, removal of the coronoid process does not prevent the development of DJD. The coronoid process and the attached annular ligament apparently impart some stability to the joint; persistent instability and incongruity contribute to the progression of DJD.

Other Noninflammatory Joint Disorders

Numerous other noninflammatory joint disorders occur in dogs and cats (see Box 21-2). Some, such as carpal instability syndrome of young dogs, are relatively common but remain poorly understood. Others, such as mucopolysaccharidosis, are quite rare. Selected references on these and other noninflammatory joint disorders are cited in Box 21-2. Traumatic joint disease has been described in Chapters 5, 8, 9, and 16. Disorders of the hip and stifle are detailed in Chapters 17 and 18, respectively. Neoplastic disease is described in Chapter 19.

INFLAMMATORY JOINT DISORDERS

Many inflammatory joint disorders occur in dogs and cats. The inflammatory disorders have been subdivided into two groups (see Box 21-2). Joint disease caused by bacteria, mycoplasma, L forms, rickettsia, spirochetes, fungi, and virus particles are classified as infectious. Idiopathic nondeforming arthritis, systemic lupus erythematosus (SLE), rheumatoid arthritis, feline progressive polyarthritis, and others are classified as noninfectious. The noninfectious diseases are further subdivided into the deforming or erosive disorders (e.g., rheumatoid arthritis) and the nondeforming or nonerosive disorders (e.g., SLE). Most of the noninfectious inflammatory joint disorders are considered to have an immune-mediated etiology. This method of classification provides an insight to the treatment and the prognosis associated with the various inflammatory disorders; the most clinically important of these are described here.

General Considerations

It is usually possible to differentiate inflammatory from noninflammatory joint disease on the basis of historical, physical, and joint fluid examinations (see Chapter 1). Multiple joint involvement and systemic signs or illness are more common with inflammatory than noninflammatory joint disease. Discrete lameness may not be present in animals with polyarticular involvement. Instead, these animals appear stiff; they have a stilted gait and seem reluctant to walk. Clinical signs of inflammatory joint disease are often abrupt in onset; inflammatory disorders are more fulminating than noninflammatory ones. Joint effusion is more likely with inflammatory than noninflammatory disease.

The complex nature of immune-mediated disease and the potentially catastrophic effects of infection pose many diagnostic and therapeutic challenges. Unfortunately, differentiating infectious from noninfectious or immune-mediated inflammatory joint disease is not always straightforward. Since the process of inflammation is central to the pathogenesis of both, the clinical features of infectious and immune-mediated disease can be quite similar. Animals in both groups may have fever and be anorectic and lethargic or have other systemic signs.

Fortunately, some clinical differences exist between infectious and immune-mediated joint disease. Infectious polyarticular arthritis is rare in all but the very young. Immune-mediated joint disease is much more prevalent than infectious arthritis in mature dogs and cats. Infectious arthritis in mature animals tends to be monoarticular, whereas polyarticular involvement is common with immune-mediated disease. Animals having polyarticular arthritis associated with septicemia are often febrile and quite ill. In comparison, animals with immune-mediated polyarticular joint disease do not generally appear as ill (per degree of fever) as the septicemic animal. Lameness associated with infection of a single joint is usually severe; the joint is quite painful. The lameness associated with multiple joint involvement is generally less discrete.

Although joint fluid analysis is probably the only definitive method of differentiating infectious from immune-mediated inflammatory joint disease, such analysis has limitations. The predominant cell type in both disorders is the neutrophil. Although huge numbers of white blood cells (WBCs) are usually present in the joint fluid of animals with bacterial arthritis, WBC counts greater than 50,000/μl^3 may occur with idiopathic nonerosive arthritis and SLE. Although toxic or degenerative changes in neutrophils suggest the presence of infection, some bacterial infections do not cause such changes.[85] Negative cultures do not eliminate the possibility of infection; positive cultures are not consistently obtained even when the joint has been inoculated with bacteria.[72]

Routine culturing techniques cannot be expected to allow detection of mycotic, mycoplasmal, rickettsial, or spirochete infections.

It is difficult for the veterinarian to differentiate between infectious and immune-mediated arthritis when joint fluid analysis is equivocal. Few other laboratory tests are specific (see Chapter 1). Peripheral WBC counts should be interpreted carefully. Although infection tends to cause the greatest elevation of WBC numbers, increased peripheral WBC counts have been associated with immune-mediated disorders as well. Most dogs with monoarticular infectious arthritis have little or no elevation in WBC numbers. Radiographic examination is of little help in early diagnosis of inflammatory joint disease because changes are nonspecific (see Chapter 1).

When doubt exists as to the etiology of polyarticular inflammatory joint disease, it seems prudent to first treat the disease as if infection is the cause. This approach is even more reasonable if an animal is being treated in an area where *Borrelia burgdorferi* or rickettsial diseases such as Rocky Mountain spotted fever and ehrlichiosis are considered endemic. At worst, the animal having immune-mediated disease does not respond, and immunosuppressive/cytotoxic therapy is delayed for 3 to 5 days. To err on the side of immune-mediated disease could have more serious consequences.

Bacterial Arthritis

Bacterial arthritis occurs relatively infrequently in dogs and cats. It is reported to develop most often in young dogs, especially large breeds of dogs. Monoarticular involvement is much more common than polyarticular infection (septicemia) in all but young pups and kittens. The large or spacious joints such as the hip, shoulder, stifle, and elbow are most frequently affected. Penetrating injury, surgery, debilitation, immunosuppression, and preexisting joint disease (e.g., DJD) are predisposing factors. Although infectious arthritis of bacterial etiology is relatively rare, the potential consequences of infection make it clinically important. Acute septic arthritis must be treated without delay if joint structure and function are to be preserved (Fig. 21-9).

Various bacteria have been isolated in cases of bacterial arthritis; staphylococci, streptococci, and coliforms are the most common.[16, 85] Infection may follow penetrating joint injury or surgery; hematogenous delivery of bacteria to the synovial membrane may occur in animals that have infection at another site. Although the source of bacteria frequently remains an enigma, hematogenous spread has been associated with umbilical infections and septicemias in pups and kittens and with bacterial endocarditis and severe periodontal disease in older animals. Only rarely does bacterial arthritis develop by spread

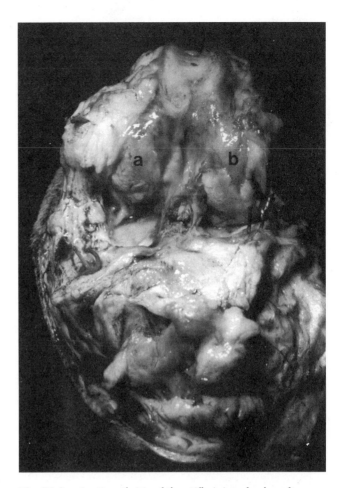

Fig. 21-9   Septic arthritis of the stifle joint of a dog after surgical intervention for multiple ligamentous injury. There is severe erosion of cartilage on the medial (*a*) and lateral (*b*) condyles of the femur; the articular surfaces are covered with fibrinous material. Recovery of satisfactory joint function is unlikely.

from adjacent osteomyelitis or soft tissue abscess. Apparently the joint capsule is an effective barrier against this type of spread. Few clinical cases of diaphyseal osteomyelitis breech an intact joint capsule and result in septic joint disease.

Diagnosis. Bacterial arthritis is usually monoarticular and results in an acute onset of lameness or reluctance to use the affected extremity. The degree of clinical dysfunction is usually severe. Infected joints are often swollen and warm and appear painful when touched or manipulated. There may be a history of previous joint trauma or preexisting joint disease. Bacterial arthritis of mature dogs frequently develops where DJD is present; there is usually a sudden increase in the intensity of lameness or a change in the character of lameness when this occurs (Fig. 21-10). Weakening of supporting soft

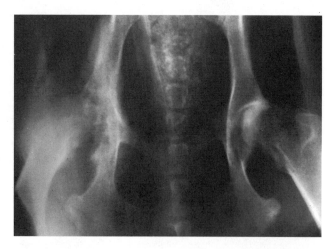

Fig. 21-10 Streptococcal arthritis and osteomyelitis of the right hip of a dog. There is extensive periosteal new bone formation along the right ilial body and the medial aspect of the right acetabulum and ischium. The subchondral margins of the right acetabulum and femoral head are irregular and difficult to identify. This dog had an acute onset of severe rear limb lameness 6 weeks before this radiograph was made. The presence of preexisting degenerative joint disease undoubtedly delayed the diagnosis of infection; in addition, it may have been a predisposing factor.

tissue structures may be associated with bacterial arthritis; rupture of the cranial cruciate ligament has been associated with infection of the stifle joint.

Dogs and cats with bacterial arthritis and septicemia appear systemically ill; they are usually febrile and have other abnormalities that suggest a septicemic state. Septicemia with polyarticular involvement is rare; it is most common in very young and sometimes in aged or debilitated animals.

Physical examination should be complete and should include a search for the underlying cause. The skin overlying the joint should be carefully examined for evidence of disruption. Ancillary diagnostic procedures such as urinalysis, microbiological examination of urine and blood, radiographs of the chest and abdomen, and hematological and biochemical testing may be indicated. The patient's status and the owner's needs and wishes determine which tests are appropriate. The limitations of a specific test should be understood; for example, blood cultures have a relatively low yield and high cost.

The early radiographic findings associated with bacterial arthritis are nonspecific. The most consistent abnormality is soft tissue swelling (see Chapter 1, Fig. 1-23). Some bacteria cause rapid destruction of articular cartilage with subsequent collapse of the joint (cartilage) space; others cause relatively little cartilage destruction.[85] Periarticular new bone formation and lysis of subchondral bone may take 2 to 3 weeks to become apparent. Early radiographic diagnosis is especially difficult when there is preexisting joint disease. Remodeling

changes associated with DJD may obscure the radiographic changes associated with infection (Fig. 21-10).

Early diagnosis of septic arthritis is essential. Since hematological, serum biochemical, and radiographic abnormalities are often nonspecific, joint fluid analysis should be performed any time the historical and physical findings suggest that infection might be present. Cytological and microbiological evaluations of synovial fluid help confirm that an infection exists and determine the etiological agent. The limitations of joint fluid analysis in diagnosis of infectious arthritis have been described (see General Considerations).

Treatment. Treatment of septic arthritis is focused on early detection, evacuation of the affected joint, and administration of antimicrobial drugs. Heroic measures are often necessary to preserve life and joint function in young and aged animals having concurrent septicemia and multiple joint involvement. The underlying cause should be sought and, when possible, treated. Fluid deficits and acid-base imbalances should be corrected. Fever and pain are treated by use of analgesic-antipyretic drugs (NSAIDs). Affected joints are evacuated and broad-spectrum bacteriocidal antimicrobial drugs administered. In pups, kittens, and older animals with multiple joint involvement, the joint capsules can be lanced and be left open to allow drainage. Unfortunately, many animals with septicemia and polyarticular infection die or continue to do poorly despite such measures. Postmortem examination of affected animals often reveals the presence of pneumonia, hepatic abscess, pyelonephritis, or other organ involvement.

Treatment of monoarticular bacterial arthritis is usually more successful. Again, the underlying cause should be sought and, if possible, treated. Considerable relief of pain can be derived from decompression of the distended joint capsule. Evacuation of joint fluid that contains bacteria, enzymes, and other substances potentially injurious to articular cartilage and intraarticular soft tissues is facilitated by repetitive lavage with sterile isotonic saline or lactated Ringer's solution. Joint lavage can be accomplished via surgical arthrotomy or closed irrigation through large-bore needles. Unfortunately, practical considerations limit the usefulness of both evacuation and lavage methods; these are most apparent when multiple joints are infected or when the fluid is inspissated or contains fibrin clots.

Drip irrigation of the joint cavity via a large-bore needle is not an effective method of lavage. Flow patterns are quickly established, which preclude complete evacuation. Alternate distention-irrigation appears to be a better method of evacuating joint contents.[50] The joint is filled with sterile isotonic fluid until the capsule is distended; the fluid is removed and the process repeated four or five times once or twice daily.

Surgical arthrotomy allows the most complete evacuation of joint contents. This method is indicated and practical when monoarticular infection exists. A drain tube may be inserted at surgery to allow continued drainage and lavage of the joint. The drain tube should be carefully maintained to prevent retrograde contamination of the joint.

Surgery allows removal of necrotic soft tissues and bone, foreign bodies, and suture materials or orthopedic implants that might have been used in the treatment of other disorders. Femoral head and neck excisional arthroplasty has been beneficial in resolving septic arthritis of the hip in animals with preexisting DJD.[91] Surgical intervention allows culture and histopathological examinations of soft tissues and bone, which is important when the cause remains in doubt. Inflammatory joint disease should be considered whenever a synovial membrane that is especially thick or hyperemic is encountered. Typically, only infection and the erosive forms of noninfectious inflammatory joint disease cause diffuse pitting/erosion of cartilage and subchondral bone (Fig. 21-11).

Antimicrobial therapy should be started immediately after fluid or tissue samples have been collected from the dog or cat suspected of having bacterial arthritis. Efficacy against staphylococci, streptococci, and coliforms is important. The use of synergists or more than one antibiotic to enhance efficacy or to broaden the antimicrobial spectrum of therapy is often warranted. Definitive antimicrobial therapy depends on clinical response and results of culture and sensitivity testing. The blood synovial fluid barrier is ineffective when the synovium is inflamed; adequate intraarticular concentrations of antibiotic will be attained if appropriate blood levels are achieved. Intraarticular administration of antibiotics does not appear to be necessary,[28,74,90] and some preparations may even contribute to the inflammatory response.

Rickettsial- and Spirochete-Associated Arthritis

Many of the clinical, diagnostic, and therapeutic features of joint disease associated with exposure to *Rickettsia rickettsii* (Rocky Mountain spotted fever), *Ehrlichia canis* (ehrlichiosis), and *Borrelia burgdorferi* (Lyme disease) are similar; these diseases are described together.

Diagnosis. Each of these organisms, whether directly or indirectly, is apparently able to cause a diverse group of clinical signs, many of which are nonspecific and vague.[103] Joint pain (lameness) has been associated with each; however, lameness is much more prevalent with borreliosis than with rickettsial infection. Clinical studies suggest that lameness associated with *B. burgdorferi*

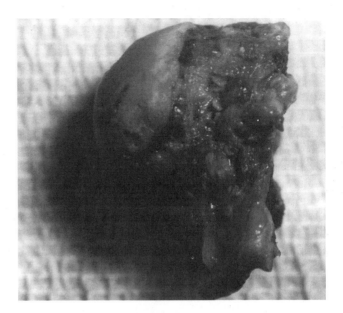

Fig. 21-11 Excised femoral head and neck taken from a dog with septic arthritis and osteomyelitis of the hip. Diffuse pitting and deep erosions involve the articular cartilage and subchondral bone of the femoral head. The bone of the adjacent femoral neck is pitted as well, and the soft tissues are thickened and discolored. Deep, discrete erosion of the articular surface is much more likely to develop with inflammatory than noninflammatory joint disease.

is usually acute in onset, is generally transient and episodic, and involves only one or a few joints.[58]

Clinical cases are most frequently diagnosed in areas considered to be endemic for the particular disease; each organism has a specific tick vector.[103] Habitat and the presence of ticks provide clues that facilitate the diagnosis of these diseases. Radiographic abnormalities are nonspecific, and although joint fluid analysis supports the diagnosis of inflammatory joint disease, the organisms are almost never identified. Thus, diagnosis of these diseases is almost always based on presumptive evidence of infection: clinical signs, knowledge of habitat, serology, exclusion of other possible causes, and response to therapy.

Laboratory confirmation of these diseases is best accomplished by indirect fluorescent antibody testing. Antibodies to *R. rickettsii* and *E. canis* become detectable 2 to 3 weeks after infection.[103] Paired samples, used to detect rising titer, are collected 2 to 4 weeks apart. The first sample is stored frozen until the second sample is collected. Both serums should be submitted and tested at the same time.[103] With Rocky Mountain spotted fever, titers less than 1:64 are considered negative; recently infected dogs usually have titers greater than 1:128.[103] Titers of 1:10 or greater are considered positive for *E. canis*.[103] The use and limitations of indirect immunofluorescent testing for confirmation of infection with *B. burgdorferi* are described in Chapter 1.

Treatment. Tetracycline, 22 mg/kg every 8 hours (10 mg/lb every 8 hours) for 14 to 21 days, has been recommended in the treatment of Rocky Mountain spotted fever, ehrlichiosis, and borreliosis. Choramphenicol, doxycycline, and other drugs have been used as well.[103] The response in acute infections is usually favorable.

Since joint disease caused by rickettsial organisms and *B. burgdorferi* can be difficult to differentiate from certain immune-mediated disorders, treating all cases of apparently sterile inflammatory arthritis in animals from endemic areas with tetracycline can be justified. If such therapy fails, immunosuppressive/cytotoxic therapy could be initiated with some confidence.[85]

Other Causes of Infectious Arthritis

Joint infections have been caused by bacterial L forms, *Mycoplasma* species, fungal organisms, and viruses. Such infections are apparently rare because few clinical cases have been reported in the veterinary literature. However, these disorders are difficult to document because the causative agents are difficult to culture or otherwise identify.

Systemic signs are often associated with these infections. Viral infections may indirectly cause arthralgia via immunostimulation and subsequent deposition of immune complexes in the joint(s). Sterile inflammatory joint disease has been observed after administration of modified live vaccines. The clinical signs are usually transient and spontaneously regress, but treatment with an immunosuppressive or cytotoxic agent may be necessary. Selected references on viral and other infectious agents are cited in Box 21-2.

Idiopathic Nondeforming Arthritis

Idiopathic nondeforming arthritis is the most common form of inflammatory joint disease, accounting for at least 50% to 60% of clinical cases.[9,82] Although the exact cause is unknown, failure to isolate microorganisms from joint fluid, failure to obtain a response with antibiotic therapy, and resolution of clinical signs after administration of immunosuppressive agents suggest an immune-mediated etiology. Although arthritis may be the sole clinical manifestation of this disorder, a similar type of nondeforming arthritis has been seen in conjunction with infection at a distant site, GI disease, and neoplastic processes. Bennett[9] has described these as idiopathic nondeforming arthritis types I to IV, respectively, whereas Pedersen and others[82,85] classify these as separate entities, that is, idiopathic nondeforming arthritis, enteropathic arthritis, and nondeforming arthritis associated with chronic infection or neoplasia. Whether all these disorders should be considered idiopathic is debatable; it certainly causes confusion. Unfortunately, the causal relationship between distant infection, GI disease, or neoplasia and development of inflammatory joint disease is not known; immune-mediated processes have been implicated.

Diagnosis. Idiopathic nondeforming arthritis most often develops in large breeds of adult dogs, such as German shepherds, Doberman pinschers, setters, retrievers, and pointers.[9,85] Approximately one half of affected dogs in one study were between 1 and 3½ years of age, and 60% of affected dogs were male.[9] The disorder occurs in small dogs as well; it is only rarely diagnosed in cats.[85]

Idiopathic nondeforming arthritis is usually associated with an acute onset of lameness or reluctance to walk. Single or multiple joints may be affected; polyarticular arthritis is most common. Animals with polyarthritis have a stiff or stilted gait, and some are reluctant to rise or walk. Physical examination often reveals that multiple joints are affected even though lameness has been observed in only one limb. Anorexia, lethargy, and fever often accompany the lameness. A waxing-waning or cyclical course is common.

Affected joints are swollen (effusion) and painful and may be warm to the touch; the degree of swelling varies and can fluctuate from day to day. Mild to moderate enlargement of peripheral lymph nodes is a common physical finding. Atrophy of muscles, especially the muscles of mastication, occurs in chronic cases.[85] Arthritis is the major and often sole manifestation of idiopathic nondeforming arthritis, as described by Pedersen and others,[85] or type I arthritis described by Bennett.[9] If one chooses to accept the classification scheme described by Bennett,[9] numerous other abnormalities have been found in dogs with this form of nondeforming arthritis (types II to IV). The possibility of local or remote infections should always be considered in animals with inflammatory joint disease. The importance of complete physical and historical examinations cannot be overemphasized.

The lack of certain clinical criteria and specific radiographic or laboratory abnormalities helps differentiate idiopathic nondeforming arthritis from other inflammatory joint disorders (e.g., SLE, rheumatoid arthritis). Radiographic abnormalities associated with idiopathic nondeforming joint disease are nonspecific. Soft tissue swelling is a consistent finding. Mild subchondral erosion and periarticular new bone formation may be seen in some dogs. The nonprogressive nature of the radiographic abnormalities helps the clinician differentiate idiopathic nondeforming arthritis from rheumatoid or rheumatoid-like arthritis.

Mild to moderate anemia, mild thrombocytopenia, and leukocytosis may be found in affected animals. Leukopenia is found less often. Likewise, serum alkaline phosphatase and liver enzymes may be elevated. In one study,[9] severe proteinuria was documented in about 30% of affected dogs. Serological abnormalities such as LE cell phenomenon, antinuclear antibody, and rheumatoid factor are insignificant or absent.[9,85] Joint fluid analysis suggests sterile inflammatory joint disease. WBC numbers are generally high, sometimes exceeding 100,000/μl[3], and neutrophils predominate. Bacteria are not seen on microscopic examination and are not cultured from the joint fluid.

Diagnosis of idiopathic nondeforming arthritis is made by a process of exclusion. The diagnosis is justified when the criteria for other forms of sterile inflammatory joint disease (e.g., SLE, rheumatoid arthritis) cannot be met. Whether arthritis associated with chronic infection, GI disease, and neoplasia should be included in this category is debatable; development and adoption of a standard classification scheme would help alleviate some of the confusion that currently exists.

Treatment. Treatment of idiopathic nondeforming arthritis generally includes the use of corticosteroids, sometimes in combination with cytotoxic agents (see Treatment of Noninfectious Inflammatory Joint Disease). In addition, potential causative factors should be sought and, if possible, eliminated or treated. Antibiotic and/or surgical therapy is indicated if there is a coexisting infection such as pyometra (type II disease). Use of immunosuppressive therapy must be carefully considered in such patients.

Response to steroid therapy is usually quick and dramatic. Short-term remission of lameness and joint swelling are quite common; long-term remission is less likely to be achieved. It appears that only 30% to 40% of dogs with uncomplicated idiopathic (type I) arthritis recover completely; the remainder experience residual stiffness and recurrences, require continuous drug therapy, or, for various reasons, are euthanized.[9,85] The prognosis is apparently similar with nondeforming arthritis associated with chronic infection or so-called type II idiopathic arthritis. Animals having arthritis associated with GI disease (type III idiopathic arthritis) generally recover. Short survival times are associated with the nondeforming arthritis associated with cancer (type IV idiopathic arthritis).[9]

Nondeforming Arthritis Associated with Chronic Infection or Neoplasia

See Idiopathic Nondeforming Arthritis.

Enteropathic Arthritis

See Idiopathic Nondeforming Arthritis.

Drug-Induced Nondeforming Arthritis

Drug-induced arthropathies have been documented in dogs and cats but are apparently rare. The development of lameness or joint swelling after administration of a drug should alert the clinician to the possibility of a drug-induced arthritis. Antibiotic drugs are the most frequent offenders. Since these are basically hypersensitivity reactions, the lameness is often accompanied by other clinical signs.[85]

Diagnosis and treatment. Drug-induced arthritis has been described in Doberman pinschers and other dogs after trimethoprim-sulfa administration.[36,85] The onset of clinical signs is often delayed. Multiple joints are usually affected; the arthritis may be accompanied by fever, myalgia/myositis, skin rashes, anemia, leukopenia, thrombocytopenia, and other abnormalities.[36] Pedersen and others[85] have observed similar signs in dogs receiving antibiotics for primary or secondary pyoderma. Although the initial skin disorder seemed to resolve, clinical signs began to recur 1 to 2 weeks later. Antibiotic therapy was continued when, in fact, the antibiotic was responsible for the recurrence of skin lesions and the development of lameness.

Thorough historical and physical examinations usually uncover clues that support the diagnosis of drug-induced arthritis. The drugs should be discontinued whenever such reactions occur; corticosteroid therapy is useful. Resolution of clinical signs after drug withdrawal helps confirm the diagnosis.

Systemic Lupus Erythematosus

SLE is a polysystemic disorder that affects dogs and, less often cats. Although canine SLE was originally described as a disease characterized by glomerulonephritis, hemolytic anemia, and thrombocytopenia, numerous other clinical signs and laboratory abnormalities have been associated with the disease.[85] A nondeforming inflammatory arthritis has been associated with SLE; in fact, arthritis appears to be the most common clinical manifestation of the disorder.[40,94] Although it is a relatively uncommon cause of lameness in dogs and cats, the systemic nature of SLE poses diagnostic and therapeutic challenges and has serious prognostic implications. Diagnosis and treatment of SLE are an expensive proposition; many systems need to be evaluated and the patient's status intermittently monitored. Complete or long-term remission is rarely achieved with the drug protocols currently in use.

The cause of SLE is unknown; genetic, environmental, infectious, hormonal, and drug-induced causes have been implicated. A myriad of autoantibodies, including antinuclear antibodies, have been identified in the sera of patients with the disease (see Chapter 1). Immune complexes appear to be primary mediators of tissue injury in SLE; sequestration of antibody-antigen complexes with activation of complement in the capillary beds of the skin, synovial membrane, kidney, and other tissues results in clinical signs.[57] Anticellular antibodies may directly or indirectly result in anemia, leukopenia, and thrombocytopenia. Diagnosis of SLE is based on identifying these autoantibodies and documenting that certain clinical or laboratory abnormalities exist. The diagnostic criteria for SLE have been established in humans; they provide a model for diagnosis of SLE in dogs and cats (Boxes 21-3 and 21-4).

Canine SLE has been diagnosed in many different breeds. It has been diagnosed most frequently in German shepherd dogs, other large breeds of dogs, and poodles; however, this may reflect breed popularity or other factors.[94] Scott and others[94] suggest that a breed predilection exists in collies, Shetland sheepdogs, and beagles. Although some reports would suggest otherwise, there is probably no sex predisposition in dogs; in humans, SLE occurs more often in females. Feline SLE appears to be similar to canine SLE; very few feline cases have been reported in the literature.[92]

Diagnosis. The historical and physical features of SLE are variable and nonspecific, they frequently imitate those of other disease states. The onset of clinical signs may be obvious or insidious depending on which tissues are affected and to what extent. Numerous combinations of clinical and laboratory abnormalities may be found.

Fever, lethargy, and anorexia are common clinical signs. The fever is nonresponsive to antibiotic therapy. Nondeforming inflammatory joint disease, usually affecting multiple joints, has been reported in 65% to 75% of dogs having SLE.[40,94] These dogs have a stiff or stilted gait and may be reluctant to rise and walk. Affected joints are usually swollen; no crepitus or deformity can usually be detected. Lameness may wax and wane, progress, or undergo variable periods of remission.[82]

From 30% to 55% of dogs with SLE have alopecia or dermatological abnormalities.[94] The dermatitis is frequently seborrheic, pruritic, and most severe on the face, ears, and limbs. The cutaneous lesions associated with SLE are pleomorphic; "classical" canine cutaneous SLE probably does not exist.[94] Scott and others[94] found that almost 40% of dogs with SLE had oral ulcers, a much higher prevalence than observed by others. Peripheral lymph node enlargement has been found in 30% of dogs having SLE.[40] Myocarditis, polymyositis, seizures, and a variety of other abnormalities have been documented, but with less frequency.

BOX 21-3
DIAGNOSTIC CRITERIA FOR SYSTEMIC LUPUS ERYTHEMATOSUS

CRITERIA

1. Malar rash
2. Discoid rash
3. Photosensitivity
4. Oral or nasopharyngeal ulcers
5. Arthritis
6. Serositis
   a. Pleuritis *or*
   b. Pericarditis
7. Renal disorder
   a. Proteinuria > 0.5 grams/day *or*
   b. Cellular casts
8. Neurologic disorder
   a. Seizures *or*
   b. Psychosis
9. Hematologic disorder, one of the following
   a. Hemolytic anemia
   b. Leukopenia
   c. Lymphopenia
   d. Thrombocytopenia
10. Immunologic disorder, one of the following
    a. Positive LE prep
    b. Antibody to DNA
    c. Antibody to SM
    d. False positive serologic test for syphilis
11. Antinuclear antibody in abnormal titer

DIAGNOSIS

Four or more are required for the diagnosis of systemic lupus erythemotosus.

From Tan EM and others: The 1982 revised criteria for the classification of systemic lupus erythematosus, *Arthritis Rheum* 25:1271-1277, 1982.

The presence of systemic signs helps the veterinarian differentiate SLE from idiopathic nondeforming (type I) inflammatory joint disease (see Idiopathic Nondeforming Arthritis). Unfortunately, systemic signs may be associated with septic polyarthritis, rheumatoid arthritis, and other immune-mediated disorders. Laboratory and radiographic evaluations help differentiate one from the other.

Hematological abnormalities are common in dogs with SLE. Anemia is seen in 35% to 60% of affected animals.[40,94] The anemia may be regenerative or nonregenerative. The direct Coombs test quantitates the amount of antibody or complement bound to erythrocyte surface membranes. If a regenerative anemia is present without evidence of detectable blood loss or autoagglutination, a direct Coombs test should be performed.[105] Overall, the direct

BOX 21-4
PROPOSED CRITERIA FOR DIAGNOSIS OF SYSTEMIC LUPUS ERYTHEMATOSUS IN DOGS

HALLIWELL

1. Skin disease with clinical/histological resemblance to SLE
2. Polyarthritis that is not rapidly progressive
3. Hemolytic anemia that is Coombs positive
4. Thrombocytopenia
5. Proteinuria

Diagnosis of SLE is justified when one or more criteria are present and there is suitable serological evidence (positive ANA, LE cells).

DRAZNER

1. Eczematous rash with/without mucocutaneous ulceration
2. Nonerosive/nondeforming arthritis
3. Hemolytic anemia
4. Thrombocytopenic purpura
5. Glomerulonephritis
6. Myositis
7. Myocarditis
8. Interstitial pneumonitis

Diagnosis of SLE is justified when one or more criteria are present and there are ANA and/or LE cells, anticell antibodies (RBCs, platelets), or anti-ribonucleic acid (anti-RNA) antibodies.

BENNETT

1. Evidence of multisystemic involvement (see above)
2. ANA detectable at a significantly high titer
3. Immunopathological features consistent with clinical disease (antibodies present to RBCs, WBCs, platelets; immune complexes demonstrable in skin, kidney, etc.)

Diagnosis of SLE is justified when all three criteria are present; if only one and two are present, probable canine SLE is diagnosed.

Data from Halliwell REW: Autoimmune disease in the dog, *Adv Vet Sci Comp Med* 22:222-263, 1978; Drazner FH: Systemic lupus erythematosus in the dog, *Comp Cont Educ* 2(3):243-254, 1980; Bennett D: Immune-based nonerosive inflammatory joint disease of the dog. 1. Canine systemic lupus erythematosus, *J Small Anim Pract* 28:871-889, 1987.

Coombs test is positive in 20% to 40% of dogs with SLE.[10,40,82] Bone marrow aspiration and evaluation are indicated in dogs with nonregenerative anemia. Leukocytosis and leukopenia have been reported to develop in canine SLE as well; both apparently develop with about equal\frequency, about 30% according to one review.[94] Thrombocytopenia is reported less frequently. Platelet factor-3 (PF-3) test can be used to detect antiplatelet antibody.[105]

Depending on the degree of renal involvement, azotemia and hypoalbuminemia may develop. Urinalysis reveals some degree of proteinuria in 40% to 50% of affected dogs.[40,94] Serum globulin levels are often elevated.

Tests for antinuclear antibody (i.e., FANA, LE prep) and synovial fluid analysis are indicated in the diagnosis of SLE (see Chapter 1). Synovial fluid analysis reveals sterile inflammatory joint disease. The radiographic abnormalities associated with SLE are minimal and nonspecific; lack of subchondral bony erosion and periarticular new bone formation helps to differentiate chronic SLE from chronic deforming or erosive joint disorders.

Treatment. Immunosuppressive/cytotoxic agents are used in treatment of SLE (see Treatment of Noninfectious Inflammatory Joint Disease). In addition, associated abnormalities such as azotemia and pyoderma may require specific treatment. Antibiotic therapy is indicated in the initial stages of treatment or whenever high dosages of corticosteroids or other immunosuppressive agents are being given.

Most authorities on SLE use a similar therapeutic approach; even so, little information exists on the long-term results of treatment of canine and feline SLE. Clinical remission is usually achieved with corticosteroid therapy alone. A few dogs experience clinical remission, and drug therapy can eventually be discontinued; however, clinical remission is usually incomplete or maintained only by long-term therapy. Use of cytotoxic agents seems to be indicated when corticosteroid therapy fails to induce or maintain remission or when the effective dose of corticosteroid is unacceptably high. Even though the use of cytotoxic agents is widespread, little objective evidence currently proves their efficacy. Careful long-term follow-up evaluations are needed to assess properly the value of the various drugs used in the treatment of SLE and the other immune-mediated joint disorders. Unfortunately, in two studies, almost one-half the dogs having SLE died of SLE-associated or drug-induced problems or were euthanized within 1 year of diagnosis.[10,94]

Rheumatoid Arthritis

Rheumatoid arthritis (RA) is a slowly progressive inflammatory joint disorder that ultimately results in pronounced joint instability and deformity. The disease is apparently rare in dogs; a prevalance of 2 in 25,000 was observed in one clinical population.[85] There is apparently no breed or sex predisposition for RA in dogs.[8] RA generally develops in middle-aged or older dogs but has been diagnosed in dogs less than 2 years of age. The small joints of the paw and the carpus and tarsus are most often affected, but RA may occur in any diarthroidal joint. The prognosis associated with RA is poor.

The etiology of RA is unknown, but immune-mediated mechanisms are thought to play a major role in its pathogenesis. Villous hyperplasia of the synovial membrane with pronounced lymphoid and plasma cell infiltrates is a characteristic pathological finding; this feature may help the pathologist distinguish RA and plasmacytic-lymphocytic arthritis from other noninfectious inflammatory disorders (see Chapter 1). Synovial hyperplasia and pannus formation are thought to play an important role in the destruction of articular structures. Articular cartilage is undermined as a result of resorption of subchondral bone adjacent to inflamed synovium. In addition, pannus extends across the surface of the articular cartilage and, perhaps by interfering with nutrition or other physiological mechanisms, results in cartilage destruction. Invasion of supporting soft tissue structures leads to instability and eventual deformity.

Diagnosis. Although clinical signs may develop acutely, RA is generally characterized by an insidious onset and slow progression of clinical signs. Initially, lameness is usually mild and intermittent and may shift from one limb to another. In early cases the lack of demonstrable swelling or deformity may conceal the diagnosis. Intermittent low-grade fever, anorexia, lethargy, and mild peripheral lymph node enlargement are common at this stage of the disease. The presence of systemic signs helps the clinician differentiate RA from noninflammatory joint disease.

As the disease progresses, joint swelling, instability, and deformity become more apparent. Joint involvement tends to be symmetrical and most severe in the distal joints of the limb. Affected joints are swollen, painful, and crepitant. As time goes by, the digits become deformed and the paws deviate outward. The animal has difficulty rising and walking. Carpal and tarsal instability may result in a palmograde/plantagrade stance (Fig. 21-12). Cranial drawer sign and patellar luxation may be detected on examination of affected stifles. On gross examination, the cruciate ligaments may be stretched, frayed, or totally disrupted. The historical features of RA and the severe deformity, instability, and destruction of joint structures distinguish advanced RA from most other joint diseases.

Unfortunately, in the early stages of disease, the radiographic abnormalities associated with RA are nonspecific. With time, erosion of subchondral bone, collapse of the joint (cartilage) space, and deformity become evident (Fig. 21-13). Subchondral erosion and cyst formation tend to be much more evident with RA than with DJD. Compared with the radiographic findings of DJD associated with chronic instability (cruciate ligament

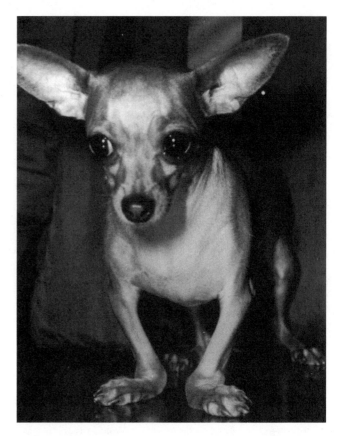

Fig. 21-12 Middle-aged Chihuahua having rheumatoid arthritis of at least 1-year duration. There is symmetrical deformity and swelling in the region of the carpus. Destruction of supporting soft tissues has resulted in a palmograde stance with valgus and rotational deviation of the paws. Notice the plantigrade stance on the right side. The hock joints were similarly affected.

rupture, hip dysplasia), periarticular new bone or osteophyte formation appears less organized and is a less prominent feature of RA.

Few clinical pathological abnormalities are associated with RA. Affected dogs may be mildly anemic and have mild leukocytosis or leukopenia and hyperfibrinogenemia. Joint fluid analysis suggests the presence of an inflammatory process. The joint fluid tends to contain fewer WBCs with a larger proportion of mononuclear cells than would be expected with infectious or the nondeforming inflammatory joint disorders. Even so, WBC numbers can exceed 80,000/μl.[8] Also, contrary to what might be expected, only a scant amount of synovial fluid may be present in affected joints. Much of the joint swelling is caused by soft tissue proliferation rather than effusion.

In humans the diagnosis of RA is largely made on the basis of fulfilling certain clinical criteria. These criteria,

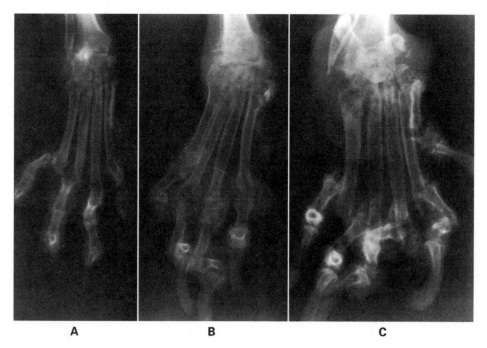

Fig. 21-13   A to **C**, Radiographic examples of rheumatoid arthritis in three dogs. The early radiographic abnormalities associated with rheumatoid arthritis (soft tissue swelling) are nonspecific (carpus, **A**) and may be difficult to detect. As time passes, erosion/dissolution of subchondral bone and articular cartilage and joint instability become more evident (carpus, **B** and **C**). Notice that the disruption of supporting soft tissues has resulted in metacarpal-phalangeal luxation and severe deformity of the digits **A** and **C**. The presence of excessively long nails suggests that the dogs are not walking properly.

with some modification, are used in the diagnosis of canine RA as well (Box 21-5). The ability to detect rheumatoid factor(s) in dogs with RA varies, ranging from about 25% in one report[81] to 70% to 90% in others.[8,75] Philosophical differences over the significance of low titers and the importance of having a positive test to diagnose the disease as well as differences in laboratory methods probably account for the large degree of variability. A large percentage of dogs having chronic progressive deforming joint disease, that is, "rheumatoid-like" disease, have no detectable titer. Rheumatoid factor testing is described in Chapter 1.

Treatment. Although the cause of RA remains obscure, treatment is directed at altering the immune reaction that apparently plays a role in the pathogenesis of the disease. Corticosteroid and cytotoxic drug therapy is indicated; recommendations are described at the end of this chapter.

Some suggest that remission can be achieved if drug therapy is instituted early. Unfortunately, many cases are diagnosed so late in the course of the disease that clinical dysfunction would continue to be evident even if the underlying pathological mechanisms could be arrested. Overall, the prognosis associated with canine RA is poor.

The clinical response to corticosteroids is usually temporary and cannot be sustained even with progressively higher dosages.[85] NSAIDs are ineffective.

Slow-acting remittive agents such as gold salts have been used for treatment of RA in humans and dogs.[76] Various adverse effects are associated with such therapy in humans. Presently, not enough information is available to support the use of gold salts in dogs, and further studies are necessary. Surgical intervention (synovectomy, arthrodesis) may not be practical or reasonable, since multiple joints are usually affected and the underlying pathological process cannot usually be controlled by these measures. Some small dogs cope reasonably despite progression of the disease. Weight control is especially important in dogs having RA.

Plasmacytic-Lymphocytic Synovitis

Plasmacytic-lymphocytic synovitis is an inflammatory joint disorder that tends to occur in small or medium-sized dogs. Monoarticular or pauciarticular involvement is most common; the stifle joint(s) is (are) most often affected.

The cause of plasmacytic-lymphocytic synovitis is not known; immune-mediated mechanisms are probably

---

BOX 21-5

REVISED CRITERIA FOR CLASSIFICATION OF RHEUMATOID ARTHRITIS (TRADITIONAL FORMAT)

CRITERIA

1. Morning stiffness
   Morning stiffness in and around the joints, lasting at least 1 hour before maximal improvement.
2. Arthritis of 3 or more joint areas
   At least 3 joint areas simultaneously have had soft tissue swelling or fluid (not bony overgrowth alone) observed by a physician. The 14 possible areas are right or left PIP, MCP, wrist, elbow, knee, ankle, and MPT joints.
3. Arthritis of hand joints
   At least 1 area swollen (as defined above) in a wrist, MCP, or PIP joint.
4. Symmetric arthritis
   Simultaneous involvement of the same joint areas (as defined in 2) on both sides of the body.
5. Rheumatoid nodules
   Subcutaneous nodules, over bony prominences, or extensor surfaces, or in juxtaarticular regions, observed by a physician.
6. Serum rheumatoid factor
   Demonstration of abnormal amounts of serum rheumatoid factor by any method for which the result has been positive in < 5% of normal control subjects.
7. Radiographic changes
   Radiographic changes typical of rheumatoid arthritis on posteroanterior hand and wrist radiographs, which must include erosions or unequivocal bony decalcification localized in or most markedly adjacent to the involved joints (osteoarthritis changes alone do not qualify)

For classification purposes, a patient shall be said to have rheumatoid arthritis if he/she has satisfied at least 4 of these 7 criteria. Criteria 1 through 4 must have been present for at least 6 weeks. Patients with 2 clinical diagnoses are not excluded. Designation as classic, definite, or probable rheumatoid arthritis is not to be made.

From Arnett FC and others: 1987 Revised American Rheumatoid Arthritis Association classification of rheumatoid arthritis, *Arthritis Rheum* 31:315-324, 1988.

---

involved. Although the disease has some distinctive features, it is probably a variant of RA.[85] As with RA, it is characterized by synovial hyperplasia with plasma cell and lymphocytic infiltration and by cartilage and subchondral erosions and joint instability. The erosive changes are much less pronounced than those associated with advanced RA and are sometimes absent. If the affected joint is unstable, bone and cartilage changes may be the result of instability rather than the underlying disease.

Diagnosis. The onset of clinical signs with plasmacytic-lymphocytic synovitis is usually insidious; however, lameness may appear to develop suddenly with an associated rupture of supportive soft tissues (cranial cruciate ligament). Clinically, only one or two joints are usually affected. The affected joint is thickened and painful. In dogs thought to have a rupture of the cranial cruciate ligament, the presence of an unusual degree of thickening or similar thickening in the opposite stifle should be a clue that some underlying disease process is present. Many cases of plasmacytic-lymphocytic synovitis are diagnosed only after surgical exploration of the cruciate deficient stifle has revealed thickening and discoloration of the synovial membrane or gross abnormalities in the joint fluid. Synovial membrane and joint fluid analysis should be performed whenever such abnormalities are seen. Failure to recognize such abnormalities may result in inappropriate therapy and rendering of an overly optimistic prognosis.

Few systemic abnormalities are associated with plasmacytic-lymphocytic synovitis. The relative lack of systemic signs and the limited number of affected joints help to differentiate plasmacytic-lymphocytic arthritis clinically from other noninfectious inflammatory disorders. Radiographic changes are usually nonspecific. Joint fluid analysis suggests inflammatory joint disease; however, unlike other inflammatory disorders, WBC numbers tend to remain relatively low (5000 to 20,000/μl) and mononuclear cells predominate.[85]

Treatment. Little information is available on the treatment of plasmacytic-lymphocytic synovitis in the dog. Specific treatment protocols have yet to be evaluated. The disorder can usually be partially controlled with the use of immunosuppressive drugs.[85] Progression to other joints occurs infrequently.

Immunosuppressive/cytotoxic drug therapy might increase the risk of dehiscence and postoperative infection in affected dogs that have undergone surgical exploration and stabilization procedures. The risk of infection may be enhanced when heavily braided or multifilament sutures have been used to effect an extracapsular stabilization of the cruciate ligament-deficient stifle. It is probably wise to wait 2 to 3 weeks before administering immunosuppressive and/or cytotoxic drugs to dogs that have had surgery.

Feline Progressive Polyarthritis

Feline progressive polyarthritis occurs only rarely in domestic cats. The disorder has been described most completely by Pedersen and co-workers.[80,83] It primarily occurs in male cats 1 to 5 years of age. Two distinct clinical syndromes are recognized. The prognosis associated with both forms of the disease is poor.

The etiology of feline progressive polyarthritis is not known. The periosteal proliferative form of the disorder appears to be linked to feline leukemia (FeLV) and feline syncytium-forming virus (FeSFV) infections.[85]

Diagnosis. The periosteal proliferative form of the disease is more common than the erosive form. The onset of clinical signs is sudden in cats with the proliferative form of feline progressive polyarthritis. Signs include high fever, severe joint pain, and stiffness. The tarsal and carpal joints are most often affected, and regional lymph nodes are enlarged.[85] All affected cats test positive for FeSFV; up to one-half test positive for FeLV.[85]

The initial radiographic abnormality associated with the periosteal proliferative form of the disease is soft tissue swelling. Osteopenia and periosteal new bone formation develop over the next 2 to 3 months (Fig. 21-14).[85] After the first few weeks, the fever slowly sub-

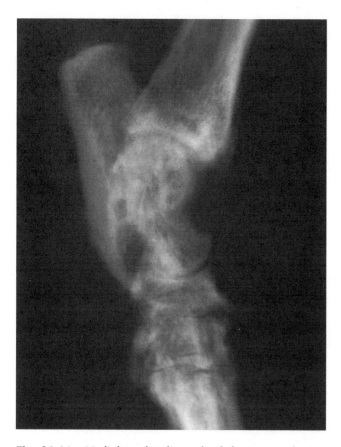

Fig. 21-14 Mediolateral radiograph of the tarsus of a cat with the periosteal proliferative form of feline progressive polyarthritis. Notice the mottled appearance of the bones (loss of normal trabecular pattern) and the diffuse periarticular new bone formation.

From Sherding RG: *The cat: diseases and clinical management*, New York, 1989, Churchill Livingstone.

sides and the disease takes a more chronic progressive course. Affected cats become emaciated and appear stiff.[85] There are bony enlargements about the joints, and ankylosis occurs.[85] The clinical features of the periosteal proliferative form of feline progressive polyarthritis are similar to those found in humans having Reiter syndrome.[11]

The erosive or deforming form of feline chronic progressive polyarthritis is clinically and histologically similar to canine RA.[85] In fact, Bennett and Nash[11] refer to this form of the disease as feline RA. The erosive/deforming form of feline progressive polyarthritis is less common than the proliferative form. It is characterized by an insidious onset and a gradually progressive course. There is usually symmetrical involvement of the joints of the feet and the carpal and tarsal joints. As the disease progresses, subchondral erosions and deformity become radiographically evident (Fig. 21-15). Joint instability and deformity occur.[85]

The two forms of feline chronic progressive polyarthritis are easily differentiated on the basis of clinical and radiographic features. In addition, joint fluid from cats affected with the periosteal proliferative form contains high numbers of neutrophils. The synovial fluid from cats having the erosive form has fewer cells and a higher proportion of mononuclear cells.[85]

Treatment: Treatment of feline progressive polyarthritis has not been rewarding. Corticosteroids and cytotoxic drugs temporarily slow the progression of clinical signs, but recurrences and refractiveness to drug therapy are common.[85] Therapeutic decisions are complicated by the relationship of periosteal proliferative arthritis to FeLV and FeSFV infection. All cats with polyarthritis should undergo FeLV testing.

Other Noninfectious Inflammatory Joint Disorders

Other noninfectious inflammatory joint disorders occur in dogs and cats. Selected references on these are cited in Box 21-2.

Treatment of Noninfectious Inflammatory Joint Disease

The use of corticosteroids and cytotoxic agents in the treatment of canine and feline noninfectious inflammatory joint disease is ubiquitous. The use of such drugs is supported by the pervasiveness of inflammatory (immune) response. Although the disorders are clinically distinct, it is quite possible that the various diseases are no more than different manifestations of the same or very similar processes; they are treated with similar drugs using similar protocols. In addition, the scope of

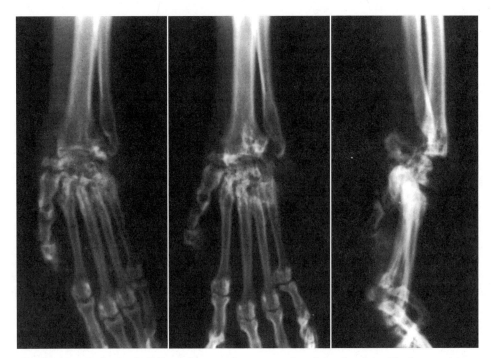

Fig. 21-15 Radiograph (*left*) of the carpal-metacarpal region of a cat with the erosive or deforming form of feline progressive polyarthritis (feline rheumatoid arthritis). There is soft tissue swelling about the carpus and disruption of the intercarpal and carpometacarpal joints. Fourteen months later (*center* and *right*), further destruction of the carpal bones and caudal subluxation of the affected joints have occurred. Such radiographic abnormalities are similar to those noted in dogs with advanced rheumatoid arthritis (see Fig. 21-13).

drug therapy has been limited to these and a few other drugs by the relative ineffectiveness of aspirin and other NSAIDs.

The principles of corticosteroid and cytotoxic drug therapy are described in an earlier section of this chapter (see Principles of Treatment, Drug Therapy). The use of these drugs remains somewhat empirical; modifications or changes in protocols are dictated by the patient's response. Some trial and error or experimentation is usually necessary before the appropriate drug or dosage is determined. Underlying or coexisting problems must be detected and appropriately managed; this is essential whenever an infection is present or predisposed by therapy or by the animal's weakened condition. Antibiotic therapy is indicated in debilitated or chronically ill patients and whenever high dosages of immunosuppressive drugs are being given.

Serial physical and historical examinations and intermittent reevaluation of therapy are essential. If any change occurs in the character or severity of clinical signs, the animal should be examined before therapy is modified or reinstituted. Owners must comply with instructions, have the ability to detect changes in the status of their pet, and be able to recognize and thus prevent the adverse effects of drug therapy. It is sad to see a dog whose joint disorder is successfully controlled with low-dose alternate-day corticosteroid therapy be overfed by a noncompliant owner and become obese.

Prednisone or prednisolone, alone or in combination with cytotoxic drugs, is the usual starting point for chemotherapy. Dosages of 1.5 to 2.5 mg/kg per day (0.75 to 1.25 mg/lb per day) are generally effective in inducing clinical remission. Cats and small dogs should be given doses on the higher side of this range and large dogs on the lower side. Cats seem to require higher doses than dogs to effect a positive response. This dosage is given for 2 to 3 weeks. Some believe that, as a general rule, the response to corticosteroids alone should be determined before any combinations or cytotoxic drugs are used. The dosage of corticosteroids is gradually tapered at 2- to 3-week intervals over 2 to 3 months as long as the response is favorable and remission appears to be maintained. Alternate-day therapy can usually be instituted after 5 to 7 weeks. The ultimate goal is to discontinue corticosteroid therapy completely or be able to maintain remission with no more than 0.5 to 1.0 mg/kg (0.25 to 0.50 mg/lb) of prednisone given once on alternate days. Serial physical examinations, owner communication, and joint fluid analysis are helpful in assessing the response to therapy. The use of tests for antinuclear antibody and rheumatoid factor to monitor response is probably not a reliable method of assessing therapy in seropositive patients.

When corticosteroid therapy fails to effect or maintain remission or when high doses are necessary to achieve a satisfactory result, cytotoxic drugs such as cyclophosphamide and/or azathioprine are indicated. Cytotoxic agents are used more often as part of induction therapy than for long-term maintenance of remission. When used alone, they do not appear to be as effective as corticosteroids in causing abatement of clinical signs.

Initially, cytotoxic drugs are usually administered in combination with prednisone or prednisolone. The dosage of prednisone is similar to that just described. The use of cytotoxic therapy may permit use of a lower initial dosage of corticosteroid; this is helpful in animals who cannot or should not receive large doses of prednisone. The reported dose of cyclophosphamide, when used to induce remission, is 1.75 to 2.5 mg/kg (0.8 to 1.2 mg/lb) given once daily for 4 consecutive days of each week for 3 to 5 weeks.[85] Again, dogs weighing less than 10 kg are given doses on the higher side of this range and dogs weighing more than 25 kg on the lower side. Alternately, azathioprine can be administered at 1.75 to 2.0 mg/kg (0.8 to 1.0 mg/lb) once daily for the first 2 to 3 weeks, then on alternate days.[85]

Pedersen and others[85] recommend serial blood cell counts be obtained when using cytotoxic drugs. The first complete blood count is performed 2 weeks after initiation of therapy and every 12 to 14 days thereafter. If the WBC or platelet counts drop to 6000 or 125,000 cells/μl, respectively, the dosage of these agents should be decreased by one-fourth. Cytotoxic drugs should be discontinued if WBC or platelet counts drop to the 4000 and 100,000 cells/μl level. Cytotoxic therapy is reinstituted at one-half the previous level 1 week after the drug is discontinued.

Remission generally occurs within 2 to 16 weeks after initiating combination drug therapy.[85] Dosages of corticosteroid are tapered as previously described. Dosage of cytotoxic agents is decreased and discontinued 1 to 2 months after remission has been induced. Azathioprine is probably better suited for long-term use than cyclophosphamide because of the problem of hemorrhagic cystitis. Cyclophosphamide should probably not be used for longer than 3 to 4 months. Azathioprine is much more toxic in cats than dogs and should probably not be used in cats without close monitoring.[85]

Unfortunately, only a few reports have documented the results of chemotherapy in the treatment of the various noninfectious inflammatory joint disorders of dogs and cats.[8-11,75,80-83,94] Although there is little proof that one drug or drug combination is any better than another, corticosteroid administration generally produces the most dramatic clinical response. Cures are often the exception rather than the rule. Control or remission of clinical signs is often temporary; drug therapy is usually required to prevent recurrence or exacerbation of clinical signs.

Overall the prognosis associated with immune-mediated joint disease tends to be better in animals having nonerosive/nondeforming arthritis than erosive/deforming disease. It is especially good when arthritis is associated with a treatable condition, that is, when arthritis is drug induced or associated with chronic infection or enteric disease. The prognosis is better when there is no or only limited systemic involvement. The prognosis associated with plasmacytic-lymphocytic synovitis or idiopathic (type I) polyarthritis is better than with SLE. Avoiding adverse effects of drug therapy while maintaining simultaneous control of all the various clinical manifestations of SLE is difficult. The prognosis associated with canine SLE is, at best, fair. The prognosis is poor with the erosive and proliferative forms of feline progressive polyarthritis and with the rheumatoid or rheumatoid-like disorders of dogs. Affected animals are often euthanized because of persistent pain and progressive disability.

REFERENCES

1. Alexander JW, Earley TD: A carpal laxity syndrome in young dogs, *J Vet Orthop* 3(1):22-26, 1984.
2. Altera KP, Bonasch H: Periarteritis nodosa in a cat, *J Am Vet Med Assoc* 149:1307-1311, 1966.
3. Axelrod L: Glucocorticoid therapy, *Medicine* 55:39, 1976.
4. Banks WJ: *Applied veterinary histology*, Baltimore, 1981, Williams & Wilkins.
5. Barnhart ER, publisher: *Physicians' desk reference*, ed 44, Oradell, NJ, 1990, Medical Economics.
6. Beale BS, Goring RL: Exposure of the medial and lateral trochlear ridges of the talus in the dog. Part I. Dorsomedial and plantaromedial surgical approaches to the medial trochlear ridge, *J Am Anim Hosp Assoc* 26:13-18, 1990.
7. Bellah JR, and others: *Ehrlichia canis*–related polyarthritis in a dog, *J Am Vet Med Assoc* 189:922-923, 1986.
8. Bennett D: Immune-based erosive inflammatory joint disease of the dog; canine rheumatoid arthritis. 1. Clinical, radiological and laboratory investigations, *J Small Anim Pract* 28:779-797, 1987.
9. Bennett D: Immune-based non-erosive inflammatory joint disease of the dog. 3. Canine idiopathic polyarthritis, *J Small Anim Pract* 28:909-928, 1987.
10. Bennett D: Immune-based non-erosive inflammatory joint disease of the dog. 1. Canine systemic lupus erythematosus, *J Small Anim Pract* 28:871-889, 1987.
11. Bennett D, Nash AS: Feline immune-based polyarthritis: a study of thirty-one cases, *J Small Anim Pract* 29:501-523, 1988.
12. Berzon JL, Quick CB: Fragmented coronoid process: anatomical, clinical and radiographic considerations with case analyses, *J Am Anim Hosp Assoc* 16:241-251, 1980.
13. Boulay JP and others: Effect of cimetidine on aspirin-induced gastric hemorrhage in dogs, *Am J Vet Res* 47:1744-1746, 1986.
14. Braun JP and others: Haematological and biochemical effects of a single intramuscular dose of 6-methylprednisolone acetate in the dogs, *Res Vet Sci* 31:236-238, 1981.
15. Brodey RS: Hypertrophic osteoarthropathy in the dog: a clinicopathologic survey of 60 cases, *J Am Vet Med Assoc* 159:1242-1256, 1971.
16. Brown SG, Newton CD: Infectious arthritis and wounds of joints. In Newton CD, Nunamaker DM, editors: *Textbook of small animal orthopaedics*, Philadelphia, 1985, Lippincott.
17. Buffington T: Obesity better prevented than treated: involve owner in treatment, *DVM Mag* 21(6):27-31, 1990.

18. Castell MJH: Acute peri-arthritis in a kennel of greyhounds, *Vet Rec* 84:652-654, 1969.

19. Chastain CB: Aspirin: new indications for an old drug, *Comp Cont Educ Pract Vet* 9:165-170, 1987.

20. Chastain CB: Use of corticosteroids. In Ettinger SJ, editor: *Textbook of veterinary internal medicine*, ed 3, Philadelphia, 1989, Saunders.

21. Chastain CB, Graham CL: Adrenocortical suppression in dogs on daily and alternate-day prednisone administration, *Am J Vet Res* 40:936-941, 1979.

22. Chrisman OD: Biochemical aspects of degenerative joint disease, *Clin Orthop Rel Res* 64:77-86, 1969.

23. Clark L and others: Longbone abnormalities in kittens following vitamin A administration, *J Comp Pathol* 80:113-120, 1970.

24. Clarke M: Osteochondritis dissecans in a Burmese cat, *Feline Pract* 15(5):6-7, 1985.

25. Daehler MH: Transmural pyloric perforation associated with naproxen administration in a dog, *J Am Vet Med Assoc* 189:694-695, 1986.

26. Davis LE: Clinical pharmacology of salicylates, *J Am Vet Med Assoc* 176:65-66, 1980.

27. Dougherty SA, and others: Juvenile-onset polyarthritis syndrome in Akitas, *J Am Vet Med Assoc* 198:849-856, 1991.

28. Drutz DJ, and others: The penetration of penicillin and other antimicrobials into joint fluid, *J Bone Joint Surg* 49A:1415-1421, 1967.

29. Ellison GW, Norrdin RW: Multicentric periarticular calcinosis in a pup, *J Am Vet Med Assoc* 177:542-546, 1980.

30. Ewing GO: Indomethacin-associated gastrointestinal hemorrhage in a dog, *J Am Vet Med Assoc* 161:1665-1668, 1972.

31. Flo GL and others: Synovial chondrometaplasia in five dogs, *J Am Vet Med Assoc* 191:1417-1422, 1987.

32. Flower RJ and others: Analgesic-antipyretics and anti-inflammatory agents: drugs employed in the treatment of gout. In Gilman AG, Goodman LS, Gilman A, editors: *The pharmacological basis of therapeutics*, ed 6, New York, 1980, Macmillian.

33. Freston JW: Cimetidine. 1. Developments, pharmacology, and efficacy, *Ann Intern Med* 97:573-580, 1982.

34. Frey HH, Rieh B: Pharmacokinetics of naproxen in the dog, *Am J Vet Res* 42:1615-1617, 1981.

35. Gibson JP, Roenigk WJ: Pseudogout in a dog, *J Am Vet Med Assoc* 161:912-915, 1972.

36. Giger U, and others: Sulfadiazine-induced allergy in six Doberman pinschers, *J Am Vet Med Assoc* 186:479-484, 1985.

37. Gilmour MA, Walshaw R: Naproxen-induced toxicosis in a dog, *J Am Vet Med Assoc* 191:1431-1432, 1987.

38. Goad DL, Goad ME: Osteoarticular sporotrichosis in a dog, *J Am Vet Med Assoc* 189:1326-1328, 1986.

39. Goring RL, Beale BS: Exposure of the medial and lateral trochlear ridges of the talus in the dog. Part II. Dorsolateral and plantarolateral surgical approaches to the lateral trochlear ridge, *J Am Anim Hosp Assoc* 26:19-24, 1990.

40. Grindem CB, Johnson KH: Systemic lupus erythematosus: literature review and report of 42 new canine cases, *J Am Anim Hosp Assoc* 19:489-503, 1983.

41. Grondalen J: Arthrosis in the elbow joint of young rapidly growing dogs. III, *Nord Vet Med* 31:520-527, 1979.

42. Haskins ME and others: Mucopolysaccharidosis in a domestic short-haired cat: a disease distinct from that seen in the Siamese cat, *J Am Vet Med Assoc* 175:384-387, 1979.

43. Haskins ME, and others: Betaglucuronidase deficiency in a dog: a model of human mucopolysaccharidosis VII, *Pediatr Res* 18:980, 1984.

44. Haynes RC, Murad F: Adrenocorticotropic hormone; adrenocortical steroids and their synthetic analogs; inhibitors of adrenocortical steroid biosynthesis. In Gilman AG, Goodman LS, Gilman A, editors: *The pharmacological basis of therapeutics*, ed 6, New York, 1980, Macmillian.

45. Hench PS and others: The effects of a hormone of the adrenal cortex (17-hydroxy-11-dehydrocorticosterone, compound E) and of the pituitary adrenocorticotropic hormone on rheumatoid arthritis, *Proc Staff Meet Mayo Clin* 24:181, 1949.

46. Herron MR: Ununited anconeal process in the dog, *Vet Clin North Am* 1:417-428, 1971.

47. Hjelle JJ, Grauer GF: Acetaminophen-induced toxicosis in dogs and cats, *J Am Vet Med Assoc* 188:742-746, 1986.

48. Hooper PT and others: Mycoplasma polyarthritis in a cat with probable severe immune deficiency, *Aust Vet J* 62:352, 1985.

49. Huxtable CR, Davis PE: The pathology of polyarthritis in young greyhounds, *J Comp Pathol* 86:11-21, 1976.

50. Jackson RW, Parsons CJ: Distension-irrigation treatment of major joint sepsis, *Clin Orthop Rel Res* 96:160-164, 1973.

51. Jeffery MS, Carson Dick W: Forward: the role of the laboratory in rheumatology, *Clin Rheum Dis* 9:ix, 1983.

52. Jezyk PF: Feline Maroteaux-Lamy syndrome (mucopolysaccharidosis VI). In Bojrab MJ, editor: *Pathophysiology in small animal surgery*, Philadelphia, 1981, Lea & Febiger.

53. Kelly MJ: Pain. In Ettinger SJ, editor: *Textbook of veterinary internal medicine*, ed 3, Philadelphia, 1989, WB Saunders.

54. Kemppainen RJ and others: Adrenocortical suppression in the dog after a single dose of methylprednisolone acetate, *Am J Vet Res* 42:822-824, 1981.

55. Kemppainen RJ and others: Adrenocortical suppression in the dog given a single intramuscular dose of prednisone or triamcinolone acetonide, *Am J Vet Med Res* 43:204-206, 1982.

56. Kemppainen RJ, and others: Effects of prednisone on thyroid and gonadal endocrine function in dogs, *J Endocrinol* 96:293-302, 1983.

57. Koffler D: The immunology of rheumatoid diseases, *Clin Symp (CIBA)* 31:6-20, 1979.

58. Kornblatt AN and others: Arthritis caused by *Borrelia burgdorferi* in dogs, *J Am Vet Med Assoc* 186:960-964, 1985.

59. Kusba JK and others: Suspected villonodular synovitis in a dog, *J Am Vet Med Assoc* 182:390-392, 1983.

60. Lanza FL and others: Endoscopic evaluation of the effects of aspirin, buffered aspirin, and enteric-coated aspirin on gastric and duodenal mucosa, *N Engl J Med* 303:136-138, 1980.

61. Lenehan TM, Van Sickle DC: Canine osteochondrosis. In Newton CD, Nunamaker DM, editors: *Textbook of small animal orthopaedics*, Philadelphia, 1985, Lippincott.

62. Lenehan TM, Van Sickle DC: Ununited anconeal process, ununited medial coronoid process, ununited medial epicondyle, patella cubiti, and sesamoidal fragments of the elbow. In Newton CD, Nunamaker DM, editors: *Textbook of small animal orthopaedics*, Philadelphia, 1985, Lippincott.

63. Lipowitz AJ, Newton CD: Degenerative joint disease and traumatic arthritis. In Newton CD, Nunamaker DM, editors: *Textbook of small animal orthopaedics*, Philadelphia, 1985, Lippincott.

64. Mahaffey E and others: Disseminated histoplasmosis in three cats, *J Am Anim Hosp Assoc* 13:46-51, 1977.

65. Marshall JL: Periarticular osteophytes: initiation and formation in the knee of the dog, *Clin Orthop Rel Res* 62:37-47, 1969.

66. Mason TA and others: Osteochondrosis of the elbow joint of young dogs, *J Small Anim Pract* 21:641-656, 1980.

67. Melby JC: Clinical pharmacology of systemic corticosteroids, *Annu Rev Pharmacol Toxicol* 17:511-527, 1977.

68. Miller RM, Kind RE: A gout-like syndrome in a dog, *Vet Med Small Anim Clin* 61:236-240, 1966.

69. Mitten RW, Hoefle WD: Ununited anconeal process: unusual presentation in two dogs, *J Am Anim Hosp Assoc* 14:595-596, 1978.

70. Miyabayashi T and others: Use of a flexed dorsoplantar radiographic view of the talocrural joint to evaluate lameness in two dogs, *J Am Vet Med Assoc* 199:598-600, 1991.

71. Moise NS and others: *Mycoplasma gateae* arthritis and tenosynovitis in cats: case report and experimental reproduction of the disease, *Am J Vet Res* 44:16-21, 1983.

72. Montgomery RD and others: Comparison of aerobic culturette, synovial membrane biopsy, and blood culture medium in detection of canine bacterial arthritis, *Vet Surg* 18:300-303, 1989.

73. Mount ME: Toxicology. In Ettinger SJ, editor: *Textbook of veterinary internal medicine*, ed 3, Philadelphia, 1989, Saunders.

74. Nelson JD: Antibiotic concentrations in septic joint effusions, *N Engl J Med* 284:349-353, 1971.

75. Newton CD and others: Rheumatoid arthritis in dogs, *J Am Vet Med Assoc* 168:113-121, 1976.

76. Newton CD and others: Gold salt therapy for rheumatoid arthritis in dogs, *J Am Vet Med Assoc* 174:1308-1309, 1979.

77. Olsewski JM and others: Degenerative joint disease: multiple joint involvement in young and mature dogs, *Am J Vet Res* 44:1300-1308, 1983.

78. Olsson SE: Pathophysiology, morphology, and clinical signs of osteochondrosis (chondrosis) in the dog. In Bojrab MJ, editor: *Pathophysiology in small animal surgery*, Philadelphia, 1981, Lea & Febiger.

79. Oxenford CJ, Middleton DJ: Osteomyelitis and arthritis associated with *Aspergillus fumigatus* in a dog, *Aust Vet J* 63:59-60, 1986.

80. Pedersen NC and others: Chronic progressive polyarthritis of the cat, *Feline Pract* 5(1):42-51, 1975.

81. Pedersen NC and others: Noninfectious canine arthritis: rheumatoid arthritis, *J Am Vet Med Assoc* 169:295-303, 1976.

82. Pedersen NC and others: Noninfectious canine arthritis: the inflammatory, nonerosive arthritides, *J Am Vet Med Assoc* 169:304-310, 1976.

83. Pedersen NC and others: Feline chronic progressive polyarthritis, *Am J Vet Res* 41:522-535, 1980.

84. Pedersen NC and others: A transient febrile "limping" syndrome of kittens caused by two different strains of feline calicivirus, *Feline Pract* 13(1):26, 1983.

85. Pedersen NC and others: Joint diseases of dogs and cats. In Ettinger SJ, editor: *Textbook of veterinary internal medicine*, ed 3, Philadelphia, 1989, Saunders.

86. Piermattei DL, Greeley RG: *An atlas of surgical approaches to the bones of the dog and cat*, ed 2, Philadelphia, 1979, Saunders.

87. Roudebush P, Morse GE: Naproxen toxicosis in a dog, *J Am Vet Med Assoc* 179:805-806, 1981.

88. Rudd RG and others: The effects of beveling the margins of articular cartilage defects in immature dogs, *Vet Surg* 16:378-383, 1987.

89. Salmon JE, Kimberly RP: Formulary (Appendix G). In Beary JF, Christian CL, Sculco TP, editors: *Manual of rheumatology and outpatient orthopedic disorders*, Boston, 1981, Little, Brown.

90. Schmid FR: Principles of diagnosis and treatment of infectious arthritis. In McCarty DJ, editor: *Arthritis and allied conditions*, ed 9, Philadelphia, 1979, Lea & Febiger.

91. Schrader SC: Septic arthritis and osteomyelitis of the hip in six mature dogs, *J Am Vet Med Assoc* 181:894-898, 1982.

92. Schrader SC, Sherding RG: Disorders of the skeletal system. In Sherding RG, editor: *The cat: diseases and clinical management*, New York, 1989, Churchill Livingstone.

93. Scott DW: Dermatologic use of corticosteroids: systemic and topical, *Vet Clin North Am* 12:19-32, 1982.

94. Scott DW and others: Canine lupus erythematosus. I. Systemic lupus erythematosus, *J Am Anim Hosp Assoc* 19:461-479, 1983.

95. Seawright AA, and others: Hypervitaminosis A of the cat, *Adv Vet Sci Comp Med* 14:1-27, 1970.

96. Shires PK, and others: Carpal hyperextension in two-month-old pups, *J Am Vet Med Assoc* 186:49-52, 1985.

97. Simon LS, Mills JA: Nonsteroidal antiinflammatory drugs. Part 1, *N Engl J Med* 302:1179-1185, 1980.

98. Sinibaldi KR, Arnoczky SP: Surgical removal of the ununited anconeal process in the dog, *J Am Anim Hosp Assoc* 11:192-198, 1975.

99. Smith MM and others: Clinical evaluation of dogs after surgical and nonsurgical management of osteochondritis dissecans of the talus, *J Am Vet Med Assoc* 187:31-35, 1985.

100. Somer T and others: Pigmented villonodular synovitis and plasmacytoid lymphoma in a dog, *J Am Vet Med Assoc* 197:877-879, 1990.

101. Spyridakis LK and others: Ibuprofen toxicosis in a dog, *J Am Vet Med Assoc* 188:918-919, 1986.

102. Stockham SL and others: Canine granulocytic ehrlichiosis in dogs from central Missouri: a possible cause of polyarthritis, *Vet Med Rev* 6(2/4):3, 1985.

103. Swango LJ and others: Bacterial, rickettsial, protozoal, and miscellaneous infections. In Ettinger SJ, editor: *Textbook of veterinary internal medicine*, ed 3, Philadelphia, 1989, Saunders.

104. Thomas NW: Piroxicam-associated gastric ulceration in a dog, *Comp Cont Educ Pract Vet* 9:1004, 1987.

105. Thompson JP: Immunological diseases. In Ettinger SJ, editor: *Textbook of veterinary internal medicine*, ed 3, Philadelphia, 1989, Saunders.

106. Wallace MS and others: Gastric ulceration in the dog secondary to the use of nonsteroidal antiinflammatory drugs, *J Am Anim Hosp Assoc* 26:467-472, 1990.

107. Wilcke JR: Principles of drug therapy. In Sherding RG, editor: *The cat: diseases and clinical management*, New York, 1989, Churchill Livingstone.

108. Wind AP: Elbow incongruity and developmental elbow disease in the dog. Part I. *J Am Anim Hosp Assoc* 22:711-724, 1986.

109. Wind AP, Packard ME: Elbow incongruity and developmental elbow diseases in the dog. Part II. *J Am Anim Hosp Assoc* 22:725-730, 1986.

110. Wisner ER and others: Osteochondrosis of the lateral trochlear ridge of the talus in 7 Rottweiler dogs, *Vet Surg* 19:435-439, 1990.

111. Woodard JC, and others: Erosive polyarthritis in 2 greyhounds, *J Am Vet Med Assoc* 198:873-876, 1991.

112. Yeary RA, Brant RJ: Aspirin dosages for the dog, *J Am Vet Med Assoc* 167:63-64, 1975.

22

Tendon, Muscle, and Ligament Injuries and Surgery

MARK S. BLOOMBERG

Injuries to the muscles, tendons, and ligaments of small animals are of low incidence in routine small animal veterinary practice. The exceptions are injuries to the cruciate and collateral ligaments of the stifle and plantar ligaments of the carpus and tarsus, which are described in other chapters in this textbook. However, veterinarians that deal with the sporting breeds of dogs, especially the racing greyhound, are often presented with patients with musculotendinous and ligamentous injuries.

The key to the proper and successful treatment of musculotendinous and ligamentous injuries is early and accurate diagnosis. This is accomplished through an accurate history, signalment, and a "hands on" physical examination of the patient. Failure to detect such injuries early in their course may result in chronic injuries that shorten athletic careers and even may result in crippling diseases. Fortunately, most musculotendinous injuries do not require surgical intervention.

This chapter describes the anatomy and physiology of tendons, ligaments, and muscles and the healing, diagnosis, classification, and treatment of muscle and tendon injuries.

PRINCIPLES OF TENDON REPAIR
Anatomy and Function

Tendons are composed of long, spiraling bundles of collagen fibers arranged in parallel rows and embedded in ground substance and extracellular fluids.[67] The cellular component of the tendon fibers is the fibroblast or tenocyte. The collagen fibers are surrounded by a woven mesh of loose areolar connective tissue termed an *endotenon*. The endotenon allows longitudinal movement of the collagen bundles and carries all the blood vessels, lymphatics, and nerves. The *epitenon* covers the entire tendon and is continuous on its undersurface with the endotenon. The free gliding motion is provided by the outer sheath of the tendon called the *paratenon*. The paratenon covers and separates other tendons from each other. The paratenon forms a synovial sheath in areas of local pressure.[48]

The blood supply enters the tendon at three locations. Blood vessels entering at the musculotendinous junction supply the proximal third of the tendon. Blood vessels penetrating longitudinally in the paratenon or synovial sheath supply the middle third, whereas the distal third is supplied by vessels entering at the osseous tendon insertion. The vascularity of the tendon varies with location.[23,48]

Tendons act to facilitate and transmit forces developed by muscles across joints. The action of tendons as they cross over joints is modified by retinacular bands that function as pulleys to alter the direction of the tendon over the joint. The elasticity of tendons also may attenuate sudden forces that allow for greater velocity of movement and prevent injury to the muscle body.

Healing of Tendons

Most tendon injuries in small animals are related to trauma. Acute trauma may result in complete or partial severance of a tendon, for example, lacerated flexor tendons of the carpus from stepping on a sharp object. Tendons can also be injured from the overwhelming force of the contraction of a muscle-tendon unit. This is especially true in deceleration injuries when the limb is extended and the muscles contract at the same time.[6] The injury may result in avulsion of the tendon from its insertion, midtendon disruption, or failure at the musculotendinous junction.

The dog differs from the horse in that lower-intensity trauma appears to be less of a problem for the dog. Strained tendons are unique to the canine athlete such as

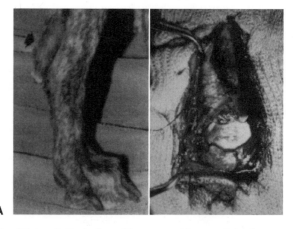

Fig. 22-1 **A**, Typical swelling seen with tear of the flexor carpi ulnaris tendon. **B**, Surgical view of the palmar aspect of the carpus demonstrating a transverse tear in the tendon of insertion of the humeral head of the flexor carpi ulnaris.

Reprinted with permission from Dee JF, and others: Injuries of high performance dogs. In Whittick WG, editor: *Canine orthopedics*, ed 2, Philadelphia, 1990, Lea & Febiger.

the racing greyhound. These are usually chronic injuries and involve the tendons of the flexor carpi ulnaris muscle near its insertion on the accessory carpal bone. Chronic injuries result in a weakened fibrotic tendon similar to the "bowed tendon" of the horse (Fig. 22-1).

The healing pattern of tendons is similar to other connective tissues. The typical stages of wound healing follow injury. Tendon injuries are frequently compound and therefore subject to a prolonged inflammatory phase of healing. Although the surgeon has no control of the wound condition before presentation, the inflammatory process can be minimized through gentle handling of tissues, meticulous wound cleansing, and thorough wound debridement.

A second important factor is whether a tendon heals without adhesions to adjacent tissues. Because tendon injuries are often accompanied by injury to surrounding tissue, healing does not take place in an isolated environment. Musculotendinous tissues attempt to heal largely by fibrosis without regard to function. This principle is referred to as the "one wound–one scar" concept of wound healing.[48] This concept refers to the early phases of repair in which undifferentiated mesenchymal cells from surrounding connective tissue migrate into the wound. These mesenchymal cells differentiate into fibroblasts and secrete ground substance and collagen, which permeate all areas of the wound. The extent of excessive fibrous tissue formation determines the degree of gliding function restored to an injured tendon. This loss of gliding function of tendons is of little consequence in small animals compared with humans.[6] However, extensive fibrosis adjacent to the carpus or tarsus may result in a limited range of motion and pain that can ultimately affect athletic performance.[21]

Tendons are divided into paratenon-covered tendons and sheathed tendons.[48] The healing of paratenon-covered tendons depends more on the extrinsic blood supply from the paratenon. A sheathed tendon depends more on its intrinsic blood supply, and thus healing is much slower. The tenocytes in a sheathed tendon have very little capacity for reproduction.[10]

During the first week after injury, the undifferentiated fibroblasts and capillary buds from the paratenon invade the injured area between the tendon ends. The fibroblasts synthesize collagen and ground substance. As the ground substance increases, the collagen polymerizes into fibrils. The thin, wavy fibers are deposited randomly in the wound during the first week after injury. In the second week of healing, the vascular reaction, fibroplastic proliferation, and collagen production reach their peak. Longitudinal orientation of the collagen fibers near the tendon ends occurs during the third and fourth weeks. However, the collagen fibers in the center of the wound remain unorganized and perpendicular to lines of stress.[48]

The final stages of wound healing involve remodeling of the wound edges. The collagen remodels, is reduced in mass, and increases in tensile strength through reorganization along lines of stress. This collagenization takes approximately 20 weeks, with the result being little histological difference between tendon and scar tissue. Return of movement and function weakens and remodels adhesions.[23,40,48]

It is important to protect surgically repaired tendons from weight bearing the first 3 to 4 weeks to minimize the gap between tendon ends. A large gap between tendon ends results in slower healing and a weaker fibrous scar. After 3 to 4 weeks of protection, gradual use of the repaired tendon is increased over the next 6 to 8 weeks. At this time the healing process is usually complete for clinical function.[10,40]

Diagnosis and Classification

Open wounds and conformational abnormalities make the diagnosis of tendon injuries easy. However, in patients with partial disruption or chronic injury, it is important to palpate the tissues carefully to make an accurate diagnosis.

Tendon injuries may occur at their origin, insertion, midsubstance, or musculotendinous junctions. The diagnosis of musculotendinous injuries depends on careful palpation. Radiographic evaluation of the affected limb assists in the diagnosis of the avulsion of a portion of the tendon's bony insertions, such as the tuber calcanei or tibial tuberosity. Diagnosis of displacement of a traction apophysis (tibial tuberosity) in the immature animal may be difficult, especially if there is minimum displacement. If in doubt, the opposite, normal anatomical location should be radiographed (Fig. 22-2).

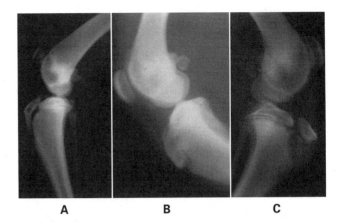

Fig. 22-2 **A**, Radiograph of an immature racing greyhound with a partial displacement of the tibial tuberosity. **B**, Normal tibial tuberosity. **C**, Avulsed tibial tuberosity.

Treatment

Surgical repair of tendon injuries. The basic principles of proper handling of tissues should be followed.* The goals of the veterinary surgeon should be to minimize adhesion formation, minimize the gap between tendon ends to provide for a strong union, and maintain proper tendon length. These principles assist in the restoration of gliding function, which is less critical in small animals.

The surgeon should have a detailed plan of repair. The skin incision, if different than the original wound, should not be made directly over the tendon to minimize adhesions. Meticulous hemostasis is important. Tourniquets may be helpful with hemostasis but may have the disadvantage of distorting the tendons because of the pressure placed on the tissues proximal to the wound

The tendon ends should be handled with straight needles or skin hooks. Any traumatized tissue should be sharply excised from the tendon ends. Accurate apposition of the tendon ends is desired.

Many types of suture material are appropriate for tenorrhaphy, but monofilament nylon is preferable; this nonabsorbable material is inert and strong and passes easily through the tissues. Suture materials such as stainless steel, nylon, polypropylene, and braided polyester are acceptable. Some of the new synthetic monofilament absorbable suture material such as PDS† or MAXON‡ also may be used when there is minimum to no gap between tendon ends. The size of the suture material should be the largest that comfortably passes through the tissues. In most small animals the suture material varies from 2-0 to no. 2

It is frequently said that the suture pattern is more important than the suture material.[6,23] A number of suture

*References 1, 2, 14, 15, 23, 40, 54, 58, 61.
†Ethicon, Inc., Somerville, NJ 08876-0151.
‡Davis-Geck, Inc., Manati, PR 00701, USA.

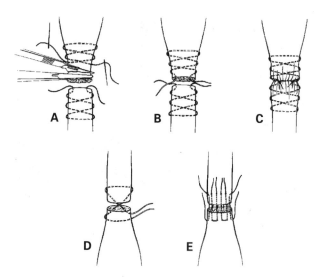

Fig. 22-3 Suture technique used for end-to-end anastomosis. **A**, **B**, and **C**, Bunnell-Mayer technique. **D**, Bunnell technique. **E**, Interrupted horizontal mattress suture technique.

Reprinted with permission from Bloomberg MS: Muscle and tendons. In Slatter DH, editor: *Textbook of small animal surgery*, ed 2, Philadelphia, 1991, Saunders.

patterns have been described in the veterinary literature, including the horizontal mattress, Bunnell, Bunnell-Mayer, locking loop (Kessler-Mason-Allen, modified Kessler), and pulley suture patterns (Fig. 22-3).[1,2,14,23,60] The locking loop and pulley suture patterns are superior because they are less constrictive to the intrinsic blood supply and provide greater tensile strength and better resistance to gap formation than the other suture patterns (Fig. 22-4).[2,4,60] The size, shape, and degree of tendon tissue available also dictate the type of suture material and pattern chosen by the surgeon.

The initial care of tendon injuries usually involves the principles of good wound management because most injuries are open wounds. The wound should be thoroughly cleansed and debrided before surgical repair. If the wound is infected, the tendon ends should be labeled with sutures to allow for later repair when the infection is under control.[15,48] The affected joint should be stabilized or coapted in flexion to allow for apposition of the tendon ends. With partial disruption of a tendon, the affected area should be placed in flexion or the animal's activity restricted to kennel rest to avoid further damage.

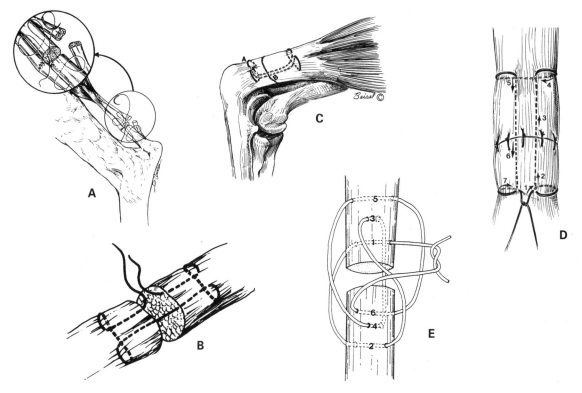

Fig. 22-4 **A** and **B**, Locking loop (Kessler-Mason-Allen) suture technique. **C** and **D**, Modified Kessler suture. These two suture patterns can be used for end-to-end tendon anastomosis. It is important that the transverse segment of either suture pattern passes just superficial to the two longitudinal segments of the suture (**D**). **E**, Three-loop pulley suture pattern. The initial loop is made when the needle passes 1 and 2 are placed in a near-far pattern. The three continuous horizontal mattress sutures or loops are positioned in separate planes approximately 120 degrees apart. Each loop is tightened before tying the knot.

A and B reprinted with permission from Tomlinson J, Moore R: Locking loop tendon suture use in repair of five calcanean tendons, *Vet Surg* 3:105-109, 1982; C and D reprinted with permission from Aron DN: A "new" tendon stitch, *J Am Anim Hosp Assoc* 17:587-591, 1981; E reprinted with permission from Berg RJ, Egger EL: In vitro comparison of the three loop pulley and locking loop suture patterns for repair of canine weightbearing tendons and collateral ligaments, *Vet Surg* 15:107-110, 1986.

Conservatively treated tendon injuries are usually limited to injuries at the musculotendinous junction or partial tears. Cage rest, restricted activity, and physiotherapy modalities such as cold laser, ultrasound, and magnetic field therapy may aid the healing process and minimize adhesion formation.

Surgical repair of several tendons. Surgical repair is the treatment of choice for most tendon injuries in small animals. This is because laceration of the tendons is more common than complete or partial rupture. The best method of restoration of several tendons is primary end-to-end tenorrhaphy.[6] This may not be possible in severely traumatized tendons or chronically injured tendons that have contracted.

When the tendon injury is accompanied by an open wound, the surgeon must decide if a primary or delayed repair should be performed. Although the "golden period" of wound healing has been described as being 6 to 8 hours, this period can be extended by means of copious lavage and meticulous debridement of the wound.[48]

If the wound is severely infected or the surrounding soft tissues are of questionable viability, the wound should be lavaged and debrided. This should be followed by the placement of nonabsorbable monofilament marker sutures in the stumps of the tendons. This allows location of the tendons when a secondary tenorrhaphy is performed after the environment of the wound improves. This technique is excellent in theory but should be reserved for situations when tissue grafts or synthetic materials will be implanted into tendon defects. Immediate, direct end-to-end anastomosis of severed tendons when possible is preferred.

Various suture patterns and anastomosis techniques have been described, but by far most injuries allow for end-to-end anastomosis.[6] Round or semiround tendons should be repaired with a locking loop or pulley-type suture pattern. Small, flat tendons may be better repaired using the Bunnell-type suture pattern or horizontal mattress sutures. Avulsion tendon injuries are best repaired by reattaching the avulsed piece of bone with a bone screw or tension-band wiring. If the tendon has torn away without a piece of bone or too small a piece of bone, it can be secured by running the suture through holes drilled in the main bone fragment (Fig. 22-5).

Following apposition of the tendon ends, the paratenon of each stump of tendon should be closed using smaller single interrupted, simple continuous, or horizontal mattress suture.[6]

Tendon lengthening. Lengthening of a tendon is usually indicated for contracture deformities caused by muscle fibrosis or chronic tendon contracture after previous injury. Surgery is seldom indicated unless there is a severe chronic lameness or conformational deformity.

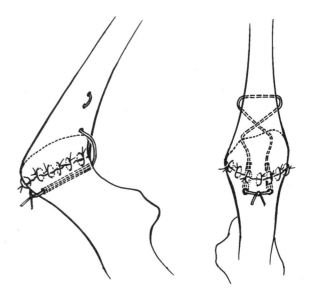

Fig. 22-5 Repair of an avulsion of the calcanean tendon from the tuber calcaneus. Bunnell suture has been woven through the tendon and then continued through two drill holes in the calcaneus and tied to itself. Sutures should be placed in the paratendinous tissue to enhance collateral stability of the tendon.

Reprinted with permission from Bloomberg MS: Muscle and tendons. In Slatter DH, editor: *Textbook of small animal surgery,* ed 2, Philadelphia, 1991, Saunders.

The most common clinical entities requiring tendon lengthening are fibrotic myopathy of the semitendinosus or semimembranosus muscles, contracture deformities of the flexor tendons of the carpus, and infraspinatus tendon contracture.* If the function of the muscle must be preserved, the tendon should be lengthened. However, if the function of the muscle can be sacrificed, the treatment of choice is incision or release of the contracted fibrotic tendon. The most common surgical methods of tendon lengthening are the techniques of Z tenotomy and accordion incision (Fig. 22-6).[6,8,15,57]

The Z tenotomy involves the half-section splitting by means of an elongated Z incision (Fig. 22-6, *A*). The tendon is first split longitudinally, then the ends of the incision are incised in the opposite direction. The ends of the tendon are separated the desired distance but left overlapping to allow for a side-to-side anastomosis. The sides of the overlapping tendons are apposed with interrupted horizontal mattress suture patterns. This is followed by closure of the paratenon in a simple continuous pattern.

The accordion technique works well in combined musculotendinous contractures, such as in fibrotic myopathy of the semitendinosus or semimembranosus muscles (Fig. 22-6, *D*). The fibrotic tissue must first be freed from the surrounding tissue. This is followed by making

---

*References 12, 23, 33, 34, 37, 41, 42, 44, 51.

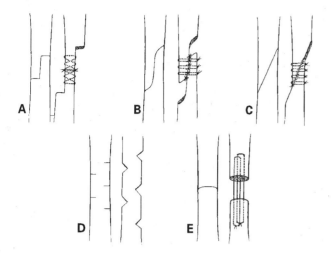

Fig. 22-6 Various tendon-lengthening techniques: **A**, Z tenotomy. **B**, Modification of the Z tenotomy. **C**, Oblique section and gliding. **D**, Accordion partial tenotomy. **E**, Lange method.

Modified from Butler HC: Tendon, muscle and fascia. In Archibald J, editor: *Canine surgery*, ed 2, Santa Barbara, Calif, 1974, American Veterinary Publications.

full-thickness incisions through approximately one-third the width of the tendon. The incisions should alternate from side to side until the desired lengthening is reached.[15] The length between the incisions varies with the tendon's size.

Tendon shortening. The techniques of tendon shortening are usually indicated for tendon injuries in which a previous repair has failed or repair was not performed, resulting in hyperextension or hyperflexion of a joint. Examples include improper healing of the Achilles mechanism or improper healing of the superficial and deep flexor tendons of the forelimb. Care must be taken to examine the animal carefully to rule out concurrent ligamentous injury.

A tendon can be shortened by several techniques.[6,10,15] The difficulty in using such techniques as the Hoffa method or doubling over the tendon is that the tendons are often thickened and fibrotic, making these techniques difficult (Fig. 22-7, *A* and *B*). In addition, the sutures may loosen prematurely, resulting in lengthening again.

The prefered technique is the Z tenotomy, which involves a similar technique as described for lengthening of the tendon, but an area of the Z incision is excised (Fig. 22-7, *C*).[6,10,15] Another technique involves simple tenectomy of a transverse section followed by an end-to-end anastomosis (Fig. 22-7, *D*).[2,15] After any lengthening or shortening of a tendon, the same postoperative management should be followed as for any type of tendon repair.

Tendon grafts. Primary end-to-end anastomosis of severely injured tendons or chronic injuries may not be feasible because of extensive loss of tendon tissue or contracture of the ends of the tendon. Although frequently

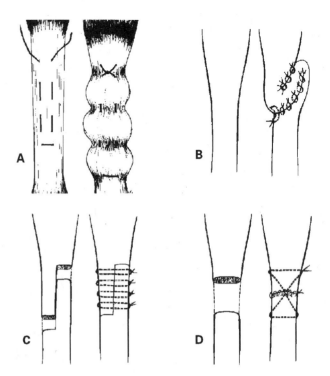

Fig. 22-7 Tendons may be shortened using the following techniques. **A**, Hoffa method. **B**, Doubling over. **C**, Z tenectomy. **D**, Segmental tenectomy.

Modified from Butler HC: Tendon, muscle and fascia. In Archibald J, editor: *Canine surgery*, ed 2, Santa Barbara, Calif, 1974, American Veterinary Publications.

used in tendon repair in human hand surgery, tendon grafts are seldom indicated in small animal tendon repair.

Large tendon defects are usually repaired with synthetic material such as polyester, dacron, carbon fibers, or other nonabsorbable surgical implant material.[6,9,63,64] The implant is used to fill the gap between the tendon ends. The graft may be woven into the ends of the tendon or used as a suture material. This implant material serves to restore function to the muscle tendon unit while acting as a scaffold for the formation of fibrous connective tissue scar.

The tensor fascia lata is an excellent source of autogenous tissue to use as a graft to fill a tendon defect.[2,9,11] The fascial graft is harvested in a strip 1 to 2 cm in width. The graft can then be sutured directly to the tendon ends with a Bunnell-Mayer or Bunnell suture pattern.[9,11] Alternatively, the graft may be used as a suture. The graft is passed through the proximal portion of the tendon defect and sutured back in itself. The graft is then passed through the distal tendon end and carried back to the proximal portion of the tendon defect. Each strip of graft should be sutured to itself. If remaining graft is available, it should be wrapped like a tube around itself (Fig. 22-8).[2]

The healing period after repair of a tendon defect using an implant is much longer than after primary repair. The repair site should be immobilized for 6 to 8

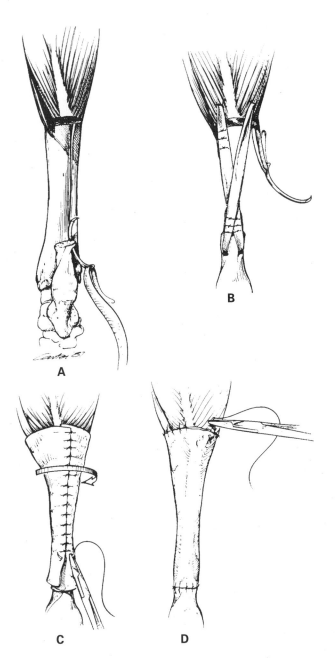

Fig. 22-8   Fascial graft technique for repair of chronic ruptures of the common calcanean tendon.

Reprinted with permission from Aron DW: Tendons. In Bojrab MJ, editor: *Current techniques in small animal surgery*, ed 3, Philadelphia, 1990, Lea & Febiger. (Modified from White RK, Kraynick BM: *Surg Gynecol Obstet* 180:117, 1959.)

weeks using external pin splintage, casts, or splints (Fig. 22-9).[2,28,50] After removal of the external support, the animal's activity should be restricted to leash or kennel activity for an additional 3 to 4 weeks.

Tendon transposition or relocation. Tendon transposition or relocation is a technique that can be used to alter the function of a muscle, stabilize a diarthrodial joint, or fill a tendon defect. With peripheral nerve paralysis, a tendon of a functioning flexor muscle can be

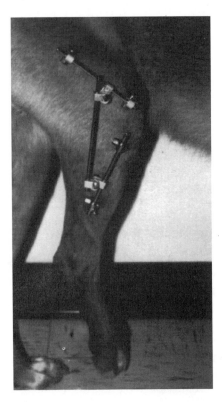

Fig. 22-9   Transarticular type I external pin splintage placed on the stifle of a dog after surgical stabilization of a deranged stifle.

transposed and anastomosed to the tendon of insertion of a paralyzed extensor muscle. For example, with paralysis of the extensors of the carpus (radial nerve) and tarsus (peroneal nerve), the tendon of the insertion of a flexor of the carpus or flexor of the tarsus can be anastomosed side by side to the respective extensor tendon (Fig. 22-10). A combination of external coaptation and physical therapy often results in restoration of limb function. These techniques have been described in detail in the veterinary literature.*

The technique of tendon transposition or relocation has been used to stabilize the shoulder, hip, and stifle joints of small animals. For example, the caudal/distal transposition of the greater trochanter (insertion of the tendon of middle gluteal muscles) has been used to stabilize the hip joint after surgical reduction of a luxated hip. Medial or lateral transposition of the tendons of origin of the bicipital tendon has been used to stabilize a luxating humeral head. Numerous techniques have been described in the literature relative to transposition of muscles and tendons in and around the stifle joint for treatment of rupture of the cruciate ligaments.

A tendon can also be transferred to restore the continuity of another tendon. An example is using the distal end of the peroneus brevis tendon to fill a defect in the common calcanean (calcaneal) tendon (Fig. 22-11).[2]

---

*References 2, 3, 27, 36, 39, 45.

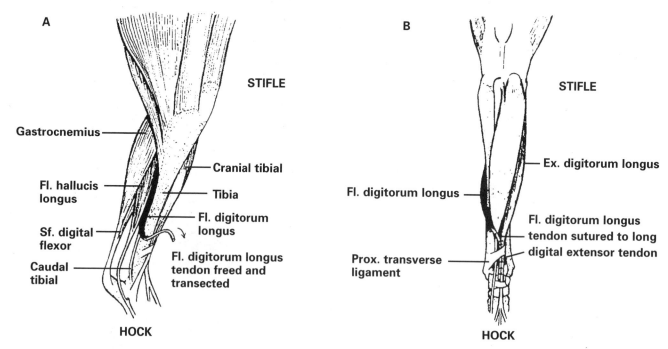

Fig. 22-10   Relocation of the flexor digitorum longus muscle for treatment of peroneal nerve paralysis. **A**, Medial aspect of the lower hind limb showing dissection of the flexor digitorum longus muscle. **B**, Cranial aspect of the lower hind limb illustrating suturing of the flexor tendon to the long digital extensor tendon.

Reprinted with permission from Bennett D, Vaughn LC: The use of muscle relocation techniques in the treatment of peripheral nerve injuries in dogs and cats, *J Small Anim Pract* 17:99-108, 1976.

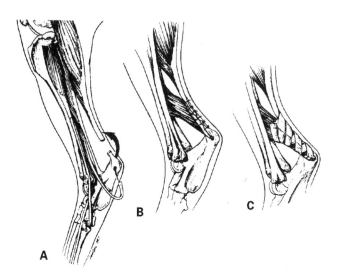

Fig. 22-11   Repair of chronic ruptures of the common calcanean tendon by transfer of the peroneus brevis tendon.

Reprinted with permission from Aron DN: Tendons. In Bojrab MJ, editor: *Current techniques in small animal surgery*, ed 3, Philadelphia, 1990, Lea & Febiger. (Modified from White RK, Kraynick BM: *Surg Gynecol Obstet* 108:117, 1959.)

Tendon displacement. The displacement of a tendon from its normal position, especially as it crosses a joint, can result in limb dysfunction and clinical lameness. The etiology of tendon displacement is usually chronic trauma to supporting ligamentous or other stabilizing connective tis-

sues. This chronic trauma causes chronic inflammation, resulting in degenerative changes to supporting structures. Examples of this type of injury include displacement of the superficial digital flexor tendon of the rear limb, tendon of origin of the long digital extensor muscle, and tendon of origin of the biceps brachii.[3,5,28,42,62] Displacement of the straight patellar tendon associated with medial or lateral patellar luxation also falls into this classification of orthopedic diseases (see Chapter 18).

Displacement of the superficial digital flexor tendon. The superficial digital flexor muscle is one of the five muscles composing the Achilles mechanism of the rear limb. The muscle originates from the lateral supracondylar tuberosity of the femur, and its tendon courses over the tuber calcanei to insert on the bases of second phalanx or P–2 of digits II, III, IV, and V. The function of the superficial digital flexor muscle is to extend the hock, flex the stifle, and flex the digits. There is a small bursa beneath where the tendon passes dorsally over the tuber calcanei. The tendon is secured laterally and medially as it passes over the tuber calcanei by dense connective tissue.[24]

Disruption of this stabilizing tissue results in displacement of the tendon laterally or medially when bearing weight on the affected limb. The lameness is usually mild and chronic in nature. The hock is slightly dropped, but not to the extent noted when the Achilles mechanism is completely disrupted.[42,65]

The skin incision should be made lateral or medial to the calcaneus rather than directly over it to avoid excessive tension. Treatment consists of the stabilization of the lateral or medial retinacular tissue using a monofilament suture material in a horizontal mattress or simple interrupted pattern. Postoperatively a soft padded bandage is applied to the operated limb, extending from the toes to midway between the hock and stifle. The bandage is left in place for 3 to 5 days, and the dog is confined to restricted or leash activity for 10 to 14 days. Prognosis for return to normal function is excellent.

Displacement of the tendon of origin of the long digital extensor muscle. Displacement of the tendon of origin of the long digital extensor muscle has been reported on rare occasions in the dog.[3,62] It usually occurs in young dogs and is evidenced by a severe chronic lameness. The tendon of origin snaps in and out of its muscular groove on the craniolateral aspect of the tibia when the stifle is flexed and extended. Treatment involves the surgical stabilization of the tendon by reconstruction of the retinacular support to the tendon. This is accomplished by the use of monofilament, nonabsorbable sutures or a metal staple placed as a roof over the tendon. As a last resort, tenotomy can be performed at the tendon's origin on the lateral femoral condyle and secured to the proximal craniolateral aspect of the proximal tibia.

Displacement of the tendon of origin of the biceps brachii muscle. Medial displacement of the tendon of origin of the biceps brachii muscle has been most frequently described in the racing greyhound but has also been reported in the miniature poodle and border collie.[28] The biceps brachii muscle is a long fusiform muscle that arises on the supraglenoid tuberosity and inserts on the proximal ends of the radius and ulna. The tendon or origin courses over the proximal cranial aspect of the humerus through the intertubercular groove. The tendon is held in place by the transverse humeral ligament that joins the lesser and greater tubercles of the humerus.[24]

Disruption of the transhumeral ligament is thought to result from a combination of chronic inflammation of the tendon and tendon sheath and the trauma of athletic competition.[28] The shoulder joint capsule acts as the tendon synovial sheath. The lameness that results is a chronic weight-bearing lameness. Palpation of the area about the tendon or origin during extension and flexion of the shoulder joint usually reveals pain and discomfort. Flexion of the shoulder joint results in medial displacement of the tendon. Extension of the elbow, with the shoulder joint held in partial flexion, may also produce medial displacement of the tendon.

Treatment of this condition in the athletically competitive dog requires surgical stabilization of the biceps tendon in the intertubercular groove. The pet dog may respond to rest and administration of nonsteroidal antiinflammatory drugs (NSAIDs).

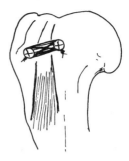

Fig. 22-12 Placement of screws at level of intertubercular groove followed by figure-eight suture pattern to mimic restoration of intertubercular ligament.

Reprinted with permission from Boemo C: Medial displacement of the tendon of origin of the biceps brachii muscle in the racing greyhound. In *Proceedings, Refresher Course on Greyhounds,* Australia:University of Sydney, 122:103-116, 1989.

Surgical treatment is accomplished through a craniomedial skin incision over the shoulder joint.[50] Extension of the shoulder joint facilitates replacement of the tendon into the groove. The chronicity of the disease may result in degenerative changes that result in a very shallow groove. If the groove is shallow, it can be deepened using a bone curette or rongeurs. Any remnants of the synovial sheath and ligament should be sutured over the tendon with monofilament, nonabsorbable suture material. Additional fixation is often necessary. This usually consists of the insertion of a bone screw on each side of the groove and the application of a figure-eight nonabsorbable suture material between the two screws and over the tendon (Fig. 22-12). Other techniques that have been used to stabilize the tendon include wire staples or a bone plate placed over the groove, forming a lid over the tendon.[28] If the tendon is too severely damaged to be replaced in the intertubercular groove, it can be incised and the tendon of origin stapled to the proximal humerus.

Postoperative care involves strict confinement with no exercise for 2 weeks. It is not necessary to place external support on the limb. This is followed by an additional 3 to 4 weeks of leash exercise, then a gradual return to normal activity.

The prognosis for return to normal function is good for the pet dog and fair for the racing greyhound.

Injury to digital extensor and flexor tendons. Disruption of the superficial and/or deep digital flexor or extensor tendons is usually caused by sharp laceration of the skin. If limb function is not compromised after trauma to these tendons, surgical intervention is not indicated. The surgeon should be less concerned about trauma to the digital extensor tendons than flexor tendons because of the many anastomoses after they branch from the main extensor tendon (Fig. 22-13).[15]

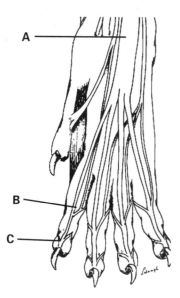

Fig. 22-13 Cranial view of the carpus of the dog. The common digital extensor tendon (**A**) has numerous anastomotic sites (**B**) before its final insertion on P-3 (**C**).

Reprinted with permission from Butler HC: Tendon, muscle, fascia. In Archibald J, editor: *Canine surgery*, ed 2, Santa Barbara, Calif, 1974, American Veterinary Publications.

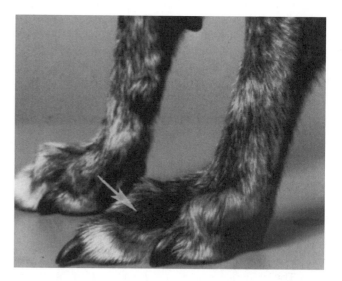

Fig. 22-14 Injury to the superficial digital flexor tendon of the fourth digit has resulted in a "dropped toe" because of inability to flex the proximal interphalangeal joint.

Courtesy of Dr. Richard Eaton-Wells, West Chermside Veterinary Clinic, Brisbane, Australia.

The most common digital tendon injury involves the severance of all or part of the superficial and deep digital flexor tendons. The insertions of the superficial and deep digital flexor tendons are on the proximal end of the second phalanx or P-2 and third phalanx or P-3 respectively. Severance of the superficial digital flexor tendon results in flattening of the digit, which is termed "dropped toe" (Fig. 22-14).[21]

The flexor tendons are more often lacerated just above or below the metatarsal or metacarpal foot pad. The animal usually has extensive hemorrhage because of surrounding soft tissue damage. Once emergency first aid has been administered, manipulation of the digits or visualization through the wound aids in the diagnosis of the injury.

If there is flattening of one or more of the digits or elevation of the toes, surgical exploration is indicated. This is especially true for athletic dogs such as the racing greyhound. It may be cosmetically indicated in the pet dog. Repair is also indicated if the foot is severely dropped to avoid excoriation of the foot pads.

Surgical exposure of the digital tendons is directly over the site of injury. If a skin laceration is present, it may be modified to provide adequate exposure. The tendon ends should be anastomosed as described earlier in the text. If the skin wound is contaminated, it should be thoroughly cleansed and debrided. Drainage should be provided if the skin edges are closed primarily. Postoperatively the foot should be placed in partial flexion in external coap-

tation for 3 to 4 weeks. After removal of the external support, activity should be restricted for 3 to 4 more weeks.

Chronic digital flexor and extensor tendon injuries carry a poor prognosis. Reattachment of the severed tendon ends is difficult because of excessive scar tissue and retraction of the tendon ends. If the ends can be isolated and mobilized, the defect can be spanned with tendon grafts, fascial grafts, or suture material.

Severed Achilles mechanism (common calcanean tendon). The Achilles mechanism is also commonly referred to as the Achilles tendon, common calcanean (calcaneal) tendon, or gastrocnemius tendon. It actually is three tendons formed from a combination of five muscles. The medial and lateral heads of the gastrocnemius muscle fuse distally to form a large tendon that inserts on the tuber calcanei. The tendon of insertion of the superficial digital flexor muscle and the common tendon of the biceps femoris, gracilis, and semitendinosus muscles are the other two tendon components of the Achilles mechanism. The function of the Achilles mechanism is to extend the tibiotarsal joint while flexing the stifle and digits.[24]

Rupture of the common calcanean tendon can occur at the musculotendinous junction, at the midsubstance, or at or near the tendon's insertion on the tuber calcanei.* The tendon is disrupted usually by sharp trauma in the pet animal or by blunt trauma combined with distractive forces, as in the racing greyhound.

---

*References 8-10, 42, 43, 54, 55, 63, 64, 66.

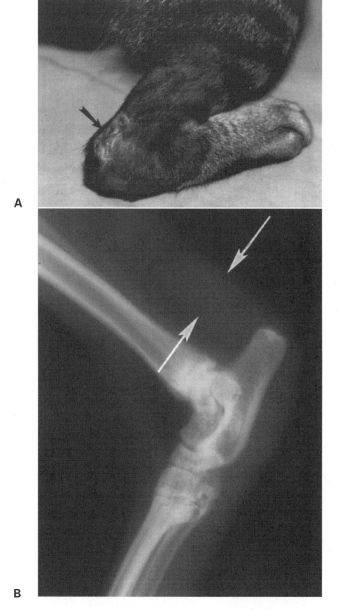

A

B

Fig. 21-15 **A**, Cat with laceration of the common calcanean tendon of its right rear leg. Note the plantigrade posture and wound on the dorsal aspect of the calcaneus. **B**, Lateral radiographic view of the rear leg demonstrating the fibrous thickening in the area of the damaged tendon.

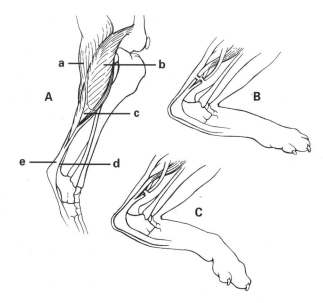

Fig. 22-16 Rupture of the gastrocnemius tendon and common tendon of the biceps femoris, gracilis, and semitendinosus muscles. **A**, Lateral view of Achilles mechanism. *a*, Semitendinosus muscle; *b*, gastrocnemius muscle; *c*, superficial digital flexor muscle; *d*, tendon of the gastrocnemius muscle; *e*, common tendon of the biceps femoris muscle, gracilis muscle, and semitendinosus muscle. **B**, Note hyperflexion of the hock with complete rupture of the common calcanean tendon. **C**, On weight bearing, the hock not only drops, but the digits flex, indicating the superficial digital flexor tendon is intact (*arrow*).

Modified from Reinke JD, Kus SP: Achilles mechanism injury in the dog, *Comp Cont Educ* 8:639-645, 1982.

Severance of the common calcanean tendon should be repaired surgically if possible. If a skin wound is present, it should be thoroughly cleansed and debrided. Depending on the location of the skin wound, the incision should be made lateral to the tendon rather than directly over the tendon and calcaneus. Each of the three tendon components should be debrided, followed by direct end-to-end anastomosis of the tendon ends. Anastomosis is enhanced by extending the tarsus. The locking loop or pulley suture pattern should be used and the wound closed as described previously (see Fig. 22-4).

If the tendon is avulsed from the calcaneus, repair can be accomplished using two methods (Fig. 22-17). If a large enough piece of bone is avulsed, it can be reattached using a bone screw and washer or a tension band. If this technique cannot be used, the tendon is reattached by first placing the suture in the proximal portion of the tendon. To incorporate all the tendon components, two sutures should be used. The ends of the sutures are then passed through two drill holes in the calcaneus and tied once the tendon is approximated to its insertion (see Fig. 22-5). The surrounding soft tissues should be sutured to

Affected animals usually demonstrate a plantigrade posture of the affected limb (Fig. 22-15). The tarsus is hyperflexed and the stifle hyperextended. If the superficial digital flexor is intact, the digits are partially flexed (Fig. 22-16).[7,9,15,54] The Achilles mechanism should be thoroughly palpated to locate the site of disruption. Radiographs should be taken of the tarsus to determine if there is an avulsion of the tendon from, or fracture of, the calcaneus.

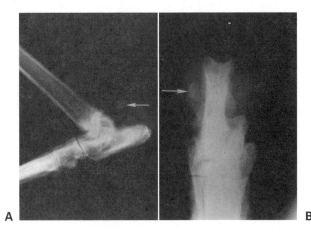

Fig. 22-17 Lateral (**A**) and "skyline" (**B**) views of the tarsus of a dog with a chronic avulsion of the insertion of the common calcanean tendon. Note the avulsed bone fragments (*arrows*) and hyperflexed tibiotarsal joint (**A**).

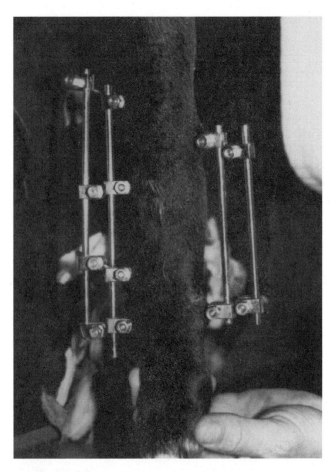

Fig. 22-18 Transarticular skeletal fixation placed across tarsal joint to immobilize the tarsus for treatment of severely comminuted calcaneal fracture.

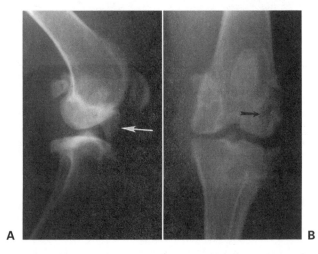

Fig. 22-19 Lateral (**A**) and craniocaudal (**B**) radiographic views of the stifle of a 5-year-old English sheepdog. Note the defect in the lateral condyle (**B**) and the avulsed piece of bone within the stifle joint (**A**). The avulsed piece of bone was excised through a lateral arthrotomy because of the chronic nature of the injury. The proximal end of the tendon was secured to the proximal lateral tibia and joint capsule.

the tendon at its insertion on the calcaneus with simple interrupted sutures. This prevents potential deviation of the tendon from the calcaneus. In chronic or severe injuries the surgeon may be unable to perform end-to-end anastomosis of the tendon. Such defects may be spanned by nonabsorbable suture, autogenous fascia, or transposition of the peroneus brevis tendon.[2]

Postoperatively the hock must be immobilized in a semiextended position for 6 to 8 weeks. This can be accomplished with an external fixator, cast, or placement of a bone screw or intramedullary pin that engages the calcaneus and the distal tibia (Fig. 22-18). Additional immobilization can be afforded by placement of a figure-eight stainless steel wire between the tuber calcanei and distal caudal tibia. The tibia tarsal joint should be immobilized at a functional angle for the breed. After removal of the immobilization device, the animal should be confined for an additional 3 to 4 weeks to leash or kennel activity.

The prognosis for recovery is good in pet dogs except for the very large breeds. The prognosis in the racing greyhound is poor for return to racing.

Avulsion of the tendon of origin of the long digital extensor muscle. The tendon of origin of the long digital extensor muscle originates intraarticularly on the lateral condyle of the femur. The tendon inserts on the extensor process of P-3 of digits II, III, IV, and V. The long digital extensor muscle's function is to extend the digits and flex the tarsus.[24]

This injury has been reported most often in immature large breeds of dogs.[34,46,51,52] The animal usually has a chronic weight-bearing lameness. Palpation of the stifle reveals some lateral swelling and pain. This injury seldom is diagnosed acutely because of the mild lameness. Radio-

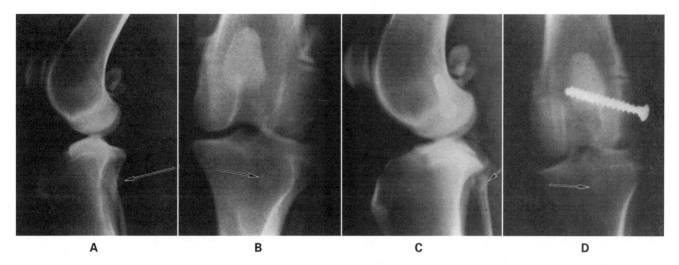

Fig. 22-20   Lateral (**A**) and craniocaudal (**B**) radiographs of the stifle showing distal displacement of the sesamoid bone of the popliteal tendon (*arrow*). Lateral (**C**) and craniocaudal (**D**) radiographs of the stifle taken immediately postoperatively. A bone screw has been placed in the lateral condyle of the femur. The arrow points to the sesamoid bone, which is located more proximally than noted preoperatively.

Reprinted with permission from Pond MJ, Losonsky JM: Avulsion of the popliteus muscle in the dog: a case report, *J Am Anim Hosp Assoc* 12:60-63, 1976.

graphic evaluation may assist early detection if a piece of bone is avulsed with the tendon (Fig. 22-19). More frequently the radiographs of the stifle reveal an avulsed segment of bone and cartilage with chronic proliferative changes. The diagnosis is confirmed by exploratory arthrotomy.

The treatment of choice is surgical reattachment of the avulsed piece of bone through a lateral arthrotomy. The avulsed segment of bone and its tendon should be reattached with a bone screw and spiked washer. If the tendon cannot be reattached, the bony fragment and intra-articular potion of the tendon should be excised. The remaining portion of the proximal tendon can be stapled or sutured extraarticularly on the proximal craniolateral aspect of the tibia.[34,51]

Postoperatively the stifle should be protected from hyperflexion by placement in a full-length half cast, modified Robert Jones dressing, or Schroeder-Thomas splint for 2 to 3 weeks. After removal of the coaptation, activity should be restricted for an additional 2 to 3 weeks. The prognosis for return to normal function is good except for very chronic cases accompanied by degenerative joint disease.

Avulsion of tendon of origin of the popliteus muscle. The tendon of origin of the popliteus muscle originates from the lateral femoral condyle just medial to the collateral ligament of the stifle. A small sesamoid bone is located in the tendon near its origin. The tendon of origin courses caudally to the stifle to blend with the popliteus muscle on the caudal aspect of the proximal tibia. The popliteus muscle functions to flex the stifle and inwardly rotate the leg.[24]

Avulsion of the tendon of origin of the popliteus muscle is a rare injury.[58] It may occur more often, but an accurate diagnosis may not be made if radiographic evaluation of the stifle is not performed (Fig. 22-20).[53] The clinical signs are very similar to other stifle injuries, such as a rupture of the anterior cruciate ligament. Radiographic evaluation of the affected stifle reveals distal displacement of the sesamoid bone of the popliteal tendon.

The treatment of choice is surgical reattachment of the avulsed tendon. The stifle joint should be approached through a lateral parapatellar skin incision.[50] After caudal reflexion of the biceps femoris muscle, the lateral joint capsule should be incised to expose the origin of the popliteal tendon medial and caudal to the collateral ligament. The avulsed tendon is usually accompanied by a portion of bone from the lateral femoral condyle. The tendon is reattached to its origin using a staple or bone screw and spiked washer. Postoperative management of this condition is similar to that of avulsion of the long digital extensor.

Avulsion of the head(s) of the gastrocnemius muscle. The two bellies of the gastrocnemius muscle are the main components of the common calcanean tendon. The muscles originate from the tendinous attachment of the lateral and medial heads on the lateral and medial supracondylar tuberosities of the posterior distal femur. Avulsion of these attachments is also an unusual injury that may go undiagnosed. Each head of the gastrocnemius muscle has a small sesamoid bone, referred to as a fabella, buried in its tendon of origin. Each fabella articulates with its respective femoral condyle and is bound to it by ligamentous tissue.[24]

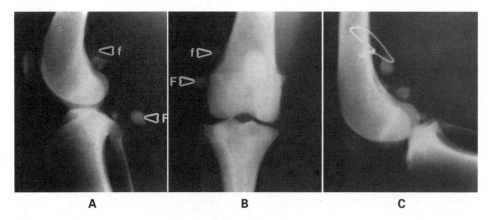

Fig. 22-21 Radiographs depicting avulsion of the lateral head of the gastrocnemius muscle. **A**, Lateral view showing that the lateral fabella has been fractured into one small proximal fragment (f). **B**, Craniocaudal view also demonstrates f in a nondisplaced position and F displaced distally. **C**, Postoperative lateral view showing that a wire has been passed around the base of the distal fracture fragment of the lateral fabella and pulled proximally into reduction.

Reprinted with permission from Reinke JD and others: Traumatic avulsion of the lateral head of the gastrocnemius and superficial digital flexor muscles in a dog, J Am Anim Hosp Assoc 18:252-256, 1982.

The clinical diagnosis is based on the presence of a rear leg weight-bearing lameness characterized by hyperflexion of the hock with weight bearing.[17,55] Radiographic evaluation of the affected stifle reveals distal displacement of the fabella (Fig. 22-21). The treatment of choice involves surgical reattachment of the head(s) of the gastrocnemius muscle. This is accomplished through a lateral or medial parapatellar skin incision, depending on the type of injury.[50] The displaced head of the gastrocnemius muscle is repositioned by placing proximal traction on the displaced fabella. This traction is made possible by securing a heavy nonabsorbable suture either around or through a drill hole in the fabella. The suture is then passed through a drill hole in the supracondylar tuberosity of the femur. Additional sutures should be placed in any remnants of tendinous insertion (Fig. 22-22). Postoperative care is similar to that for other tendon injuries described in this chapter.

Avulsion of the tendon of origin and insertion of the biceps brachii muscle. The function of the biceps brachii muscle is described earlier in this chapter. The tendon of origin originates from the supraglenoid tuberosity of the scapula. The tendon inserts on the proximal radius and ulna. Avulsion of the origin of the biceps brachii has been described primarily in young, large breeds of dogs, whereas avulsion of the insertion has been reported in the racing greyhound.[21]

The clinical signs include a weight-bearing lameness. There is pain on flexion and extension of the shoulder or elbow, depending on whether the origin or the insertion of the tendon is involved. Treatment of both conditions involves the reattachment of the avulsed tendon and accompanying piece of bone using a bone screw, bone

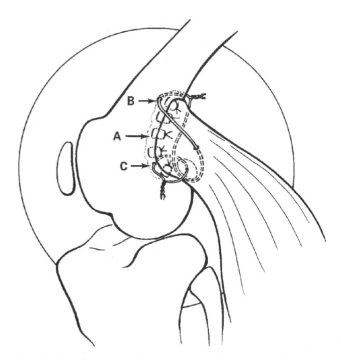

Fig. 22-22 Depiction of various methods of repair of an avulsion of the head of the gastrocnemius muscle. The muscle may be reattached by primary suture of the tendinous tissue of origin (**A**), figure-eight wire suture around the fabella and through drill hole in distal femur (**B**), wire suture through caudodistal femur and the fabella (**C**), or any combination of these methods.

Reprinted with permission from Bloomberg MS: Muscles and tendons. In Slatter DH, editor: *Textbook of small animal surgery*, ed 2, Philadelphia, 1991, Saunders.

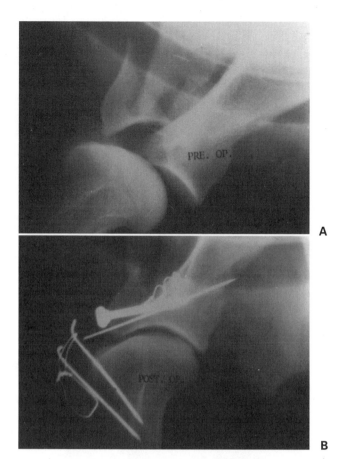

Fig. 22-23 **A**, Lateral radiographic view of a dog with a comminuted scapular fracture. The supraglenoid tubercle has been distracted by the pull of the origin of the biceps brachii muscle. **B**, Repair technique using a lag screw and K wire. Note that surgical exposure was enhanced after osteotomy of the greater tubercle of the humerus. The osteotomy was also repaired with a pin and tension-band wire.

Courtesy of Dr. Robert Parker, University of Florida, Gainesville.

screw and washer, or Kirschner (K) wires and tension-band wire (Fig. 22-23).[42] The surgical approaches have been described in detail for craniomedial shoulder joint and the elbow joint.[50]

Postoperative care consists of bandaging the front leg with the shoulder in extension and the elbow flexed. The external support should be left in place for 2 to 3 weeks, followed by 3 to 4 weeks of kennel confinement or limited leash exercise. The prognosis for return to function is excellent if the fixation does not fail prematurely.

LIGAMENT INJURIES

An injury to a ligament is termed a sprain.[13,25] Although the "crimp" in ligaments provides for limited elasticity, when fibers become elongated by 10% or more, disruption occurs.[13,67]

Ligamentous injuries have been classified as three types of sprains.[13,25] A *first-degree sprain* is a mild dis-

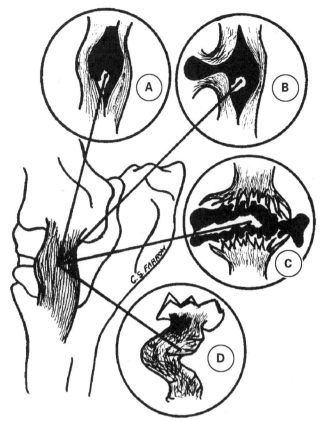

Fig. 22-24 Sprain classification schemes generally focus on the qualitative aspects of the ligamentous injury. First-degree sprain injury involves minimum tearing of ligament and associated fibers, as well as a varying degree of internal hemorrhage (**A**). Second-degree sprain usually results in definite structural breakdown as a result of partial tearing. Hemorrhage is both internal and periligamentous, with inflammatory edema being moderately extensive (**B**). Third-degree sprain is most severe and often involves complete rupture of the ligament body (**C**). Avulsion at the points of origin or insertion usually results in one or more small bone fragments, which may often be identified radiographically (**D**).

From Farrow CS: Sprain, strain, and contusion, *Vet Clin North Am* 8(2):169-182, 1978.

ruption of the ligamentous tissues resulting from a moderate force (Fig. 22-24, *A*). Minimum damage to collagen fibers, little loss of function, and minimum instability of the involved joint occur. An inflammatory process ensues with the formation of hematoma and edema. This type of injury heals rapidly with minimum or no treatment. A *second-degree sprain* is moderate in its severity (Fig. 22-24, *B*). Compared with the first-degree sprain, a more extensive disruption of collagen fibers and greater inflammatory reaction occur. As a result, there is more soft tissue swelling in the area of the injury and greater functional disability and joint instability. The ligament remains functionally intact, and healing proceeds well without surgical treatment. A *third-degree sprain* is the most severe ligamentous injury because it involves a partial or complete interstitial disruption of the ligament or avulsion of the bony insertion of the ligament (Fig. 22-24, *C* and *D*). The affected joint is unstable, and function is completely lost. Surgical restoration of the ligament is generally required to restore joint function. Conservative treatment may result in joint instability that results in chronic degenerative joint disease and lameness.

Anatomy and Physiology

Ligaments are highly specialized, dense connective tissue structures that connect bones to other bones. Ligaments provide stability to joints and serve to guide joint motion. There is also evidence that ligaments have a neurosensory role in supplying proprioceptive information and act as transducers of dynamic information to muscles.[67]

Ligaments consist of water, types I and III collagen, several proteoglycans, elastin, and various other substances. They are relatively hypocellular, with the predominant cells being the fibroblasts in the main substance of the ligament and more chondroid cells near the insertion of the ligaments. Ligaments are less elastic than tendons. Their limited elasticity is enhanced by the periodic wave of the collagen fibers known as its "crimp." The tensile strength of ligaments varies with age. As an animal matures, a ligamentous injury is more likely to involve the midsubstance. In the immature animal, a ligament is more likely to fail by avulsion.[13,25] The gross configuration of ligaments varies from flat bands to round structures. The configuration thus dictates the type of suture pattern chosen for repair.

Healing of Ligaments

Ligamentous tissues are similar to tendons in that they are relatively avascular. Injury to ligaments is followed by the classical stages of inflammation. The degree of inflammatory response depends on the extent of damage to surrounding soft tissues and degree of joint instability. A common cause of ligamentous injuries in small animals is shearing injuries of the carpus and tarsus. This type of injury results in open, contaminated wounds with severe joint instability (Fig. 22-25). The stages of healing are very similar to those of tendons; however, the healing process requires 3 to 4 weeks more than for tendon healing. In first- and second-degree sprains, the gap in the ligamentous tissue is replaced by a weaker fibrous scar tissue unless the ends of the ligament are reunited. It has been demonstrated in humans and animals that passive motion and partial weight bearing during the early phases of ligament healing result in a rapid regeneration of ligamentous tissue and more correct anatomical alignment of the collagen fibers, as well as a ligament that heals with more strength.[66] However, veterinary patients are not cooperative, and optimum healing depends on

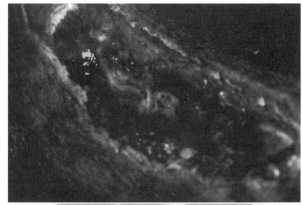

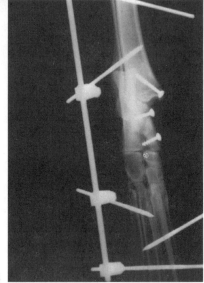

Fig. 22-25 A, Lateral view of the tarsus of a dog with a shearing injury. Note the gross debris and destruction of ligamentous support to the medial aspect of the tarsal joints. **B**, Craniocaudal radiographic view showing stabilization of the tarsal joints with bone screws and external pin splintage.

early immobilization of the affected joint for 4 to 6 weeks followed by gradual return to activity over the next 8 to 12 weeks.[13]

Diagnosis

The initial treatment of any ligamentous injury must be preceded by a diagnosis. The animal will usually have a history of acute trauma with varying degrees of lameness and soft tissue swelling in the area of the injury. Unless there is a third-degree sprain, no joint instability is demonstrated. If an acute ligamentous injury is suspected, it is important to palpate carefully for joint instability as soon as possible after the injury. If physical examination is delayed, the subsequent soft tissue swelling and discomfort to the animal make all but severe ligamentous injuries difficult to detect. The degree of lameness, pain, and swelling is directly related to the severity of the sprain.

Physical examination is often enhanced by the administration of tranquilizers or analgesics. The affected joint should be carefully palpated and taken through a full range of motion to detect any instability or crepitus. The joint should be stressed in cranial and caudal directions as well as in lateral and medial directions.

Physical examination should be followed by radiographic evaluation of the affected area. Mild and moderate sprains usually have roentgenographic changes reflective of soft tissue swelling. Third-degree or severe sprains may show articular fractures or bony avulsions of the ligamentous insertions as well. Stressed radiographic views of the affected joint are also important in the assessment of the degree of instability.

Treatment

The initial treatment of ligamentous injuries involves the basic principles of first aid, that is, cold and immobilization. After the initial injury, the swollen area should have cold water or melting ice (hand-held ice cube or ice on a popsicle stick works well) placed on the area two or three times per day for 15 to 20 minutes. After 24 to 48 hours, the cold treatment should be replaced with the application of heat via warm water, liniments, or various physiotherapy techniques that generate heat, that is, ultrasound, diathermy, and so on. A soft, padded bandage should be applied from the tip of the toes to above the affected joint to minimize soft tissue swelling. If joint instability is present, more secure coaptation splinting is indicated.

For first-degree sprains, treatment consists of enforced rest for 7 to 10 days. A padded bandage may be helpful for the first 3 to 4 days. This is followed by 7 to 10 days of leash exercise and then return to normal activity.

Second-degree sprains should be treated by immobilization of the affected joint for 2 to 3 weeks and strict confinement. This is followed by 2 to 3 weeks in a soft, padded bandage and leash exercise only. If joint instability is present, these times should be doubled. After removal of the splint, the animal is gradually returned to restricted exercise. Return to normal activity should not occur before 10 to 12 weeks after injury.

Surgical treatment of second- or third-degree ligamentous injuries is indicated if marked joint instability exists. Surgical treatment of a moderate sprain involves the imbrication or plication of the stretched ligament in a functional position followed by external support. Surgical repair of torn ligaments involves a direct approach over the injured tissue. This is followed by careful exploration of the affected joint if the capsule is disrupted or the radiographs indicate bony damage. The suture patterns and suture materials described for tendon repair are used for ligamentous repair as well. The amount and configuration of the ligament dictate the type of suture pattern and size of suture material used. If its integrity is severely damaged such that the ligament will not hold

suture materials, it can be augmented with nonabsorbable suture materials. Braided polyester-type materials are preferred because they allow for more normal excursion of the joint and tend to fail less frequently than monofilament nonabsorbable materials such as nylon or stainless steel. The veterinary surgeon should be aware that placement of braided nonabsorbable suture materials in open, contaminated wounds may result in suture fistulas requiring removal at a subsequent date. The suture material should be secured around bone screws or through bony tunnels. The bone screws should be anatomically correct in their placement so as to mimic as much as possible the ligament's origin and insertion (see Fig. 22-25). Preplacement of K wires allows the surgeon to identify the correct site for screw placement. The suture material is wrapped in figure-eight fashion around the anchor screws. The material should be tight enough to provide normal cranial and caudal motion and stabilize any lateral or medial instability. Adjacent ligamentous or fascial tissue should be apposed adjacent to or over the prosthetic repair for reinforcement.

If the ligament is avulsed with a piece of bone, the insertion should be reattached using a bone screw and spiked washer or stainless steel wire secured in a tunnel in the bone. Avulsion fractures can also be secured with K wire(s) and a tension-band wire.

Postoperative management is similar to that of second-degree sprains. It is important not to keep the affected joint in a cast or splint for longer than 4 to 6 weeks to avoid stress shielding of the ligament.[13] After removal of the cast or splint, the dog's activity should be restricted for an additional 6 to 8 weeks while allowing weight bearing. Weight bearing promotes maturation of the fibrous scar to resemble more the original ligament and results in stronger healed tissue. Joint motion also provides nutrition to the cartilage and restores pliability of the periarticular tissues.

Postoperative immobilization of ligamentous repair can also be accomplished with external fixators. These devices are especially helpful in shearing injuries of the carpus and tarsus and allow easy access for wound treatment postoperatively.

Chronic third-degree sprains may result in varying degrees of degenerative changes to the joint surface because of instability. As described in Chapter 23, partial or complete arthrodesis of the affected joint is the usual treatment of choice.

MUSCLE INJURIES

Injuries to skeletal muscles are the result of trauma from normal activity, athletic competition, or surgical trauma when approaching a bone or body cavity. Muscle injuries, unless they are severe spontaneous disruptions, are usually not as dramatic as tendon or ligament injuries. These injuries may vary from contusions (bruising) to partial or complete disruption.

Racing greyhounds place extreme pressures and strains on their muscle tendon units as they race at speeds of 35 to 40 miles per hour in groups of seven or eight around various-shaped race tracks. It is easy to understand that such exertion results in injuries to muscles and tendons that vary from acute bruises, contusions, tears, avulsions, and ruptures to chronic atrophy and fibrous scarring. Injury to the muscle tendon unit is termed a strain and may occur within the muscle belly, at the musculotendinous junction, or at the muscle's insertion or origin. An accurate history and thorough physical examination are paramount to detect such injuries as promptly as possible. Failure of early recognition and delayed treatment can mean subpar performance or a premature end to the athlete's racing career.

Anatomy and Physiology

Striated or skeletal muscle comprises approximately one-third to one-half the total body weight of mammals.[24] Muscle mass of the racing greyhound accounts for up to 57% of its body weight.[59] Muscles function to provide the power for almost all body functions.

Skeletal muscle consists of long cylindrical fibers. Each fiber contains elongated multinuclear cells. These fibers are organized into distinctive bundles that are surrounded by connective tissue sheaths or envelopes. The outermost sheath is the epimysium and surrounds the entire muscle. The fiber bundle is surrounded by the perimysium and the individual fibers by the endomysium. The fibrous connective tissue envelopes contain the blood vessels and nerve fibers and function to allow movement between fibers, bundles, and muscles.[29,42]

Each muscle fiber is composed of individual myofibrils, which in turn are composed of several hundred thick and thin myofilaments. Muscle contraction is initiated by a nerve impulse that causes shortening of the interdigitating myofilaments.

Skeletal muscles attach to their origins or insertions by dense connective tissue in the form of a tendon, flat aponeurosis, or expanded fleshy attachment directly to bone. The proximal portion of the muscle is termed its origin and the distal part its insertion. The belly is the expanded fleshy part of the muscle; the origin is the head; and minor insertions are called slips. The nerve supply usually enters the muscle near its origin on the muscle's deep surface. In general the blood supply is close to the nerve supply.[24]

Healing of Muscles

The initial insult to the muscle results in damage to local blood vessels and, depending on the severity of the injury, to muscle fibers and the muscle sheath. Hematoma formation is followed by tissue swelling caused by extravasation of blood and extracellular fluids. This is followed within the next 6 to 12 hours by the infiltration of white blood cells (WBCs), enzyme release, and phagocytosis. Within 48 hours the repair process begins, as evidenced by capillary invasion and myoblast proliferation. This is followed by the formation of myofibers. By days 4 to 6, proliferation of fibroblasts and collagen formation result in the formation of fibrous scar tissue. By day 10 the damaged area is filled with a collagen network. The myofibrils continue to proliferate and penetrate the collagen network. The muscle's ability to heal histologically normal depends on how well the muscle edges are opposed. The tissue strength increases rapidly over 2 weeks, then slows.[26]

Stages I and II muscle injuries heal without surgical intervention by means of regeneration of muscle cells and fibrosis.[16] Stage III muscle injuries are best treated by surgery if in the acute or subacute stage. If stage III muscle injuries are left untreated, they heal by fibrous scarring. This fibrous scar can result in muscle elongation and decreased muscle action and strength.

Diagnosis and Incidence

In general, animals are very stoic, and muscle soreness often goes unnoticed. The diagnosis of musculotendinous injuries can be very subjective. Consequently, many lay people (trainers, etc.) are involved with the diagnosis and treatment of these injuries. The veterinarian may be very hesitant to challenge the opinion of an experienced dog trainer.[19,26]

It has been demonstrated that muscle soreness can be directly correlated with disruption of contractile proteins of muscle. Other indications of muscle injury include elevation of creatinine phosphokinase levels in the blood and myoglobinuria.[30] It is not unusual for a muscle injury to result from abnormal forces being placed on a limb because of the concurrent presence of another orthopedic injury. For example, during a race, a greyhound uses the right hind leg for propulsion on the curves and the left hind leg on the straightaways. If either leg has a previous injury, it may result in overcompensation by the other leg.

Muscle injuries have been divided into three stages.[30] Stage I is myositis or simple bruising or contusion. Stage II involves myositis and tearing of the sheath. Stage III involves tearing of the fascial sheath, disruption of muscle fibers, and hematoma formation. One stage may progress to another stage if proper treatment is not instituted after injury. The diagnosis of muscle injuries is by visual examination, careful palpation, and history. The greyhound is a very hardy animal and will often walk without evidence of a limp after a severe muscle injury. The history is important because the animal may present without frank lameness, but rather a poor racing performance or a subtle gait abnormality.

It has been said that dogs with persistent limps have pad, joint, or bone problems rather than muscle injuries.[26] This is supported by the fact that stage I or II muscle injuries may not result in marked lameness 24 hours after injury, although the animal may exhibit a stiff gait for the first 3 to 4 minutes of walking. A critical time to evaluate a dog for lameness is when it is turned out for exercise the morning after a race or stressful workout. Radiographs should be taken of the affected area to rule out fractures or avulsion chips. Acute strains, if examined before much swelling occurs, are often readily detectable by the presence of:

1. Localized pain
2. Inability to resist firm palpation
3. Minimum to no loss of function
4. Minimum to no heat

As the injuries advance in severity to stage II, the clinical signs become more severe with:

1. Localized swelling
2. Localized pain and slight heat
3. Some palpable tissue disruption
4. Marked pain on palpation
5. Slight loss of function
6. Variable lameness
7. Weakness
8. Asymmetry

Stage I and II injuries are usually seen in the power group of muscles such as triceps, biceps femoris quadriceps, fascia lata, semitendinous, and semimembranosus. A dog that appears to have routine muscle soreness following a race is classified with a stage I muscle injury.

Stage III muscle injuries usually present with the following clinical signs:

1. Marked lameness
2. Marked pain, swelling, and hematoma formation
3. Subcutaneous hemorrhage
4. Palpable disruption of tissues
5. Marked asymmetry

Stage III muscle injuries most often involve the long head of the triceps, gracilis (origin and insertion), gastrocnemius, and tensor fascia lata muscles.

A variety of musculotendinous injuries have been described and include damage to:

Forelimb

1. Long head of the triceps muscle
2. Insertion of the biceps brachii muscle
3. Origin of the pectoralis muscle

4. Infraspinatus tendon contracture
5. Insertion of the flexor carpi ulnaris muscle
6. Origin of infraspinatus muscle
7. Insertion of the rhomboideus thoracis muscle

Hind limb

1. Origin and insertion of the gracilis muscle
2. Origin and insertion of the tensor fascia lata
3. Origin of the pectineus muscle
4. Origin of the external abdominal oblique muscle
5. Anterior portion of the sartorius muscle
6. Achilles mechanism injury

General Principles of Treatment

The initial treatment of muscle injuries involves efforts to decrease the inflammation and reduce the swelling. The reduction in swelling results in a decrease in pain and improves local circulation. The application of cold may be in the form of ice packs, chemical packs, cold water baths, or melting ice. The area should be treated for 15 to 20 minutes two or three times per day for the first 48 hours.[6,19,26,30]

If anatomically feasible, a light compression bandage should be placed over the injured area. This restricts movement and prevents further enlargement of the hematoma. Bandaging is more appropriate for distal limb muscle injuries.[20,26]

Antiinflammatory medications may also be used to decrease the inflammation of myositis. The veterinarian must be knowledgeable of the side effects and the withdrawal times necessary to clear the drug from the serum or urine of the dog before racing. Corticosteroids can be used for the treatment of myositis when given locally or systemically. Injection of long-acting corticosteroids into muscles or tendons should be avoided. The veterinarian should be aware of the side effects of corticosteroids.[6,18,26]

The NSAIDs are very effective in treating the pain of myositis. Again, the veterinarian must be aware of the required withdrawal times of the medication. NSAIDs may be given orally or systemically. The most common side effects are vomiting and diarrhea.

Topical antiinflammatory agents such as DMSO can be applied to promote circulation and reduce edema. Ultrasound and magnetic field therapy can also be used to decrease the inflammatory response.

Another treatment modality involves physiotherapy techniques. Such techniques include electrical modalities, massage, exercise, laser and acupuncture, and needling and acupuncture. The electrical modalities may involve ultrasound, diathermy, magnetic field therapy, and microwave therapy. All these modalities increase the temperature of the treated area and thus should not be used before 48 hours following injury.

Massage of the injured tissues helps remove tissue edema and reduce adhesion formation. This technique should be used in subacute and chronic conditions. A good lubricant should be applied to the area before massage.

Exercise is an important part of therapy to prevent adhesions and allow more rapid return to function. The initiation of exercise varies with the injury but may be begun once most of the pain has subsided (5 to 10 days). The initial exercise involves walking only.

The cold laser functions by stimulating cells and has found wide use in the treatment of muscle injuries. The usual treatment regimen involves a 2- to 3-minute treatment daily. The use of acupuncture has been very successful. However, it is a time-consuming therapy that requires extensive training to administer successfully.

Stage I and II muscle tears are usually treated conservatively, which involves various combinations of ultrasound, massage, NSAIDs and 5 to 10 days of rest followed by gradual return to training.

Advanced stage II and stage III muscle injuries require immediate surgery. The clinician should allow 2 to 3 days for inflammation and hemorrhage to subside and then repair surgically. Surgical repair consists of evacuation of the hematoma, debridement of the damaged muscle, and placement of appositional sutures of synthetic absorbable suture material to reestablish continuity of the muscle. Apposition of the ends of muscle or tendon/muscle junction can be enhanced by manipulation of the affected limb, that is, adduction and addition of stints to aid in purchase of the sutures deep in the muscle tissue (Figs. 22-26 and 22-27). When possible, the anastomosis should be reinforced with horizontal mattress sutures placed in muscle fascial sheaths.

The dog should begin walking in 7 to 10 days, with return to running in 3 to 4 weeks. Some stage III muscle injuries that heal with conservative therapy allow the dog to return to competitive racing; however, the dog may drop a grade in race caliber. An example of such an injury is a torn long head of the triceps muscle. It is imperative that the veterinarian does a thorough physical examination of the injury at 3 to 4 weeks after injury before returning the dog to training.

Specific Muscle Injuries

Injuries to specific individual muscles of the dog are more common in the racing greyhound than other breeds. The basic principles of muscle repair are discussed earlier in the text. However, the unique characteristics of each individual muscle injury are briefly described here.[19,20,26,30]

Rupture of the serratus ventralis. Traumatic rupture of the serratus ventralis muscle has been reported in the

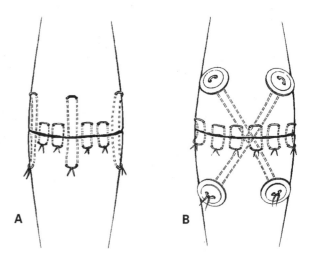

Fig. 22-26   Suture techniques for anastomosis of muscle. **A**, Interrupted horizontal mattress sutures placed deep and superficial in an attempt to penetrate any available fascial sheaths within the muscle. **B**, Interrupted horizontal mattress sutures have been bolstered by the addition of button tension sutures.

Modified from Milton JL, Henderson RA: Surgery of muscles and tendons. In Bojrab MJ, editor: *Current techniques in small animal surgery,* ed 2, Philadelphia, 1983, Lea & Febiger.

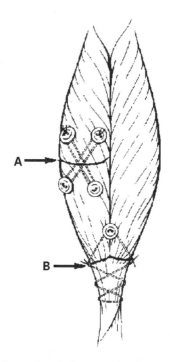

Fig. 22-27   **A**, Surgical repair of a rupture of the muscle belly of the gastrocnemius using tension button technique. **B**, Musculotendinous rupture of the distal end of the gastrocnemius muscle repaired with button tension technique and Bunnell-Mayer suture patterns.

Modified from Reinke JD, Kus SP: Achilles mechanism injury in the dog, *Comp Cont Educ* 8:639-645, 1982.

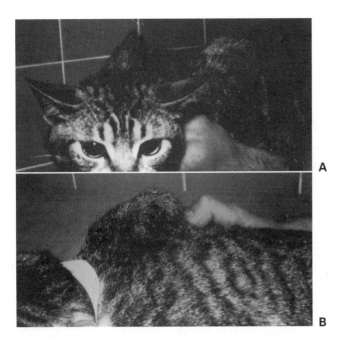

Fig. 22-28   Cat with a tear of the serratus ventralis muscle resulting in upward displacement of the scapula.

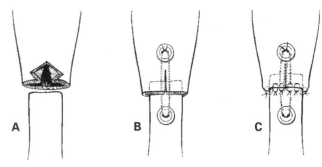

Fig. 22-29   Anastomosis of muscle at musculotendinous junction. **A**, Muscle has been slit for 2 to 3 cm, creating a bed for implantation of the tendon end. **B**, Tendon end has been implanted in the bed and secured with button tension sutures. **C**, After implantation, the fascial sheath of the muscle has been sutured to the paratenon of the tendon with simple interrupted horizontal mattress sutures of nonabsorbable material.

Modified from Braden TD: Tendon and muscles. In Bojrab MJ, editor: *Current techniques in small animal surgery*, Philadelphia, 1975, Lea & Febiger.

dog and cat.[15,31,42] It results in upward displacement of the scapula (Fig. 22-28). The condition is usually unilateral and manifests itself by upward displacement of the scapula and forelimb lameness. The diagnosis of the condition may be missed if other injuries to the forelimb prevent weight bearing on the affected limb and subsequent gross displacement is present. Consequently, such injuries as scapular fractures should be carefully evaluated to detect injury to the serratus ventralis muscle.

This condition can be treated conservatively if diagnosed acutely by placing the affected limb in a shoulder sling or some other non-weight-bearing coaptation for 3 to 4 weeks. However, animals more often have a more chronic injury. This requires surgical exposure of the torn muscle through a dorsal and caudal skin incision. This allows for exposure of the torn muscle, which can then be sutured. In addition, if repair of the muscle is not possible, the scapula may be wired to one of the ribs.

The prognosis for return to function is excellent.

Rupture of the Achilles mechanism. Disruption of the muscular or musculotendinous portion of the Achilles mechanism has been described primarily in mature dogs of the working or racing breeds. The muscle may be injured by sharp trauma, parasitic diseases, or more frequently the forces generated when the animal lands on the rear with the stifle fixed in extension. The condition is usually unilateral but may be bilateral.*

---

*References 8-10, 42, 43, 47, 54, 55, 57, 63, 64, 66.

The clinical presentation is that of an animal demonstrating tarsal hyperflexion and stifle hyperextension (see Fig. 22-15). The degree of lameness and limb deformity depends on the degree of muscle disruption. The diagnosis of Achilles mechanism injury is made by postural changes, flaccidity of the calcanean tendon, and palpation of the muscle and tendon for continuity. Careful palpation of the gastrocnemius muscle usually reveals a deficit in the muscle where it is torn or has fibrous scarring. Radiographs should be taken of the stifle and tarsus to rule out other orthopedic injuries. All three musculotendinous units must be disrupted before excessive tarsal hyperflexion is present.

Rupture of the musculotendinous junction of the Achilles mechanism should be treated surgically. A posterolateral incision should be made over the musculotendinous junction of the middle third of the tibia. The muscle and tendon tissues are anastomosed as described earlier in the text (Figs. 22-27 and 22-29).

Postoperatively the hock should be rigidly fixed in a functional position using techniques described under tendon repair in this chapter. Postoperative care is as described for repair of the calcanean tendon.

Chronic injuries to the Achilles mechanism may be treated by shortening the calcanean tendon to reestablish the function of the gastrocnemius and superficial digital flexor muscles.

Disruption of the muscle belly at midsubstance occurs infrequently. This type of injury can be treated surgically or conservatively. If a conservative approach is used, the tibiotarsal joint must be stabilized as described early in this section.

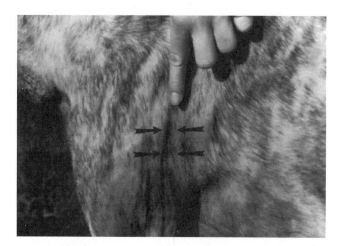

Fig. 22-30 Classical "dropped muscle" of the front leg of a racing greyhound. The finger is pointing to the defect where the insertion of the long head of the triceps muscle has torn away from the posterior scapula.

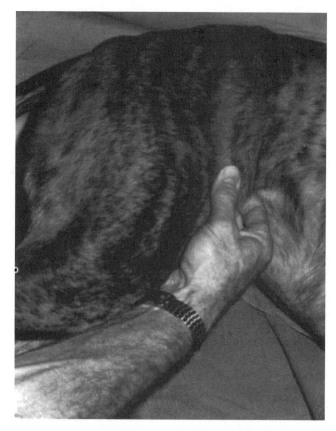

Fig. 22-31 Palpation of right flank of a racing greyhound to detect torn tensor fascia lata muscle. The torn tensor fascia lata muscle is evidenced by a depressed area dorsal and caudal to the veterinarian's thumb.

Courtesy of Dr. Robert Taylor, Alameda East Veterinary Hospital, Denver.

Rupture of long head of the triceps. Avulsion of the origin of the long head of the triceps is the classical dropped muscle in the foreleg of the racing greyhound. The muscle usually tears from its origin on the posterior edge of the scapula. It appears as a hollow, depressed area posterior and distal to the scapula (Fig. 22-30). Although this injury responds well to conservative therapy, the dog may drop a grade when it returns to racing because of decreased range of motion of the shoulder. Early surgical repair offers the best results. Repair involves the reattachment of the muscle's origin to the caudal scapula.

Injury to the flexor carpi ulnaris. The flexor carpi ulnaris muscle consists of two bellies, a humeral head, and ulnar head. The ulnar head inserts on the accessory carpal bone in a cordlike fashion.[23] The humeral head fans out on the posterior aspect of the accessory carpal bone and may have transverse tears.[21] Injury to the insertion of the flexor carpi ulnaris tendon is commonly referred to as "bowed tendon" (see Fig. 22-1). The onset of this injury is insidious, with poor performance the first sign. With successive races, the injury becomes more obvious and the area becomes bruised and swollen. The insertion of the ulnar head pulls away and may cause variously sized avulsion fractures. The transverse tears should be surgically repaired and have a good prognosis. The avulsion of the ulnar head should be likewise repaired. The chip should be reattached by wire or bone screw if large and excised if too small. Return to normal athletic function is guarded, depending on how much range of motion is restored to the carpal joint. This injury is less severe than an avulsion fracture off of the ventral and articular portions of the accessory carpal bone ac-

companied by injury to the distal accessory carpal or short radial lateral ligament. Many of these injuries are chronic and progressive, which negates surgical repair. Treatment at this stage should be 2 to 3 months' rest, physiotherapy, and possibly sclerosing agents.

Injury to the tensor fascia lata. Injury to one or both portions of the tensor fascia lata muscle is readily palpable if acute.[19,20,30,59] It most often involves the left rear leg. A depression is visible and palpable in the proximal cranial area of the thigh (Fig. 22-31). The tear usually occurs at the musculotendinous junction. Primary surgical repair is recommended (Fig. 22-32). Postoperative care is the same as for any other muscle injury. Prognosis for return to athletic performance was once thought to be poor, but with primary surgical repair, it is good.

Rupture of the gracilis. Rupture of the gracilis muscle is the classical "dropped back muscle" of the rear leg of the greyhound (Fig. 22-33). The gracilis muscle is an

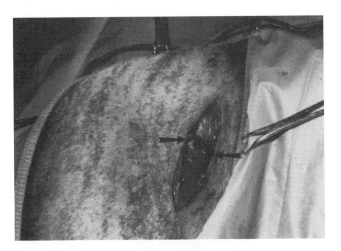

Fig. 22-32   Surgical repair of tensor fascia lata muscle.
Courtesy Dr. Robert Taylor, Alameda East Veterinary Hospital, Denver.

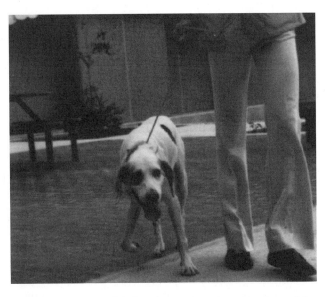

Fig. 22-34   Dog with infraspinatus muscle contracture of the right front leg. Note the characteristic way the dog carries its carpus and elbow.
Courtesy Dr. Robert Parker, University of Florida, Gainesville.

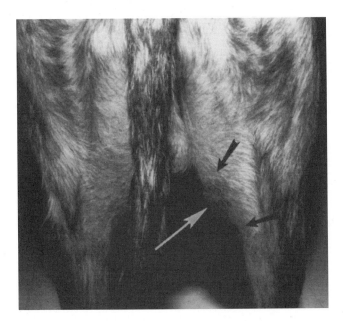

Fig. 22-33   Classical "dropped muscle" of the right rear leg of a racing greyhound. The gracilis muscle has been torn from its insertion. Note the bruising of the medial thigh.
Courtesy Dr. Robert Taylor, Alameda East Veterinary Hospital, Denver.

Muscle Contractures and Fibrosis

Infraspinatus contracture. Contracture of the infraspinatus muscle and tendon of insertion has been described primarily in the working breeds of dogs.[32,49,63] The animal has a history of having been worked, followed soon after by a painful front leg lameness.[42] The animal progressively improves, but the lameness never completely resolves. As a result, the animal is usually presented to the veterinarian with a lameness characterized by an outward rotation and adduction of the elbow and abduction of the distal forelimb with a carpal flip (Fig. 22-34). It is postulated that trauma to the shoulder area results in a progressive fibrosis and contracture of the infraspinatus muscle over 2 to 4 weeks.[49] The dog also demonstrates limited range of motion of the shoulder and abduction of the humerus. There is usually disuse atrophy of the shoulder muscles, as evidenced by a pronounced prominence of the scapular spine. The condition is usually unilateral, but I have seen it bilaterally in a Labrador retriever.

The treatment of choice is surgical excision of the contracted tissue. A lateral or caudolateral approach to the shoulder joint is used to expose the contracted infraspinatus muscle as it courses across the shoulder joint.[50] Using blunt and sharp dissection, the scarred musculotendinous area is incised. Care should be taken to remove all fibrotic tissue. Once the fibrotic muscle and tendon are incised completely, the forelimb easily moves into a more normal adduction positon. Postoperatively the animal should be allowed to bear weight on the limb immediately, with gradual return to normal activity in 10 to 14 days. The prognosis for full recovery is excellent.

adductor of the thigh and extender of the hip and hock.[24] Thus, it is a very important muscle in racing performance. Injury results in a great deal of hemorrhage, swelling, and hematoma formation. Injury to the muscle may occur at the origin, belly, or insertion. Primary surgical repair is the treatment of choice, followed by 2 to 3 months of strict rest. Rupture of the gracilis muscle can be a devastating injury, and the prognosis for returning to racing is fair to good. If the tendon of insertion is partially intact, this injury can be treated conservatively.

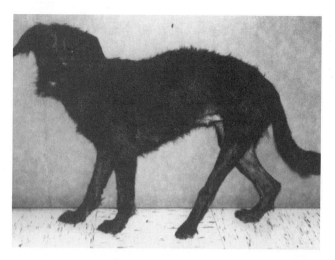

Fig. 22-35 Dog has assumed the classic "walking stick" posture with the right rear leg. The dog had a Salter-Harris II fracture of the distal femoral physis complicated by osteomyelitis.

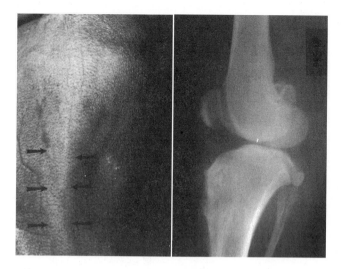

Fig. 22-36 Lateral radiographic view of a dog with chronic quadriceps muscle contracture. Note the hyperextension of the stifle and the extensive degenerative joint disease and fibrous thickening of periarticular tissues.

Quadriceps contracture. Contracture of the quadriceps group of muscles is frequently associated with fracture repair in young animals. It is usually associated with inadequate fracture repair, osteomyelitis, severe trauma, or overzealous handling of tissues surrounding the femur.[15,35,42,48,61] Prolonged immobilization of the rear leg in extension and failure to bear weight early after internal fixation also contribute to the development of this condition. A congenital form of quadriceps contracture has been reported in puppies.[56]

The pathological process involves a traumatic incident to the femur that results in inflammatory process involving the bone and periosteum as well as the stripping of muscular attachments. With or without the surgeon's intervention, this inflammatory and healing process results in adhesions between the quadriceps muscle and the distal femur. The animal is reluctant to use the affected leg and holds it in extension (Fig. 22-35). The extension may be severe enough that the stifle is curved backward in a position of genu recurvatum. With the stifle extended, the hock is extended as well. The rear leg becomes very stiff and serves as a "walking stick" for locomotion. As time progresses, the muscles of the thigh become atrophied, taut, and adhered to the femur. If left untreated, the periarticular and intraarticular tissues also become fibrotic, and degenerative joint disease develops in the stifle (Fig. 22-36). No specific surgical procedure offers a good prognosis in advanced cases.

The objective of surgery is to restore motion to the stifle joint.[15,35,42,62] This is accomplished through a lateral parapatellar skin incision.[49] The adhesions must be broken down between the quadriceps muscle group and distal femur. The stifle should be explored to release any fibrous tissue. The quadriceps mechanism, specifically the sartorius and rectus femoris, can be mobilized using a sliding myopathy or Z myoplasty.[47] Gel foam may be placed between freed muscle groups and the bone to prevent recurrence of the adhesions.[68] After freeing the fibrotic tissues, the stifle joint should be flexed as much as possible to assist in the release of fibrous tissue. Care should be taken, especially in animals with open growth plates, not to cause a Salter fracture of the distal femoral or proximal tibial physis.

Regardless of the surgical procedure used, the postoperative goal is to prevent recurrence of extension and initiate physiotherapy to improve the stifle's range of motion. This can be accomplished best by application of transarticular external pin splintage. The fixator can be connected by heavy rubber bands to assist in flexion, or the animal can be periodically anesthetized, the external fixator loosened, and the stifle flexed and extended.

The best approach to this disease is prevention. Repair of femoral fractures in young animals should be rigid enough and reduction accurate enough to allow for early ambulation. A figure-eight sling can be put on the operated leg for 7 to 10 days to assist in prevention of hyperextension. In addition, animals with this type of fracture should be rechecked at least every 10 to 14 days after surgical repair. If the animal is exhibiting clinical signs of hyperextension, an external fixator can be placed across the stifle to maintain the leg in a functional position. The alternatives to surgical treatment of quadriceps contracture are arthrodesis of the stifle or amputation.

Fibrotic myopathy. Fibrotic myopathy has been reported involving the supraspinatus, gracilis, quadriceps, and semitendinosus muscles of small animals.[37,44] This condition may be the result of direct trauma to or disruption of the specific muscle, especially if left untreated. Other possible etiologies may be a primary neuropathy

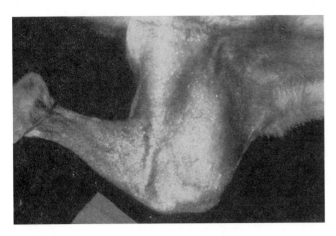

Fig. 22-37   Chronic tear of the semitenbranosus resulting in a fibrous "cording" of the medial thigh.

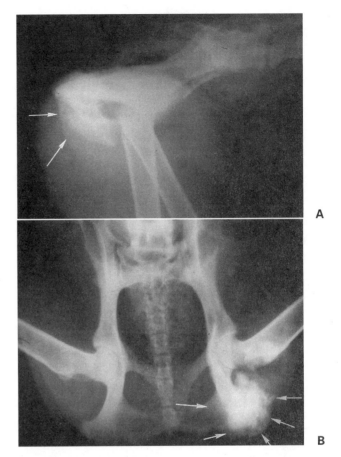

Fig. 22-38   Lateral (**A**) and ventrodorsal (**B**) radiographic views of the pelvis of an adult Doberman pinscher depicting a well-defined calcified mass typical of myositis ossificans involving the ischial tuberosity (*arrows*). Surgical excision of the calcified tissue resulted in recovery with no recurrence.

Courtesy of Dr. Robert Parker, University of Florida, Gainesville.

or myopathy, frequent intramuscular injections, exercise induced, or congenital. The pathological changes result in replacement of the muscle fibers by dense collagenous connective tissue, resulting in a taut fibrous band (Fig. 22-37). The presence of clinical lameness depends on the muscle involved and the extent of the fibrosis.

The most frequently affected muscle is the semitendinosus.[37] Clinically affected dogs have a lameness characterized by external rotation of the hock and internal rotation of the stifle when a rear limb is carried forward. The foot of the affected limb is flipped forward with each stride.

The treatment of choice is surgical release of the fibrotic tissue.[37,44] This may involve tenotomy, myotenotomy, Z-plasty, or complete excision of the fibrotic tissue. Surgical release usually restores a normal range of motion and resolves the lameness. Surgical treatment carries a poor prognosis because the condition usually recurs within a few months. As a result, the prognosis remain guarded.

Myositis ossificans. Myositis ossificans has been reported to occur in similar locations in humans and animals. The condition is a progressive generalized or localized calcification of muscles around the hip joints.[22,38] It has also been reported in the supraspinatus muscle of the forelimb. The exact cause is unknown but may be the result of a local initiating factor resulting in proliferation of mesenchyme to bone. Proposed causes include ossification of hematomas, infectious process, and trauma.[47] The animal may exhibit clinical signs of chronic lameness accompanied by atrophy, possible neurological deficits, and pain after exercise. Radiographically the lesion is represented as a well-defined calcified mass that may have a centralized area of transparency (Fig. 22-38).

Surgical excision of the calcified mass frequently permanently resolves the clinical signs. When possible, the etiology of the condition should be identified and eliminated. Dueland, Wagner, and Parker[22] reported on five cases of osteochondrofibrosis in Doberman pinschers associated with below-normal levels of von Willebrand factor antigen.

REFERENCES

1. Aron DN: A "new" tendon stitch, *J Am Anim Hosp Assoc* 17:587-591, 1981.
2. Aron DN: Tendons. In Bojrab MJ, editor: *Current techniques in small animal surgery*, ed 3, Philadelphia, 1990, Lea & Febiger.
3. Bennett D, Vaughn LC: The use of muscle relocation techniques in the treatment of peripheral nerve injuries in dogs and cats, *J Small Anim Pract* 17:99-108, 1976.
4. Berg RJ, Egger EL: In vitro comparison of the three loop pulley and locking loop suture patterns for repair of canine weightbearing tendons and collateral ligaments, *Vet Surg* 15:107-110, 1986.
5. Bernard MA: Superficial digital flexor tendon injury in the dog, *Can Vet J* 18:105-107, 1977.
6. Bloomberg MS: Muscle and tendons. In Slatter DH, editor: *Textbook of small animal surgery*, ed 2, Philadelphia, 1991, Saunders.

7. Bloomberg MS, Hough JD, Howard DR: Repair of severed Achilles tendon in a dog: a case report, *J Am Anim Hosp Assoc* 12:841-843, 1977.

8. Bone DL, Govin MD: Myositis ossificans in the dog: a case report and review, *J Am Anim Hosp Assoc* 21:135-138, 1985.

9. Braden TD: Musculotendinous rupture of the Achilles apparatus and repair using internal fixation only, *Vet Med Small Anim Clin* 69:729-735, 1974.

10. Braden TD: Tendons and muscles. In Bojrab MJ, editor: *Current techniques in small animal surgery*, Philadelphia, 1975, Lea & Febiger.

11. Braden TD: Fascia lata transplants for repair of chronic Achilles tendon defects, *J Am Anim Hosp Assoc* 12:800-805, 1976.

12. Braund KG: Hereditary myopathy in Labrador retrievers, *Calif Vet* 39:18-22, 1985.

13. Brinker WD, Piermattei DL, Flo GL: *Handbook of small animal orthopedics and fracture treatment*, ed 2, Philadelphia, 1990, Saunders.

14. Bunnell S: Primary repair of several tendons: the use of stainless steel wire, *Am J Surg* 47:502-516, 1940.

15. Butler HC: Tendon, muscle, and fascia. In *Canine surgery*, Archibald ed 2, Santa Barbara, Calif, 1974, American Veterinary Publications.

16. Carlson BM: The regeneration of skeletal muscle: a review, *Am J Anat* 137:119-150, 1973.

17. Chaffee VW, Knecht DC: Avulsion of the medial head of the gastrocnemius in the dog, *Vet Med Small Anim Clin* 70:929-931, 1955.

18. Davies JV, Clayton-Jones DG: Triceps tendon rupture in the dog following corticosteroid injection, *J Small Anim Pract* 23:779-786, 1982.

19. Davis PE: Examination of the greyhound for soundness. In *Proceedings, Refresher Course on Greyhounds*, Australia: University of Sydney, 64:601-611, 1983.

20. Dee JF: Soft tissue surgery in the racing greyhound. In *Proceedings, Refresher Course on Greyhounds*, Australia: University of Sydney, 122:527-535, 1989.

21. Dee JF, Dee LG Eaton-Wells RD: Injuries of high performance dogs. In Whittick WG, editor: *Canine orthopedics*, ed 2, Philadelphia, 1974, Lea & Febiger.

22. Dueland RT, Wagner SD, Parker RB: von Willebrand heterotopic osteochondrofibrosis in Doberman pinschers: five cases (1980-1987), *J Am Vet Med Assoc* 197:383-388, 1990.

23. Early TD: Tendon disorders. In Bojrab MJ, editor: *Pathophysiology of small animal surgery*, Philadelphia, 1981, Lea & Febiger.

24. Evans HE, Christensen GC: *Miller's anatomy of the dog*, ed 2, Philadelphia, 1979, Saunders.

25. Farrow CS: Sprain, strain and contusion, *Vet Clin North Am* 8:169-182, 1979.

26. Ferguson RG: The treatment of soft tissue injuries in the racing greyhound. In *Proceedings, Refresher Course on Greyhounds*, Australia: University of Sydney, 122:103-116, 1989.

27. Gleeson LN: Treatment of traumatic lesions of tendo-Achilles by joint fixation with a Stader splint, *Vet Med* 41:442, 1946.

28. Goring RL, Parker RB, Dee L: Medial displacement of the tendon of origin of the biceps brachii muscle in the racing greyhound, *J Am Anim Hosp Assoc* 20:933-938, 1984.

29. Ham AW: *Histology*, ed 8, Philadelphia, 1980, Lippincott.

30. Hill FWG: Muscle injuries, their extent and therapy in the racing greyhound. In *Proceedings, Refresher Course on Greyhounds*, Australia: University of Sydney, 298-303, 1977.

31. Hoerlein BF, Evans LE, Davis JM: Upward luxation of the canine scapula: a case report, *J Am Vet Med Assoc* 136:258-259, 1960.

32. Hufford T, Olmstead ML, Butler HC: Contracture of the infraspinatus muscle and surgical correction in two dogs, *J Am Anim Hosp Assoc* 11:613-618, 1975.

33. Kramer JW and others: A muscle disorder of Labrador retrievers characterized by deficiency of type II muscle fibers, *J Am Vet Med Assoc* 169:817-820, 1976.

34. Lammerding JJ and others: Avulsion fracture of the origin of the extensor digitorum longis muscle in 3 dogs, *J Am Anim Hosp Assoc* 12:764-767, 1976.

35. Leighton RL: Muscle contractures in the limbs of dogs and cats, *Vet Surg* 10(3):132-135, 1981.

36. Lesser AS: Tendon transfer for treatment of sciatic paralysis. In Bojrab MJ, editor: *Current techniques in small animal surgery*, Philadelphia, 1990, Lea & Febiger.

37. Lewis DD: Fibrotic myopathy of the semitendinosus muscle in a cat, *J Am Vet Med Assoc* 193:240-241, 1988.

38. Liu SK, Dorfman HD: A condition resembling human localized myositis ossificans in two dogs, *J Small Anim Pract* 17:371-377, 1976.

39. Malnati GA: Deep digital flexor tendon transposition for rupture of the calcanean tendon in a dog, *J Am Anim Hosp Assoc* 17:451-454, 1981.

40. Mason ML, Allen HS: The rate of healing of tendon: an experimental study of tensile strength, *An Surg* 113:424-459, 1941.

41. McKerrell RE, Braund KG: Hereditary myopathy in Labrador retrievers: clinical variations, *J Small Anim Pract* 28:479-489, 1987.

42. Milton JL, Henderson PA: Surgery of muscles and tendons. In Bojrab MJ, editor: *Current Techniques in small animal surgery*, ed 2, Philadelphia, 1983, Lea & Febiger.

43. Mitchell M: Spontaneous repair of a ruptured gastrocnemius muscle in a dog, *J Am Anim Hosp Assoc* 16:513-516, 1980.

44. Moore RW, and others: Fibrotic myopathy of the semimembranosus muscle in four dogs, *Vet Surg* 10:169-174, 1981.

45. Morshead D, Leeds EB: Kirschner-Ehmer apparatus immobilization following Achilles tendon repair in six dogs, *Vet Surg* 13:11, 1984.

46. Olmstead ML, Butler HC: Surgical correction of avulsion of the origin of the long digital extensor muscle in the dog: a case report, *Vet Med Small Anim Clin* 71:608-610, 1976.

47. Parker RB, Cardinet GH: Myotendinous rupture of the Achilles mechanism associated with parasitic myositis, *J Am Anim Hosp Assoc* 20:115-118, 1984.

48. Peacock EE, Van Winkle WV: *Surgery and biology of wound repair*, ed 3, Philadelphia, 1984, Saunders.

49. Pettit GD and others: Studies on the pathophysiology of infraspinatus muscle contracture in the dog, *Vet Surg* 7:8-11, 1978.

50. Piermattei DL, Greeley RG: *An atlas of surgical approaches to the bones of the dog and cat*, ed 2, Philadelphia, 1979, Saunders.

51. Pollock S, Franklin GA, Wagner BM: Clinical significance of trauma, myositis ossificans, and malignant mesenchymoma in the dog: report of an unusual case, *J Am Anim Hosp Assoc* 14:237-242, 1978.

52. Pond MJ: Avulsion of the extensor digitorum longus muscle in the dog: a report of four cases, *Small Anim Pract* 14:785-796, 1973.

53. Pond MJ, Lasonsky JE: Avulsion of the popliteus muscle in the dog: a case report, *J Am Anim Hosp Assoc* 12:60-63, 1976.

54. Reinke JD, Kus SP: Achilles mechanism injury in the dog, *Comp Cont Educ* 4(8):639-645, 1982.

55. Reinke JD, Kus SP, Owens JM: Traumatic avulsion of the lateral head of the gastrocnemius and superficial digital flexor muscles in a dog, *J Am Anim Hosp Assoc* 18:252-256, 1982.

56. Rudy RL: Stifle joint. In *Canine surgery*, Archibald ed 2, Santa Barbara, Calif, 1974, American Veterinary Publications.

57. Smith KW: Achilles tendon surgery for correction of hyperextension of the hock joint, *J Am Anim Hosp Assoc* 12:848-849, 1976.

58. Srugi S, Adamson JE: A comparative study of tendon suture material in dogs, *Plast Reconstruct Surg* 50:31-35, 1972.

59. Taylor RA: Surgical diseases of skeletal muscle. In Bojrab MJ, editor: *Mechanisms of disease in small animal surgery*, Philadelphia, 1992, Lea & Febiger.

60. Tomlinson J, Moore R: Locking loop tendon suture use in repair of five calcanean tendons, *Vet Surg* 11:105-109, 1982.

61. Urbaniak JR, Cahill JO, Mortenson RA: Tendon suturing methods: analysis of tensile strength. In American Academy of Orthopedic

Surgeons: *Symposium on Tendon Surgery of the Hand*, St Louis, 1975, Mosby.

62. Vaughn LC: Muscle and tendon injuries in dogs, *J Small Anim Pract* 20:711-736, 1979.

63. Vaughn LC: Tendon injuries in dogs, *Calif Vet* 34:15-19, 1980.

64. Vaughn LC, Edwards GB: The use of carbon fibers (Grafil) for tendon repair in animals, *Vet Rec* 102:287-288, 1978.

65. Vaughn LC, Faull WB: Correction of a luxated superficial digital flexor tendon in a greyhound, *Vet Rec*, 67:335-336, 1955.

66. Vierheller RC: Surgical repair of severed tendons and ligaments in the dog, *Mod Vet Pract* 53:35-38, 1972.

67. Woo SL-Y, Buckwalter JA: In *Symposium on Injury and Repair of the Musculoskeletal Soft Tissues,* Chicago, 1988, American Academy of Orthopaedic Surgeons.

68. Wright JR: Correction of quadriceps contractures, *Calif Vet* 34:7-9, 1980.

V

SALVAGE PROCEDURES

23

Arthrodesis

KENNETH A. JOHNSON

Arthrodesis refers to the surgical procedure designed to induce fusion of a diarthrodial joint, as well as the solid bony union that ultimately develops. A successful arthrodesis completely eliminates joint motion but restores limb function by stabilizing the diseased joint and rendering it pain free. By contrast, *ankylosis* is the pathological stiffening or immobilization of a joint by osteophytosis, enthesophytosis, intraarticular fibrosis, periarticular fibrosis, capsular adhesion, or musculotendinous contracture. In addition, articular hyaline cartilage in ankylosed joints degenerates, and there is narrowing of the joint space and subchondral bone sclerosis. Ankylosed joints are invariably painful. A failed attempt at surgical arthrodesis may result in either painful ankylosis or nonunion.

Arthrodesis is often categorized as a salvage procedure, but this should not imply that it is an inferior procedure. Although arthrodesis should never be performed instead of an appropriate primary joint reconstruction, it is a valuable procedure in properly selected patients. Arthrodesis can be performed in all the appendicular diarthrodial joints except the hip. Limb function is the main limitation on the success of an arthrodesis. In humans, prosthetic joint replacements are available for most of the diarthrodial joints and represent a real alternative to arthrodesis. In small animals, however, this is not the case. The canine hip is the only joint for which a prosthesis is currently available commercially. So for now, arthrodesis remains a standard and very acceptable treatment for a variety of severe joint injuries, diseases, and conditions.

INDICATIONS
Congenital Luxation

When functional reduction is impossible and limb use is significantly compromised, arthrodesis may be indicated. Complete or partial agenesis of a bone may contribute to the luxation. Some congenital luxations become clinically apparent at a few months of age. If possible, arthrodesis should be delayed until after the physes have closed.

Physeal Fractures

Physeal fractures that heal with malunion and those that result in an asymmetrical Salter-Harris type V premature closure cause distortion of the overlying articular surface and subluxation. Condyles may be misshapen, articular surfaces tilted, or joint spaces widened. Early diagnosis and treatment of physeal injuries are the ideal approaches (see Chapter 13). Late recognition of a physeal injury may result in loss of the joint with osteoarthritis, for which arthrodesis may be the only treatment.

Third-Degree Sprains

Arthrodesis is appropriate when ligament repair is not feasible or when ligament repair has failed or is likely to fail. Traumatic ruptures of ligaments (e.g., palmar carpal ligaments) that have a principal role in support of low-motion joints are treated by immediate arthrodesis of the affected joints without any attempt at ligament repair. Satisfactory techniques for primary repair of these ligaments have yet to be developed. Unfortunately, these joints are often otherwise normal, except for the sublux-

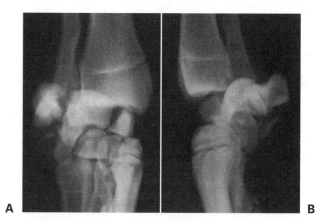

Fig. 23-1 **A** and **B**, Fracture/luxation of the radial carpal bone, combined with intraarticular fractures of the ulnar and accessory carpal bones, which were subsequently treated by carpal arthrodesis.

Courtesy The University of Sydney.

ation, but they subsequently develop osteoarthritis secondary to mechanical instability.

Intraarticular Fractures

Comminuted intraarticular fractures with multiple small fragments or missing bone and articular cartilage may be irreparable and salvageable only by arthrodesis (Fig. 23-1).

Open Traumatic Fractures/Luxations

Joints that develop septic arthritis and subchondral osteomyelitis are candidates for arthrodesis once the infection is quiescent. Immediate debridement, lavage, chemotherapy, and stabilization of acute open fractures/luxations with the goal of preserving the joint constitute the preferred approach. However, once articular cartilage is destroyed by trauma or degraded by inflammatory processes and bacteria, arthrodesis is indicated.

Contracture

Contracture of musculotendinous groups, ligaments, and joint capsule secondary to disuse, limb immobilization, and denervation may force the limb into a stiff and functionless position. Although the stiffened joints may be essentially normal, transection of scar tissue and arthrodesis of involved joints in a functional position are one possible treatment option.

Peripheral Nerve Injuries

Traumatic injuries involving the radial or tibial nerve, in which the animal is unable to bear weight on the limb

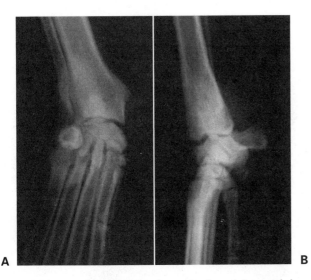

Fig. 23-2 **A** and **B**, Chronic traumatic shear injury with loss of bone from the ulnar styloid process and ulnar carpal bone, which resulted in a marked valgus deviation and osteoarthritis of the carpal joints.

Courtesy The University of Sydney.

because of loss of extension of the carpus or tarsus, respectively, are potential indications for arthrodesis. Absence of cutaneous sensory innervation to digits and pads is an absolute contraindication to arthrodesis. Dragging the leg and the self-trauma of licking and chewing will cause mutilation of the paw.[16] Tendon transposition may be an alternative to arthrodesis.[2,24]

Osteoarthritis

Painful, chronic, and intractable osteoarthritis is an indication for arthrodesis. The osteoarthritis rarely is the primary condition. More often, it is secondary to subluxation, sepsis, trauma, or developmental disorders such as osteochondritis dissecans (Fig. 23-2).

Cortical Bone Alloimplants

Massive bone defects in the juxtaarticular metaphyseal region caused by traumatic bone loss, severe comminution, or resection of primary bone tumors may be bridged with a cortical allograft and stabilized by plating in conjunction with arthrodesis of the adjacent joint.[23]

PRINCIPLES

Thorough assessment of the patient and radiographs, an informed client, and precise presurgical planning are essential prerequisites for a successful outcome in arthrodesis, as in any surgical procedure. Principles and procedures somewhat unique to arthrodesis, but generally applicable to any joint, are considered here.

Patient Selection

Other than the joint that is to have an arthrodesis, the rest of the limb and the contralateral limb ideally should all be normal. Arthrodesis imposes extra stresses on the adjacent normal joints and bones. After arthrodesis, there is a slightly increased risk of fracture in that limb, and breakdown of joints more distal to the arthrodesis can occur. In growing animals, arthrodesis is best postponed until the physes adjacent to the involved joint have closed, since surgical trauma or bridging by internal fixation of an open physis may cause premature physeal closure and undesired limb shortening. Multiple joint arthrodeses in an animal with an intractable, immune-mediated polyarthropathy are feasible but usually inadvisable.

Postarthrodesis Limb Function

After arthrodesis of joints that normally have limited movement, such as the carpometacarpal, proximal intertarsal, and tarsometatarsal joints, dogs can return to hunting, sheep and cattle herding, hiking, and racing. However, arthrodesis of a high-motion joint such as the elbow or stifle severely impedes activity. Negotiation of uneven terrain and stairs is very difficult and can cause exercise intolerance.

Angle of Fusion

Joints should be fused at an angle that allows functional limb use. Specific recommendations on angles are made in the sections on individual joints. Before surgery, the normal standing angle of the contralateral joint is measured with a goniometer, taking into consideration the effect of the additional weight being taken on this leg. A correction for varus, valgus, or rotation may be necessary, especially with intraarticular fracture, intraarticular fracture malunion, and subluxation secondary to physeal injury (Fig. 23-3). Resection of the joint surfaces in arthrodesis surgery causes some limb shortening. This is more significant in smaller dogs. It can be corrected by a slight increase in the angle of arthrodesis. Dogs can adapt to some hind limb shortening by extension of the normal joints. In the forelimb, however, shortening and overextension of the shoulder or elbow are not well tolerated.

Surgical Exposure

The surgical exposure of the joint needs to be sufficiently extensive to allow visualization of most of the articular cartilage and permit application of the internal fixation.[28] Joint capsule and collateral ligaments can be transected or resected to give adequate surgical access. Slow gain in tensile strength of transected collateral ligaments, which

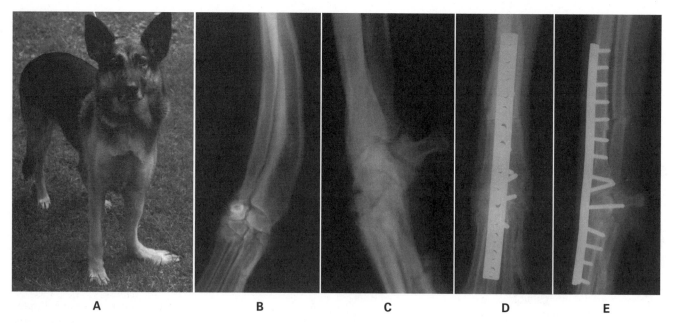

Fig. 23-3 A, Seven-year-old German shepherd dog with longstanding forelimb deviation caused by premature distal ulnar physeal closure. **B**, Marked radial curvature and relative shortening of the ulna developed after premature distal ulnar physeal closure at 6 months of age. **C**, Osteoarthritis of the carpal joints with osteophytes, caused by incongruity of the antebrachiocarpal joint and abnormal mechanical loading of the joint. **D** and **E**, Corrective closing wedge osteotomy combined with carpal arthrodesis. At 7 weeks after surgery, there is healing of the osteotomy and bridging of joint spaces in the arthrodesis.

B to **E**, Courtesy The University of Sydney.

is usually a concern, is irrelevant because the joint will be immobilized by the internal fixation. Tendons that span the joint and insert more distally in the limb or digits must be protected. If necessary, the tendon sheath is opened longitudinally to allow the tendon to be moved aside. Tendons that insert on a bony prominence adjacent to the joint undergoing arthrodesis may be either transected or mobilized by an osteotomy and reflected with a bone fragment. An example of this procedure is osteotomy of the olecranon to reflect the triceps muscle and tendon. Osteotomy of a bony prominence may also facilitate contouring of a plate across a joint. Tendon transection is acceptable when the primary function of the musculotendinous unit is to flex or extend the joint being arthrodesed.

Neurovascular bundles and other soft tissues crossing the joint are protected and preserved. Hemorrhage during arthrodesis surgery can be troublesome. Angiogenic response in the tissues around chronically inflamed joints causes profuse capillary bleeding, which obscures the surgical field and slows surgery. Wrapping the entire limb tightly from distal to proximal with a sterile elasticized bandage (Vetrap) as an Esmarch bandage helps with hemostasis in arthrodesis of distal joints. Problems are that the bandage restricts joint mobility during surgery, has a tendency to slip distally, and causes greater postoperative swelling of the distal limb. Judicious use of the elec-

troscalpel for blended cutting and vessel coagulation is a better way of dealing with troublesome hemorrhage.

Articular Cartilage Excision

Articular cartilage must be removed from all contact regions of the joint surface to expose viable, vascular subchondral or cancellous bone to facilitate a solid osseous union for arthrodesis. Although rigid immobilization of a normal joint causes thinning and degeneration of the articular cartilage, the joint cavity is invaded and bridged only by fibrous tissue, not bone (Fig. 23-4). After several months the internal fixation begins to loosen and fail, with the clinical result being an unstable, painful ankylosis.

Articular cartilage can be removed with an air-driven bur, Volkmann bone curette, osteotome, or oscillating saw (Fig. 23-5). In young animals in which the cartilage is thick and the bone soft, the curette or osteotome is a suitable instrument for this purpose. In adult animals, however, the subchondral bone plate is dense and thick, and an air-driven bur works better. Copious irrigation of the joint with saline to minimize burning of the bone during burring is mandatory. Flutes in the burs need to be kept clean with a steel brush and dull burs replaced with new ones. After cartilage removal, forage of dense subchondral bone with a 1.5 mm drill bit opens up channels for metaphyseal vessels to invade and vascu-

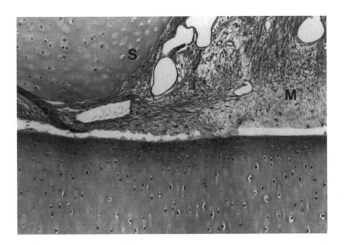

Fig. 23-4 Undifferentiated mesenchymal tissue (M) invading the joint space in an experimental carpal arthrodesis after 12 weeks. Articular cartilage was not removed by curettage. Articular cartilage erosion and degeneration, marked by chondrocyte loss in the superficial zone (S) and cloning, are evident. However, no new bone has formed to bridge the arthrodesis. (Hematoxylin-eosin stain, × 100 magnification.)

Reprinted with permission from Johnson KA, Bellenger CR: The effects of autologous bone grafting on bone healing after carpal arthrodesis in the dog, *Vet Rec* 107:126-132, 1980.

larize the healing arthrodesis. In the congruent joints such as carpus, tarsus, and elbow, simple removal of articular cartilage and preservation of joint surface contours work best. However, in the incongruent joints such as the stifle, there is limited contact, and resection with an oscillating saw to produce two flat surfaces gives better bone-to-bone contact across the arthrodesis. Once the two cuts are made, the angle of the arthrodesis is determined, so careful planning with goniometer and Kirschner guide pins is essential. A minor disadvantage of the resection technique is that it causes limb shortening.

Bone Grafts

Autogenous cancellous bone grafts (see Chapter 5) are used to stimulate osseous union in an arthrodesis so that joint fusion occurs before implant loosening or failure (Fig. 23-6). Delayed union and implant loosening are common sources of failure in arthrodesis. Cancellous bone may be packed into the joint cavity between the denuded joint surfaces and into voids and defects around the arthrodesis and under the plate after stabilization is complete. Increasing the cross-sectional dimensions of the arthrodesis produces a stronger union that is more resistant to late fracture and breakdown.

The proximal metaphyses of the ipsilateral humerus and tibia are good collection sites. Some additional cancellous bone may be harvested from resected articular condyles, such as the distal femur. In cats and small dogs,

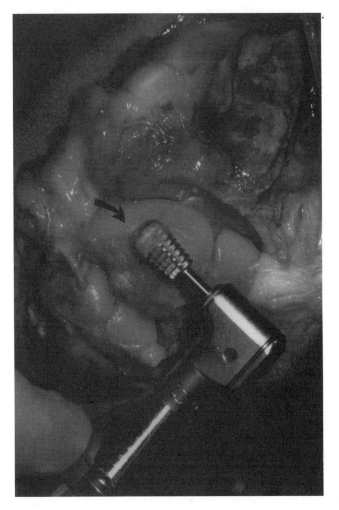

Fig. 23-5 Articular cartilage removal with an air-driven bur from the radial carpal bone (*arrow*) during carpal arthrodesis.

a composite corticocancellous graft from ilium or rib, cut up into small fragments, is the next best choice for graft material when insufficient cancellous bone exists. Fresh autogenous bone grafts promote new bone formation by introducing osteoblasts and osteogenic precursor cells (osteogenesis), by release of growth factors that induce osteogenic differentiation in mesenchymal tissue at the graft bed (osteoinduction), and by acting as a scaffold on which new bone can be deposited (osteoconduction).

Bone grafting is of greatest benefit in joints in which the articular cartilage has been removed from the subchondral bone by burring or curetting, leaving dense subchondral bone. In chronic osteoarthritis, thickening of the subchondral bone plate is particularly notable, and being less vascular and cellular than cancellous bone, union at these arthrodeses is delayed. Also, in the compound tarsal and carpal joints, the small cuboidal bones are devitalized by surgical resection of the joint capsule containing blood supply and by the trauma of burring. Bone grafting to stimulate healing is particularly important

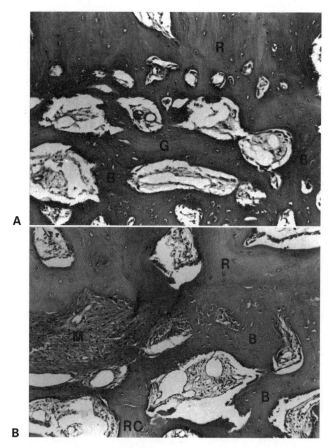

A

B

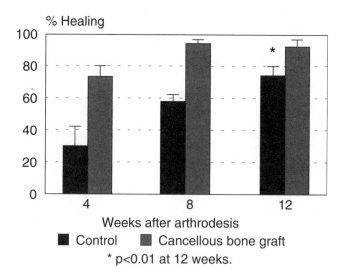

Fig. 23-7 Percentage width (mean +/− standard error) of the antebrachiocarpal joint united by new bone trabeculae in sagittal histological sections (depicted in Fig. 23-6) after experimental carpal arthrodesis performed with autogenous cancellous bone graft and without a graft (control).

Modified from Johnson KA, Bellenger CR: The effects of autologous bone grafting on bone healing after carpal arthrodesis in the dog, *Vet Rec* 107:126-132, 1980.

Fig. 23-6 **A**, Union at 4 weeks at the level of the antebrachiocarpal joint of an experimental carpal arthrodesis in which autogenous cancellous bone graft had been inserted. The distal radius (R) and grafted cancellous bone (G) are identified by empty osteocytic lacunae. New bone trabeculae (B), formed on the distal radius and grafted bone, completely bridge the arthrodesis. (H-E stain, × 100.) **B**, Control carpal arthrodesis at 4 weeks in which no bone graft was inserted. The arthrodesis gap between the distal radius (R) and radial carpal bone (RC), is incompletely united by new bone trabeculae (B), with undifferentiated mesenchymal tissue (M) present in the remaining gap. (H-E stain, × 100.)

Reprinted with permission from Johnson KA, Bellenger CR: The effects of autologous bone grafting on bone healing after carpal arthrodesis in the dog, *Vet Rec* 107:126-132, 1980.

Stabilization

in each of these circumstances. With cancellous bone grafting, osseous union of arthrodeses occurs in 4 to 8 weeks, whereas without a graft, union is less predictable and takes in excess of 12 weeks[20,21] (Fig. 23-7).

When metaphyseal cancellous bone has been exposed by resection with an oscillating saw and these two flat surfaces are brought into apposition, as in stifle arthrodesis, there does not seem to be a significant benefit from interposing cancellous bone graft. However, bone grafts can be packed into voids around the periphery of the arthrodesis. If the arthrodesis is stabilized with interfragmentary compression, direct primary cancellous bone healing occurs within 4 weeks.[7]

Secure fixation of the bone with interfragmentary compression is mandatory if arthrodesis is to be reliably achieved. Usually, internal fixation with a plate is most appropriate. Occasionally, tension-band wiring is indicated. In open fracture/luxation and joint sepsis, where further damage to blood supply and the introduction of foreign material (implants) into the fracture are concerns, a transarticular external fixator is the fixation of choice. Kirschner wires or Steinmann pins driven across the joint are an excellent method of providing intraoperative alignment, but this cannot solely be relied on to provide arthrodesis fixation.

Weight-bearing loads and muscle contraction acting on an arthrodesis are a mixture of compressive, tensile, bending, and torsional forces. These must be neutralized by the internal fixation; otherwise, interfragmentary motion leads to bone resorption, implant loosening, loss of stability, and nonunion. Of these forces, craniocaudal bending is the most significant in causing disruption of an arthrodesis. With few exceptions, most joints are fused at an angle between 90 and 180 degrees, but rarely 180 degrees. Therefore, bending forces acting on these joints may be greater than those acting on an anatomically reduced diaphyseal fracture. Ideally, plates are positioned on the tension surface of the joint, that is, the convex surface. Provided interfragmentary compression exists between the bones, the plate will be loaded in tension and protected from cyclical bending and fatigue failure (Fig. 23-8, *A*). Soft tissues may preclude the application of a

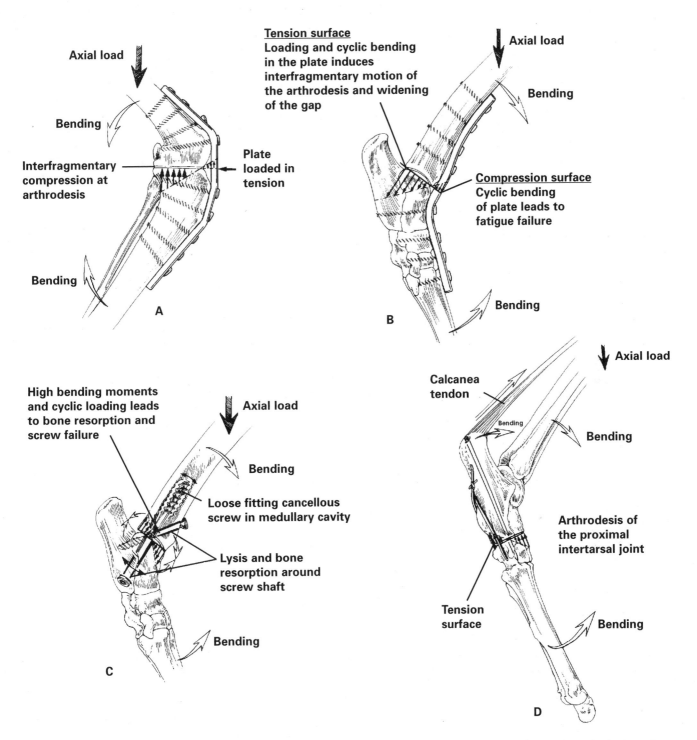

Fig. 23-8 **A**, Bone plate applied across the cranial (tension) surface of a stifle joint arthrodesis. Weight bearing on the limb produces interfragmentary compression of the arthrodesis, and the plate is loaded in tension. The plate tolerates tensile loads well and is relatively resistant to cyclical fatigue failure. **B**, Bone plate applied to the compression surface of a tarsocrural arthrodesis. With weight bearing on the limb, the plate carries most of the load and the arthrodesis very little. Cyclical bending of the plate at the arthrodesis may result in fatigue failure. Bending of the plate reduces interfragmentary compression, induces interfragmentary motion, and widens the gap at the arthrodesis. **C**, Tarsocrural arthrodesis stabilized with transarticular lag screws poorly resists axial loading and resultant bending forces that are concentrated at the arthrodesis. Repeated cyclical bending loads at the arthrodesis may cause loosening of the screws because of resorption of surrounding bone, bending of the screws as they cross the arthrodesis, and metal fatigue and screw breakage. Transarticular cancellous screws inserted into the tibial medullary cavity provide little resistance to bending if the screw thread diameter is less than that of the medullary canal. **D**, Tension-band wire fixation of a proximal intertarsal arthrodesis. Bending forces acting on the arthrodesis, generated by axial load and avulsion of the calcaneus by the calcaneal tendon, are counteracted by tension in the figure-eight wire, which in turn produces interfragmentary compression at the arthrodesis.

plate to the tension surface of some joints, in which case the plate ends up being applied on the concave surface (Fig. 23-8, *B*). A plate applied in this position absorbs most of the bending load; the bone absorbs almost none. Therefore the plate must be stiffer than usual and well secured by screws (three to five in each main bone fragment) to resist implant failure. Lag screws or Kirschner wires used alone for arthrodesis stabilization are subject to fatigue by cyclical bending forces that are concentrated at the arthrodesis (Fig. 23-8, *C*). Being more flexible than plates and not as well secured to the bone on each side of the arthrodesis, these wires or screws frequently fail by breaking or loosening.

Some small joints between the cuboidal bones are principally subjected to tensile-avulsive forces. Therefore these arthrodeses are stabilized by tension-band wiring (Fig. 23-8, *D*). Provided the tension-band fixation is positioned to effectively counteract tensile loading by the soft tissues, as well as axial and bending loads of weight bearing, interfragmentary compression between the bones at the arthrodesis is maintained.

Postoperative Management and Adjunctive Splinting

Arthrodesis surgery causes more trauma to the soft tissues and bone than does internal fixation of a fracture. The resultant inflammation produces significant postoperative swelling and compromised circulatory drainage of the distal parts of the limb. Flunixin meglumine (1.1 mg/kg intramuscularly or intravenously) given once perioperatively is beneficial in reducing this inflammatory response. In addition, narcotics are administered for postoperative analgesia.[30] Hot packing of the surgical area and distal limb and a padded Robert Jones dressing help to control and dissipate swelling.

Adjunctive splinting of the limb with a fiberglass cast or lateral splint for 4 to 8 weeks protects the internal fixation from excessive loading until osseous union of the arthrodesis occurs. The stiffness of the splint and the duration of application are influenced by the body weight and demeanor of the animal. Activity is strictly curtailed until osseous union is achieved.

Healing of Arthrodeses

Healing of an arthrodesis is monitored by physical examination and radiology. The acute inflammatory response begins to subside after 5 days. This is replaced by a firm swelling of the tissues because of scar tissue, periosteal new bone, and internal fixation implants. Normally an animal should begin partial weight bearing on the limb after 1 to 2 weeks and be capable of full pain-free weight bearing after 2 to 4 months. No instability should be detectable on palpation at any time, since this indicates loosening of the internal fixation and interfragmentary motion between the bones. Such a finding warrants immediate radiographic examination.

Radiographic examination is currently the best available means of monitoring arthrodesis healing. Radiographs taken immediately after surgery before any bandage or splint has been applied allow an assessment to be made of the angle and alignment of the arthrodesed joint and implant placement. These initial radiographs are an essential reference point for comparison with subsequent radiographs to assess healing. No two arthrodeses look exactly alike immediately postoperatively because of preexisting pathological changes and minor variations in joint alignment and width of joint spaces. Changes in radiographic appearance with healing may be quite subtle, so similarly positioned views need to be repeated every 4 to 6 weeks, at least until 12 weeks postoperatively, or until completion of healing.

Within the joint space or spaces of an arthrodesis, the pattern of osseous union is influenced by the method of articular cartilage excision and width of the gap. When articular cartilage is removed with curette or bur so that the contours of the joint surfaces are maintained, remnants of dense subchondral bone plate frequently remain and can be appreciated radiographically (Fig. 23-9, *A*). Some joint spaces may collapse, especially if interfragmentary compression is used. When cancellous bone graft is inserted into the joint cavities at surgery, there is a hazy or patchy radiodensity in the joint spaces, depending on how much graft was used. In the first 4 to 8 weeks after surgery, there is a progressive and uniform increase in opacity of the joint spaces as they become bridged by new bone trabeculae in response to the graft.[20] The dense subchondral bone is progressively resorbed and remodeled during this time, but complete disappearance of subchondral bone is not essential to healing and may take 6 to 12 months[19] (Fig. 23-9, *B*). With time the cancellous bone adjacent to the metaphysis becomes continuous with that bridging the arthrodesis. When healing is disturbed, delayed, or arrested, the joint space remains radiolucent and widens if instability causes resorption.

When the joint surfaces are cut off flat with an oscillating saw and compressed together, there is direct cancellous bone-to-bone contact and no joint space. This is achievable when the osteotomies are carefully planned, the two surfaces are accurately apposed, and the arthrodesis is stabilized with interfragmentary compression. Healing is by primary cancellous bone union, with apposition of new bone onto the existing trabeculae, thereby bridging the arthrodesis.[7] This mode of healing causes bone within 1 or 2 cm of the arthrodesis to appear sclerotic 4 to 8 weeks after surgery (Fig. 23-9, *C*). This may be

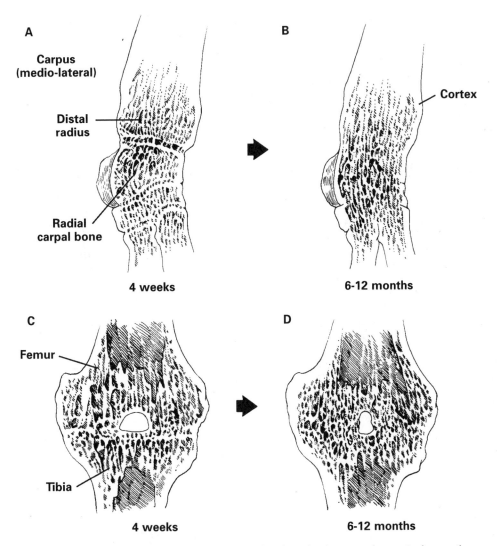

Fig. 23-9 Schematic radiological features of arthrodesis healing. **A**, When articular cartilage has been removed with a bur, any remaining dense subchondral bone is evident radiographically for at least 4 to 8 weeks after arthrodesis. A progressive increase in bone density occurs within the arthrodesis gap and is associated with the graft and new bone formation. **B**, Six to 12 months after arthrodesis, metaphyseal trabecular bone is continuous across the arthrodesis. **C**, Articular condyles resected with an oscillating saw to produce two flat surfaces compressed together heal by primary cancellous bone union. Radiographically, cancellous bone at the arthrodesis and immediately adjacent to it appears more sclerotic after 4 to 8 weeks. **D**, Six to 12 months after arthrodesis, bone in the region of the arthrodesis has remodeled, and trabecular bone from one metaphysis is continuous across the arthrodesis into the distal bone.

the only radiographic change evident, and it is similar to healing of metaphyseal fractures fixed with stable interfragmentary compression.[15] When fully healed, cancellous bone of one metaphysis is continuous with that of the other bone (Fig. 23-9, *D*). There is no evidence of the original joint except for the external contours.

Most arthrodeses heal with minimum external callus around the periphery of the joint, unless some was pres-

ent before surgery or extensive bone grafting was used. Lack of external callus seems to be related to stable internal fixation and the normal absence of periosteum at joints. However, it is not unusual to see periosteal and endosteal new bone along the diaphysis around the plate (Fig. 23-10). This may be caused by the surgical trauma to the periosteum or alterations in diaphyseal cortical bone strains induced by stiffness of the plate and the fused joint.

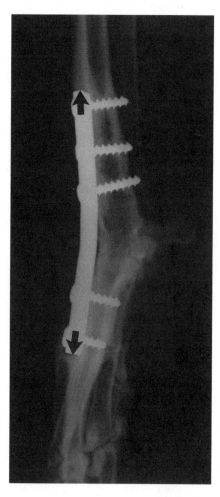

Fig. 23-10   Healed arthrodesis at 12 months. Original external contours of the distal radius and carpal bones are maintained, whereas trabecular bone is continuous across the carpus with little evidence of the original joint spaces. In the radial and metacarpal diaphyses, new periosteal and endosteal bone has formed at the ends of the plate (*arrows*).

Courtesy The University of Sydney.

COMPLICATIONS AND FAILURES

The most common complication is failure to achieve complete osseous union at the arthrodesis, resulting in a painful ankylosis or nonunion. Principal features of a failed arthrodesis are continued instability at the joint, widening of the joint space caused by resorption of bone, and sometimes sclerosis of metaphyseal bone. Implants may break, loosen, or migrate out of the bone. In animals that were originally being treated for subluxation or osteoarthritis, the pain and instability of a failed fusion can be greater than the original disease process. Correction of a failed arthrodesis requires a surgical procedure that is at least as involved as a properly performed initial arthrodesis. Identification of the specific factor(s) responsible for failure is essential, since repeat surgery on a failed arthrodesis without correcting the underlying mistake will probably result in another failure. Important causes of failure to consider, together with several other complications, are discussed here.

Inadequate Reduction

Removal of articular cartilage by pathological processes and surgery distorts the joint surfaces and may result in poor bone-to-bone apposition. Accurate intraoperative alignment and elimination of gaps by using autogenous cancellous bone grafting and dynamic compression plate fixation, when possible, are the ideal approaches.

Persistence of Articular Cartilage

Failure to remove articular cartilage prevents osseous fusion. Fibrous tissue invades the joint space, and cartilage slowly degenerates because of the effects of immobilization and pressure. Invariably, however, the internal fixation fails before cartilage is completely degraded.

Failure to Bone Graft

Insertion of autogenous cancellous bone into the joint after cartilage has been removed with a bur decreases time to osseous fusion by 4 to 8 weeks.[21] Although fusion may occur without a graft, it takes longer, and premature implant loosening and failure are more likely to occur.

Infection

Osteomyelitis following an open fracture/luxation, as well as septic arthritis, may complicate an arthrodesis if the initial arthrodesis was performed without proper planning. There is an increased risk of iatrogenic osteomyelitis in arthrodeses in the distal parts of extremities.

Fixation Failures

Loosening of the internal fixation may result from a technical mistake made in applying the fixation originally or may follow delayed union for any of the reasons previously mentioned. Some common causes of implant failure are application of the plate in a mechanically disadvantageous position, too few screws on each side of the arthrodesis, too narrow a plate, reliance on transarticular pins and lag screws alone, and insufficient adjunctive immobilization of the limb or patient (Fig. 23-11). Restriction of activity and adequate splinting of the limb to protect the fixation from acute overload are mandatory in large or active patients, when the fixation by necessity has been placed on the nontension side of the joint, or when some of the smaller joints have not been immobilized by the internal fixation.

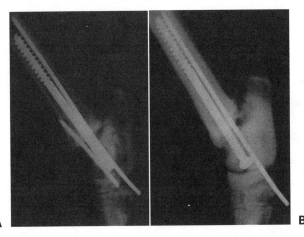

Fig. 23-11 **A,** Tarsocrural arthrodesis, stabilized with a 6.5 mm cancellous screw and two Steinmann pins, immediately after surgery. **B,** Transarticular screw and pin fixation failed to stabilize this arthrodesis adequately. Nonunion or ankylosis is the outcome after 1 year.

Courtesy The University of Sydney.

Diaphyseal Fractures

When the diaphyses of the two bones involved in the arthrodesis are greatly disparate in size, fracturing of the smaller bone by insertion of "oversized" screws can occur. This is mostly a problem in the metacarpal and metatarsal bones. Diaphyseal fractures at the end of the plate at any time after surgery, irrespective of the state of union of the arthrodesis, are a constant risk. Not only is there an abrupt change in material stiffness at the end of the plate, but the normal shock-absorbing capacity of the joint is abolished.

Late Implant Loosening

Screws that loosen and back out of the bone may cause pain, lameness, and intermittently discharging sinuses in the soft tissues over the implants. This tends to become a problem approximately 6 months after arthrodesis of a carpal or tarsal joint when the plate has been secured to a metacarpal or metatarsal bone. Staphylococci and other cutaneous pathogens can usually be isolated. Provided the arthrodesis has healed, implant removal resolves the problem.

SHOULDER ARTHRODESIS

Although not frequently performed, arthrodesis of the shoulder is a successful procedure for resolution of selected shoulder joint injuries and conditions. Shoulder arthrodesis alters but does not significantly impair forelimb function.[14,23] The scapular-thoracic musculature permits increased scapular mobility postoperatively, with a 150-degree arc of scapular motion in flexion and extension after complete recovery from surgery.[14] Some dogs tend to abrade the dorsum of the foot after prolonged exercise or occasionally skip on the leg while running.[14,34]

Indications

Indications for shoulder arthrodesis include chronic luxation, comminuted intraarticular fractures, nonunion and malunion of intraarticular fractures, and osteoarthritis. For acute luxations, stabilization with a tendon transposition procedure or capsule imbrication is the preferred management (see Chapter 16). In congenital medial luxation and chronic posttraumatic luxation, there are erosion of the glenoid rim and flattening of the humeral head. These conditions are not usually amenable to primary surgical stabilization, and arthrodesis may be indicated. Also, irreparable comminuted fractures of the glenoid, scapular neck, or humeral head are candidates for shoulder arthrodesis. Chronic secondary osteoarthritis is another valid indication for arthrodesis when pain cannot be alleviated medically. Proximal humeral alloimplants inserted following large resections for bone neoplasia and comminuted fractures are arthrodesed proximally to the scapula.[23]

Surgery

Internal fixation with a plate is the preferred method of stabilization for shoulder arthrodesis.[4,5,14] A craniolateral surgical approach is made to the shoulder, with the skin incision extending from the midpoint of the scapular spine distally to the midhumerus. Attachments of the trapezius and omotransversarius muscles on the scapular spine are transected, and together with the brachiocephalicus muscle, they are retracted craniomedially. The origin of the acromial head of the deltoid muscle is transected, or the acromion process is osteotomized, to allow the acromial head to be reflected distally. The greater tubercle of the humerus is osteotomized, and the supraspinatus muscle is reflected proximally. Additional exposure can be obtained by tenotomy of biceps brachii, infraspinatus, and teres minor (Fig. 23-12).

Articular cartilage is removed using rongeurs, bur, or curette so the normal contours of the joint surfaces are preserved. Cancellous bone graft from the proximal humerus is packed into the joint space. Alternatively, the humeral head and glenoid cavity are osteotomized with an oscillating bone saw to produce two flat surfaces. The plane of the osteotomies must be carefully planned so that the joint is arthrodesed at an angle of 105 to 110 degrees. The tendency to remove too much bone from the scapular glenoid and neck, thereby compromising screw holding power, must be avoided. After alignment of the joint, temporary fixation is made with one or two

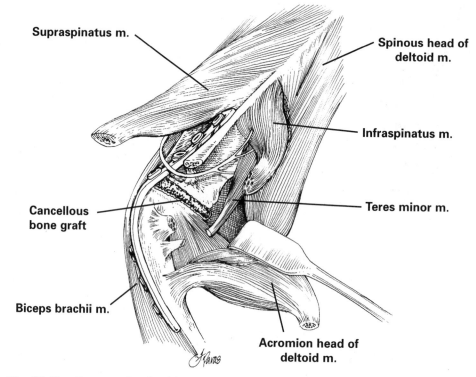

Supraspinatus m.

Spinous head of deltoid m.

Infraspinatus m.

Cancellous bone graft

Teres minor m.

Biceps brachii m.

Acromion head of deltoid m.

Fig. 23-12 Exposure for shoulder arthrodesis obtained by acromial osteotomy and distal reflection of the acromion head of the deltoid muscle. The greater tubercle of the humerus is osteotomized and the supraspinatus muscle reflected from the distal half of the scapular spine. Additional exposure is obtained by tenotomy of the biceps brachii, infraspinatus, and teres minor. Fixation is with a dynamic compression plate or reconstruction plate, which is applied along the spine of the scapula and cranial aspect of the humerus. Additional cancellous bone graft is packed around the arthrodesed joint.

Reproduced with permission from Brinker WO, Piermattei DL, Flo GL: *Handbook of small animal orthopedics and fracture treatment,* ed 2, Philadelphia, 1990, Saunders.

Kirschner wires, and AO-ASIF* pointed reduction forceps. A seven- to ten-hole, 2.7 mm or 3.5 mm plate is selected for the fixation, depending on the dog's size. The plate is contoured by bending and twisting so that it lies in the cranial angle made by the spine and blade of the scapula, then crosses the region of the greater tubercle, and extends down the cranial aspect of the humerus (Fig. 23-12). A reconstruction plate is easier to contour than the regular dynamic compression plate, and although weakened by the notches, it provides adequate stability because it is loaded mainly in tension.[29] The suprascapular nerve should be protected and preserved and the plate positioned under it. One or two of the plate screws or independent screws are lagged across the shoulder joint (Fig. 23-13). At least three plate screws are placed into the scapula and angled carefully to maximize holding power. Bone in this region of the scapula is very thin, and premature screw loosening in the scapula is a potential problem. Additional cancellous bone is packed around the arthrodesis.

Lag screw fixation alone is an alternative method that is only recommended for toy breeds of dogs.[34] The lag screw is inserted in the area of the supraglenoid tuberosity of the scapula, angled across the joint, and anchored into the humeral head and proximal humeral metaphysis. For added stability, a second lag screw is inserted from the region of the greater tubercle, across into the scapular glenoid. If the joint is stabilized with a lag screw alone, care should be taken to ensure that the shoulder is not too straight; excessive extension results in poor limb use.

For closure, the greater tubercle is reattached just lateral to the plate with two or three Kirschner wires. The acromion is reattached with a small tension band. Although plate fixation provides quite secure stabilization, the shoulder is immobilized with a spica splint for 3 to 4 weeks to protect the implants from excessive loading and loosening.[5,34]

---

*Arbeitsgemeinschaft für Osteosynthesefragen and Association for the Study of Internal Fixation.

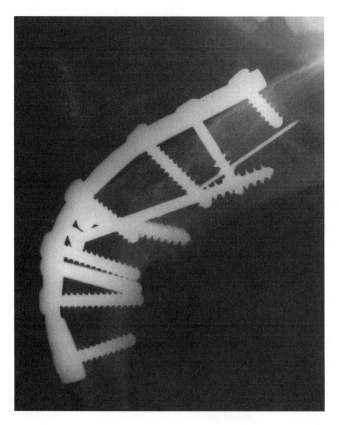

Fig. 23-13 Shoulder arthrodesis with a 3.5 mm dynamic compression plate and 4.0 mm cancellous transarticular lag screw is completely healed at 7 months.

Courtesy RT Dueland.

ELBOW ARTHRODESIS

Elbow arthrodesis impairs forelimb function significantly and produces a choppy gait. Therefore it is reserved for cases that are not amenable to specific surgical correction or medical management or cases in which these measures have failed. After elbow arthrodesis, shoulder, scapular-thoracic, and trunk movements become exaggerated. Animals with an elbow arthrodesis have great difficulty negotiating stairs and rough terrain.

Indications

Arthrodesis is indicated for severe osteoarthritis caused by a fragmented medial coronoid process, nonunited anconeal process, osteochondritis dissecans, nonunion or malunion of an intraarticular fracture, congenital luxation, chronic posttraumatic luxation, and asynchronous radius-ulna growth. Premature closure of the distal ulnar physis or distal radial physis that goes unrecognized for months can result in severe subluxation, joint deformity, and osteoarthritis (see Chapter 13). In some of these patients, elbow arthrodesis may be the only treatment option. Arthrodesis of the elbow and ipsilateral carpus is in-

frequently indicated in cases of asymmetrical closure of the distal radial physis, where both the radiocarpal and the elbow joints are subluxated.

Surgery

Arthrodesis at an angle of 110 degrees has been recommended, but in each case the angle will be influenced by the animal's species, breed, and conformation.[5] If the arthrodesis angle is too flexed, the animal tends to carry the leg, whereas with too much extension the toenails and digits are abraded in the swing phase of gait. Deficiency or malformation of bone resulting from traumatic loss, premature physeal closure, malunion, and osteomyelitis may have caused an angular or rotational deformity of the elbow, which needs to be accounted for in the planning stages.

Bone plate fixation is the optimum technique of stabilization. Lag screw fixation alone has advantages of speed, ease, and economy, but it is not recommended because high bending forces at the arthrodesis are poorly tolerated, and screw loosening, bending, and breakage lead to instability and painful ankylosis. Transarticular external fixator stabilization is indicated in open fractures and sepsis.[3]

A caudal transolecranon approach to the elbow is made. This exposure is extended proximally into a caudolateral approach to the distal humerus and distally into a caudal approach to the proximal ulna.[28] The radial and ulnar nerves are identified and protected, and the olecranon is osteotomized (Fig. 23-14). Size and shape of the olecranon may be quite abnormal in cases such as premature closure of the distal ulnar physis. However, the olecranon fragment needs to be just of sufficient size to allow for its subsequent reattachment to the humerus, along with the triceps tendon. Further resection and shaping of the olecranon and proximal ulna are done with a saw or rongeurs to produce a smooth, curved surface on which is contoured the bone plate. An arthrotomy is performed by subperiosteal elevation of the anconeus muscle from the humerus and ulna. The origin of the ulnaris lateralis muscle is elevated from the humerus, and the lateral collateral ligament is transected to allow the joint to be hinged open. This provides enough access for removal of articular cartilage. Articular cartilage is removed with a curette, air-driven bur, or osteotome to expose bleeding cancellous bone. In chronic osteoarthritis, eburnated subchondral bone on the condyle is relatively avascular and may be a barrier to successful fusion. It is disrupted with a curette to expose cancellous bone or foraged with multiple 1.5 mm drill holes to allow ingrowth of repair tissues.

Cancellous bone harvested from the proximal metaphysis of the humerus is placed between the joint surfaces, and then the fusion angle is determined with a goniometer. Temporary fixation of the joint is provided

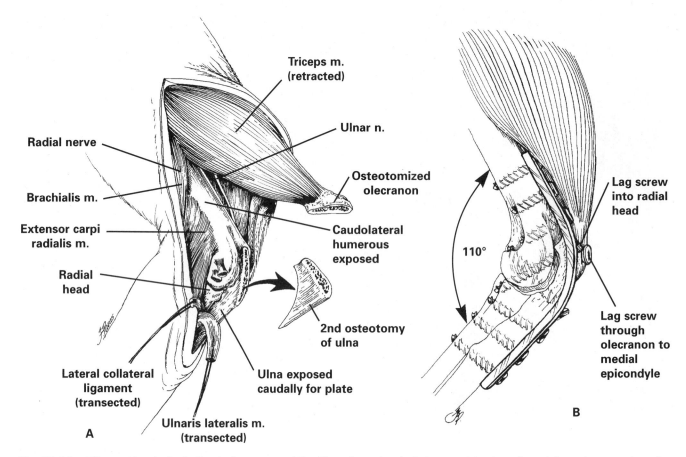

Triceps m.
(retracted)

Ulnar n.

Radial nerve

Osteotomized
olecranon

Brachialis m.

Caudolateral
humerous
exposed

Extensor carpi
radialis m.

Radial
head

2nd osteotomy
of ulna

Lateral collateral
ligament
(transected)

Ulna exposed
caudally for plate

Ulnaris lateralis m.
(transected)

A

110°

Lag screw
into radial
head

Lag screw
through
olecranon to
medial
epicondyle

B

Fig. 23-14 Elbow arthrodesis. **A**, Surgical exposure of the elbow for arthrodesis is a combination of caudolateral approach to the distal humerus, an olecranon osteotomy, and a caudal approach to the proximal ulna. Additional bone is removed from the olecranon to allow smooth contouring of the plate. Lateral collateral ligament is transected, articular cartilage is curetted from the joint, and cancellous bone graft is inserted. **B**, Stabilization of an elbow arthrodesis at an angle of approximately 110 degrees with a dynamic compression plate. The olecranon is reattached to the medial epicondyle.

Reproduced with permission from Brinker WO, Piermattei DL, Flo GL: *Handbook of small animal orthopedics and fracture treatment*, ed 2, Philadelphia, 1990, Saunders.

with pointed bone-holding forceps and Kirschner wires from the medial epicondyle into the radial head and from the olecranon into the humeral condyles. An 8- to 12-hole dynamic compression plate is contoured to the caudal surface of the humerus, elbow, and ulna (Fig. 23-14). Because of the shape of the involved bones, the plate is bent to an angle that is 10 to 20 degrees more acute than the desired angle of the elbow fusion. The plate is not prestressed by overbending because subsequent application of the plate forces the joint into a more flexed position. In addition to bending, some twisting of the plate is necessary to conform it to the ulnar diaphyseal cortex. A minimum of four screws in the humerus and four in the ulna-radius are recommended. In large dogs, more screws are used (Fig. 23-15). A plate hole directly over the supracondylar fossa should be avoided, since this predisposes to implant breakage. At the elbow joint, one of the plate screws is lagged through the plate and humerus into the radial head, and another is lagged through the plate and ulna into the humeral condyles. After the plate is applied,

Kirschner wires may be removed and replaced with lag screws. Remaining cancellous bone graft is packed into defects and around the joint. The olecranon is fixed to the medial epicondyle. To ensure good bone-to-bone contact, soft tissue is excised, and the epicondyle is flattened using an osteotome. The olecranon is fixed with a lag screw and Kirschner wire. A tension-band wire fixation can also be employed.

Aftercare includes a padded bandage for 10 to 14 days and then a lateral spica splint for another 4 weeks. Activity is strictly limited for a total of 8 to 10 weeks, by which time healing should have occurred.

CARPAL ARTHRODESIS

Arthrodesis is performed more often in the carpus than any other joint. The reasons are that severe palmar carpal sprain is a common injury, such injuries respond poorly to treatments other than arthrodesis, and limb function is not adversely affected by arthrodesis.

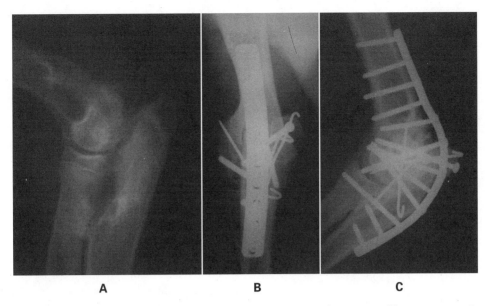

Fig. 23-15 **A,** Humeroulnar subluxation and painful osteoarthritis caused by posttraumatic premature closure of the distal ulnar physis in a 1-year-old Rottweiler. **B** and **C,** Twelve-hole, broad, 3.5 mm dynamic compression plate and Kirschner wire stabilization of the arthrodesis, immediately after surgery. The olecranon is reattached to the medial epicondyle with a lag screw and Kirschner wire.

Courtesy The University of Sydney.

The normal dorsal angle of the carpus in dogs while weight bearing varies from 140 to 180 degrees, depending on the breed. Extension beyond the upright 180-degree position normally occurs at the antebrachiocarpal joint. Normal range of flexion of the antebrachiocarpal joint is 100 degrees, whereas the middle carpal joint allows 40 degrees of flexion and the carpometacarpal joint 10 degrees.[36] Primary stabilizers of the carpus during weight bearing are the complex array of small palmar intercarpal ligaments, the overlying palmar fibrocartilage that blends with these ligaments, and the accessorometacarpal IV and V ligaments that form a stay apparatus from the tip of the accessory carpal bone to the metacarpal bones.[12]

Carpal Sprain Injury

In sprain injury a ligament may be disrupted in its midsubstance, torn from its insertion on bone, or rendered functionless by a sprain-avulsion fracture of the bone at an insertion. Midsubstance sprains are further classified as being an interstitial hematoma (grade 1, mild), partial rupture (grade 2, moderate), or complete rupture (grade 3, severe).[13] Hyperextension injuries of the carpus are the most common and devastating of the carpal sprains.[5] Invariably, multiple injuries occur to the palmar ligaments, palmar fibrocartilage, and accessorometacarpal ligaments. Falling or jumping from heights or moving vehicles is the usual cause, and about 10% of dogs have bilateral injury. Acutely there is considerable carpal swelling,

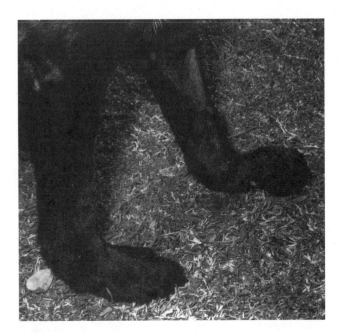

Fig. 23-16 Bilateral plantigrade stance in Labrador with chronic grade 3 palmar ligament sprains and carpometacarpal subluxation.

and the degree of subluxation apparent can vary from a slight increase in hyperextension to a complete plantigrade stance with a dorsal carpal angle of 90 degrees (Fig. 23-16). The degree of hyperextension depends on the severity of injury to individual ligaments and the

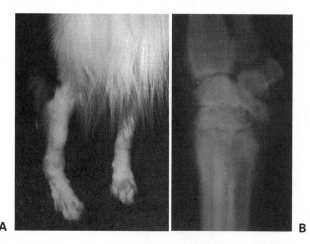

Fig. 23-17 **A**, Chronic carpal sprain injury caused by trauma in a collie with carpal hyperextension and a varus deviation. **B**, Osteoarthritis of all the carpal joints, with extensive osteophytosis.

B, Courtesy The University of Sydney.

number of ligaments damaged. After an acute injury, the severity of hyperextension tends to increase as inflammatory swelling and pain diminish, and weight bearing increases. Rupture of the short radial collateral and medial middle carpal ligaments may complicate palmar sprains, in which case both carpal valgus deviation and hyperextension are evident.

Carpal radiographs usually show only soft tissue swelling and sprain avulsion fractures. Fractured fragments may correspond with known insertion sites of supporting palmar ligaments and the fibrocartilage. Chip fractures along the dorsal margins of the joints, produced by impingement during the hyperextension injury, may be seen. Occasionally there is complete luxation or an intraarticular fracture of a carpal bone. Chronic carpal sprains have osteophytes and other signs of osteoarthritis (Fig. 23-17). Radiographs taken in the mediolateral projection with the carpus stressed into forced hyperextension (mimicking weight bearing), as well as dorsopalmar views with valgus and varus stress applied, are needed to demonstrate which of the carpal joints are subluxated.[13] Severe sprains are readily diagnosed by the subluxation seen on stressed radiographs, but grade 1 and 2 sprains are not always apparent until signs of osteoarthritis develop subsequently. Fracturing and proximal displacement of the accessory carpal bone and accessoroulnar joint subluxation occur frequently in hyperextension injury. These findings indicate disruption of the accessorometacarpal ligament stay apparatus. More than 80% of the hyperextension injuries involve the middle carpal joint, the carpometacarpal joint, or both.[5,19] Often there is no detectable injury to the antebrachiocarpal joint, although grade 1 and 2 sprains of this joint can be difficult to exclude.

Indications

Severe carpal sprain is the main indication for arthrodesis. Treatment of grade 1 and 2 sprains that have no appreciable hyperextension with splinting in flexion is occasionally successful. However, treatment of grade 3 hyperextension sprains by splinting invariably fails because of the slow gain in tensile strength of healing ligaments and their subsequent breakdown once splints are removed. Palmar ligament repair with wire and fascial strip reconstruction has been described, but long-term studies of outcome are needed.[11] Arthrodesis is the recommended treatment because it is invariably successful in restoring limb function.[19,27,35] It is performed as soon as a diagnosis of severe hyperextension injury is made; trial periods of splinting are futile. Injuries confined to the middle carpal and carpometacarpal joints can be treated by partial carpal arthrodesis of these joints, preserving the antebrachiocarpal joint. Pancarpal arthrodesis is indicated for any injury or disease involving the antebrachiocarpal joint. Partial arthrodesis of the antebrachiocarpal joint alone, preserving the middle carpal and carpometacarpal joints, is not considered worthwhile because these two distal joints are relatively immobile.[36]

Other indications for arthrodesis include secondary osteoarthritis, intraarticular fractures, open fractures (see Chapter 10), antebrachiocarpal subluxation following premature closure of the distal radial physis (see Chapter 13), septic arthritis, and immune-mediated joint disease (Fig. 23-18).

Pancarpal Arthrodesis

For pancarpal arthrodesis, a surgical exposure of the distal fourth of the radius, all the carpal joints, and the diaphysis of metacarpal bone III is needed. The skin incision is longitudinal and slightly dorsomedial. It commences at the bifurcation of the accessory cephalic and cephalic veins and continues medial and parallel to the accessory cephalic vein, extending distally along the diaphysis of metacarpal bone II. The accessory cephalic vein and accompanying proximal radial collateral artery (lateral branch) and superficial radial nerve (lateral branch) are preserved. If necessary, more exposure of the radial diaphysis is gained by undermining and elevating the cephalic vein as it branches to the medial side of the antebrachium. The abductor pollicis longus muscle is either elevated from the radius and moved medially or is transected. The tendon sheath of the extensor carpi radialis is opened longitudinally, and its insertions on metacarpal bones II and III are transected. Similarly, the tendon sheath of common digital extensor overlying the distal radius and dorsal carpus is opened longitudinally. This incision continues along the medial border of the common digital extensor tendon II, then all the digital extensor

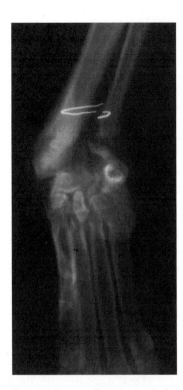

Fig. 23-18 Chronic fracture/luxation of the antebrachio-carpal joint. Initially an open shearing injury caused extensive bone loss from the distal radius and separation of the radial and ulnar diaphyses. Open wounds were debrided and allowed to heal by second intention, and the radius and ulna were united with cerclage wires. Carpal arthrodesis is indicated to correct the resultant osteoarthritis and joint instability.

Courtesy The University of Sydney.

tendons are displaced laterally and preserved. The carpus is flexed, and joint capsules of the antebrachiocarpal, middle carpal, and carpometacarpal joints are incised transversely. Articular cartilage is removed completely from all three joints, as well as the vertical intercarpal joints, with an air-driven bur (Fig. 23-19, *A*). Insertion of a small narrow Hohmann retractor can greatly facilitate exposure of the palmar compartment of each joint.

For most dogs, a seven-hole 3.5 mm dynamic compression plate, with three screws in the distal radius, one in the radial carpal bone, and three in metacarpal bone III, is the fixation of choice (Fig. 23-19, *B*). For large breeds of dogs, an eight-hole plate with four screws in the radius is used. The broad 3.5 mm dynamic compression plate is used for giant breeds of dogs and the 2.7 mm plate for very small dogs. The plate is contoured to the distal end of the radius, across the radial carpal bone, and down metacarpal bone III. The carpus is positioned in 10 degrees of extension, but not more, since bending stresses on the plate can lead to implant failure. The first hole is drilled in the radial carpal bone, and this screw is inserted so that the "middle" of the plate lies distal to this screw (Fig. 23-19, *B*). Holes for screws in metacarpal bone III and the distal radius are drilled in the load position, measured, and tapped (Fig. 23-19, *B*). Bone graft collected from the ipsilateral proximal humerus is packed into the joint cavities. Insertion of screws into the previously drilled holes in the radius and metacarpal bone III produces interfragmentary compression at the carpus. Application of the plate is completed with insertion of

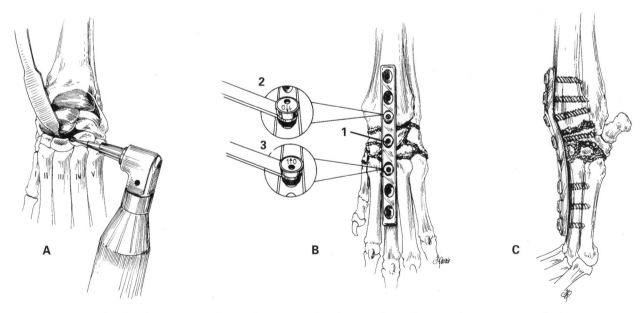

Fig. 23-19 Pancarpal arthrodesis. **A**, Articular cartilage removal with an air-driven bur. A Hohmann retractor facilitates exposure of the joint compartments. **B**, Seven-hole 3.5 mm dynamic compression plate applied to the distal radius, radial carpal bone, and metacarpal bone III. The initial screw (1) is inserted into the radial carpal bone. Screws into the distal radius (2) and metacarpal bone III (3) are inserted in the load position to produce interfragmentary compression in the arthrodesis. **C**, Precontouring of the plate positions the carpus in approximately 10 degrees of extension.

the remaining screws in neutral position (Fig. 23-19, *C*). Care is needed to avoid fracturing the metacarpal bone during screw insertion. Residual bone graft is placed on the dorsal surface of the carpus, adjacent to the plate. Bone grafts induce healing of the arthrodesis by 4 to 8 weeks, whereas union without a graft takes more than 12 weeks, by which time the plate may fatigue and break or screws may loosen.[21]

External coaptation for 6 to 12 weeks is indicated, with longer periods for large, active dogs and bilateral arthrodesis. Considerable swelling of the distal limb follows this surgery, but it can be controlled by soft padded bandages and hot packing, applied for the first 4 to 7 days. After swelling subsides, external coaptation with a splint is needed to protect against implant failure, to immobilize carpal and metacarpal bones not secured by screws, and to protect against fracturing of metacarpal bone III distal to the plate. Beyond 6 months postoperatively, loosening of the screws in metacarpal bone III can be associated with draining sinuses, which only resolve after implant removal (Fig. 23-20). Plate removal at this time is safe, provided that the fusion is solid, which is usually the case.

Partial Carpal Arthrodesis

The surgical exposure for partial carpal arthrodesis is the same as for pancarpal arthrodesis, except that it does not extend so far proximally, the abductor pollicis longus muscle is not elevated, insertions of the extensor carpi radialis muscle are preserved, and antebrachiocarpal joint arthrotomy may be unnecessary. Articular cartilage is removed from the middle carpal, carpometacarpal, and intercarpal joints with an air-driven bur. Internal fixation is with two pins[35] or a T plate.[5,31]

Pinning is the usual method of fixation (Fig. 23-21). Slots are burred in the dorsal cortex of metacarpal bones III and IV, just proximal to the metacarpophalangeal joint. Trocar-point intramedullary pins, 1.6 or 2.0 mm in diameter, are curved slightly and driven normograde by hand up the medullary canal of the metacarpal bones using a pin chuck. Before complete insertion of the pins, cancellous bone graft harvested from the ipsilateral humerus is packed into the joint cavities. The pins are then advanced farther through the distal row of numbered carpal bones and seated into the radial carpal bone.[5] During final seating of the pins, the carpus is held

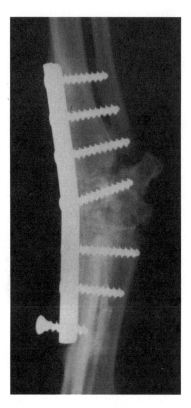

Fig. 23-20 Healed carpal arthrodesis at 6 months in the collie shown in Fig. 23-17. Screw loosening may cause lameness and draining tracts. These signs resolve with implant removal.

Courtesy The University of Sydney.

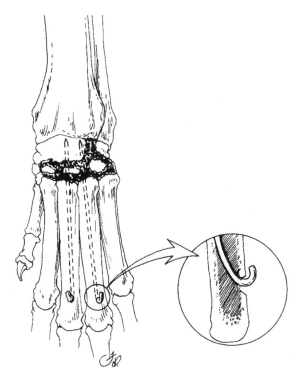

Fig. 23-21 Partial carpal arthrodesis with pins. Articular cartilage is removed from the middle and carpometacarpal joints, autogenous cancellous bone is packed into the joint cavities, and intramedullary pins inserted in slots made distally are driven up metacarpal bones III and IV, to be seated into the radial carpal bone.

in 90 degrees of flexion to ensure that the joints are not fixed in a hyperextended position. Pins must not be advanced into the antebrachiocarpal joint. Pin placement can be monitored intraoperatively by premeasuring pin length or by direct inspection via a small antebrachiocarpal arthrotomy. Once pins are finally seated, the distal ends may be bent over and cut off.

T plate fixation is an alternative to pinning.[4,5,31] The same techniques of surgical exposure, articular cartilage removal, and cancellous bone grafting described for pin fixation are employed before T plate application. Several AO-ASIF T plates that vary in screw size and number of screw holes in the plate are suitable for this application. The T plate is applied to the radial carpal bone with two to three screws and to metacarpal bone III with three to five screws (Fig. 23-22). Impingement of the distal end of the radius onto the edge of the plate during weight bearing causes osteoarthritis of the antebrachiocarpal joint and can be a problem with this method of fixation. Positioning the plate more distally on the radial carpal bone minimizes this complication. Because these plates are generally intended to function as metaphyseal buttress plates, they are thinner than a dynamic compression plate and thus susceptible to bending.

After partial arthrodesis with pins or a T plate, the internal fixation must be protected by immobilization of

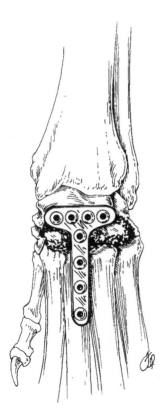

Fig. 23-22 Partial carpal arthrodesis with a T plate applied to the proximal row of carpal bones and to metacarpal bone III.

the carpus in flexion. Initially a thick padded bandage is applied until swelling subsides, then a thinner bandage reinforced with a lateral fiberglass slab is applied. This is maintained until fusion is apparent radiographically, usually at 6 to 10 weeks.[35]

Although the antebrachiocarpal joint is intentionally preserved in this procedure, range of motion of the antebrachiocarpal joint after complete fusion of the middle and carpometacarpal joints is approximately half of normal.[31,35] Reasons for this may include alteration in antebrachiocarpal joint kinesiology by fusion of the two distal joints, extraarticular fibrosis caused by occult sprain injury of the antebrachiocarpal joint and surgery, and loss of extensor tendon gliding function as a sequela to surgery. In one study of 45 partial carpal arthrodeses, hyperextension persisted in 11%, and 15% developed antebrachiocarpal joint osteoarthritis, but no dog needed to have panarthrodesis at a later date.[35] In 68% the lameness was eliminated by partial carpal arthrodesis, and in the rest it was improved.[35]

METACARPOPHALANGEAL ARTHRODESIS

Arthrodesis of the metacarpophalangeal or metatarsophalangeal joints is performed rarely. Amputation is a satisfactory solution to serious diseases or injuries involving a single digit, but digit preservation by arthrodesis becomes essential when several digits are injured or other digits are missing already.

Indications

Specific indications are chronic septic arthritis with osteomyelitis,[33] unstable luxations, open fracture/shearing injuries, and comminuted intraarticular fractures. Another indication is correction of hyperextension of the digits after chronic transection of the digital flexor tendons, in which tenorrhaphy has previously failed (Fig. 23-23).

Surgery

A dorsal paramedian longitudinal incision is made over the joint, the extensor tendon mobilized and reflected laterally, and the joint capsule incised transversely. Articular surfaces are excised with an oscillating saw to produce two flat surfaces. Osteotomies are angled to allow the joint to be fused with a dorsal angle of 110 to 170 degrees, corresponding to the position of normal contralateral digits. The two palmar sesamoid bones are excised. A five-hole 2.7 mm dynamic compression plate or 2.0 mm plate is applied to the dorsal surface, and autogenous cancellous bone graft is packed around the joint (Fig. 23-23). After surgery, a splint is applied for 6 to 8 weeks to protect the fixation until fusion has occurred.

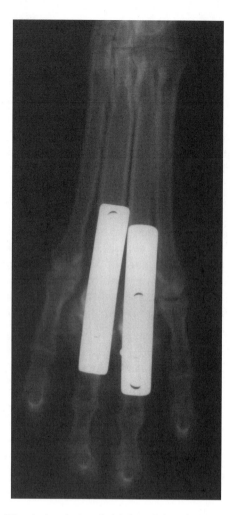

Fig. 23-23 Arthrodesis of third and fourth metatarsophalangeal joints with 2.7 mm dynamic compression plate fixation. Courtesy The University of Sydney.

PROXIMAL INTERPHALANGEAL ARTHRODESIS

Arthrodesis of the proximal interphalangeal joint may be an alternative to digit amputation. Normally, amputation of one digit is well tolerated, but digit preservation is desired when other digits of the involved foot are abnormal or have been amputated previously. Arthrodesis of this joint is not usually performed, but experience with a limited number of cases indicates that the surgical procedure usually results in a solid fusion; once fusion of the joint is complete, there is no appreciable loss of limb function or residual lameness. Greyhounds have returned to racing after proximal interphalangeal arthrodesis in the forelimb, but attempts at arthrodesis of this joint in the hind limb have been unsuccessful.[10] Arthrodesis of the distal interphalangeal joint has not been described, and severe injuries of this joint are managed by amputation of the distal phalanx.[10]

Indications

Luxations of the proximal interphalangeal joint with rupture of one collateral ligament can be corrected by suturing the ligament and joint capsule.[10] However, with rupture of both collateral ligaments, there is often concurrent disruption of the superficial digital flexor insertion, torn dorsal joint capsule–extensor tendon complex, avulsion fractures at the insertions of these soft tissues, or a combination of these injuries. These injuries permit complete luxation, and either arthrodesis or amputation is indicated because attempts at primary repair invariably fail.

Comminuted intraarticular fractures not amenable to internal fixation or chronic luxations and intraarticular fractures with painful osteoarthritis are candidates for arthrodesis. In traumatic degloving injuries to the digits and open fractures/luxations, appropriate wound management (see Chapter 10) and secondary arthrodesis of the proximal interphalangeal joint may preserve the digit. Neurovascular injury is a potential complication of these injuries and requires careful assessment.

Surgery

The joint is exposed by a longitudinal incision, slightly off midline, on the dorsomedial or dorsolateral surface of the proximal and middle phalanx. The extensor retinaculum is incised longitudinally, and the extensor tendons and sesamoid cartilage are reflected to one side. The joint capsule is incised transversely, and articular cartilage is removed with rongeurs or a curette. The palmar angle of the joint is approximately 120 degrees in digits III and IV and 135 degrees in digits II and V. The joint is stabilized in a position that allows normal contact of the digital pad and nail with the ground while weight bearing. A Kirschner wire is driven obliquely through the distal end of the proximal phalanx, into the medullary cavity of the middle phalanx, and stabilized with a dorsal figure-eight tension-band wire[10,18] (Fig. 23-24, A). More rigid fixation is obtained with a four- or five-hole plate, which is contoured and applied to the joint's dorsal surface (Fig. 23-24, B). The 2.7 mm dynamic compression plate is suitable for very large dogs, whereas the miniplate with 2.0 or 1.5 mm screws is appropriate for all others. Careful planning is needed to ensure that none of the screw holes in the plate remains empty because of the risk of implant fatigue failure, and one of the plate screws should be lagged across the arthrodesis for improved stability.[18]

Alternatively, articular cartilage and bone ends may be resected with an oscillating saw to produce two flat surfaces (Fig. 23-24, C). This results in some shortening of the digit, and the palmar angle of the joint needs to be increased to compensate for this shortening. If osteotomies are angled at 75 degrees to the long axis of each

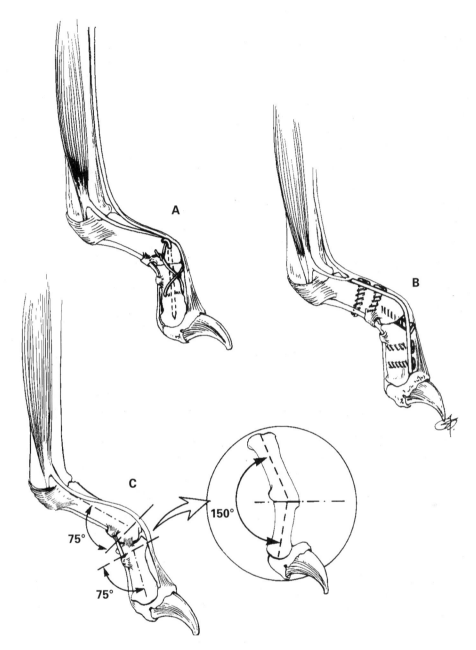

Fig. 23-24 Proximal interphalangeal arthrodesis. **A,** Stabilization of a proximal interphalangeal arthrodesis with a Kirschner wire and dorsal figure-eight tension-band wire. **B,** Five-hole plate fixation of a proximal interphalangeal arthrodesis. One plate screw is lagged across the arthrodesis. **C,** Articular surfaces may be resected with an oscillating saw for arthrodesis. Presurgical planning determines the osteotomy and arthrodesis angles.

bone, the joint will be fused at an angle of 150 degrees. When comminution, lysis, or trauma has caused severe bone loss, the joint is fused at 180 degrees, in which case a straight plate may be applied to the dorsal or lateral aspect. A cancellous bone graft from the proximal humerus is packed around the joint.

After surgery, a thick padded bandage protects the digit for 5 to 10 days. Subsequently, a lightweight fiberglass cast or splint is applied for 4 more weeks.

STIFLE ARTHRODESIS
Indications

Arthrodesis of the stifle joint may be indicated when primary repair, reconstruction, or correction of severely comminuted fractures, ligamentous rupture, grade 4 patellar luxation, and chronic nonunion or malunion of intraarticular fractures are not feasible or have failed. Severe osteoarthritis after chronic rupture of the cranial cruciate ligament and repeated surgical procedures for joint stabilization are a difficult problem. Stifle arthrodesis initially appears to be a solution to painful osteoarthritis, and many factors favor a good outcome. The femoral condyles and tibial plateau provide two large surfaces of cancellous bone that can be brought into apposition for bone union. Also, the plate is applied on the tension surface of the knee. However, a major problem is that postoperative function may be poor.[8] When the stifle joint is fused, hock joint flexion is precluded by tension in the gastrocnemius muscle that spans both joints. Because of limited stifle and hock joint mobility, the limb is advanced by circumduction in the swing phase of the gait. Animals with a stifle arthrodesis may be unable to negotiate stairs without assistance. Because of the overall rigidity of the hind limb, minor falls have occasionally resulted in fracturing of the tibia distal to the plate.

Surgery

The angle for the joint fusion should be about 10 degrees less than the normal standing angle to allow easier ambulation. Suggested angles of fusion are 135 to 140 degrees for dogs and 120 to 125 degrees for cats. Preoperative radiographs and tracings made of the radiographs with a felt-tip pen on acetate sheets are useful for precise planning of osteotomy angles[5] (Fig. 23-25, A).

The surgical approach is by a craniolateral exposure, with a large osteotomy of the tibial crest and tuberosity to increase exposure and allow subsequent placement of the plate. The quadriceps muscles are reflected medially off the distal femur. Remnants of the cruciate ligaments and meniscal cartilages are resected. The long digital extensor tendon and collateral ligaments are preserved. These provide some joint stability before plate application.

The stifle joint is positioned at the desired angle of fusion with the aid of a goniometer, and Kirschner wires are inserted in the midsagittal plane into the distal femur and proximal tibia to mark the alignment for the osteotomies[5] (Fig. 23-25, A and B). The first osteotomy is made in the proximal tibia, removing a 20-degree wedge of proximal tibia, which increases in thickness caudally. This particular orientation of the osteotomy assists in achieving sufficient flexion in the fusion. Before osteotomizing the femur, the condyles are brought into reduction to ensure that the femur and tibia are axially aligned. If there is bone loss or deformity of the condyles, as occurs in grade 4 medial patellar luxation, a correction for valgus or varus is made by angling the osteotomy in a medial-to-lateral direction. With the stifle at the chosen angle of fusion, and using the Kirschner wire as a guide, the femoral osteotomy is made parallel to the tibial osteotomy. Care is taken to avoid lacerating the popliteal artery that lies between the two femoral condyles, just external to the joint capsule caudally. After the osteotomies are made in the tibia

and femur and the resected pieces removed, the two cut surfaces of bone are brought into apposition (Fig. 23-25, B). The initial trial reduction of the arthrodesis is maintained with AO-ASIF pointed bone-holding forceps. The angle of arthrodesis is then measured again with a goniometer. A careful evaluation of the whole limb is made to ensure that the tibia is correctly aligned with respect to rotation, valgus, and varus. It may be necessary to reposition the tibia or to resect more bone off the distal femur to correct for malalignment. Once a satisfactory reduction is achieved, two Kirschner wires are inserted in the frontal plane, from each femoral epicondyle, diagonally across the joint. These stabilize the bones while the plate is being applied.

Before applying the plate, the tibial crest may be resected to allow easier contouring of the plate. Excessive bone should not be removed because this weakens the tibia and reduces the holding power of plate screws. Although it is not necessary to remove any of the articular cartilage from the trochlear groove, the trochlear ridges and osteophytes can be flattened off with an oscillating saw, rongeurs, or osteotome to position the plate in better contact with the bone. An 8- to 10-hole dynamic compression plate is contoured to the cranial aspect of the stifle joint (Fig. 23-25, C). The bend in the plate will be more acute than the predetermined angle for the arthrodesis because of convexity in the distal femur and proximal tibia. If the plate is not sufficiently contoured, the arthrodesis tends to open up caudally, and the arthrodesis ends up being too straight. The plate's distal end is twisted so that it comes to lie on the craniolateral surface of the tibial diaphysis. The plate should be positioned such that the central portion of the plate is lying over the junction between the two bones. The screws proximal and distal to the plate's center can be angled and lagged across the arthrodesis to increase interfragmentary compression (Fig. 23-25, C). Remaining plate screws are inserted in the neutral position. Insertion of plate screws in the load position increases interfragmentary compression immediately under the plate but tends to cause gaping of the arthrodesis caudally. Cancellous bone harvested from the resected femoral condyles is packed into the intercondylar region, into the space under the plate, and into any other defects. Additional bone graft can be collected from the usual sites. The tibial tuberosity is reattached with lag screws or tension-band wiring.

Postoperatively, a thick padded bandage is applied to the limb to control swelling, which can be extensive after this surgery. This support can be removed after 2 to 4 weeks. Because the plate is applied to the tension surface of the stifle, it is biomechanically very stable.

Stabilization with a transarticular external fixator is indicated when arthrodesis is being performed to resolve septic arthritis or osteomyelitis.[3] Proximally the fixator is

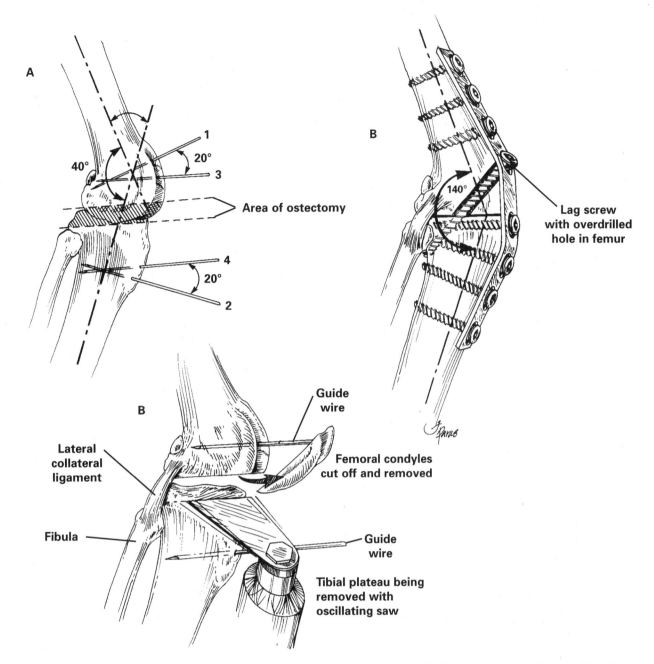

Fig. 23-25   Stifle arthrodesis stabilized with a dynamic compression plate. **A**, Presurgical planning. Kirschner wires 1 and 2 are inserted perpendicular to the femoral and tibial diaphyses. The arthrodesis angle of 140 degrees has a complement of 40 degrees. Halving the complementary angle gives 20 degrees, which is the angle of pins 3 and 4 to pins 1 and 2. Pins 3 and 4 indicate the directions of osteotomies. **B**, Femoral condyles and tibial plateau osteotomized with an oscillating saw. **C**, Stabilization of stifle arthrodesis with a plate on the cranial tension surface. Plate screws adjacent to the arthodesis can be angled and lagged across the arthrodesis

A, Reproduced with permission from Brinker WO, Piermattei DL, Flo GL: *Handbook of small animal orthopedics and fracture treatment*, ed 2, Philadelphia, 1990, Saunders.

a type I applied to the lateral aspect of the distal femur and a type II in the frontal plane in the proximal tibia. Premature loosening of the pins is a significant problem with external fixators applied in this location because of the large muscles that are transfixed by the fixation pins.

Muscle movement around the pins leads to tissue necrosis, pin tract infection, and pin loosening. After resolution of osteomyelitis, the fixator may need to be replaced with a plate to provide enough stability for osseous fusion of the arthrodesis.

TARSAL ARTHRODESIS

Arthrodesis of the entire tarsal joint complex is occasionally indicated, but more often a partial arthrodesis is performed, which has the advantage of preserving some normal joint motion. The three main types of arthrodesis are tarsocrural, proximal intertarsal, and tarsometatarsal.

Tarsocrural Arthrodesis

Arthrodesis at this level involves fusion of both the talocrural and the talocalcaneal joints. Normally the talocrural joint allows the greatest range of motion in the tarsus, and the more distal joints are relatively immobile.[12] However, inclusion of the talocalcaneal joint in the tarsocrural fusion is advisable. Insertion of screws into the calcaneus and the relatively smaller talus provides more secure internal fixation and also prevents secondary painful talocalcaneal joint instability. Dogs with a well-arthrodesed tarsocrural joint have acceptable limb function. Loss of mobility in these joints can be accommodated by the stifle joint. Tarsocrural arthrodesis would be performed more often if not for the difficulty in obtaining secure internal fixation of the arthrodesis and a robust, complete, pain-free bony fusion. Surgical failure rates in the order of 50% have been a deterrent to recommending the procedure.[22] However, this success rate can probably be improved by using stronger, more biomechanically stable internal fixation and providing external support until fusion is complete.

Indications. Specific indications for tarsocrural arthrodesis are chronic fracture/luxation of the talocrural joint with instability and osteoarthritis, osteoarthritis secondary to talar osteochondritis dissecans, irreparable intraarticular fractures, and chronic irreparable injuries or deficiencies of the common calcaneal tendon. Other indications are open shearing injuries and open fracture/luxations when greater than one third of the distal tibia or talus articular surface has been lost or when sepsis has destroyed articular cartilage.

Surgery. The surgical approach is dictated by the type and placement of fixation, as well as wounds, shearing injuries, and open fractures/luxations. For medial exposure, the medial malleolus of the tibia is osteotomized in the sagittal plane and discarded because the stability of the medial collateral ligament is no longer needed. All articular cartilage of the talocrural joint is removed using a curette or air-driven bur so that the joint contours are preserved. A less desired alternative is to osteotomize the distal tibia perpendicular to the tibial axis and osteotomize the talus at a predetermined angle that allows fusion of the joint at an angle of 135 to 145 degrees in dogs and 115 to 125 degrees in cats.[5] Osteotomy of the distal

tibia to remove the cochlea and expose cancellous bone involves removal of considerable bone and some limb shortening. Also, ostectomy of the talus can compromise stability.

Additionally, articular cartilage and soft tissues between the talus and calcaneus are curetted and resected, and subsequently both the talocrural and the talocalcaneal joints are bone grafted. Internal fixation of tarsocrural arthrodeses with a plate applied cranially, laterally, or caudally across the joint has been described.[5,25,32] Caudal plate application is the most biomechanically stable because the plate acts as a tension band, but the surgical approach is complicated and digital flexor tendons are adversely affected. Therefore, cranial plate application represents the best compromise.[9,17]

For cranial application of the plate, the distal tibia and tarsus are exposed with a longitudinal incision medial to the long digital extensor and cranial tibialis tendons. Additional exposure is gained by transection of the cranial tibialis tendon at its insertion on metatarsal bone II. A five- to eight-hole dynamic compression plate is contoured to the distal tibia and talus. One screw is inserted as a positional screw through the distal tibia and into the calcaneus[5] (Fig. 23-26). A gliding hole is not drilled, and bone in the distal tibia and the calcaneus is tapped. This positional screw minimizes bending stresses on the plate.[5] Ideally the plate does not extend beyond the proximal intertarsal joint, but a limitation of this technique is that only two screws engage the talus. For increased stability, a longer plate extending down to the central and third tarsal bones or to metatarsal bone III is usually applied

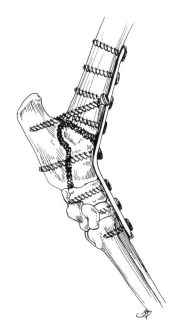

Fig. 23-26 Tarsocrural arthrodesis with a dynamic compression plate on the cranial aspect.

(Fig. 23-26). Bridging of several normal tarsal joints is the compromise accepted for an increase in security of plate attachment distally. Although there is normally little motion in the distal joints and minimum functional loss, this motion eventually causes screw loosening, which necessitates implant removal.

Lateral application of a plate for tarsocrural arthrodesis has advantages in that the plate is loaded on edge and is more resistant to bending loads than a cranial plate.[32] A lateral approach is made by ostectomy of the distal third of the fibula. A 2.0/2.7 mm AO-ASIF veterinary cuttable plate is contoured to the lateral surface of the distal tibia and around the distal plantar surface of the calcaneus. The plate is applied with 2.0 or 2.7 mm cortical screws. Advantages of this plate are that the screw holes are at 6 mm centers, allowing three to five fixation screws to be inserted in the calcaneus and talus. Also, stacking two plates provides extra stiffness. The most distal plate screw, or another independent screw, is lagged from the calcaneus through the talus into the distal tibia to provide interfragmentary compression.

Transarticular external fixator stabilization and arthrodesis of the talocrural joint or entire tarsus are primarily indicated in open fractures/luxations and shearing injuries (see Chapter 10). The goal is to allow management of the open wound, stabilize the soft tissues, and prevent reluxation. Initially the soft tissues are debrided and irrigated. A type II transarticular configuration of external fixator is applied[3] (Fig. 23-27). A primary arthrodesis can be performed, but in case of infection, it is better to wait until healthy granulation tissue is formed and then curette the articular cartilage and use a bone graft as a delayed procedure.

Proximal Intertarsal Arthrodesis

Indications. Rupture of the plantar ligaments of the proximal intertarsal joint, with consequent joint instability, is the main indication for proximal intertarsal arthrodesis. Shetland sheepdogs and collies are at increased risk for this injury,[6] and a collagen disorder is suspected to be the underlying cause. In these breeds the subluxation usually develops without overt trauma and is often bilateral. Affected animals may also exhibit carpal hyperextension. Traumatic luxation of the proximal intertarsal joint is often the result of an injury sustained while jumping over a fence. A hind foot becomes entrapped in wire mesh or wooden pickets, then the animal falls to the other side of the fence. In racing greyhounds with injury to this joint, the calcaneoquartal joint subluxates with concomitant calcaneal avulsion-fractures, whereas the talocentral joint may be normal.[26]

Mechanical instability of the joint causes lameness, but beyond the acute injury phase, it is not very painful, although osteoarthritis develops subsequently. Physical ex-

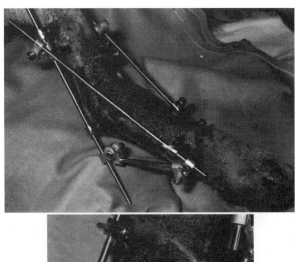

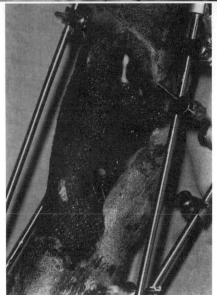

Fig. 23-27 Type II transarticular external fixator stabilization of an open shearing injury of the tarsus after 14 days. After infection was resolved, tarsocrural articular surfaces were curetted and bone grafted. The external fixator maintained stability until arthrodesis occurred. **A,** Craniolateral aspect of the right tarsus, with fixation pins in the distal tibial, calcaneus, and metatarsal bones. Stabilization against bending forces is achieved by triangulating the connecting bars on each side of the limb. **B,** Granulation tissue and exposed bone seen from craniomedial aspect.

amination may reveal palpable joint instability, soft tissue swelling, and a convex curvature of the tarsus while weight bearing. With severe joint angulation, increased tension in the digital flexor tendons causes the digits to be hyperflexed in a clawlike position. Diagnosis is confirmed with a mediolateral radiograph while the tarsus is hyperflexed to demonstrate instability. Treatment of these injuries with rest and extended periods of external coaptation is invariably unsuccessful. The only satisfactory treatment is arthrodesis. Open shearing injury is another indication for arthrodesis of this joint, and it may be performed in conjunction with tarsocrural arthrodesis.

Surgery. Arthrodeses of the proximal intertarsal joint can be stabilized by tension-band wiring, a laterally applied plate, or an external fixator.

A calcaneoquartal arthrodesis is stabilized with tension-band wiring (Fig. 23-28), preserving the unaffected talocentral joint.[1] A plantarolateral longitudinal skin incision is made from the calcaneal tuber to the tarsometatarsal joint. Deep fascia and retinaculum of the superficial digital flexor tendon are incised, and the digital tendon is retracted medially. The articular surfaces are exposed by flexing the joint, and cartilage is removed with an air-driven bur or curette. A figure-eight wire is placed through transverse drill holes in the base of the calcaneus and the fourth tarsal bone. A pilot hole for the Steinmann pin is drilled axially through the calcaneus, starting from the distal articular surface and emerging through the proximal tip of the calcaneus. Because the calcaneus is composed of very dense compact bone, predrilling facilitates Steinmann pin insertion and minimizes bone burning and necrosis. Autogenous cancellous bone graft is packed into the joint space. A 1.2 or 2.0 mm pin is inserted normograde through the calcaneus and seated into the fourth tarsal bone. The pin is either cut off short and countersunk into the bone or bent over to minimize damage to the superficial digital flexor tendon.[4,26] The tension-band wire is tightened by even twisting on each side of the bone, and the ends are cut off and turned over (Fig. 23-28). Additional cancellous bone is packed around the periphery of the arthrodesis before closure.

Lateral plate stabilization is indicated for complete luxation of the proximal intertarsal joint. Before plate application, both the calcaneoquartal and the talocentral joints are debrided of cartilage and bone grafted, as described for tension-band wiring. A 2.0 or 2.7, or 3.5 mm dynamic compression plate is contoured to the lateral surface of the calcaneus, fourth tarsal bone, and metatarsal bone V. Because the plate is loaded on edge when applied in this way, it resists bending forces. After surgery, a thick padded bandage and splint are applied until swelling subsides, after which a short leg fiberglass cast is applied for 6 to 8 weeks, by which time there should be radiographic evidence of fusion of the arthrodesis. Loosening of plate screws occurs after 4 to 6 months because of the mobility of the nonfused joints bridged by the plate. For open shearing injuries, the external fixator is the preferred means of stabilizing the joint for arthrodesis.

Tarsometatarsal Arthrodesis

The primary indication for arthrodesis of the tarsometatarsal joint is rupture of the plantar ligaments and fibrocartilage and luxation. Although occurring less often than proximal intertarsal luxation, this injury is also sustained traumatically when a hind leg is caught in wire mesh or pickets as an animal jumps over a fence. Automobile trauma is another cause of this injury. Treatment with rest and immobilization of the limb in external coaptation invariably fails, and arthrodesis is the only successful treatment. The clinical signs are similar to proximal intertarsal luxation, except that the swelling and instability are located more distally. The diagnosis is confirmed by a stressed mediolateral radiograph taken with the tarsus and metatarsus forced into full flexion.

Surgery. A longitudinal plantarolateral skin incision is made to expose the fourth tarsal bone, the tarsometatarsal joint, and metatarsal bone V. Articular cartilage is removed from the joint surfaces with an air-driven bur, and autogenous cancellous bone is packed into the joint cavity. In chronic cases, osteophytes, callus, and periosteal new bone impede exposure and reduction of the joint and need to be resected. The arthrodesis is stabilized with a 2.7 mm dynamic compression plate applied to the lateral surface of the calcaneus, fourth tarsal bone, and metatarsus[4] (Fig. 23-29). Screws inserted distally normally only engage metatarsal bones IV and V because of the arrangement of these bones in a curved arcade. Excessive interfragmentary compression of the joint, produced by loading several plate screws, is undesired because it induces a valgus deviation of the metatarsus. After surgery, a thick padded bandage is applied until

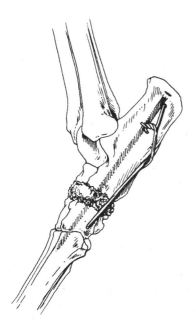

Fig. 23-28 Stabilization of calcaneoquartal arthrodesis with intramedullary pin and tension-band wire.

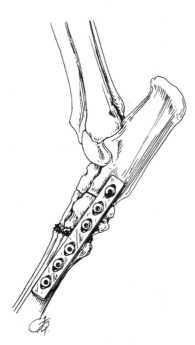

Fig. 23-29 Tarsometatarsal arthrodesis stabilized with a dynamic compression plate on the lateral surface of the calcaneus, fourth tarsal bone, and metatarsal bone V.

swelling subsides, then a short leg fiberglass cast is applied for 6 to 8 weeks until radiographic evidence of healing is seen. Loosening of screws caused by movement of the metatarsal bone may cause lameness and draining fistulas 4 to 6 months after surgery. By this time, healing of the arthrodesis should be complete, and the problem is resolved by implant removal.

REFERENCES

1. Allen MJ, Dyce J, Houlton JEF: Calcaneoquartal arthrodesis in the dog, *J Small Anim Pract* 34:205-210, 1993.
2. Bennett D, Vaughan L: The use of muscle relocation techniques in the treatment of peripheral nerve injuries in dogs and cats, *J Small Anim Pract* 17:99-108, 1976.
3. Bjorling DE, Toombs JP: Transarticular application of the Kirschner-Ehmer splint, *J Vet Surg* 11:34-38, 1982.
4. Brinker WO, Hohn RB, Prieur WD: *Manual of internal fixation in small animals*, Berlin, 1984, Springer-Verlag.
5. Brinker WO, Piermattei DL, Flo GL: *Handbook of small animal orthopedics and fracture treatment*, ed 2, Philadelphia, 1990, Saunders.
6. Campbell JR, Bennett D, Lee R: Intertarsal and tarsometatarsal subluxation in the dog, *J Small Anim Pract* 17:427-442, 1976.
7. Charnley J, Baker SL: Compression arthrodesis of the knee: a clinical and histological study, *J Bone Joint Surg* 34B:187-199, 1952.
8. Cofone MA, and others: Unilateral and bilateral stifle arthrodesis in eight dogs, *J Vet Surg* 21:299-303, 1992.
9. DeCamp CE, Martinez SA, Johnston SA: Pantarsal arthrodesis in dogs and a cat: 11 cases (1983-1991), *J Am Vet Med Assoc* 203:1705-1707, 1993.
10. Dee JF, Dee LG, Eaton-Wells RD: Injuries of high performance dogs. In Whittick WG, editor: *Canine orthopedics*, ed 2, Philadelphia, 1990, Lea & Febiger.
11. Earley T: Canine carpal ligament injuries, *Vet Clin North Am* 8:183-199, 1978.
12. Evans HE, Christensen GC: *Miller's anatomy of the dog*, ed 2, Philadelphia, 1979, Saunders.
13. Farrow CS: Sprain, strain, and contusion, *Vet Clin North Am* 8:169-182, 1978.
14. Fowler DJ, Presnell KR, Holmberg DL: Scapulohumeral arthrodesis: results in seven dogs, *J Am Anim Hosp Assoc* 24:667-672, 1988.
15. Francis DJ, Johnson KA: Interfragmentary stability influences healing of intraarticular fractures: a radiographic study of canine femoral condyle fractures repaired with lag screws, *Vet Comp Orthop Traumatol* 3:71-77, 1990.
16. Frost WW, Lumb WV: Radiocarpal arthrodesis: a surgical approach to brachial paralysis, *J Am Vet Med Assoc* 149:1073-1078, 1966.
17. Gorse MJ, Earley TD, Aron DN: Tarsocrural arthrodesis: long-term functional results, *J Am Anim Hosp Assoc* 27:231-235, 1991.
18. Heim U, Pfeiffer KM: *Small fragment set manual*, ed 2, Berlin, 1982, Springer-Verlag.
19. Johnson KA: Carpal arthrodesis in dogs, *Aust Vet J* 56:565-573, 1980.
20. Johnson KA: A radiographic study of the effects of autologous cancellous bone grafts on bone healing after carpal arthrodesis in the dog, *Vet Radiol* 22:177-183, 1981.
21. Johnson KA, Bellenger CR: The effects of autologous bone grafting on bone healing after carpal arthrodesis in the dog, *Vet Rec* 107:126-132, 1980.
22. Klause SE, Piermattei DL, Schwarz PD: Tarso-crural arthrodesis: complications and recommendations, *Vet Comp Orthop Traumatol* 3:119-124, 1989.
23. LaRue SM, and others: Limb-sparing treatment for osteosarcoma in dogs, *J Am Vet Med Assoc* 195:1734-1744, 1989.
24. Lesser AS: The use of a tendon transfer for the treatment of a traumatic sciatic nerve paralysis in the dog, *J Vet Surg* 7:85-89, 1978.
25. Newton CD: Arthrodesis of the stifle, tarsus and interphalangeal joints. In Newton CD, Nunamaker DM, editors: *Textbook of small animal orthopaedics*, Philadelphia, 1985, Lippincott.
26. Ost PC, and others: Fractures of the calcaneus in racing greyhounds, *J Vet Surg* 16:53-59, 1987.
27. Parker RB, Brown SG, Wind AP: Pancarpal arthrodesis in the dog: a review of 45 cases, *J Vet Surg* 10:35-43, 1981.
28. Piermattei DL: *An atlas of surgical approaches to the bones of the dog and cat*, ed 3, Philadelphia, 1992, Saunders.
29. Richards RR and others: Shoulder arthrodesis using a pelvic-reconstruction plate, *J Bone Joint Surg* 70A:416-421, 1988.
30. Short CE: Pain, analgesics, and related medications. In Short CE, editor: *Principles and practice of veterinary anesthesia*, Baltimore, 1987, Williams & Wilkins.
31. Smith MM, Spagnola J: T-plate for middle carpal and carpometacarpal arthrodesis in a dog, *J Am Vet Med Assoc* 199:230-232, 1991.
32. Sumner-Smith G, Kuzma A: A technique for arthrodesis of the canine tarsocrural joint, *J Small Anim Pract* 30:65-67, 1989.
33. Van Ee RT, Blass CE: Arthrodesis of metatarsophalangeal joints in a dog, *J Am Vet Med Assoc* 194:82-84, 1989.
34. Vasseur PB: Arthrodesis for congenital luxation of the shoulder in a dog, *J Am Vet Med Assoc* 197:501-503, 1990.
35. Willer RL and others: Partial carpal arthrodesis for third degree carpal sprains: a review of 45 carpi, *J Vet Surg* 19:334-340, 1990.
36. Yalden DW: The functional morphology of the carpal bones in carnivores, *Acta Anat* 77:481-500, 1970.

24

Amputations

STEVEN C. BUDSBERG

Amputation is a procedure that produces irreversible anatomical changes in the patient. In general, amputation should be considered only when no alternative exists that would allow retention of normal function. Amputation is a decision based on medical, emotional, and financial factors. Medical indications include severe trauma (often with massive tissue loss), neoplasia, chronic infection, severe neurological dysfunction, or other diseases in which the prognosis is poor for return of acceptable function. Patient morbidity and mortality are low and functional results and client satisfaction are high when amputation is properly considered and performed. It is important to remember that the ultimate and best decision is made by a well-informed owner.

The position or level of the amputation is an important consideration in each patient. For the forelimb, the most common options are complete forequarter removal, including the scapula, or disarticulation at the scapulo-humeral joint. A proximal-humeral procedure has recently been advocated, but this is not yet widely accepted. For the hind limb, the most common approach is a mid-femoral procedure, which produces the most acceptable cosmetic outcome. Coxofemoral disarticulation is usually reserved for patients with primary tumor or chronic osteomyelitis in or near the proximal femur. For the digits or tail, the level is determined by the pathology needed to be removed or, when done for cosmetic reasons, by breed standards.

PREOPERATIVE CONSIDERATIONS

When considering an amputation, a complete assessment of the patient's physical status is mandatory. It is important to realize that in most cases an amputation is an elective procedure that need not be hurried. The patient should be adequately evaluated and stabilized before surgery. Laboratory data at least should include a complete blood count and a urinalysis. A chemical profile should be performed when indicated and is recommended for all patients older than 3 to 4 years. Dehydration, anemia, or infection should be addressed before surgery. Fluid balance is important not only for anesthetic management, but also because of the possibility of blood loss and subsequent hypovolemia that may occur during surgery. If neoplastic disease exists, chest radiographs to evaluate metastases are necessary before amputation. If a limb is under consideration for amputation, careful examination of the other three limbs is necessary to ensure that the patient will be able to function. In large dogs this almost always entails pelvic radiographs to assess presence and/or progression of dysplastic changes in the coxofemoral joints.

If the surgeon is uncertain whether the patient will be functional on three limbs, the limb in question can simply be placed in a non-weight-bearing sling (i.e., Velpeau for the forelimb and Ehmer on the rear limb) and the patient evaluated for a few days to assess its ability to resume normal daily activities.

GENERAL SURGICAL PRINCIPLES

In all patients, a balanced electrolyte solution should be given intravenously throughout the preoperative period, beginning before and continued 6 to 12 hours until the patient recovers completely from anesthesia. A wide surgical site preparation is necessary for surgery, since generous skin incisions should be made to allow for large skin flaps for closure. At closure, redundant skin can easily be trimmed if needed. Sharp dissection is maintained whenever possible and unnecessary undermining of skin or fascial planes should be avoided. Major arteries and veins are double-ligated separately to help prevent arte-

riovenous fistula. Sharp transection of nerves is recommended. The use of prophylactic antibiotics in amputations is generally not indicated; however, certain cases may warrant such treatment.

FORELIMB AMPUTATION

Complete forequarter amputation (including the scapula) is the easiest and most common procedure performed. Other procedures are scapulohumeral disarticulation and humeral osteotomy. For any of the forelimb procedures, patient positioning is lateral recumbency with the affected leg hung and then draped-in completely.

Forequarter Amputation

Procedure. The skin incision should be made in an inverted Y or T design, beginning above the dorsal border of the scapula and running distal along the scapular spine to a point just distal to the acromion (Fig. 24-1).

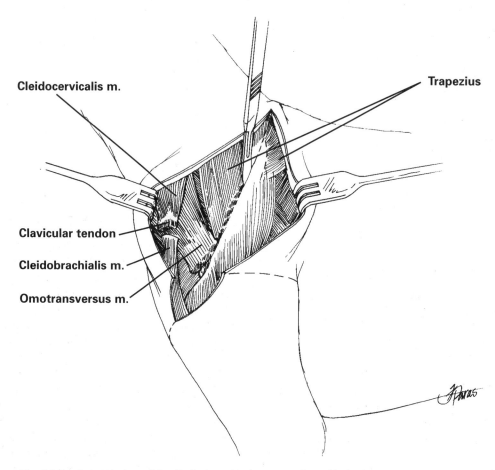

Cleidocervicalis m.

Trapezius

Clavicular tendon

Cleidobrachialis m.

Omotransversus m.

Fig. 24-1 Lateral view of forelimb denoting location of initial skin incision and superficial muscle dissection. Skin incision can be an inverted T or Y with the medial aspect at the level of the fold of the axilla (broken line). Only the vertical portion of the incision must be done to proceed with deeper dissection. Incision of muscles is performed at their insertions on the scapula and clavicular tendon.

The incision is then made cranially and caudally in a circular fashion at the level of the greater tubercle around the limb. The medial aspect of the incision should be at the level of the fold of the axilla. It is not necessary to complete the entire medial part of the incision until near the end of the procedure. Sharp dissection is preferred, leaving the subcutaneous tissue and cutaneous trunci muscle attached to the skin and thus minimizing the undermining of tissue and formation of excessive dead space. This also protects the vasculature to the skin and avoids placing excessive tension on the skin sutures.

The axillobrachial and omobrachial veins are identified and double ligated. Then the brachiocephalicus muscle (made up of three muscles) is identified and transected at the level of the clavicular tendon (Fig. 24-1). Distal to the clavicular tendon is the cleidobrachialis muscle, and proximal to the tendon are two muscles, the cleidocervicalis and, deeper, the cleidomastoideus muscle. (*Note*: Some

descriptions of this procedure vary in describing these muscle names and thus can be confusing.) The origin of the omotransversarius muscle is incised from the cranial aspect of the scapular spine. Moving dorsally on the scapular spine, the insertion of the trapezius muscle is identified and incised from the craniodorsal and caudodorsal aspects of the spine.

Retraction of this first layer of muscles, which have been removed, now allows visualization of the next group of structures to be addressed (Fig. 24-2, *A*). Retraction of the trapezius reveals the insertion of the three bellies of the rhomboideus muscle on the dorsomedial aspect of the scapula (Fig. 24-2, *B*). Sharp dissection of the muscles at their insertion on the scapula can help limit the hemorrhage. Rotating the scapula and limb lateral and caudal helps the exposure for the dissection (Fig. 24-3). At its caudal region of attachment, the rhomboideus muscle group begins to blend in with the latissimus dorsi muscle.

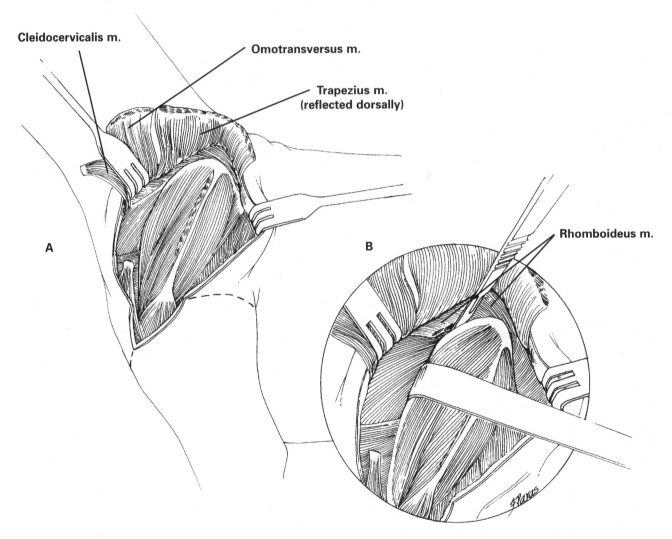

Fig. 24-2   A, Following incision of the omotransversarius and trapezius muscles from their origins on the scapular spine, they are reflected dorsally. **B,** After retraction, the rhomboideus is identified and the insertion of the three bellies is incised from its insertion on the dorsomedial aspect of the scapula.

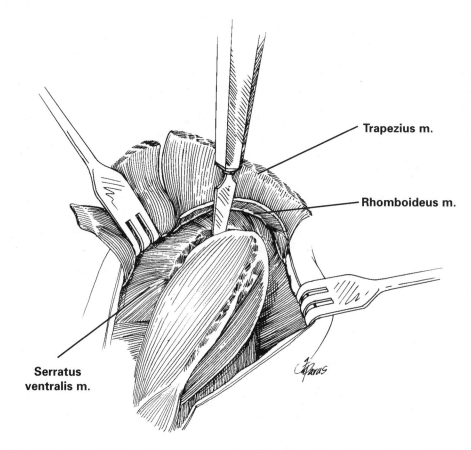

Trapezius m.

Rhomboideus m.

**Serratus
ventralis m.**

Fig. 24-3 Superficial muscles are retracted to allow dissection of serratus ventralis from craniomedial aspect of scapular body. Note: rhomboideus muscle group has previously been incised from the scapular body in a similar fashion.

Retraction of the rhomboideus exposes the insertion of the serratus ventralis muscle on the dorsomedial third of the scapula. Periosteal elevation or sharp dissection of the serratus ventralis at its insertion is performed.

Caudally the latissimus dorsi muscle is then identified and severed at its insertion on the major teres tuberosity of the humerus. The thoracodorsal artery and vein should be visible at this time and should be identified, double-ligated, and severed (Fig. 24-4, *A*). The thoracodorsal nerve is then sharply severed. The axillary lymph node(s) can be easily identified just under the insertion of the latissimus dorsi to the humerus. The limb vessels and nerves of the brachial plexus can now be easily seen. The axillary artery should be approached first and double-ligated proximally and ligated once distally before transection (Fig. 24-4, *B*). One of the two proximal sutures should be a transfixation suture. The axillary vein is then isolated and double-ligated and severed. The nerves of the brachial plexus are then individually severed with a scalpel blade.

Next, moving cranially, the limb is externally rotated (Fig. 24-5). The tendinous insertion of the superficial pectoral muscle on the greater tubercle of the humerus is identified and severed. The deep pectoral muscle and its insertion on

the greater and lesser tubercle of the humerus are identified, and the insertion is severed. At this point, the suprascapular artery and vein should be identified, ligated, and severed. Also, the suprascapular nerve should be sharply transected. Continuance of the skin and subcutaneous incision medially completes the amputation.

Closure. Closure of the muscle bellies is facilitated by using inverting suture patterns (Lembert, etc.) in the fascial sheaths to reattach them to the body. The deep pectoral is attached to the scalenus muscle and the ventral border of the latissimus dorsi muscle (Fig. 24-6, *A*). The fasciae of the rhomboideus, trapezius, and omotransversarius are sutured to the dorsal border of the latissimus dorsi and ventrally to the pectoral muscles (Fig. 24-6, *B*). Closure of the subcutaneous tissues and skin is routine. The use of drains is optional, but with atraumatic technique, proper hemostasis, and closure of dead space, the use of drains should be unnecessary.

Postoperatively a padded bandage applied with some pressure should be placed over the incision site. Administration of analgesics immediately postoperatively varies and should be done as necessary.

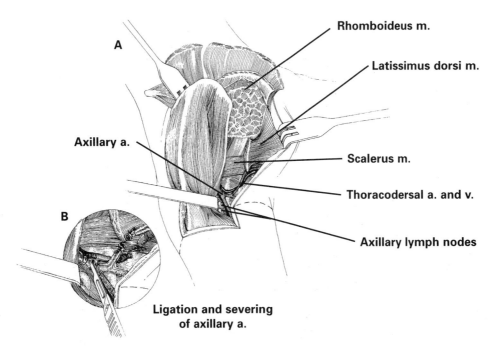

Fig. 24-4 **A,** Rotate scapula and limb cranially to visualize latissimus dorsi and sever its insertion on the teres major tuberosity of the humerus. The thoracodorsal artery, vein, and nerve should now be visible. Double ligate and sever the vessels, and sharply divide the nerve. **B,** The brachial plexus can now be identified. Axillary artery and vein should be approached first and double ligated distally prior to dissection.

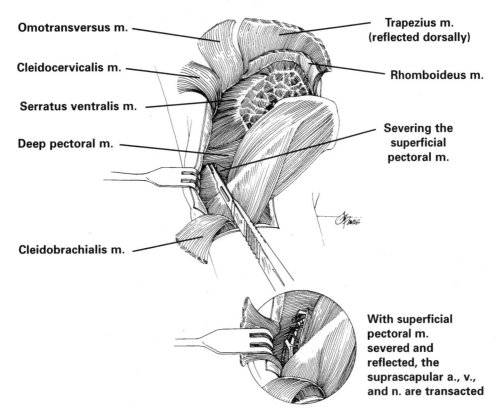

Fig. 24-5 To complete muscle dissection, move to cranial aspect of limb and identify superficial and deep pectoral muscles. Transection of these muscles reveals the suprascapular vein, artery and nerve. Following ligation and transection of these structures, the amputation is completed by continuing medial incision through skin and subcutaneous tissues.

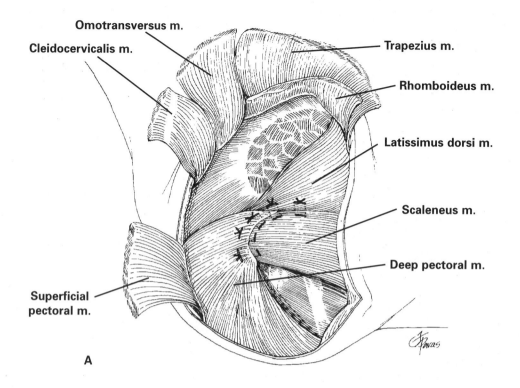

Omotransversus m.

Cleidocervicalis m.

Trapezius m.

Rhomboideus m.

Latissimus dorsi m.

Scaleneus m.

Deep pectoral m.

Superficial pectoral m.

A

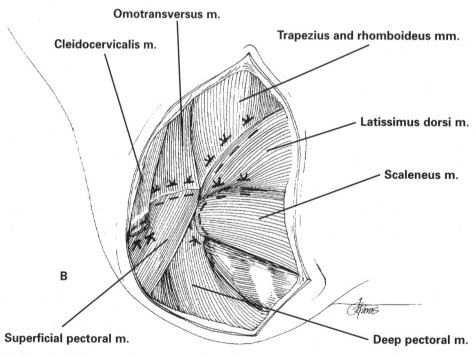

Omotransversus m.

Cleidocervicalis m.

Trapezius and rhomboideus mm.

Latissimus dorsi m.

Scaleneus m.

Superficial pectoral m.

Deep pectoral m.

B

Fig. 24-6 **A,** Closure of deep pectoral muscles to scalenus muscle and ventral border of latissimus dorsi muscle. Suture pattern used should be appositional or inverting. **B,** Fascia of the rhomboideus, trapezius, and omotransversarius muscles are sutured to the dorsal edge of the latissimus dorsi and the ventral border of the pectorals. The cleidocervicalis is reattached to the cranial border of the superficial pectoral at the level of the clavicular tendon. Routine closure of subcutaneous tissues and skin completes the amputation.

Scapulohumeral Disarticulation

Procedure. A lateral semicircular incision is made from the greater tubercle (point of the shoulder) caudodistally to the midhumeral region and then caudoproximally to the caudal angle of the axillary fold (Fig. 24-7). This provides a skin flap of sufficient quantity to cover the stump. On the medial aspect a similar incision is made; however, this one does not have to project as distal on the humerus. The cleidobrachialis muscle is identified and severed just below the clavicular tendon. The cephalic vein lies in this region and must be isolated, ligated, and cut. Next, the acromial head of the deltoid muscles is severed at its insertion on the deltoid tuberosity of the humerus. The lateral and long heads of the triceps muscle group are separated from the caudal border of the humerus and the brachialis muscle. The triceps is isolated and the tendon of insertion cut just above its insertion on the olecranon (Fig. 24-7). The limb is externally rotated to expose the pectoral muscles. The insertion of the superficial pectoral muscle on the greater tubercle of the humerus is severed. Next, the deep pectoral muscle is severed from its insertion on the greater and lesser tubercles of the humerus. The insertion of the supraspinatus muscle on the greater tubercle is transected (Fig. 24-8).

Retraction of these muscles exposes the nerves of the brachial plexus and the associated vasculature (Fig. 24-8). The brachial artery is isolated and double-ligated below the level of the subscapular artery. The same procedure is repeated for the brachial vein. The nerves of the plexus are sharply transected. Moving back to the lateral aspect of the limb, dorsal retraction of the deltoids and supraspinatus allows visualization and transection of the tendons of the infraspinatus, teres minor, and the biceps

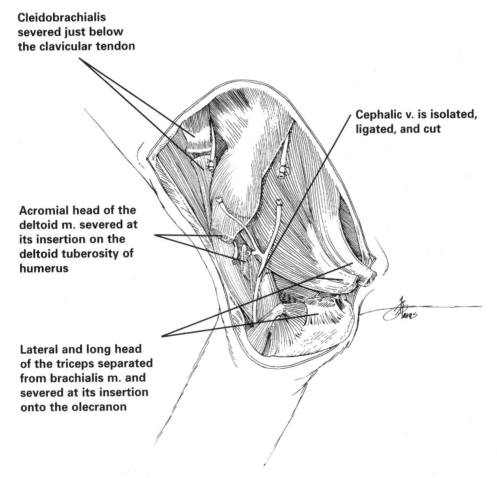

Cleidobrachialis severed just below the clavicular tendon

Cephalic v. is isolated, ligated, and cut

Acromial head of the deltoid m. severed at its insertion on the deltoid tuberosity of humerus

Lateral and long head of the triceps separated from brachialis m. and severed at its insertion onto the olecranon

Fig. 24-7   Lateral view of approach for scapular humeral disarticulation. Skin incision is in a curvilinear fashion from greater tubercle to axillary fold. Cleidobrachialis is severed below clavicular tendon. Cephalic vein is identified, ligated, and transected. Next, acromial head of deltoideus muscle is severed from insertion on deltoid tuberosity of the humerus. Long and lateral heads of the triceps are separated from brachialis muscle and then transected just proximal to the olecranon.

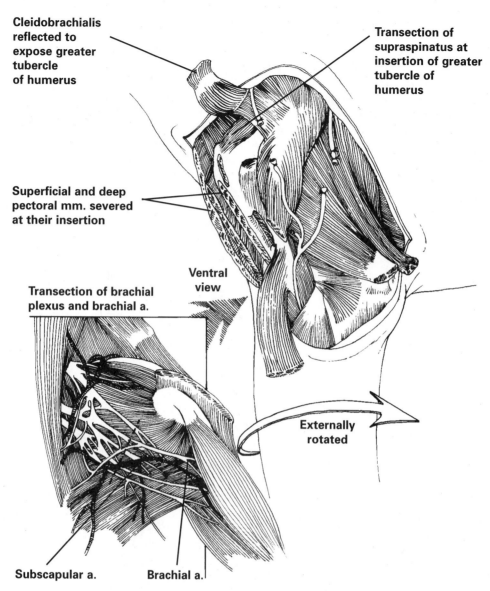

Cleidobrachialis reflected to expose greater tubercle of humerus

Transection of supraspinatus at insertion of greater tubercle of humerus

Superficial and deep pectoral mm. severed at their insertion

Ventral view

Transection of brachial plexus and brachial a.

Externally rotated

Subscapular a.   **Brachial a.**

Fig. 24-8 Externally rotate the limb. Sever the insertions of the superficial and deep pectorals from the greater and lesser tubercles. Next, transect the supraspinatus muscle at its insertion on the greater tubercle. Retraction of these muscles allows visualization of the brachial plexus and associated vasculature. Double ligate the brachial artery and vein distal to the level of the subscapular artery.

brachii muscles (Fig. 24-9). The insertions of the latissimus dorsi, teres major, and cutaneous trunci muscles are severed on the humerus at the teres tubercle. The joint capsule is opened laterally and the opening continued around the medial aspects, at which time the tendons of the coracobrachialis and subscapularis muscles are concurrently severed. The amputation is complete.

Closure. Closure is accomplished by suturing the fascial sheaths in which the brachiocephalic, teres major, infraspinatus, supraspinatus, and deltoid muscles are brought

together to meet the triceps, latissimus, and pectoral muscles; the two muscle masses are sutured together. The subcutaneous and skin tissues are closed routinely.

REAR LIMB AMPUTATION

Rear limb amputation is performed most often at the level of the proximal femur because of cosmetic concerns and because it is technically easier than a higher amputation. Coxofemoral joint disarticulation is usually reserved for cases in which wider tissue margins are needed, such as

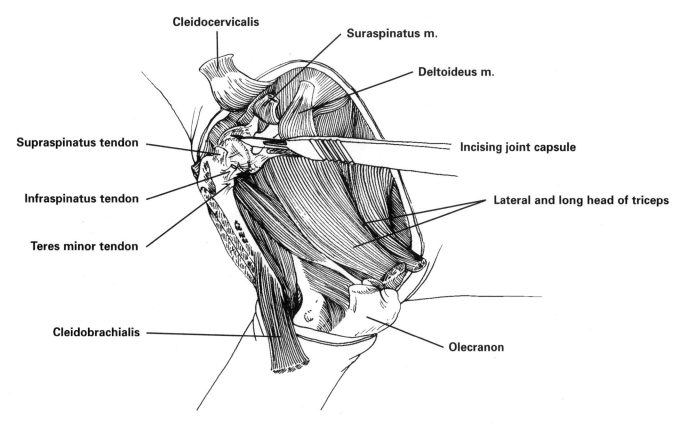

Fig. 24-9 Lateral view of the limb. Retract deltoideus and supraspinatus muscles dorsally and visualize the infraspinatus, teres minor and biceps brachii muscles. Transect the tendons of these muscles. Open the joint capsule laterally and continue medially at which time the tendons of the coracobrachialis and subscapularis are identified and severed.

when a bone tumor is present or tissue pathology extensively involves the proximal part of the limb. No amputations should be performed below the middle to proximal femur, since this may allow the animal to traumatize the stump during daily activity.

For either of the hind limb procedures, lateral recumbency with the affected leg hung and completely draped-in is recommended. Sandbags may also be placed underneath the down leg so as to position the hindquarters slightly more toward dorsal recumbency. This procedure allows for easier access to the medial aspect of the limb to be amputated.

Proximal Femoral Amputation

Procedure. A lateral semilunar skin incision extending from the fold of the flank to the tuber ischii is made. The middle of the incision should be at the level of the middle to distal femur (Fig. 24-10). The medial incision should mimic the lateral incision but does not have to extend beyond midfemur. The lateral skin is preserved in a larger flap, since it provides a more cosmetic closure than the thin, unhaired skin of the proximal medial thigh. The dissection is initially done on the leg's medial aspect. The

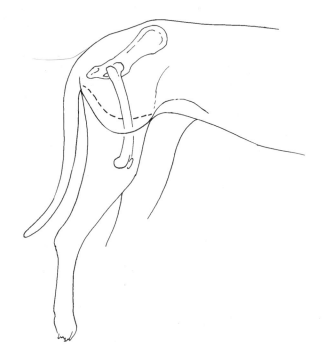

Fig. 24-10 Lateral semilunar skin incision extending from fold of the flank to the tuber ischii. Dotted line illustrates corresponding medial incision.

femoral triangle (located between the caudal belly of the sartorius muscle cranially and the pectineus and adductor muscles caudally) is located to aid in identification of the femoral artery. The artery is double-ligated just proximal to the branching of the proximocaudal femoral artery (Fig. 24-11). The femoral vein is then ligated and the saphenous nerve sharply transected.

The cranial and caudal sartorius muscles are incised at the level of the midfemur. The gracilis and pectineus muscles are then transected near their insertions distally. A second option is to transect the muscle belly proximal to the insertion, but this usually entails more hemorrhage. On the medial aspect, the adductor magnus et brevis muscle can be transected through the muscle belly or subperiosteally elevated from the caudal aspect of the femoral shaft (Fig. 24-12).

On the lateral aspect of the limb, the tensor fascia lata muscle and the biceps femoris are transected near their fascial insertions on the femur (Fig. 24-13). Alternatively, a midbelly muscle transection may be chosen. Enough muscle must be left to allow for adequate closure over the bone stump. With the biceps femoris reflected, the quadriceps muscle group (vastus medialis, vastus lateralis, vastus intermedius, rectus femoris) is visualized and transected (Fig. 24-14); the more distal the transection, the less hemorrhage and the larger the flap of muscle available for closure. The sciatic nerve should be sharply transected at the level of the proximal femur just as it appears from medial to the greater trochanter.

The caudal muscles of the limb are severed. The semimembranosus and semitendinosus muscles should be transected at the level of the middle to distal femur

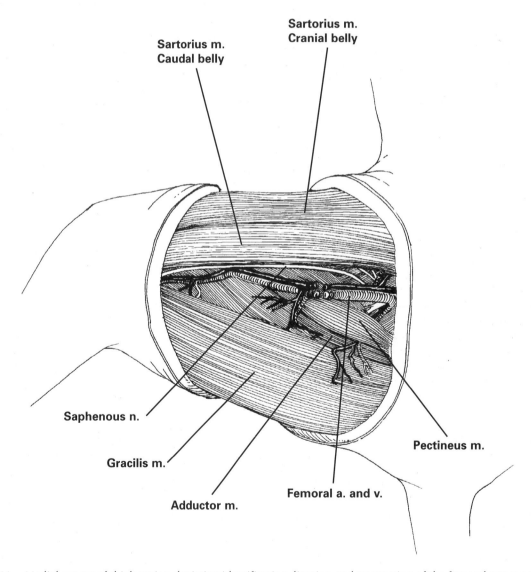

Fig. 24-11 Medial aspect of thigh region depicting identification, ligation and transection of the femoral artery and vein and the saphenous nerve.

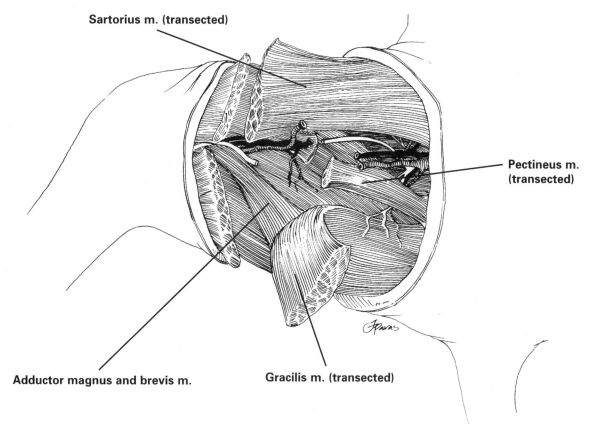

Fig. 24-12   Retraction of the gracilis and pectineus muscles reveals the adductor magus et brevis. Transect or subperiosteally elevate from femoral shaft.

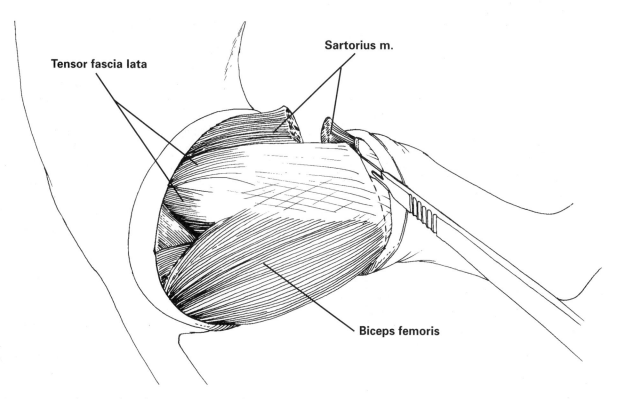

Fig. 24-13   Lateral aspect describing transection of the tensor fascia lata and biceps femoris near their fascial insertions of the femur.

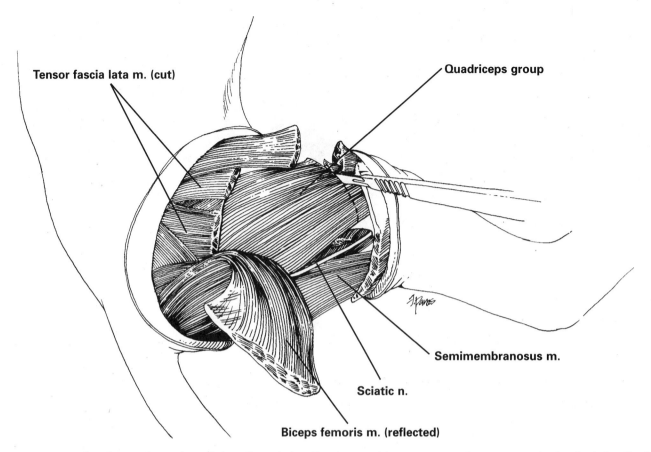

Fig. 24-14 Reflect biceps femoris caudodorsally and visualize the quadriceps group and transect at the level of the distal humerus. Identify and sharply divide the sciatic nerve.

(Fig. 24-15, *A*). The femur is cut with either an oscillating or wire saw at the level of the junction of the middle and proximal femur. Hemorrhage from the femoral marrow canal can be controlled with bone wax, but this is not always needed.

Closure. Closure entails the apposition of the muscle bellies to each other to cover the stump of the femur. The quadriceps group and the cranial sartorius are sutured caudally to the semitendinosus and semimembranosus muscles (Fig. 24-15, *B*). The biceps femoris is then closed to the gracilis, adductor, and caudal belly of the sartorius muscle. Additional sutures can be placed to complete the stump closure, from the semitendinosus and semimembranosus to the biceps femoris and from the quadriceps group to the gracilis and adductor muscles. The most popular suture pattern used in the closure is the horizontal mattress pattern, but many suture patterns are acceptable. Subcutaneous, subcuticular, and skin closure are routine but must be carefully done to eliminate dead space. The use of drains is optional.

Coxofemoral Disarticulation

Procedure. The skin incision is begun laterally and extends from the fold of the flank caudodistally in a semicircular fashion to the midfemoral region and then progresses craniodistally to the ischial tuberosity. A similar incision is made on the medial aspect of the leg; however, this incision does not need to curve as far distal as the lateral incision. After dissection of the subcutaneous tissue, the leg should be abducted to better expose the medial aspect and the femoral triangle. The femoral artery is located, double-ligated, and severed proximal to the branching of the lateral circumflex femoral artery. The femoral vein should be ligated and severed at the same spot. The superficial circumflex iliac artery should then be addressed similarly (see Fig. 24-11).

The cranial and caudal bellies of the sartorius are transected at or near their origin on the iliac crest and ventral aspect of the ilium. The pectineus and the group of muscles including the gracilis, adductor longus, and adductor magnus et brevis are removed from their insertions on the iliopectineal eminence and pelvic symphysis, respectively.

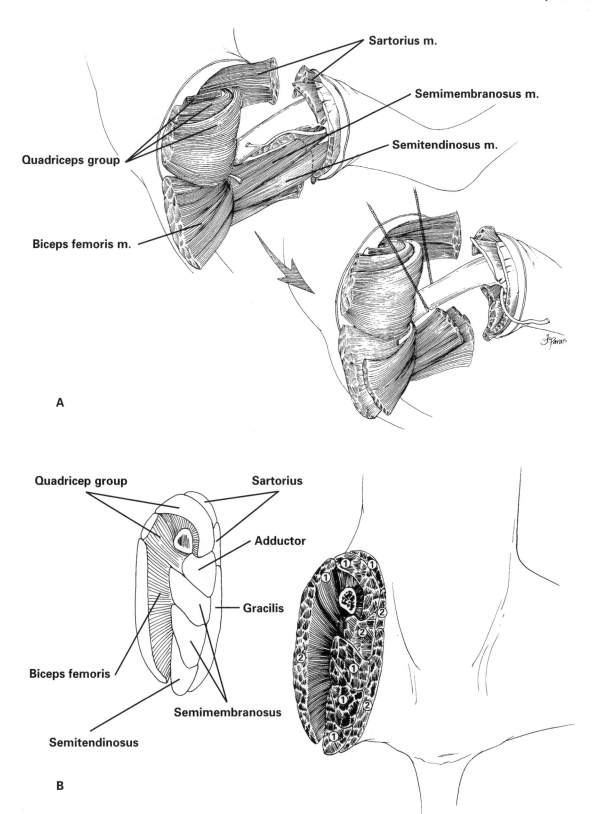

A, Retract quadriceps group, visualize, and transect semimembranosus and semitendinousus muscles distally. Cut the femur proximally (junction of mid and proximal femur). **B,** Ventral to dorsal view of remaining musculature and femur. Muscles labeled with a (1) are closed to each other in a cranial to caudal orientation. Muscles labeled with a (2) are then closed to each other laterally to medially completing the stump.

Fig. 24-15

Alternatively, they can be transected at the level of their tendons of origin just after arising from the pelvis. The medial circumflex femoral artery and vein should now be exposed, identified, and double-ligated as they pass lateral to the retracted pectineus muscle (Fig. 24-16).

The limb is adducted to continue the dissection of the lateral aspect. The tensor fascia lata and biceps femoris muscles are transected at the level of the proximal femur or can be elevated from their respective origins on the pelvis. The elevation technique is more difficult but may be necessary when wide tissue margins are required. Reflecting the biceps femoris and tensor fascia lata allows for visualization of the vastus lateralis, semimembranosus, and semitendinosus muscles (Fig. 24-17). The semimembranosus and semitendinosus are transected through

their tendons of origin. The vastus group need not be transected because these muscles are removed with the leg. The sciatic nerve should be sharply transected. The tendons of insertion of the superficial, middle, and deep gluteal muscles are severed on the third and greater trochanters of the femur, respectively. Proximal retraction of the semimembranosus and semitendinosus allows access to the insertions of the gemelli, internal obturator, and quadratus femoris muscles on the femur. Each should be transected at the level of insertion (Fig. 24-18). The joint capsule is then opened, the round ligament severed, and the amputation is complete.

Closure. Closure is begun by apposition of the gluteal muscles to the adductor muscles and continued with the

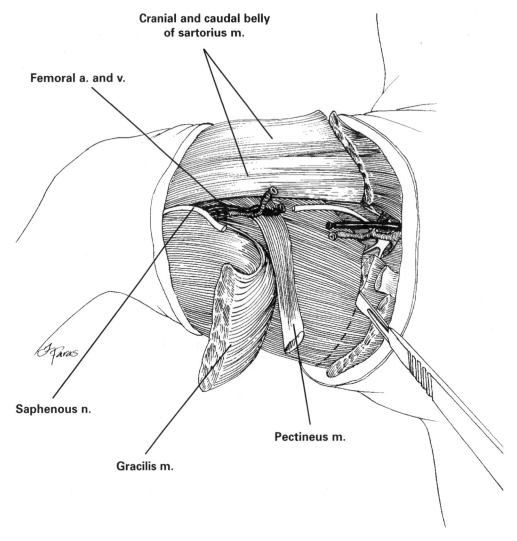

Cranial and caudal belly of sartorius m.

Femoral a. and v.

Saphenous n.

Gracilis m.

Pectineus m.

Fig. 24-16 Medial view: The sartorius, pectineus, and gracilis muscles have been incised at their insertions and reflected distally. The adductor muscle is now incised, which reveals the medial circumflex femoral artery and vein.

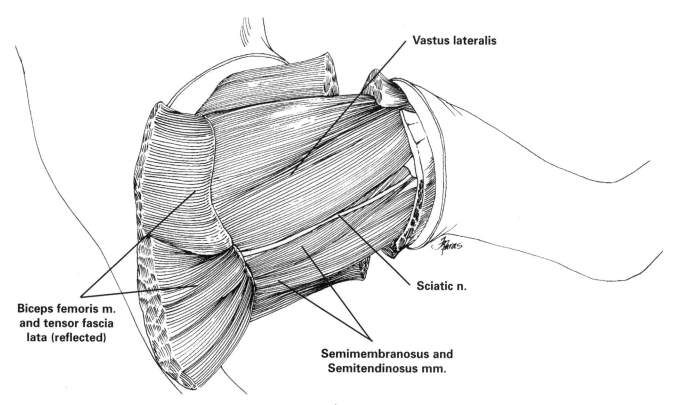

Fig. 24-17   Lateral view: Deep musculature. Reflection of superficial muscles allows visualization of vastus lateralis, semimembranosus, and semitendinosus muscles and sciatic nerve.

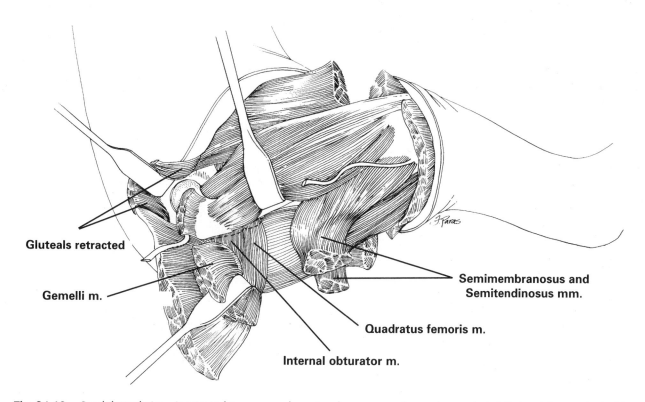

Fig. 24-18   Caudolateral view: Semimembranosus and semitendinosus muscles are transected at their origins on the ischium and reflected distally. The insertions of the gemelli, internal obturator, and quadratus femoris are visualized and excised off the femur. The tendons of insertion of the superficial, middle, and deep gluteal muscles are severed from the femur and retracted craniodorsal. The joint capsule and the ligament of the head of the femur are severed and the limb is removed.

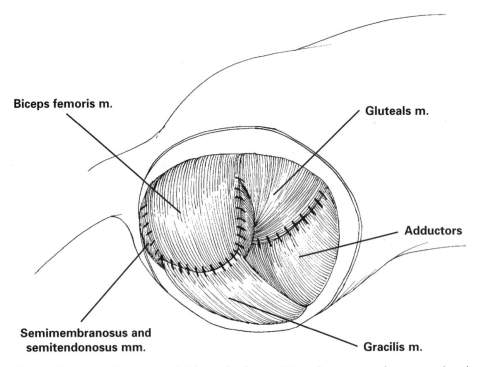

Fig. 24-19 Lateral view: Superficial muscle closure. Biceps femoris muscle is sutured to the gracilis ventrally. The remnants of the semimembranosus and semitendinosus are sutured to the biceps and gracilis caudoventrally.

biceps femoris muscle sutured to the gracilis, semimembranosus, and semitendinosus (Fig. 24-19). Strict adherence to the closure of dead space is necessary in closing the subcutaneous tissue. Subcuticular tissue and the skin are closed routinely. The use of drains is left to the surgeon's discretion. Application of a padded bandage is advised for 2 to 3 days, although it is more difficult to apply and manage than on a forelimb amputation site. Complications primarily include wound infections and seroma formation.

DIGIT AMPUTATION

Indications for amputation of digits and, when necessary, associated metacarpal/metatarsal bones include neoplasia, chronic nonresponsive osteomyelitis, and severe trauma. Dewclaws are removed for cosmetic reasons in some breeds shortly after birth according to breed standards. Another consideration that is occasionally encountered is the sacrifice of a normal digit, removing the bone structures, and use of the associated excess skin as a graft to close a defect in an adjacent area of tissue loss.

The level of amputation is not as critical as with entire limb removal. Successful amputation can occur at any level up to disarticulation and removal of the metacarpal/metatarsal bones. One word of caution in removing metacarpal bones: removal of the proximal base of the second and fifth metacarpals causes instability and prob-

ably deviation of the carpal joint. This results from the multiple ligamentous attachments from the carpal bones to these metacarpals, which provide the stability to the joint. Arterial supply to the digits comes from the dorsal common digital and the palmar (forepaw) and plantar (hind paw) digital arteries. When amputating only the third phalanx, it is paramount to save the pad.

General Digit Amputation

Depending on the level of the amputation, a variety of incisions may be used. The key points regarding the incision are that adequate exposure is allowed for the procedure and that enough skin is preserved to allow for closure over the stump (Fig. 24-20, *A*). Isolation and ligation of the arterial supply constitute the next step. However, because of the size of the vessels, they are often cut and may hemorrhage before ligation. Disarticulation at the level just proximal to the digit to be removed is performed. Closure entails first suturing deep fascia and subcutaneous tissue together to close dead space, followed by subcuticular and skin sutures (Fig. 24-20, *B*).

Dewclaw Removal

Removal of a digit is usually performed on the first digit. This is commonly termed "dewclaw amputation"; however, the term *dewclaw* should only be applied to the

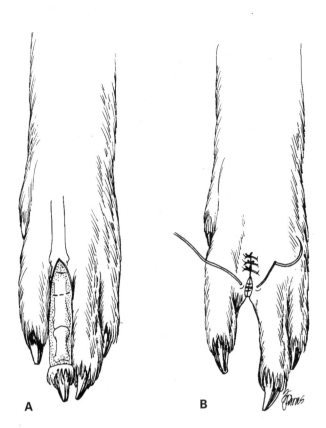

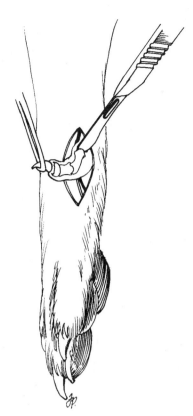

Fig. 24-20   **A,** Dorsal view of the inverted Y skin incision of the digit amputation. **B,** Closure of the inverted Y incision following digit removal.

Fig. 24-21   Medial view of elliptical dewclaw skin incision. Note disarticulation at the level of proximal P1.

variably developed first digit of the hind paw. The first digit appendage, although often rudimentary, is always present in the forelimb. One major difference between the fore and hind first digits is that the first metacarpal bone is always present, whereas the first metatarsal bone is usually atypical and the proximal phalanx may be absent. Arterial supply to the first digits is identical to that of other digits, but during amputation, only one of these arteries produces significant hemorrhage that requires ligation.

In the first few days of life, amputation is often done with scissors and the skin closed over the incision. In the older animal the surgical procedure is more involved. An elliptical incision is made around the base of the digit, and the dissection is carried down to the level of attachment of the carpometacarpal or tarsometatarsal joint (Fig. 24-21). It is easier to identify and ligate the artery before incising it. Once the disarticulation is complete, the wound is closed routinely. Application of a padded bandage is advisable for the first 12 to 24 hours.

TAIL AMPUTATION (CAUDECTOMY)

Indications for performing tail amputations include severe trauma and tissue loss, neurological dysfunction, and per-

sistent trauma. High tail amputations are required for the management of tail fold pyoderma and have been advocated as an adjunct procedure for the treatment of perianal fistulas. Amputations may also be done for cosmetic purposes or to meet individual breed standards for show purposes.

Anatomical considerations in performing a tail amputation primarily concern proper incision allotment of skin for closure and identification of the arterial supply. The median caudal artery is present on the most ventral aspect of the tail, and the paired lateral caudal arteries lie on each side of the vertebra. Disarticulation is performed proximal to the level of damage.

Skin incisions are made on the dorsal and ventral surfaces of the tail in semicircular fashion. This allows for a skin flap to cover the stump after amputation (Fig. 24-22, A). The vessels are identified and ligated proximal to the coccygeal vertebra that is to be removed (Fig. 24-22, B). Disarticulation and transection of the coccygeal muscle are performed. The subcutaneous tissue and skin are then advanced over the stump and sutured (Fig. 24-22, C).

Postoperatively, a small, snug bandage is placed over the incision for 2 to 3 days. This bandage may need to remain longer if the reason for amputation is recurrent mutilation.

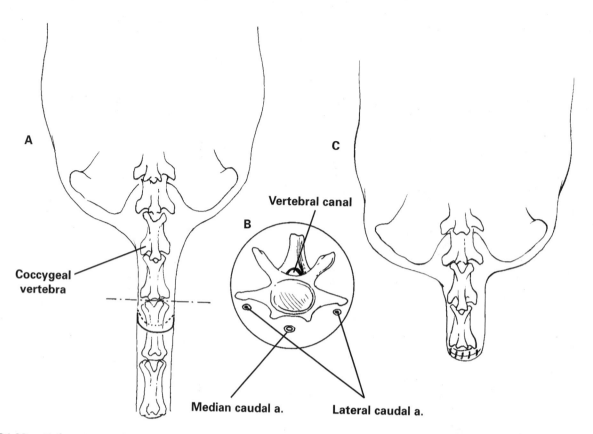

Fig. 24-22 Tail amputation. **A,** Skin incision in a semicircular fashion. The skin flap should extend one coccygeal vertebra distal to the level of the intended amputation. **B,** Cross sectional view of a coccygeal vertebra depicting the lateral caudal and median caudal arteries. **C,** Skin closure of stump.

SUGGESTED READINGS

Bone DL, Aberman HM: Forelimb amputation in the dog using humeral osteotomy, *J Am Anim Hosp Assoc* 124:525-529, 1988.

Carberry CA, Harvey HJ: Owner satisfaction with limb amputation in dogs and cats, *J Am Anim Hosp Assoc* 23:227-232, 1987.

Knapp DW: Amputation and disarticulation of the rear leg. In Bojrab MJ, editor: *Current techniques in small animal surgery*, ed 3, Philadelphia, 1990, Lea & Febiger.

Stone EA: Amputation. In Newton CD, Nunamaker DM, editors: *Textbook of small animal orthopedics*, Philadelphia, 1985, Lippincott.

Van Ea RT, Palminteri A: Tail amputation for treatment of perianal fistulas in dogs, *J Am Anim Hosp Assoc* 23:95-100, 1987.

Weigel, JP: Amputations. In Slatter DH, editor: *Textbook of small animal surgery*, Philadelphia, 1985, Saunders.

Index

A

Osteoclasts
  access to mineralized bone surface of, 36
  active, 36
  defined, 28
  derivation of, 38
  inactive, 36
  role in resorption of bone and release of calcium salts of, 28, 362-63
  ruffled (brush) border of, 38-39
Osteocyte
  defined, 28, 37
  housed in lacuna, 64-65
  role in resorption of bone and release of calcium salts of, 28, 37
  septa resorbed by, 31
Osteocyte-osteoblast pump, 37-38
Osteocytic osteolysis, 38
Osteodystrophy, hypertrophic, 263
Osteoid
  defined, 28
  deposited by osteoblasts on the cartilage core, 31
  mineralization of, 148
Osteolysis
  at anode from electric stimulation, 288
  of bone surrounding corroding implant, 262
  osteocytic, 38
Osteomalacia
  diagnosis of, 433
  treatment of, 433
Osteomedullography, 285
Osteomyelitis, 261-75
  acute
    alterations in hemograms in, 269
    antibiotics alone indicated for treatment of some, 270
    diagnosis of, 268
    transition to chronic from, 266
  appearance of, 459
  causes of, 179-80, 248, 261, 289
  chronic
    causes of, 267, 521
    diagnosis of, 261, 268-69
    low-grade, 44
    nonresponsive, 546
    recurrence of, 269, 274
    selection of antibiotics for, 273
    signs of, 266-67
    spiculated periosteal new bone typical of, 264, 267
    treated by en bloc resection of the infection, 270
    vascularized muscle flaps transferred or rotated during treatment of, 263
  clinical signs of, 266-67
  cortical deficits caused by, 272
  defined, 261
  diagnosis of, 267-69
    bacteriology in, 268
    cytology in, 268
    hematology in, 269
    histopathology in, 268-69
    radiology in, 267-68

Osteomyelitis—Cont'd
  etiology of, 261-63
  as indication for stifle arthrodesis, 327
  infection in
    bacterial, 261, 262
    fungal, 42, 262-63
    nonunions and, 289
    routes of, 262
    viral, 263
  origin of, 41
  pathogenesis of, 261
  pathophysiology of, 263-66
  perpetuating triad of, 264
  postoperative, 261
  posttraumatic, fracture disease seen after, 319
  recurrence of, 274
  refractoriness of, 266
  treatment of, 269-74
    antibiotics in, 273
    antimicrobial therapy as, 265-66
    debridement and drainage of wound in, 270-71, 274
    decision trees of options for, 268-69
    irrigation of wounds in, 271
    skin grafts and compound myocutaneous flaps in, 273
Osteon
  as basic structural unit of cortical bone, 34, 64-65
  defined, 28
Osteonecrosis, 40-41, 362-65
Osteonization, 33
Osteopenia
  developing during course of feline progressive polyarthritis, 467
  healing of fractures affected by, 281
Osteophytes
  around femoral head and neck, 368
  on medial and lateral trochlear ridges in chronic injury to the cranial cruciate ligament, 405
  periarticular
    production of, as feature of degenerative joint disease, 447-48
    proximal to the anconeal process in chronic fragmented coronoid process, 454
    removal of, 449
  as proliferations undergoing endochondral ossification, 51
Osteophytosis, 503
Osteoporosis
  as contributing to nonunion of fracture, 284-85
  of cortices, 267
  disuse, 320-21, 324
  as postoperative complication, 83
Osteosarcoma. See Neoplasia and Soft tissue sarcomas (STSs)
Osteosynthesis
  bone plate, 67
  distraction, 289
  function of implants in, 68-73
Osteotome
  to cut bone during osteotomy, 154, 156
  to excise articular cartilage, 506
  to remove periarticular osteophytes, 449
  in tibial tuberosity transposition, 400-401